PROGRESS IN BRAIN RESEARCH

VOLUME 73

BIOCHEMICAL BASIS OF FUNCTIONAL NEUROTERATOLOGY
Permanent Effects of Chemicals on the Developing Brain

Recent volumes in PROGRESS IN BRAIN RESEARCH

PROGRESS IN BRAIN RESEARCH

VOLUME 73

BIOCHEMICAL BASIS OF FUNCTIONAL NEUROTERATOLOGY
Permanent Effects of Chemicals on the Developing Brain

Proceedings of the 15th International Summer School of Brain Research, held at the Royal Netherlands Academy of Arts and Sciences, Amsterdam, The Netherlands, from August 31 to September 4, 1987

EDITED BY

G. J. BOER, M. G. P. FEENSTRA, M. MIRMIRAN,
D. F. SWAAB and F. VAN HAAREN

Netherlands Institute for Brain Research,
Meibergdreef 33, 1105 AZ Amsterdam, The Netherlands

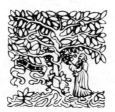

ELSEVIER
AMSTERDAM — NEW YORK — OXFORD
1988

m773

© 1988, Elsevier Science Publishers B.V. (Biomedical Division)

ISBN 0-444-80970-8 (volume)
ISBN 0-444-80104-9 (series)

Published by:
Elsevier Science Publishers B.V.
(Biomedical Division)
P.O. Box 211
1000 AE Amsterdam
The Netherlands

Sole distributors for the USA and Canada:
Elsevier Science Publishing Company, Inc.
52 Vanderbilt Avenue
New York, NY 10017
USA

Printed in The Netherlands

11/16/88

List of Contributors

Z. Annau, Department of Environmental Health Sciences, The Johns Hopkins University, Baltimore, MD 21205, USA

R. E. Baker, Netherlands Institute for Brain Research, Meibergdreef 33, 1105 AZ Amsterdam ZO, The Netherlands

R. Balázs, Developmental Neurobiology Unit, Medical Research Council, 1 Wakefield Street, London WCIN 1PJ, UK (present address: Netherlands Institute for Brain Research, Meibergdreef 33, 1105 AZ Amsterdam ZO, The Netherlands)

J. Barks, Department of Pediatrics, 1120 Neuroscience Laboratory Building, 1103 East Huron Street, The University of Michigan, Ann Arbor, MI 48104, USA

J. M. Bell, Department of Pharmacology, Duke University Medical Center, Durham, NC 27710, USA

H. K. Berry, Institute for Developmental Research, Children's Hospital Research Foundation, Cincinnati, OH 45229, USA

G. J. Boer, Netherlands Institute for Brain Research, Meibergdreef 33, 1105 AZ Amsterdam ZO, The Netherlands

N. P. A. Bos, Netherlands Institute for Brain Research, Meibergdreef 33, 1105 AZ Amsterdam ZO, The Netherlands

J. Campbell, Department of Anatomy, School of Medicine, University of California, Los Angeles, CA 90024, USA

C. Carlsson-Skwirut, Karolinska Institute, Department of Psychiatry, St. Göran's Hospital, Box 12500, 11281 Stockholm, Sweden

M. L. De Ceballos, Department of Neuropharmacology, Cajal Institute, CSIC, 28006 Madrid, Spain

E. R. De Kloet, Rudolf Magnus Institute for Pharmacology, University of Utrecht, Vondellaan 6, 3521 GD Utrecht, The Netherlands

J. Del Rio, Department of Neuropharmacology, Cajal Institute, CSIC, 28006 Madrid, Spain

F. A. Dijcks, Department of CNS-Pharmacology, Organon, P. O. Box 20, Oss, The Netherlands

M. G. P. Feenstra, Netherlands Institute for Brain Research, Meibergdreef 33, 1105 AZ Amsterdam ZO, The Netherlands

E. Fride, Department of Pharmacology, The Hebrew University, Hadassah Medical School, 91010 Jerusalem, Israel

A. J. Friedhoff, Department of Psychiatry, Millhauser Laboratories, New York University School of Medicine, New York, NY 10016, USA

T. Greenamyre, Department of Neurology, 1120 Neuroscience Laboratory Building, 1103 East Huron Street, The University of Michigan, Ann Arbor, MI 48104, USA

G. E. Handelmann, Central Nervous System Diseases Research, G. D. Searle & Company, AA5C, St. Louis, MO 63198, USA

R. Hertzberg, Department of Pharmacology, The Hebrew University, Hadassah Medical School, 91010 Jerusalem, Israel

H. J. Huisjes, Department of Obstetrics and Gynaecology, University Hospital Groningen, Oostersingel 59, 9713 EZ Groningen, The Netherlands

M. V. Johnston, 1120 Neuroscience Laboratory Building, 1103 East Huron Street, The University of Michigan, Ann Arbor, MI 48104, USA

C. K. Kellogg, Department of Psychology, University of Rochester, Rochester, NY 14627, USA

H. B. W. M. Koëter, Department of Biological Toxicology, TNO-CIVO Toxicology and Nutrition Institute, PO Box 360, 3700 AJ Zeist, The Netherlands

R. M. Kostrzewa, Department of Pharmacology, Quillen-Dishner College of Medicine, East Tennessee State University, Johnson City, TN 37614, USA

J. M. Lauder, Department of Anatomy, University of North Carolina, School of Medicine, Chapel Hill, NC 27514, USA

B. E. Leonard, Pharmacology Department, University College, Galway, Republic of Ireland

S. Levine, Department of Psychiatry, Stanford University, Stanford, CA 94305, USA

P. D. Lewis, Department of Histopathology, The Royal Postgraduate Medical School, Hammersmith Hospital, DuCane Road, London W12 OHS, UK

W. Lichtensteiger, Institute for Pharmacology, University of Zurich, Gloriastrasse 32, CH-8006 Zurich, Switzerland

M. Manthorpe, Department of Biology, M-001 School of Medicine, University of California at San Diego, La Jolla, CA 92093, USA

B.S. McEwen, Laboratory of Neuroendocrinology, The Rockefeller University, 1230 York Avenue, New York, NY 10021, USA

J.C. Miller, Department of Psychiatry, Millhauser Laboratories, New York University School of Medicine, New York, NY 10016, USA

D.R. Minck, Institute for Developmental Research, Children's Hospital Research Foundation, Cincinnati, OH 45229, USA

M. Mirmiran, Netherlands Institute for Brain Research, Meibergdreef 33, 1105 AZ Amsterdam ZO, The Netherlands

D. Montero, Department of Neuropharmacology, Cajal Institute, CSIC, 28006 Madrid, Spain

B. Odermatt, Institute for Pharmacology, University of Zurich, Gloriastrasse 32, CH-8006 Zurich, Switzerland

J.W. Olney, Department of Psychiatry and Pathology, Washington University, School of Medicine, St. Louis, MO 63110, USA

A.J. Patel, MRC Developmental Neurobiology Unit, Institute of Neurology, 1 Wakefield Street, London WC1N 1PJ, UK

P. Perkins, Department of Anatomy, School of Medicine, University of California, Los Angeles, CA 90024, USA

B.D. Perry, Department of Psychiatry, Division of Child and Adolescent Psychiatry and The Harris Center for Developmental Studies, The University of Chicago School of Medicine, 5841 S. Maryland Ave., Chicago, IL 60637, USA

B. Pettmann, Department of Biology, M-001 School of Medicine, University of California at San Diego, La Jolla, CA 92093, USA

P. Rakic, Yale University School of Medicine, New Haven, CT 06510, USA

U. Ribary, Institute for Pharmacology, University of Zurich, Gloriastrasse 32, CH-8006 Zurich, Switzerland

P.M. Rodier, Department of Obstetrics and Gynecology, University of Rochester, School of Medicine and Dentistry, 601 Elmwood Avenue, Rochester, NY 14642, USA

P. Rosenfeld, Department of Psychiatry, Stanford University, Stanford, CA 94305, USA

V.R. Sara, Karolinska Institute, Department of Psychiatry, St. Göran's Hospital, Box 12500, 11281 Stockholm, Sweden

M. Schlumpf, Institute for Pharmacology, University of Zurich, Gloriastrasse 32, CH-8006 Zurich, Switzerland

F. Silverstein, Department of Pediatrics and Neurology, 1120 Neuroscience Laboratory Building, 1103 East Huron Street, The University of Michigan, Ann Arbor, MI 48104, USA

T.A. Slotkin, Department of Pharmacology, Box 3813, Duke University Medical Center, Durham, NC 27710, USA

F.G.M. Snijdewint, Netherlands Institute for Brain Research, Meibergdreef 33, 1105 AZ Amsterdam ZO, The Netherlands

W. Sutanto, Rudolf Magnus Institute for Pharmacology, University of Utrecht, Vondellaan 6, 3521 GD Utrecht, The Netherlands

D.F. Swaab, Netherlands Institute for Brain Research, Meibergdreef 33, 1105 AZ Amsterdam ZO, The Netherlands

A. Vaccari, Department of Neurosciences, University of Cagliari, Via Porcell 4, 09124 Cagliari, Italy

S. Varon, Department of Biology, M-001 School of Medicine, University of California at San Diego, La Jolla, CA 92093, USA

J.A.M. Van Eekelen, Rudolf Magnus Institute for Pharmacology, University of Utrecht, Vondellaan 6, 3521 GD Utrecht, The Netherlands

F. Van Haaren, Netherlands Institute for Brain Research, Meibergdreef 33, 1105 AZ Amsterdam ZO, The Netherlands

C.V. Vorhees, Institute for Developmental Research, Children's Hospital Research Foundation, Cincinnati, OH 45229, USA

M. Weinstock, Department of Pharmacology, The Hebrew University, Hadassah Medical School, 91010 Jerusalem, Israel

B. Weiss, Environmental Health Sciences Center and Department of Biophysics, University of Rochester School of Medicine and Dentistry, Rochester, NY 14642, USA

H.R. Widmer, Institute for Pharmacology, University of Zurich, Gloriastrasse 32, CH-8006 Zurich, Switzerland

Preface

The Netherlands Institute for Brain Research in Amsterdam, founded in 1909, has a successful tradition of organizing Summer Schools for Brain Research. The topics which are discussed have always been related to the institute's programme, highlighting the international progress made in a particular field of brain research. Proceedings of these meetings have always been published as a volume in the Progress in Brain Research series. The topic of the 15th Summer School was "Neurochemistry of functional neuroteratology; permanent effects of chemicals on the developing brain". It was chosen to broaden our understanding of an increasingly important branch of brain research generally called 'behavioral teratology'. Rather than on gross abnormalities in development as encountered in classical teratology, this field focusses on the subtle but long-lasting changes found in the brain due to deleterious chemical and environmental factors experienced during neurogenesis and maturation. Until recently, this research field has predominantly been the domain of scientists in toxicologic and public health departments. Moreover, mainly the behavioral consequences of such perturbations have attracted attention. This is, for instance, evident by looking at the recently issued Handbook of Behavioral Teratology (Eds. E.P. Riley and C.V. Vorhees, Plenum Press, New York, 1986). The behavioral studies can be very sensitive parameters for functional changes of the brain and are probably highly relevant in view of the etiology of mental retardation, learning disabilities, emotional disturbances and social interaction problems. However, behavioral studies only focus on one expression of the anomalies induced, and, although Werboff and Gottlieb (Obstet. Gynecol., 18: 420–423, 1963), who introduced the term behavioral teratology, already recognized the chemical counterpart of the changes, it would be more appropriate to speak about 'functional neuroteratology'. Secondly, behavioral outcomes do not explain how chemicals or environment interfere with normal brain development, nor do such studies provide us with cues on how to prevent such effects or, when possible, how the impaired situation can be improved in later life. An important step into such basic questions was made at a Symposium organized in 1982 during which toxicologists and behaviorologists were brought together with pharmacologists (Application of Behavioral Pharmacology in Toxicology; Eds. G. Zbinden, V. Cuomo, G. Racagni and B. Weiss, Raven Press, New York, 1983). The 15th Summer School has tried to go one step beyond that by bringing together those who study the behavioral dysfunction in relation with the neurochemical abnormalities of the brain and those who influence brain development experimentally so as to investigate the mechanism of normal brain development. Since the subtle but long-lasting changes in brain function should have their origin in altered quantitative or qualitative measures of neurochemistry, it was our initiative to discuss the biochemistry of functional neuroteratology.

The intention of the 15th Summer School was to present high-level didactic reviews of important lines of investigation within the above-mentioned field. The present proceedings provide a series of reviews which outline functional neuroteratology, including clinical and governmental regulation aspects (section 1), followed by chapters that discuss the lasting effects in the brain induced by exposure to hormonal imbalances (section 2), neuroactive drugs (section 3) and food and environmental factors (section 4) during the period of brain development. Finally, some basic neurochemical mechanisms are reviewed which might underlie the changes seen in functional neuroteratology (section 5). This set of reviews was not meant to cover the entire field of functional neuroteratology; the reviewers were primarily chosen to stimulate and initiate the discussion on the way in which the chemical imprinting of the developing brain of laboratory animals can manifest itself and can permanently alter the organization and function of the nervous system. This would help to point the way as to how clinical studies on functional neuroteratogens should be performed and interpreted.

The editors would like to express their gratitude to Ms. Wanda Chen-Pelt and Ms. Tini Eikelboom, who both took part in the organization committee of the Summer School and without whose organizational skill the planning of this event would have been less enjoyable and the process of compiling the present proceedings impossible.

Gerard J. Boer
Matthijs G. P. Feenstra
Majid Mirmiran
Dick F. Swaab
Frans van Haaren

Acknowledgements

The Fifteenth International Summer School of Brain Research could not have been organized without the financial support of:

Ayerst Laboratories Research, Inc., Princeton (USA)
Beecham Pharmaceuticals Research Division, Surrey (UK)
Dr. Saal van Zwanenberg Foundation, Oss (The Netherlands)
Duphar B.V., Weesp (The Netherlands)
Foundation "C.J. Van den Houtenfonds", Amsterdam (The Netherlands)
Foundation "Het Remmert Adriaan Laanfonds", Amsterdam (The Netherlands)
Foundation Benefit Fund Society of Parents of Mentally Disabled Persons, Maarssen (The Netherlands)
Genootschap ter Bevordering van Natuur-, Genees- en Heelkunde, Amsterdam (The Netherlands)
I.E. Du Pont de Nemours & Company, Newark (USA)
Ministry of Welfare, Public Health and Culture, Rijswijk (The Netherlands)
Organon International B.V., Oss (The Netherlands)
Royal Netherlands Academy of Arts and Sciences, Amsterdam (The Netherlands)
Shell Centre, London (UK)

Contents

SECTION I

Outlines of Functional Neuroteratology

G.J. Boer, M.G.P. Feenstra, M. Mirmiran, D.F. Swaab and F. Van Haaren
Progress in Brain Research, Vol. 73
© 1988 Elsevier Science Publishers B.V. (Biomedical Division)

CHAPTER 1

Concept of functional neuroteratology and the importance of neurochemistry

Dick F. Swaab, Gerard J. Boer and Matthijs G. P. Feenstra

Nederlands Instituut voor Hersenonderzoek, Meibergdreef 33, 1105 AZ Amsterdam, The Netherlands

Interest in congenital malformations may be traced back to the Assyrians, Babylonians and Egyptians. In ancient Greek mythology, too, cyclops and other types of malformations are mentioned. However, a causal link with chemicals during development was not made in those days, as far as we know. Until a century ago, factors other than chemicals were generally thought to be the causes of congenital defects, e.g., excess or paucity of semen, undersized uterus, abdominal trauma during pregnancy or the influence of devils and demons (Paré, 1537, see Health Council report, 1985). Only alcohol was considered as a potential danger. Consumption of alcohol on wedding days was prohibited even in ancient Carthage, out of fear that an abnormal child might be begotten (cf. Jones and Smith, 1975).

It was only in the last century that Etienne Geoffry de Saint-Hilaire was able to induce experimentally anencephaly and spina bifida and coined the term teratology (cf. Schmid, 1987). The concept that more subtle behavioural or functional defects might be due to chemicals during pregnancy was put forward for the first time by Werboff and Gottlieb (1963), who introduced the term behavioural teratology in scientific literature. Neurochemical alterations in relation to functional teratology were reported soon after these observations (e.g., Eiduson, 1966; Tonge, 1972; Huttunen, 1971).

Functional neuroteratology is, consequently, quite a new concept in neuro*sciences*. Yet, the *idea* that emotions of the mother might affect the fetus is certainly much older as is evident from old wives' tales. The birth of the Siamese twins Judith and Helena, who were exhibited in The Netherlands during fairs from 1701 to 1723 was thought to be due to the copulating dogs their mother had watched during pregnancy ('verzien', Naaktgeboren, 1985).

For the acceptance of the importance of the concept of behavioural teratology catastrophes, e.g., in Minamata Bay and Iraq (Weiss, 1988) and the description of the fetal alcohol syndrome have been important. Lemoine et al. (1968) were the first to report disturbed brain development in children following alcohol use by the pregnant mother. Such an effect had, in fact, been suggested as early as in the beginning of the eighteenth century (cf. Warner et Rosett, 1975) and in a more recent past by Huxley, when he described in '*Brave New World*' how 'Gammas' were created by dosing the eggs almost to death with alcohol during the 'Bokanovsky Process' ("They say somebody made a mistake when he was still in the bottle – thought he was a Gamma and put alcohol into his blood surrogate. That is why he is so stunted." (Huxley, 1932)). Lemoine's findings were published in French and had, therefore, to be rediscovered and published in English by Jones et al. (1973) before it became known as 'the fetal alcohol syndrome', which is in serious cases characterized by microcephaly and mental retardation.

Alcohol now appears to be only one example of the many compounds that may cause functional teratology. Such effects may also be due to, e.g., opiates, marihuana, caffeine and nicotine (for references see Butler and Goldstein, 1973; Vorhees, 1986a; Tanaka et al., 1987; Swaab and Mirmiram, 1988), to medicines (e.g., the kinds of medicine that 80% of pregnant Dutch women seem to use; Eskes et al., 1983), to radiation from atomic bomb explosions (Miller and Blott, 1972) or X-ray examinations (Granroth, 1979), to food additives (Olney, 1988; Weiss, 1988), to heavy metals (Annau, 1988) or other environmental chemicals.

Functional neuroteratology, the iceberg under the classical teratological tip?

Some chemicals may cause only classic teratology (e.g., limb malformations), while others cause only functional teratological defects but no gross CNS malformations (Hutchings, 1983; Leonard, 1981). However, increasing numbers of chemicals appear to have the capacity of causing both functional neuroteratological and classical teratological birth defects. On the one hand, various well-established functional teratogens, such as alcohol, are also found to increase the frequency of gross morphological birth defects (Vorhees, 1986a). In general, the causal relationship between chemicals and classical teratological defects is, however, often hard to prove because of the extremely high number of exposed individuals that is needed in order to result in statistically significant numbers of affected children. On the other hand, compounds known as classical teratogens also seem capable of inducing functional defects.

It is still not well established whether or not preconceptional or early gestational exposure to sex hormones may induce teratogenic defects, but dysmorphic features have been reported in the offspring of mothers using such compounds (Lorber et al., 1979). The enormous attention the diethylstilboestrol (DES) catastrophy has received was mainly based upon the small chance (1:10000) that DES daughters would develop cervical or vaginal carcinomas (Herbst et al., 1981). However, functional defects seem to be more common. About 25% of the DES daughters and sons might develop functional, reproductive defects (Bercel and Colwell, 1981; Stenchever et al., 1981). The reported 5- to 7-times increased chance that DES daughters become bi- or homosexual (Ehrhardt et al., 1985) are of a similar order to the reproductive defects, and in any case much more frequent than the chance of gross morphological birth defects.

There is a growing concern that valproate may cause spina bifida in about 1% of exposed pregnancies (Robert and Guibaud, 1982; Bjerkedal et al., 1982). This compound is also teratogenic in rat and mouse (Trotz et al., 1987). However, valproic acid may be a functional teratogen even at lower doses that do not induce such gross malformations (Chapman and Cutler, 1984; Vorhees, 1987).

Corticosteroids, which may be teratogenic in high doses (Baxter and Fraser, 1950; Warrel and Taylor, 1968; Schardein, 1985) may inhibit psychomotor development (Marton and Szondy, 1982) or affect behaviour when given during pregnancy at much lower dose levels (cf. De Kloet et al., 1988).

In conclusion, some compounds are capable of causing both gross morphological CNS birth defects and functional teratological defects. Such compounds might seem to induce functional defects at a higher frequency and lower dose level than the classical malformations. Consequently, for such compounds functional teratology seems a more sensitive way to find their effects than the study of classical teratological defects.

What compounds might cause functional neuroteratology?

An increasing number of chemicals is reported to affect the developing brain. In fact, all those chemical compounds which are capable of influencing adult brain function may also affect brain development (Swaab, 1980). At the present time this principle has been established, e.g., for sex hormones, corticosteroids and thyroid hormones, for neurotransmitters, i.e., acetylcholine, biogenic amines, amino acids and peptides, for stimulating compounds (alcohol, nicotine, caffeine, marihuana), anaesthetics and metals. Exogenous substances which alter the balance of any of the endogenous neuroactive compounds seem to act on the formation of the materials of the brain, e.g., cell number, migration, connections and receptors. They are therefore capable of altering brain development in a permanent way (for review see Swaab and Mirmiran, 1988). When peripherally administered compounds are 'neuro'-active in adulthood, they are evidently capable of easily crossing biological barriers such as the placenta and will readily reach the fetal brain. Their level in the fetal brain might even be higher than in the maternal circulation (Mirkin and Singh, 1976) and might persist in the fetus for a much longer time than in the maternal tissues (Madsen et al., 1981; Simmons et al., 1983). Compounds which are not neuroactive in adulthood because of poor blood-brain barrier (BBB) penetration may be neuroactive in development as the fetal and neonatal BBB are known to be open for many more chemicals than the adult one (Werboff and Gottlieb, 1963).

By what mechanisms do these compounds act?

Drugs taken by the pregnant mother may impair the developing child's brain in different ways.

Firstly, this action may be *indirect*, i.e., not by a direct action on brain cells. This is e.g., the case with aspirin which, when taken by the pregnant mother, may result in a higher incidence of intracranial bleeding (Collins, 1981; Rumack et a., 1981). Another action of this kind is the alcohol-induced impairment of umbilical circulation producing hypoxia and acidosis in the fetus (Mukherjee and Hodgen, 1982). Prenatal expo-

sure of barbiturates might also influence brain development indirectly by altering liver metabolism of sex hormones (Reinisch and Sanders, 1982).

Secondly, drugs may affect brain development by interacting *directly* with the formation of the neuronal and glial network, e.g., by affecting cell division, cell death, cell migration or the formation of neurites, synapses of the synthesis of transmission-related molecules such as receptors. Most, if not all, medicines in fact appear to affect several of these processes.

Cell acquisition is reported to be slowed down by a number of medicines, both in vivo and in vitro. Barbiturates were found to cause a 30% reduction in the number of cerebellar Purkinje cells and a 15% reduction in hippocampal pyramidal cells. Other compounds which have similar deleterious effects include, e.g., corticosteroids, chlorpromazine, alcohol, reserpine, thyroid hormone and sex hormones (for references see Swaab and Mirmiran, 1984; Patel and Lewis, 1988; Vaccari, 1988). Indirect evidence for decreased brain cell division is provided by the smaller head circumferences which have been found at birth following maternal treatment with sex hormones (Huisjes, personal communication), alpha-methyldopa, propranolol or diphenylhydantoin, or by the use of alcohol during human pregnancy (for references see Swaab and Mirmiran, 1984).

Cell death is augmented by nicotine (Kraus et al., 1981), accelerated by alcohol exposure prior to birth in the rat (Yanai, 1981), and delayed by morphine in the chick embryo (Meriney et al., 1985).

Cell migration may be disturbed by alcohol (Jones et al., 1976), anticonvulsants (Trice and Ambler, 1985) and monosodium glutamate (Marani et al., 1982).

Formation of neurites and synapses is known to be affected by sex hormones, corticosteroids, morphine, methadone, anticonvulsive agents and by alcohol (for references see Swaab and Mirmiran, 1984).

Receptors may also be permanently altered by neuroactive compounds given during development. Just to mention a few examples, haloperidol, which blocks dopamine receptors, induced in this way a persisting decrease in the number of dopamine receptors in the striatum (Rosengarten and Friedhoff, 1979), whereas L-Dopa, which increases dopamine synthesis, enhanced receptor density (see Miller and Friedhoff, 1988). Prenatal morphine exposure in the rat increases the adult number and affinity of spinal cord opiate receptors (Kirby, 1984), and prenatal exposure to diazepam results in enduring reductions of its binding sites in the rat thalamus (Livezey et al., 1985).

It might be good to point out that only recently has it become clear that paternal factors may be of importance as well (Soyka and Joffe, 1980). The mechanism of action of such factors might be similar to maternal factors, as is true, e.g., in case of passive smoking. On the other hand, not-yet-revealed mechanisms of action on the gametes (Campbell and Perkins, 1988) might also exist, e.g., in the case of developmental defects in the offspring in case of paternal alcohol abuse, or in the adverse effects on the offspring of male rats pretreated with opiates, lead, ethanol, caffeine, thalidomide, anaesthetics and cigarettes before mating (Soyka and Joffe, 1980).

The biochemical basis of functional neuroteratology

All effects of neuroactive compounds on the developing brain will ultimately be based upon biochemical mechanisms, whether the effect involves cell death, cell migration, cell division, cellular outgrowths or subcellular mechanisms. With the emergence of functional neuroteratology as a scientific discipline, its biochemical basis has attained attention. It is striking in this respect that the early reviewers on this field (Barlow and Sullivan, 1975; Coyle et al., 1976) already treated the subtle morphological, biochemical and behavioural disturbances as parts of one complex, in which morphological and biochemical changes underlie the behavioural changes. In addition, it was suggested that biochemical measurements might be more sensitive than behavioural screening procedures. However, the discovery of underlying chemical mechanisms has only recently obtained momentum. In this respect one may wonder whether the term 'behavioural teratology' (Werboff and Gottlieb, 1963) is still useful. The term 'functional teratology' may be more appropriate.

Knowledge of the anatomy and chemistry of neurotransmission has increased enormously in the last decades and has made clear that many neuroactive compounds interact selectively with particular neurotransmitter systems in the brain. It is tempting to suggest that these compounds produce long-term or lasting effects on the developing brain by disturbing the neurochemical processes that they are known to affect in adulthood. Studies following this approach in development have reported both similarities and differences in the mechanisms of action as compared with the adult brain. This is of interest not only because of the relation to the mechanism by which neuroteratological effects are produced, but also since it gives information relevant to the developmental biology of the nervous system and to the study of chronic treatments with neuroactive drugs in adulthood (e.g., Miller and Friedhoff, 1988; Kellogg, 1988; Del Rio et al., 1988).

As stated by Hutchings (1980, 1983), the trade-off between human and animal neurobehavioural studies cross-validates both. Meaningful neurochemical data are difficult to obtain in the human situation, making a neurochemical cross-validation at present impossible. In the future, neurochemical measurements may certainly contribute to our knowledge of neonatal neuropathology, in particular with the emergence of non-invasive techniques. However, in our opinion the importance of neurochemistry to functional neuroteratology lies not in the detection of abnormalities in the human condition, but rather in the elucidation of the mechanism by which neuroactive compounds have produced these abnormalities. It is generally accepted that Wilson's principles of teratology (Wilson, 1977) apply to functional neuroteratology (Vorhees, 1986b) and that it is not only the developmental phase which defines the outcome of the teratological action of a chemical, but also the access, dose, chemical nature and, above all, the mechanism of action of that compound (Coyle et al., 1976; Leonard, 1981; Hutchings, 1983). Only knowledge of the mechanism of action will enable us to predict from animal studies the teratological potential of chemicals and this will be of great importance not only for the development of safer medicines, but also for unravelling the chemical steps that are essential for optimal brain development.

In which developmental period do chemicals affect the developing brain?

A central principle in teratology is that the various stages of development provide critical periods in which the developing organism is more vulnerable than in other stages. Because of the thalidomide tragedy, our awareness of the dangers of drug ingestion has cautioned us against the indiscriminate use of medicines mainly during the initial stage of pregnancy. However, although later in gestation medicines do not cause any gross physical malformations, they may cause permanent behavioural or other functional deviations. Literature suggests that at present there is not only a potential health hazard of chemicals during the second half of gestation, but during lactation as well (e.g., PCPs; Schardein, 1985). This is also an important item in relation to the increasing amounts of chemicals that are prescribed during lactation.

It seems logical that permanent alterations may be induced as long as brain areas are still developing. Recent observations of ours on the sexual differentiation of the human hypothalamus suggest that the sensitive period for functional teratology might even extend into the first postnatal

years. Observations in rat have indicated that the sexually dimorphic nucleus (SDN) of the hypothalamus is sensitive to sex hormones during the period that the sexual dimorphy of this area is just arising, i.e., during the first postnatal week (Gorski, 1984). It has been presumed that in humans this vulnerable phase of sexual differentiation would take place during mid-gestation. The SDN has been localized in the human hypothalamus as well, and in adulthood contains twice as many cells in man as in woman (Swaab and Fliers, 1985). However, in a recent developmental study (Swaab and Hofman, in prep.), the SDN appeared not to become sexually dimorphic during mid-gestation, but only after several years postnatally. This suggests that, at least for a few postnatal years, this process might be affected by chemicals.

A postnatal vulnerable period is also a relevant consideration for compounds other than sex hormones, e.g., in children suffering from minimal brain dysfunction, who are often subjected to extremely high doses of imipramine- or amphetamine-like drugs (for review see Gross and Wilson, 1974), despite the fact that improvement often occurs even in the absence of any medication whatsoever. The same concerns may be expressed with respect to the treatment of nocturnal enuresis by means of antidepressants (Huygen, 1979), about steroids used in order to inhibit growth in extremely tall boys and girls (Van der Werff ten Bosch and Bot, 1981: Van der Werff ten Bosch et al., 1986), about clonidine treatment of children for short stature (Pintor et al., 1987) and about oxytocin used to induce lactation (Boer and Kruisbrink, 1984).

When might symptoms of functional teratology occur?

One of the main problems of recognizing symptoms of functional teratology is the long time interval between the moment that chemicals are acting upon the developing brain and the occurrence of symptoms. Often, the first occasion that altered functions may become apparent is at school-going age. This has been reported, e.g., for smoking by the pregnant mother, which affects the school performance of the child (Butler and Goldstein, 1973; Abel, 1980). It goes without saying that, for this reason, it is often hard to prove a relationship between early exposure to chemicals and functional defects. Effects might even occur very late in life. In a study on the effect of clonidine on the development of rat brain and behaviour, this compound appeared to affect masculine sexual behaviour in adulthood (Mirmiran et al., 1983). Many other chemicals, when given during development might affect reproduction (for references see Swaab and Mirmiran, 1988). If such reproductive effects would also hold for human subjects, the time interval between the use of chemicals and the appearance of symptoms might be as long as several decades in humans. The observation that the effects of prenatal stress or chemicals administered during development might even be carried over to following generations (Friedler, 1974; Pollard, 1986; Campbell and Perkins, 1988) has added a new dimension to this long time interval.

What symptoms belong to functional neuroteratology?

Another set of clinical problems of functional neuroteratology is that chemical compounds do not generally give rise to a syndrome in the child that can easily be recognized by the clinician as being specific to a particular compound. In fact the symptoms, e.g., cognitive disturbances, mental retardation, reproductive or motoric defects, disturbed language development or sleep disturbances, may have so many different causes that one usually does not even make the connection between symptoms and chemicals at all. For instance, sexual differentiation of the brain may be affected not only by sex hormones, but also by serotonin, noradrenaline, dopamine-related drugs, nicotine, alcohol, cimetidine, morphine barbiturates, and maternal stress (for references

see Swaab and Mirmiran, 1988). In addition, one compound, such as alcohol, may cause many different symptoms, e.g., prematurity (Berkowitz et al., 1982; Kaminski et al., 1981), cognitive disturbances and mental retardation (Spaans and Verspreet, 1981), language disturbances (Gusella and Fried, 1984) and disturbances of sexual differentiation (McGivern et al., 1984), possibly depending on the stage of development in which it was acting on the fetal brain (cf. Rodier, 1988).

A third problem in functional teratology is that clinicians do not find defects caused by chemicals during development, because they do not know whet symptoms exactly they should look for. The sleep disturbances in 6- to 8-year-old children whose mothers had been treated with clonidine (Huisjes et al., 1986) were only found because Mirmiran et al. (1983) had described sleep defects before in rat, after early postnatal treatment with the same compound. In this respect animal experiments might be very valuable in focussing the clinician's attention to a particular set of symptoms to look for in relation to functional teratology.

A fourth problem is that functional teratology might contribute to more-or-less circumscribed neurologic or psychiatric disease entities that at present are generally considered to be multicausal. One of such diseases is *schizophrenia*. Jakob and Beckmann (1986) described histological alterations in limbic regions, e.g., heterotopic displacement of nerve cells in entorhinal cortex, suggesting a disturbance of neuronal migration during mid-gestation in which environmental factors might play a role. The *autistic* brain might also have been affected during development (Bauman and Kemper, 1984; Sanua, 1986). Pregnancy and birth complications have repeatedly been mentioned as possible causes of infantile autism. However, unexpected differences in preconceptional histories of the families of autistic children have been reported as well. An increased incidence of exposure to chemicals of the parents of such children was noted in a retrospective study (Coleman, 1979). In a follow-up study of 40 babies who had died of *sudden infant death syndrome* (SIDS) Einspieler and Kenner (1985) found that 78% of the mothers concerned had labour induced by oxytocin. Others have related SIDS to the use of cigarettes or barbiturates by the mother (cf. Naeye, 1980). It has been suggested that the *hyperactive child syndrome* is an effect of maternal alcohol use during pregnancy (Warner and Rosett, 1975). *Depression* and *anxiety* have been found to be more frequent in the sons and daughters of women who had been treated with DES during pregnancy than in controls (Vessey et al., 1983; Meyer-Bahlburg and Ehrhardt, 1987).

Of course, most possible relationships between functional teratological effects of chemicals and certain disease entities are at present highly speculative. However, the idea certainly seems worthy of a follow-up. It should be noted that there might also occur unexpected seemingly positive functional teratological effects. Maternal alcohol ingestion was associated with a decreased risk of respiratory distress syndrome (Ioffe and Chernick, 1987), and psychological development in children born to mothers treated with bromocriptine appeared to be more precocious (Raymond et al., 1985). However, the presence of yet undetected disadvantageous effects in such children should certainly be considered.

May animal experiments predict functional teratology in man?

Functional neuroteratological effects are, for various reasons, often hard to prove in humans (see before). Confirmation of effects in experimental animals may, therefore, be a crucial step in the establishment of such effects. On the other hand, the question whether animal experiments might provide good models for predicting functional teratological effects, e.g., of new chemicals, is of course of great importance too.

The few experimental animal and human investigations that have studied related phenomena owing to chemicals in development, indicate that animal experiments may indeed give useful predictions in this field. Clonidine administered during the first postnatal weeks in rat caused, among other defects, sleep disturbances in adulthood (Mirmiran et al., 1983). A recent follow-up study examined the effects of prenatal clonidine treatment of hypertensive mothers on the development of their children, who were then 6–8 years of age. Compared to non-treated hypertensives a seven-times-as-high excess of sleep disturbances was observed in the exposed group (Huisjes et al., 1986).

In the mistaken belief that it would prevent miscarriages, 1–4.5 million pregnant American women used DES. The observation that DES daughters have an increased incidence of bisexuality and homosexuality (Ehrhardt et al., 1985) could have been suspected from the masculinizing effect of DES on brain differentiation (Döhler et al., 1986). The dysmorphic facial changes of the fetal alcohol syndrome can be mimicked in animal experiments (Leonard, 1988). The same is true for the smaller head circumference due to alpha-methyl dopa (Swaab and Mirmiran, 1984).

These few examples illustrate that animal experiments in the field of functional teratology might give useful clues concerning the defects that clinicians have to look for in children exposed to chemicals in development by means of long-term follow-up studies. Of course, species differences in sensitivity to the chemicals should be taken into consideration. However, in contrast to what is generally believed, humans are often more sensitive than animals to the teratogenicity of drugs (Council on Environmental Quality, 1981).

Summary and conclusions

Functional neuroteratology – i.e., the existence of behavioural or other functional defects owing to the effect of chemicals during brain development – is a quite new development in the neurosciences with important fundamental and clinical consequences. The classical gross morphological birth defects owing to the effects of chemicals during the first months of pregnancy appear to form only the tip of the teratological iceberg. Functional teratological defects may generally be induced at lower dose levels and higher frequencies than the classical birth malformations. All neuroactive compounds may affect brain development, e.g., sex hormones, corticosteroids, thyroid hormones, neurotransmitters, addictive and stimulating compounds, anaesthetics and organometals.

Chemicals might affect the developing nervous system indirectly (e.g., by affecting the umbilical cord circulation) or directly by affecting cell division, cell death, cell migration, the formation of neurites, synapses or the synthesis of transmission-related molecules. A paternal factor may be of importance too. Functional teratological effects are generally due to chemicals taken after the first trimester of gestation. The possibility, though, that such mechanisms are still present during lactation, and even later in development, seems to exist.

The use of medicines during pregnancy and lactation and prior to conception should therefore be strictly limited to therapeutic necessity. For such cases a list of relatively safe medicines should be made, and the children exposed to such chemicals should be followed up carefully for a long-term period, using indications on the type of possible defects derived from animal experiments.

Clinical recognition of functional teratological defects may be hampered by the long time interval (up to decades) between the administration of chemicals and the occurrence of the symptoms. In addition, symptoms are not specific to certain chemicals and may include cognitive disturbances, mental retardation, reproductive or motoric defects, disturbed language development or sleep disturbances, while one compound may cause different symptoms. Moreover, one process, such as sexual differentiation, might be affected by many compounds.

In addition, functional teratology may contribute to multicausal disease entities, e.g. schizophrenia, autism, SIDS, hyperactive child syndrome, depression or anxiety. An additional problem is that clinicians generally do not know what symptoms of functional teratology they have to look for. In this respect, animal experiments may provide both a selection of the right functions to be studied in human follow-ups as well as a suggestion of the underlying biochemical mechanisms. This means that systematic searching for functional teratological effects and mechanisms of chemicals should be encouraged. On the other hand, as we have learned from the thalidomide tragedy, species differences in sensitivity to chemicals might exist. This means that safety of a compound can never be proved by animal experiments. Consequently, information must be obtained from children exposed to chemicals in prospective trials as well. This concerns not only clinical follow-up studies on possible developmental defects. Also, systematic neuropathological investigation of the exposed newborn might contribute considerably to our knowledge. Last but not least, functional teratology may give very valuable clues concerning the chemical processes that are crucial in normal brain development. This aspect is one of the ultimate purposes of the present volume.

Acknowledgement

We want to thank Aad Janssen for his secretarial help.

References

Abel, E. (1980) Smoking during pregnancy: a review of effects on growth and development of offspring. *Hum. Biol.*, 52: 593–625.

Annau, Z. (1988) Organometals and brain development. Ch. 19 this volume.

Barlow, S.M. and Sullivan, F.M. (1975) Behavioural teratology. In C.L. Berry and D.E. Poswillo (Eds.), *Teratology. Trends and Applications.* Springer, Berlin, pp. 103–120.

Bauman, M.L. and Kemper, T.L. (1984) The brain in infantile autism: a histoanatomic case report. *Neurology*, 34: 275.

Baxter, H. and Fraser, F.C. (1950) Production of congenital defects in offspring of female mice treated with cortisone. *McGill Med. J.*, 19: 245–249.

Bercel, V. and Colwell, L. (1981) Randomized trial of high doses of stilboestrol and ethisterone therapy in pregnancy: long-term follow-up of the children. *J. Epidem. Community Hlth*, 35: 155–160.

Berkowitz, G.S., Holford, T.R. and Berkowitz, R.L. (1982) Effects of cigarette smoking, alcohol, coffee and tea consumption on preterm delivery. *Early Hum. Dev.*, 7: 239–250.

Bjerkedal, T., Czeizel, A., Goujard, J., Kallen, B., Mastroiacova, P., Nevin, N., Oakley, G.Jr. and Robert, E. (1982) Valproic acid and spina bifida. *Lancet*, November 13: 1096.

Boer G.J. and Kruisbrink, J. (1984) Effects of continuous administration of oxytocin by an Accurel device on parturition in the rat and on development and diuresis in the offspring. *J. Endocrinol.*, 101: 121–129.

Butler, N.R. and Goldstein, H. (1973) Smoking in pregnancy and subsequent child development. *Br. Med. J.*, 4: 573–575.

Campbell, J.H. and Perkins, P. (1988) Transgenerational effects of drug and hormonal treatments in mammals: A review of observations and ideas. Ch. 33, this volume.

Chapman, J.B. and Cutler, M.G. (1984) Sodium valproate: effects on social behaviour and physical development in the mouse. *Psychopharmacology* (Berlin), 83: 390–396.

Coleman, M. (1979) Studies of the autistic syndromes. In R. Katzman (Ed.) *Congenital and Acquired Cognitive Disorders*. Raven Press, New York, pp. 265–275.

Collins, E. (1981) Maternal and fetal effects of acetaminophen and salicylates in pregnancy. *Obstet. Gynecol., N.Y.*, 58 (Suppl 578): 57S–62S.

Council on environmental quality (1981) *Chemical hazards to human reproduction*. Prepared by Clement Association Inc. for the Council on Environmental Quality, Government Printing Office, Washington.

Coyle, I., Wayner, M.J. and Singer, G. (1976) Behavioral teratogenesis: A critical evaluation. *Pharmacol. Biochem. Behav.*, 4: 191–200.

De Kloet E.R., Rosenfeld, P., Van Eekelen, J.A.M., Sutanto, W. and Levine, S. (1988) Stress, glucocorticoids and development. Ch. 8, this volume.

Del Rio, J., Montero, D. and De Ceballos, M.L. (1988) Long-lasting changes after perinatal exposure to antidepressants. Ch. 12, this volume.

Döhler, K.D., Coquelin, A., Davis, F., Hines, M., Shryne, J.E. and Gorski, R.A. (1986) Aromatization of testicular androgens in physiological concentrations does not defeminize sexual brain functions. *Monogr. Neural Sci.*, 12: 28–35.

Ehrhardt, A.A., Meyer-Bahlburg, H.F.L., Rosen, L.R., Feldman, J.F., Veridiano, N.P., Zimmerman, I. and McEwen, B.S. (1985) Sexual orientation after prenatal exposure to exogenous estrogen. *Arch. Sexual Behav.*, 14: 57–75.

Eiduson, S. (1966) 5-Hydroxytryptamine in the developing chick brain: its normal and altered development and possible control by end product repression. *J. Neurochem.*, 13: 993–932.

Einspieler, C., Kenner, T. (1985) A possible relation between oxytocin for induction of labor and sudden infant death syndrome. *New Engl. J. Med.*, 313: 1660.

Eskes, T.K.A.B., Nijdam, W., Buys, M.J.R.M. and Van Rossum, J.M. (1983) Drug therapy during pregnancy. Effects on mother, fetus and newborn. In: T.K.A.B. Eskes and M. Finster (Eds.) *Drug Therapy During Pregnancy*. Butterworths, London, Boston, Wellington etc., pp. 1–8.

Friedler, G. (1974) Long-term effects of opiates. In: J. Dancis and J.C. Hwang (Eds.), *Perinatal Pharmacology: Problems and Priorities*, Raven Press, New York, pp. 207–219.

Granroth, G. (1979) Defects of the central nervous system in Finland. IV. Association with diagnostic x-ray examinations. *Am. J. Obstet. Gynecol.*, 133: 191–194.

Gorski, R.A. (1984) Critical role for the medial preoptic area in the sexual differentiation of the brain. In: G.J. De Vries, J.P.C. De Bruin, H.B.M. Uylings and M.A. Corner (Eds.), *Sex Differences in the Brain. Prog. Brain Res.*, Vol. 61, Elsevier, Amsterdam, pp. 129–146.

Gross, M.B. and Wilson, W.C. (1974) *Minimal Brain Dysfunction*. Brunner/Mazel, New York.

Gusella, J.L. and Fried, P.A. (1984) Effects of maternal social drinking and smoking on offspring at 13 months. *Neurobehav. Toxicol. Teratol.*, 6: 13–17.

Health Council of the Netherlands (1985) *Report on the Evaluation of the Teratogenicity of Chemical Substances*. No. 1985/6E, the Hague, The Netherlands.

Herbst, A.L., Hubby, M.M., Azizi, F. and Makii, M.M. (1981) Reproductive and gynecologic surgical experience in diethylstilbestrol-exposed daughters. *Am. J. Obstet. Gynecol.*, 141: 1019–1028.

Huisjes, H.J., Hadders-Algra, M. and Touwen, B.C.L. (1986) Is clonidine a behavioural teratogen in the human? *Early Hum. Dev.*, 13: 1–6.

Hutchings, D.E. (1980) Neurobehavioral effects of prenatal origin: Drugs of use and abuse. In R.H. Schwartz and S.J. Yaffe (Eds.) *Drugs and Chemical Risks to the Fetus and Newborn. Prog. Clin. Biol. Res.*, Vol. 36, Alan R. Liss Inc., New York, pp. 109–114.

Hutchings, D.E. (1983) Behavioral teratology: a new frontier in neurobehavioral research. In: E.M. Johnston and D.M. Kochlar (Eds.), *Handbook of Experimental Pharmacology*, Vol. 65, Springer Verlag, Berlin, pp. 207–235.

Huttunen, M.O. (1971) Persistent alteration of turnover of brain noradrenaline in the offspring of rats subjected to stress during pregnancy. *Nature*, 230: 53–55.

Huygen, F.J.A. (1979) De behandeling van enuresis nocturna. *Ned. Tijdschr. Geneesk.*, 123: 748–752.

12

Huxley, A. (1932) *Brave New World*. Grafton Books, London, Great Britain.

Ioffe, S. and Chernick, V. (1987) Maternal alcohol ingestion and the incidence of respiratory distress syndrome. *Am. J. Obstet. Gynecol.*, 156: 1231–1235.

Jakob, H. and Beckmann, H. (1986) Prenatal development disturbances in the limbic allocortex in schizophrenics. *J. Neural Transm.*, 65: 303–326.

Jones, K.L., Smith, D.W., Ulleland, C.N. and Streissgut, A.P. (1973) Pattern of malformation in offspring of chronic alcoholic women. *Lancet*, i: 1267–1271.

Jones, K.L. and Smith, D.W. (1975) The fetal alcohol syndrome. *Teratology*, 12: 1–10.

Jones, K.L. and Smith, D.W. and Hanson, J.W. (1976) The fetal alcohol syndrome: clinical delineation. *Ann. N.Y. Acad. Sci.*, 273: 130–137.

Kaminski, M., Franc, M., Lebouvier, M., Du Mazau-Brun, C. and Rumeau-Rouquette, C. (1981) Moderate alcohol use and pregnancy outcome. *Neurobehav. Toxicol. Teratol.*, 3: 173–181.

Kellogg, C.K. (1988) Benzodiazepines: Influence on the developing brain. Ch. 14, this volume.

Kirby, M.L. (1984) Alterations in fetal and adult responsiveness to opiates following various schedules of prenatal morphine exposure. In: J. Yanai (Ed.) *Neurobehavioral Teratology*. Elsevier, Amsterdam, pp. 235–248.

Kraus, H.F., Campbell, G.A., Fowler, A.C. and Farber, J.P. (1981) Maternal nicotine administration and fetal brain stem damage: a rat model with implications for sudden infant death syndrome. *Am. J. Obstet. Gynecol.*, 140: 743–746.

Lemoine, P., Haronsseau, H., Borteyru, J.-P. and Menuet, J.-C. (1968) Les enfants des parents alcooliques; anomalies observées à propos de 127 cas. *Ouest Méd.* 25: 476–482.

Leonard, B.E. (1988) Alcohol as a social teratogen for the developing brain. Ch. 20, this volume.

Leonard, B.E. (1981) Effect of psychotropic drugs administered to pregnant rats on the behaviour of the offspring. *Neuropharmacology*, 20: 1237–1242.

Livezey, G.T., Radulovacki, M., Isaac, L. and Marczynski, T.J. (1985) Prenatal exposure to diazepam results in enduring reductions in brain receptors and deep slow wave sleep. *Brain Res.* 334: 361–365.

Lorber, C.A., Cassidy, S.B. and Engel, E. (1979) Is there an embryo-fatal exogenous sex steroid exposure syndrome (efesses)? *Fert. Steril.*, 31: 21–24.

Madsen, J.R., Campbell, A. and Baldessarini, R.J. (1981) Effects of prenatal treatment of rats with haloperidol due to altered drug distribution in neonatal brain. *Neuropharmacology*, 20: 931–939.

Marani, E., Rietveld, W.J. and Boon, M.E. (1982) Monosodium glutamate accelerates migration of hypothalamic perikarya at puberty. *Histochemistry*, 75: 145–150.

Marton, I.S. and Szondy, M. (1982) Possible neuroendocrine hazards of prenatal steroid exposure. In: Endröczi et al. (Eds.), *Neuropeptides, Neurotransmitters and Regulation of Endocrine Processes*. Akademia Press, Budapest, pp. 535–543.

McGivern, R.F., Clancy, A.N., Hill, M.A. and Noble, E.P. (1984) Prenatal alcohol exposure alters adult expression of sexually dimorphic behavior in the rat. *Science*, 224: 896–898.

Meriney, S.D., Gray, D.B. and Pilar, G. (1985) Morphine-induced delay of normal cell death in the avian ciliary ganglion. *Science*, 228: 1451–1452.

Meyer-Bahlburg, H.F.L. and Ehrhardt, A.A. (1987) A prenatal-hormone hypothesis for depression in adults with a history of fetal DES exposure. In: U. Halbreich (Ed.), *Hormones and Depression*. Raven Press, New York, pp. 325–338.

Miller, J.C. and Friedhoff, A.J. (1988) Prenatal neurotransmitter programming of postnatal receptor function. Ch. 31, this volume.

Miller, R.W. and Blott, W.J. (1972) Small head size after in utero exposure to atomic radiation. *Lancet*, ii: 784–787.

Mirkin, B.L. and Singh, S. (1976) Placental transfer of pharmacologically active molecules. In: B.L. Mirkin (Ed.) *Perinatal Pharmacology and Therapeutics*. Academic Press, New York, pp. 1–69.

Mirmiran, M., Scholtens, J., Van de Poll, N.E., Uylings, H.B.M., Van der Gugten, J. and Boer, G.J. (1983) Effects of experimental suppression of active (REM) sleep during early development upon adult brain and behavior. *Dev. Brain Res.*, 7: 277–286.

Mukherjee, A.B. and Hodgen, G.D. (1982) Maternal ethanol exposure induces transient impairment of umbilical circulation and feral hypoxia in monkeys. *Science*, 218: 700–702.

Naaktgeboren, C. (1985) Over waarneming en verklaring in de verloskunde. Deel II: 'Het verzien'. *Tijdschr. Verloskundigen*, 10: 329–341.

Naeye, R.L. (1980) Sudden infant death. *Sci. Am.*, 242: 52–58.

Olney, J.W. (1988) Excitotoxic food additives: functional teratological aspects. Ch. 18, this volume.

Patel, A.J. and Lewis, P.D. (1988) Brain cell acquisition and neurotropic drugs with special reference to functional teratogenesis. Ch. 25, this volume.

Pintor, C., Cella, S.G., Loche, S., Puggioni, R., Corda, R., Locatelli, VI and Müller, E.E. (1987) Clonidine treatment for short stature. *Lancet*, May 30: 1226–1230.

Pollard, I. (1986) Prenatal stress effects over two generations in rats. *J. Endocrinol.*, 109: 239–244.

Raymond, J.P., Goldstein, E., Konopka, P., Leleu, M.F., Merceron, R.E. and Loria, Y. (1985) Follow-up of children born of bromocriptine-treated mothers. *Hormone Res.*, 22: 239–246.

Reinisch, J.M. and Sanders, S.A. (1982) Early barbiturate exposure: the brain, sexually dimorphic behavior and learning. *Neurosci. Biobehav. Rev.*, 6: 311–319.

Robert, E. and Guibaud, P. (1982) Maternal valproic acid and congenital neural tube defects. *Lancet*, 23: 937.

Rodier, P.M. (1988) Structural-functional relationships in experimentally-induced brain damage. Ch. 22, this volume.

Rosengarten, H. and Friedhoff, A.J. (1979) Enduring changes in dopamine receptor cells of pups from drug administration to pregnant and nursing rats. *Science*, 203: 1133–1135.

Rumack, C.M., Guggenheim, W.R., Rumack, B.H., Peterson, R.G., Johnson, M.L. and Braithwaite, W.R. (1981) Neonatal intracranial hemorrhage and maternal use of aspirin. *Obstet. Gynecol., N.Y.*, 58: 52S–56S.

Sanua, V.D. (1986) The organic etiology of infantile autism: a critical review of the literature. *Int. J. Neurosci.*, 30: 195–225.

Schardein, J.L. (1985) *Chemically Induced Birth Defects*. Marcel Dekker, Inc., New York and Basel.

Schmid, B. (1987) Old and new concepts in teratogenicity testing. *TIPS*, 8: 133–138.

Simmons, R.D., Miller, R.K. and Kellogg, C.K. (1983) Prenatal diazepam: distribution and metabolism in perinatal rats. *Teratology*, 28: 181–188.

Soyka, L.F. and Joffe, J.M. (1980) Male mediated drug effects on offspring. In: R.H. Schwarz and S.J. Yaffe (Eds.), *Drug and Chemical Risks to the Fetus and Newborn. Prog. Clin. Biol. Res., Vol. 36*. Alan R. Liss, New York, pp. 49–66.

Spaans, C. and Verspreet, F.A.M. (1981) Het foetale alcohol-syndroom: vier patiënten in één gezin. *Ned. Tijdschr. Geneesk.*, 125: 452–454.

Stenchever, M.A., Williamson R.A., Leonard, J., Karp, L.E., Ley, B., Shy, K. and Smith, D. (1981) Possible relationship between in utero diethylstilbestrol exposure and male fertility. *Am. J. Obstet. Gynecol.*, 140: 186–193.

Swaab, D.F. (1980) Neuropeptides and brain development: a working hypothesis. In: C. Di Benedetta, R. Balazs, G. Gombos and P. Procellati (Eds.), *A Multidisciplinary Approach to Brain Development*. Proceedings of the International Meeting, Selva di Fasano. Elsevier/North Holland Biomedical Press, Amsterdam, pp. 181–196.

Swaab, D.F. and Fliers, E. (1985) A sexually dimorphic nucleus in the human brain. *Science*, 228: 1112–1115.

Swaab, D.F. and Mirmiran, M. (1984) Possible mechanisms underlying the teratogenic effects of medicines on the developing brain. In: J. Yanai (Ed.), *Neurobehavioral Teratology*. Elsevier, Amsterdam, pp. 55–71.

Swaab, D.F. and Mirmiran, M. (1988) Permanent effects of chemicals on the developing brain; functional or behavioral teratology. In: M.I. Levere, M.J. Bennett and J. Punt (Eds.) *Fetal and Neonatal Neurology and Neurosurgery*. Churchill, Livingstone, United Kingdom, in press.

Tanaka, H., Nakazawa, K. and Arima, M. (1987) Effects of maternal caffeine ingestion on the perinatal cerebrum. *Biol. Neonate*, 51: 332–339.

Tonge, S.R. (1972) Permanent changes in brain monoamine metabolism induced by the administration of psychotropic drugs during the pre- and neonatal periods in rats. *J. Pharm. Pharmacol.*, 24, Suppl.: 149P–150P.

Trice, J.E. and Ambler, M. (1985) Multiple cerebral defects in an infant exposed in utero to anticonvulsants. *Arch. Pathol. Lab. Med.* 109: 521–523.

Trotz, M., Wegner, Chr. and Nau, H. (1987) Valproic acid-induced neural tube defects: reduction by folinic acid in the mouse. *Life Sci.*, 41: 103–110.

Vaccari, A. (1988) Teratogenic mechanisms of dysthyroidism in the central nervous system. Ch. 6, this volume.

Van der Werff ten Bosch, J.J. and Bot, A. (1981) Growth of tall girls without and during oestrogen treatment. *Neth. J. Med.*, 24: 52–57.

Van der Werff ten Bosch, J.J., Bot, A. and Goslings, B.M. (1986) Growth of tall boys without and during androgen treatment. *Neth. J. Med.*, 29: 73–78.

Vessey, M.P., Fairweather, D.V.I., Norman-Smith, B. and Buckley, J. (1983) A randomized double-blind controlled trial of the value of stilboestrol therapy in pregnancy: long-term follow-up of mothers and their offspring. *Br. J. Obstet. Gynaecol.* 90: 1007–1017.

Vorhees, C.V. (1986a) Origins of behavioral teratology. In: E.P. Riley and C.V. Vorhees (Eds.), *Handbook of Behavioral Terotatology*. Plenum Press, New York and London, pp. 3–22.

Vorhees, C.V. (1986b) Principles of behavioral teratology. In: E.P. Riley and C.V. Vorhees (Eds.), *Handbook of Behavioral Terotatology*. Plenum Press, New York, pp. 23–48.

Vorhees, C.V. (1987) Behavioral teratogenicity of valproic acid: selective effects on behavior after prenatal exposure to rats. *Psychopharmacology* (Berlin), 92: 173–179.

Warner, R.H. and Rosett, H.L. (1975) The effects of drinking on offspring. *J. Stud. Alcohol*, 36: 1395–1420.

Warrel, D.W. and Taylor, R. (1968) Outcome for the fetus of mothers receiving prednisolone during pregnancy. *Lancet*, i: 117–118.

Weiss, B. (1988) Implications of behavioral teratology for assessing the risks posed by environmental and therapeutic chemicals. Ch. 3, this volume.

Werboff, J. and Gottlieb, J.S. (1963) Drugs in pregnancy: behavioral teratology. *Obstet. Gynecol. Surv.*, 18; 420–423.

Wilson, J.G. (1977) Current status of teratology: General principles and mechanisms derived from animal studies. In: J.G. Wilson and F.C. Fraser (Eds.), *Handbook of Teratology, Vol. 1, General Principles and Etiology*, Plenum Press, New York, pp. 47–74.

Yanai, J. (1981) Comparison of early barbiturate and ethanol effects on the CNS. *Substance Alcohol Actions/Misuse*, 2: 79–91.

14

Discussion

A.J. Patel: Your results indicate that an increase in cell number in the sexually dimorphic nucleus (SDN) is similar in both males and females up to about 2 to 5 years. Thereafter, in comparison with males, the cell number decreases much faster in females. Do you think that the reduction of cell content of the SDN is due to cell death and more so in females? Furthermore, I would appreciate your comments on testosterone, which is believed to be associated with reduction in cell formation or cell death, as a missing trophic factor in females.

D.F. Swaab: The most probable explanation for the equally high SDN cell number in boys and girls and the major diminution in cell numbers later in female is indeed that testosterone is preventing pre-programmed cell death in the SDN in a similar way as has been reported for the spinal nucleus of the bulbocavernosus (SNB) (Breedlove, 1984). The sexual dimorphy of the SNB also concerns neurons. However, an influence via steroid receptors of the muscle in which these SNB neurons terminate can certainly not be excluded. It is also not clear whether the SDN neurons contain steroid receptors themselves, or are innervated by steroid sensitive neurons.

B.S. McEwen: Could the late appearance of the sex difference in the human sexually dimorphic nucleus (SDN) be due to the second, postnatal surge of testosterone secretion in the human male, rather than the first, prenatal testosterone peak?

D.F. Swaab: Indeed, in the first postnatal months high sex hormone levels have been reported in human neonates. This is also the period in which we find the SDN increasing rapidly in cell number, whereas its cells show signs of high activity. The nucleus of SDN cells is larger in this period than in any other period in life. Although it is tempting to assume a direct relationship between the hormone levels and SDN alterations, it will of course be hard to prove its possible causal nature.

Z. Annau: The ultimate effect of chemicals on the offspring may be related very significantly to the stress (hormonal) effects induced in the mother by these chemicals, at doses which do not cause overt toxicity.

D.F. Swaab: In principle such an interaction seems quite possible.

G.J. Boer: You distinguished between direct and indirect effects of chemicals on brain development by assuming either direct or indirect effects on brain cells. But are there not many teratogens that have general effects on maturing or proliferating cells as such? This would mean that a distinction between direct and indirect effects specifically on brain cells might sometimes not exist.

D.F. Swaab: It is true that one chemical might have various effects. For instance, alcohol might affect the developing brain indirectly by causing constriction of the umbilical cord *and* directly by affecting cell division, migration, formation of neurites, etc. In fact, most chemicals seem to act by various mechanisms, being direct or indirect.

B. Weiss: Carcinogenesis is almost the only endpoint in toxicology for which we conduct lifetime studies. Yet, longitudinal studies with neurotoxicants are rare. Apart from methylmercury, I cannot think of any cogent studies. Are you aware of any such studies?

D.F. Swaab: Dr. Kellogg has made an important start into this direction by showing alterations in the rat offspring at 24 months of age following benzodiazepine treatment in development (Kellogg, 1988). It seems logical to expect effects on the ageing process when the organism has been exposed to chemicals during development. For such a study one would need rats around the age of 32 months. This would not only be an extremely time-consuming type of experiment, but also an extremely expensive one, since such rats cost a few thousand dollars each.

References

Breedlove, S.M. (1984) Steroid influences on the development and function of a neuromuscular system. In G.J. De Vries, J.P.C. De Bruin, H.B.M. Uylings and M.A. Corner (Eds.) *Sex Differences in the Brain. The Relation between Structure and Function, Progress in Brain Research, Vol. 61*, Elsevier, Amsterdam, pp. 147–170.

Kellogg, C.K. (1988) Benzodiazepines: influence on the developing brain. Ch. 14, this volume.

G.J. Boer, M.G.P. Feenstra, M. Mirmiran, D.F. Swaab and F. Van Haaren
Progress in Brain Research, Vol. 73

CHAPTER 2

Defects of neuronal migration and the pathogenesis of cortical malformations

Pasko Rakic

Yale University School of Medicine, New Haven, CI O6510, USA

Introduction

I am thankful and deeply honored to have been selected the first Ariëns Kappers lecturer. He was an important and influential figure for many brain scientists of my generation. His classic volume on 'Comparative Anatomy of the Nervous System of Vertebrates Including Man' (Ariëns Kappers et al., 1936) has frequently been used as an authoritative encyclopedia with reliable data on the evolutionary aspects of brain development. For many of us, his work demonstrated that comparative neuroanatomy can be both esthetically and intellectually appealing. It also showed

Dr. P. Rakic was invited to deliver the first C.U. Ariëns Kappers lecture on the last day of the 15th International Summer School of Brain Research, September 4, 1987, 110 years after Ariëns Kappers was born at Groningen. During his medical training Ariëns Kappers was inspired by the neurologist Prof. C. Winkler to take up brain research. Prof. Winkler was one of the founders of the Netherlands Institute for Brain Research. When Ariëns Kappers was still a student at the University of Amsterdam his research abilities were honored with a gold medal for a study on myelin sheets. In 1904 he obtained his PhD with a thesis on a comparative neuroanatomical subject and he continued to work in this field of research ever after. This choice was strongly reinforced by his appointment in 1906 as 'Abteilungsvorsteher' in the institute of the famous neurologist and comparative neuroanatomist Prof. Dr. L. Edinger in Frankfurt am Main.

Meanwhile, the International Association of Academics had decided that brain research should be placed on an international footing, resulting in 1904 in an International Committee for Brain Research, which stated that 'the time is not far distant when the study of millions of brain cells will have to be divided amongst researchers in the way that astronomers have been obliged to divide the millions of stars into various groups', and proposed 'to organize a network of institutions throughout the civilized world, dedicated to the study of the structure and functions of the central organ...' The first country to respond to this ambition was The Netherlands, where the Central Institute for Brain Research was opened in 1909. Ariëns Kappers became the first director and held this position until his death in 1946. He made the Institute into an internationally renowned place by his excellent work (the 1936 book entitled 'The Comparative Anatomy of the Nervous System of Vertebrates including Man', which he wrote together with G.C. Huber and E.C. Crosby, is still well cited), his journeys all over the world and a visiting Professorship at Peking Union Medical College in China from 1923 to 1924.

The international character of the Institute is underlined by the fact that during Ariëns Kapper's directorship 69 foreign scientists paid a working visit to the Amsterdam Institute as well as by the Honorary Doctorate of Sciences he received from Yale University in 1928. In 1929 Ariëns Kappers held his inaugural lecture as 'extraordinary professor' at the medical faculty of the University of Amsterdam.

We are glad that Dr. P. Rakic has accepted our invitation to deliver the first C.U. Ariëns Kappers lecture in honour of this exceptional scientist and hope that it will be the first in a long series of most stimulating lectures in the field of brain research.

D.F. Swaab

Source: B. Brouwer (1946) In Memoriam Prof. Dr. Cornelius Ubbo Ariëns Kappers, Psychiatrische en Neurologische Bladen, pp. 1–16.

how far-reaching conclusions, many of which eventually proved to be correct, can be made from the data obtained by rather crude methods and simple experimental tools. I also should mention that C. U. Ariëns Kappers and his contemporaries posed most of the important and interesting questions concerning mechanisms of ontogenetic and phylogenetic development, many of which they were aware could not be reliably answered at the time (Ariëns Kappers, 1929). Now, we are at the point when many modern neurobiological methods can be applied to answer some of these longstanding queries, and reveal concepts and mechanisms that could not have been suspected just a few years ago. However, it is also fair to say that we are still at the beginning of this new era. The field of neuropathology of human brain malformations in general, and neuroteratology in particular, has just begun to feel the impact of modern neurobiology.

I have chosen to talk about normal and abnormal development of the cerebral neocortex because this issue is relevant to both the legacy of the work by C. U. Ariëns Kappers on development and evolution, and to the main topic of the conference on neurochemistry of functional neuroteratology. Just how and by what mechanisms a mass of neurons generated near the ventricular layer undergoes that orderly proliferation, migration, sorting out and differentiation which provide the cortex with its parcellation into diverse cytoarchitectonic fields and its complex synaptic circuitry is still one of the most obscure and challenging problems in biology. In the last two decades, research on this problem has gained momentum and I believe it is safe to state that during this period we have learned more about cortical organization and development than in all of man's previous history. Ever more sophisticated methods and experiments reveal the inner workings of mechanisms involving cells and molecules that basically supplement the descriptive studies of C. U. Ariëns Kappers and his contemporaries.

All of us working in this field of biology have witnessed remarkable progress in understanding how precise genetic codes imprinted into DNA produce the complex multicellular organization of the brain and transfer information about precise structural details from generation to generation. However, in recent years, several lines of evidence from experiments carried out mostly in the vertebrate nervous system have accumulated against a concept of immutable determination of neuronal phenotypes, their rigid prespecification into functional areas and fixed synaptic circuits. Data from various studies seem to support the concept of neuronal development as a complex piecemeal process in which originally equipotential cells are progressively transformed by a sequence of surface-mediated cell-cell interactions. Although these interactions proceed according to definite genetic instructions, they can be regulated by external factors that include various substances from the environment. This regulation is the important link between contemporary developmental neurobiology and neuroteratology.

New methods of developmental neurobiology, particularly quantitative techniques, can also uncover minute changes in brain organization or chemical composition that are not detectable by routine neuropathological examination. These advances have opened new possibilities for exploration of a large number of abnormalities that were, until recently, beyond our reach. For example, it has been reported that about one-third of all institutionalized retardates have no identifiable abnormalities detectable by post-mortem examination at the gross or light microscopic level (Freytag and Lindenberg, 1967). One can suspect that among these are probably many deficits in mentation caused by salient changes in cell position and mismatches in the synaptic pattern occurring as a result of faulty neuronal migration, which is the main subject of this paper. I selected to focus on this relatively narrow subject among many types of abnormalities of the central nervous system because I believe that defects of cell movement are particularly susceptible to environmental factors. However, most examples given below will come from dramatic and obvious cortical malformations produced either experimentally or occurring spontaneously. In particular, I will emphasize defects in neuronal movement that result in neuronal malpositions and ectopias that are visible at light and electron microscopic levels. This choice is made with the conviction that such examples provide an illustrative model for less dramatic, more subtle changes. Finally, I will try to interpret some cortical malformations and functional deficits occurring in the human brain in the context of our present understanding of mechanisms of normal migration and in light of the radial unit hypothesis of cortical development.

Definition of the migratory phenomenon

Neurons of the mammalian neocortex, like most neurons in the central nervous system of vertebrates, are generated in sites different from those in which they permanently reside. The intervening process is termed neuronal migration. This term denotes the displacement of a neuronal cell body from its site of origin – the final cell division – in the proliferative zone to its final destination in the mature brain (Rakic, 1972; Sidman and Rakic, 1973). It is important to emphasize that neuronal migration should be distinguished from the extension and movement of axonal and dendritic tips during formation of neuropil and establishment of synaptic connections. Formation of neuronal connections commonly occurs at later developmental stages after most neurons have attained their final positions, and it is governed by different cellular and molecular mechanisms (Rakic and Goldman-Rakic, 1982).

Neuronal migration, as defined here, is particularly prominent in the large mammalian cerebrum and occurs, as a rule, only after the final mitotic division of the neuronal progenitors in the proliferative centers. The length of the migratory pathway may range from less than 300 microns in the mouse telencephalon to several thousand microns in some areas of the human cerebrum.

Despite these vast differences in length of trajectory, the size of migratory neurons is approximately the same in both species. Migration begins with dislocation of postmitotic cells from the other elements in the proliferative ventricular zone, with which it initially forms strong structural bonds (Levitt et al., 1983; Molgard et al., 1987). It is followed by active movement of undifferentiated neurons which change position in relation to the surrounding cellular milieu. This movement of neurons proceeds along specific pathways, occurs according to a well-defined time schedule, and stops at precisely defined locations (Rakic, 1978, 1985, 1988).

This paper focuses on cell movements during corticogenesis, but is should be recognized that the phenomenon of neuronal migration is not confined to the telencephalon. Actually, it has been observed in most regions of the developing vertebrate nervous systems (Rakic, 1985; Sidman and Rakic, 1973). However, I would like to emphasize that neuronal migration can assume a variety of forms, proceed along different routes, be guided by variable substrates, and be mediated by a diverse set of adhesion and recognition molecules. In terms of orientation and directionality of cell movement, migration can be classified into radial – proceeding from the ventricular to the pial surface – and tangential – running parallel to the surface of developing brain (Rakic, 1987). Several lines of evidence from both in vivo and in vitro analysis indicate that contact interaction between migrating neurons and the surfaces of neighboring cells plays a crucial role in selecting migratory pathways, and in the orienting, displacing and stopping displacement of neurons. With regard to pathway selection, migrating neurons fall into three major categories: (i) gliophilic cells which follow elongated glial fibers and bypass other neurons that are encountered within the sphere of their trajectory; (ii) neurophilic cells which follow neuronal, particularly axonal surfaces, and bypass nearby glial shafts; and (iii) biphilic cells which display temporal or regional affinities towards either glial or neuronal surfaces (Rakic, 1987).

18

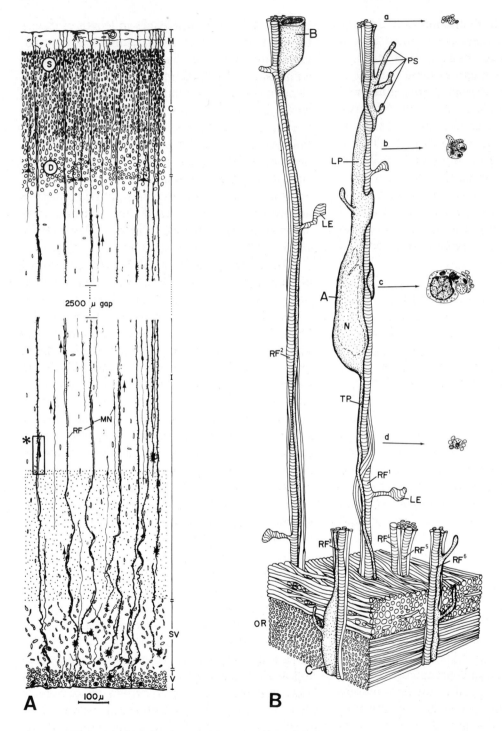

Fig. 1 A. Camera lucida drawing of the occipital lobe of the cerebral wall of a monkey fetus at midgestation. Composite illustration is derived from a Golgi section (black profiles of cell images) and from an adjacent section counterstained with toluidine blue (outline profiles of cell nuclei). The rectangle marked with an asterisk shows the approximate position of the three-dimensional reconstruction in Fig. 2B. C, cortical plate; I, intermediate zone; M, molecular layer; MN, migrating neuron;

The gliophilic mode of migration along radial glial fibers occurs in the mammalian telencephalon during formation of the neocortex and hippocampus. The relationship between migrating neurons and elongated glial fibers, which serve as a substrate for their movement, is illustrated at relatively late stages of cortical development in rhesus monkeys (Fig. 1). All cortical neurons are produced in the proliferative zone situated near the lateral cerebral ventricle (Rakic, 1974). Following their last division, postmitotic cells embark on a journey that, in the monkey fetus, may be several thousand microns long (Rakic, 1972). In human fetuses at the end of the second half of gestation, this migratory pathway is considerably longer and more torturous (Rakic, 1978).

The neurons setting out for the cortex assume a bipolar shape with a more voluminous leading process and a thin trailing process that are, in combined length, only a fraction of the distance that cells must traverse. The terrain which has to be crossed is highly complex, composed of a variety of cellular elements. The leading process follows elongated radial glial fibers which at midgestation span the entire thickness of the cerebral wall (Fig. 1A). On the basis of Golgi, electron microscopic and immunocytochemical evidence, this transient population of glial cells is a form of primitive astrocyte (Rakic, 1972; Schmechel and Rakic, 1979; Levitt and Rakic, 1980; Levitt et al., 1981).

Mechanism of cell displacement

Electron microscopic analysis shows that during their migration, neurons are invariably apposed to the membrane surface of neighboring radial glial fibers (Fig. 1B). The strong affinity between neuronal and glial cell surfaces is implied by the failure of migrating cells to follow any of a myriad of differently oriented cellular processes that they encounter during their journey to the cortex (Rakic, 1972; Rakic et al., 1974). Radial glial fibers, thus, impose lateral constraints and provide guidelines facilitating cell migration to the distant cortical plate through the complex assembly of closely packed cells and processes that compose the developing cerebral wall. After the migration of cortical neurons has been completed, radial glial scaffolding disappears as some of these glial cells degenerate, while others re-enter the mitotic cycle and transform into protoplasmic and fibrous astrocytes (Schmechel and Rakic, 1979).

An apparent problem in understanding mechanisms of neuronal movement is that migrating neurons and radial glial fibers display a strong affinity for each other while at the same time allowing the movement of the first along the latter. In order to reconcile this apparent contradiction, our working hypothesis has been that the apposing membranes of migrating neurons and radial glial shafts are fixed at any one point along their interface, and that migrating neurons move simply by adding new membrane components to the leading process (Rakic, 1981b). Neurons move

RF, radial fiber; SV, subventricular zone; V, ventricular zone. B. Three-dimensional reconstruction of migrating neurons, based on electron micrographs of semiserial sections of the occipital lobe of the monkey fetus (cf. rectangle in A). The lower portion of the diagram contains uniform, parallel fibers of the optic radiation (OR) and the remainder is occupied by more irregularly disposed fiber systems; the border between the two systems is easily recognized. Except for the lower portion of the figure, most of these fibers are deleted from the diagram to expose the radial fibers (striped vertical shafts, RF[1–6]) and their relation to the migrating cells A, B and C, and to other vertical processes. The soma of migrating cell A, with its nucleus (N) and voluminous leading process (LP), is situated within the reconstructed space, except for the terminal part of the attenuated trailing process and the tip of the vertical ascending pseudopodium. Cross-sections of Cell A in relation to the several vertical fibers in the fascicle are drawn at levels a–d at the right side of the figure. The perikaryon of cell B is cut off at the top of the reconstructed space, whereas the leading process of cell C is shown just penetrating between fibers of the optic radiation (OR) on its way across the intermediate zone. LE indicates lamellate expansions; PS indicates pseudopodia. From Rakic (1972).

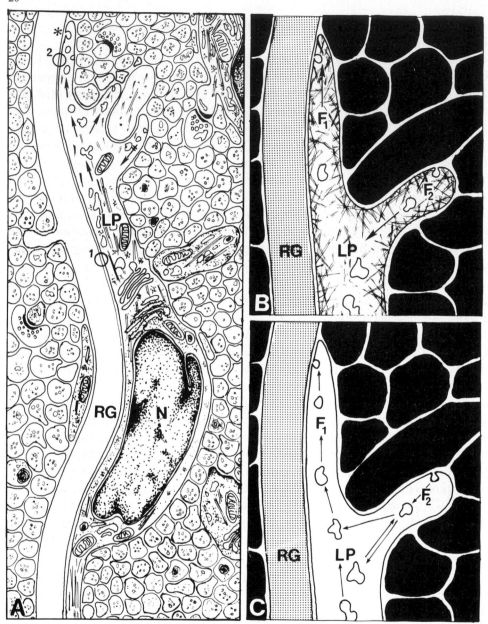

Fig. 2 A. Semi-schematic drawing of a cross-section through a migrating neuron (N) and its leading process (LP) as it moves along a radial glial shaft (RG) through terrain densely packed with various other cells and their processes. The membrane segments formed near the nucleus are transported toward the tip (arrows) within the leading process via rough and smooth endoplasmic reticulum and vesicles in order to be inserted (asterisk) at the surface of the filopodia. The leading process continues to grow along the surface of radial glial cells, while the filopodia apposed to other surfaces withdraw (crossed arrow). B. Sketch of a possible mechanism for the advancement of filopodia (F_1), alignment of the glial shaft (RG), and regression of filopodia (F_2) which have contact with less adhesive surfaces of other cells. The uniform pooling of contractile fibers within the cytoplasm would result in withdrawal of processes with lesser adhesion and preferential elongation along the surface with higher adhesion. C. Sketch of how a higher rate of endocytosis in the filopodia associated with less adhesive surfaces (F_2) could result in withdrawal, while a net increase in exocytosis in the filopodia associated with the more adhesive surface (F_1) produces selective outgrowth of the leading process (LP) along a radial glial fiber (RG). Further explanation can be found in the text. From Rakic (1985).

when their nucleus and surrounding cytoplasm transfer to a new position within the extended leading process. Although individual cells have contact with other cells, the most firmly bound filopodium would be the most likely to succeed in steering the growth of the leading process, while the filopodia less attracted to the surrounding elements would retract. Several observations reviewed below give credence to such a mechanism.

Numerous tissue culture observations indicate that neuronal processes grow preferentially along surfaces to which they adhere more strongly (Letourneau, 1975; Hatten et al., 1984). It seems contraintuitive, but the strong bond between neuronal and glial surfaces in vivo would promote rather than interfere with neuronal migration. According to our model, the migrating cell could move by adding new membrane components to its growing tip and, as a consequence, the leading process would progressively extend along the preferred substrate while the nucleus and surrounding cytoplasm subsequently become transferred to a new position within the newly formed segment of the leading process (Fig. 2A). The bonds formed between the leading process and the glial shaft (e.g., circle 1 in Fig. 2A) do not have to be broken since new bonds are formed continuously at the more distal segments (circle 2 in Fig. 2A), allowing growth of the leading tip and subsequent translocation of the entire cell.

The rate of movement of migrating neurons in the primate central nervous system, which varies between 0.5 and 10 μm/h, is compatible with the generation and insertion of new membrane components along the leading process. Several other observations give credence to this mechanism of neurite extension, including the ultrastructural composition of the leading tip (Rakic, 1972), the finding of a continuous increase in the surface areas of migrating cells as they approach the target structure (Rakic et al., 1974), and the predominant growth of neurites at their leading tips (Bray, 1973). The additional membrane needed for rapid growth can be provided by the retraction of filopodia that have been extended transiently along less adhesive surfaces.

At present, our understanding of the phenomenology at the cellular level of neuronal cell migration exceeds our knowledge of molecular mechanisms involved in the process of cell translocation. However, most investigators agree that glial and neuronal cell surfaces contain some sort of binding molecules. Many adhesive proteins are present in extracellular matrices outside of the central nervous system (Rouslahti and Pierschbacher, 1987) and several candidate molecules have been isolated directly from embryonic chick, mouse and human brain (McClain and Edelman, 1982; Edelman, 1983; Hatten and Mason, 1986; Lindner et al., 1986; Antomicek et al., 1987). Since such a molecule promotes cell-to-cell binding, lack of a molecule, its alteration or a failure in local surface modulation may result in migratory defects. The first step toward testing this hypothesis of cortical development is the identification and characterization of unique radial glial cell plasmalemmal components from the telencephalic radial glial cells and migrating neurons. Although considerable progress has been made in this area, most available candidate molecules do not have properties that can fully explain all aspects of the migratory phenomenon (see review by Rakic, 1988). The second step is to provide a test for the functional relationship between the unique molecules involved in neuronal migration. The dissociated culture system consisting of glial cells and early postmitotic neurons has been highly valuable (e.g., Hatten and Mason, 1986), but ultimately the function of molecules has to be tested in vivo. The use of slice preparations from the developing cerebral wall has considerable promise for achieving this goal (e.g., Hemendinger and Caviness, 1988).

The retraction of filopodia that grow along less adhesive surfaces may be achieved by two basic mechanisms or by their combination. One mechanism assumes uniform contraction of actin filaments, which are as abundant in the leading tips of migrating neurons as they are in growing neurites (Johnston and Wessells, 1980). It can be expected that indiscriminate retraction of the plasma membrane toward the center of the cell would eventually result in involution of those filopodia that have weaker bonds with surrounding cells (e.g., F_2 in Fig. 2B) while filopodia with stronger bonds (F_1 in Fig. 2B) would be retained. A cumulative effect of this process would result in extension of the filopodia aligned along the most adhesive surface. This possibility is also attractive because there is evidence that many adhesion proteins and their receptors connect the cytoskeleton (Rouslahti and Pierschbacher, 1987).

Another mechanism that could also contribute to the retraction of supernumerary filopodia is a higher rate of endocytosis of membrane patches that lack strong bonds with adjacent cells (Fig. 2C). It has been proposed that the endocytic cycle may play a role in the locomotion of fibroblasts (Bretscher, 1984), and a similar mechanism may apply to migrating nerve cells. A model of neuronal migration that depends on the ratio between insertion and intake of membrane at the leading tip is attractive since it takes into account the rate of membrane biosynthesis that is ultimately controlled by both the genome of individual cells and by their interaction with adjacent cells. The membrane components containing specific binding or receptor molecules may be generated only during the restricted period of time when the cell is displaying migratory behavior. Studies of the migration of cerebellar granule cells in vitro indicate that the length of the period during which an individual cell is capable of migration is intrinsically predetermined and, in this case, lasts about four days (Trenkner et al., 1984). In the monkey cerebrum, this period must be considerably longer since, at the end of corticogenesis, some neurons still need another two weeks or more to reach their appropriate layer (Rakic, 1975a). After reaching their final destinations, individual cells lose their ability to move, suggesting that neurons may change surface properties by stopping biosynthesis of specific membrane components.

Although both the selective and self-propelling capacities of the migrating cell can be explained by contact recognition of adhesion proteins and their receptors, contractile proteins within the cytoplasm must provide for the displacement of the nucleus and surrounding organelles within the elongated leading process. The presence of such molecules has been detected in immature brain cells (Goldberg, 1982), but their role in neuronal migration has not been clarified. According to the proposed model, the contractile properties of cytoplasm may be essential for both the retraction of filopodia as well as for the completion of nuclear displacement, but they are not expected to play a crucial role in the selection of appropriate pathways or the determination of an individual neuron's destination (Rakic, 1985).

Studies carried out in my laboratory during the last decade reveal that a cohort of neurons, originating from the same site in the ventricular zone (proliferative unit), migrate along a common glial guide, eventually forming an ontogenetic radial column within the developing cortex (Rakic, 1978, 1981b). Under normal conditions, each neuron in a given ontogenetic column takes a position distal (external) to its predecessor and, as a result, cells of cortical layers accumulate from the inside, outwardly, at progressively later times (Rakic, 1974). Although this phenomenon, known as an inside-out gradient of neurogenesis, has been observed in the neocortex of a variety of species (e.g., Angevine and Sidman, 1961; Luskin and Shatz, 1985), it is particularly sharp in primates (Rakic, 1974). Permanent positioning of neurons within the cortical plate is therefore a part of migratory events, but the exact site and time for cessation of movement may be regulated independently of the preceding process (Rakic, 1975a; Caviness and Rakic, 1978). Several lines of evidence indicate that the correct position attained by an individual migrating neuron within the target structure may be determined by its interaction with local milieu which includes previously generated cells and their processes. For example, in a neurological mutant mouse (reeler), cortical cells appear to migrate normally towards the cortical plate but are unable to bypass previously generated cells (Caviness and Rakic, 1978; Caviness, 1982). It has been suggested that faulty interaction between radial glia and migrating neurons at the termination of their journey may be the cause of cell malposition (Pinto-Lord et al., 1982; Caviness and Rakic, 1978). On the other hand, it is possible that the leading tip of a migrating cell fails to produce a sufficient amount of proteolytic enzymes such as plasminogen activator serine proteases (Moonen et al., 1982) which may be essential for breaking the bonds between migrating neurons and their glial guides near the site of their final destination.

Radial unit hypothesis of neocortical development

In the previous section, I mainly discussed the role of glial substrates for the movement of neurons along vertical (radial) vectors. The existence of radial glial cell scaffolding and pattern of its distribution have another important implication for the establishment of normal neocortical organization. In the telencephalon of all mammalian species, but most prominently in primates, the cortical surface is parcelled into a large number of cytoarchitectonic areas that have a characteristic biochemical composition, explicit cellular constellations, distinctive inputs and outputs, intricate local circuits and specific functional correlates (e.g., Brodmann, 1909; Rakic and Goldman-Rakic, 1982; Peters and Jones, 1984; Rakic and Singer, 1988). These cytoarchitectonic areas retain a topographic relation to one another that is consistent from individual to individual and is, to some extent, also preserved across species. However, there are considerable interspecies and intraspecies differences in the relative and absolute size of cytoarchitectonic areas. Several basic developmental questions concerning cortical parcellation remain unsolved. To what extent is the number of neurons destined for each cytoarchitectonic area innately determined? Do any environmental factors such as functional activity, experience, nutrition, and extrinsic agents (toxins, irradiation, etc.) play a role in this process? Since the migration of each postmitotic cell from the proliferative zone to the cortical plate is constrained to the given radial vector by the glial guides, it follows that the ventricular surface of the developing cerebrum itself may be parcelled as a protomap of the future cytoarchitectonic map in the cortex (Rakic, 1978, 1981c).

Parcellation of the cortical plate into cytoarchitectonic areas can be explained by the radial unit hypothesis if we assume that the ventricular zone is a mosaic of proliferative units containing the fate map (Rakic, 1978, 1981c). The terms 'fate map' or 'protomap' simply refer to the empirical fact that neurons originating from a given part of the proliferative zone, under normal circumstances, form a specific cytoarchitectonic area (Rakic, 1988). According to this concept, neurons produced within individual proliferative units align themselves along a radial glial fascicle and enter the developing cortical plate where they form ontogenetic columns (Fig. 3). Our best approximation at the present time is that in the fetal monkey telencephalon, the number of proliferative units in the ventricular zone about equals the number of ontogenetic columns in the cortical plate (Rakic, 1988). It is not known whether each unit initially (before postconceptual day 40 in the monkey) starts with a single cell, which would imply clonal relation. At the developmental stages that we have examined in the monkey, each individual proliferative unit is a polyclone, which may contain several dividing stem cells. The number of stem cells in the proliferation unit ranges from 3 to 5 in younger monkey embryos, up to about 10 at midgestation (Rakic, 1988).

Ontogenetic columns in the cortex widen considerably in the course of pre- and postnatal development as individual neurons grow, differentiate, and acquire synaptic connections from local and extrinsic sources. However, we still know little about the possible anatomical or physiological relationships between the developmentally defined ontogenetic columns and cortical columns (Mountcastle, 1979) or disjunctive terminal fields of afferent fiber systems of the

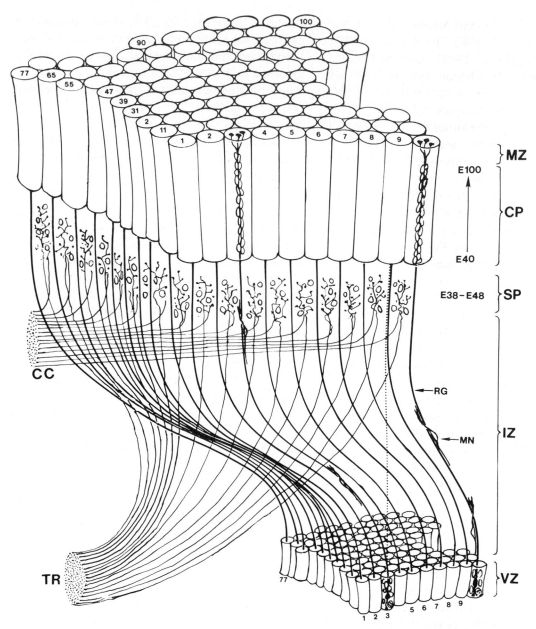

Fig. 3 The relationship between a small patch of the proliferative, ventricular zone (VZ) and its corresponding area within the cortical plate (CP) in the developing cerebrum. Although the cerebral surface in primates expands during prenatal development, resulting in a shift between the VZ and CP, ontogenetic columns (outlined by cylinders) remain attached to the corresponding proliferative units by the grid of radial glial fibers. Cortical neurons produced between embryonic day 40 and 100 by a given proliferative unit migrate in succession along the same radial glial guides (RG) and form a single ontogenic column. Each migrating neuron traverses the intermediate (IZ) and subplate (SP) zones, which contain 'waiting' afferents from the thalamic radiation (TR) and callosal and intrahemispheric fasciculi (CC). After entering the cortical plate, each wave of migrating neurons bypasses previously generated neurons and assumes a position at the interphase between the CP and marginal zone (MZ). As a result, proliferative units 1–100 produce ontogenetic columns 1–100 in the same relative position to each other. The glial scaffolding prevents a mismatch between proliferative unit 3 and ontogenic column 9 (dashed line). Thus, the specifications of topography and/or modality depend on the spatial distribution of proliferative units, while the phenotype of neurons within each unit depends on its time of origin. From Rakic (1988).

adult cortex (Goldman and Nauta, 1977; Eccles, 1984; Szenthagothai, 1983; Hubel and Wiesel, 1977; Goldman-Rakic, 1981). Use of the gene transfer method for labeling cells of common origin in conjunction with anatomical and immunocytochemical analyses of neuronal circuitry directly in the cortex promises to provide an answer to this important question. At present, we can only state that the composition of each ontogenetic column in the fetal neocortex presents the endproduct of the sequential migration of several generations of neurons, all of which have arrived along common glial fascicles from a single proliferative unit (Rakic, 1978). Furthermore, as proliferative units have matching ontogenetic columns in the cortical plate, the protomap of the ventricular zone and expanding cortex remains basically preserved in spite of considerable morphogenetic changes in the shape and size of the cerebral surface.

The major tenet of the radial unit hypothesis is that the ventricular zone contains a protomap of the prospective cytoarchitectonic areas and that glial grids serve to assure reproduction of this map onto the expanding and curving cortical mantle. We found that a similar structural relationship exists during formation of the hippocampal region (Nowakowski and Rakic, 1979) including early stages of the dentate plate (Eckenhoff and Rakic, 1984), indicating that this basic model may be applicable to other structures. However, the radial unit hypothesis can explain only how neurons acquire proper positions; it does not give a clue as to what initiates and governs their subsequent differentiation including the course of synaptogenesis. Each cytoarchitectonic area acquires its final cytological and synaptic organization by a combination of intrinsic genetic properties of the constituent neurons and uniqueness of axonal inputs from the subcortical structures during migration or after cell arrival at the cortex. Thus, the final characteristics of cytoarchitectonic fields depend on multiple factors, but the existence of glial guides and compartmentalization of the telencephalic wall into radial units seem to minimize the amount of information needed for the transfer of cells and initial construction of the neocortex (Rakic, 1978, 1988).

Experimental manipulation of cytoarchitectonic areas

How can individual and species-specific differences in the size of cytoarchitectonic areas be explained by the radial unit hypothesis? One obvious possibility is that cortical parcellation is controlled by genes that provide instruction for changes in the protomap of the ventricular surface and, therefore, effectively determine the size of each cytoarchitectonic area already at early stages. Another possibility is that all proliferative units are the same and that they produce neurons that are initially equipotential. According to this hypothesis, areal specificity is determined exclusively by afferent systems that arrive on the scene at much later developmental stages (Creutzfeldt, 1977; Mountcastle, 1979). The third possibility is that proliferative units produce cohorts of neurons which have considerable area-specific competence, but the number of ontogenetic columns devoted to a given area can be further regulated by afferents from other cortical and subcortical areas (Rakic, 1988).

To test which of the three possibilities cited above is the correct one, the amount of specific thalamo-cortical or cortico-cortical connections should be altered at early embryonic stages, and then the effect of this manipulation on the distribution and size of cytoarchitectonic areas examined. The problems in successfully carrying out such experiments are not trivial, but the visual cortex can again serve as a useful and promising model to address these issues. For example, we have recently found that binocular enucleation performed on monkey embryos in the first half of gestation diminished the number of neurons in the lateral geniculate nucleus to less than half of the normal level (Rakic, 1988; Rakic and Williams, 1986). Thus, we have an animal that has undergone a selective decrease in afferent input to the

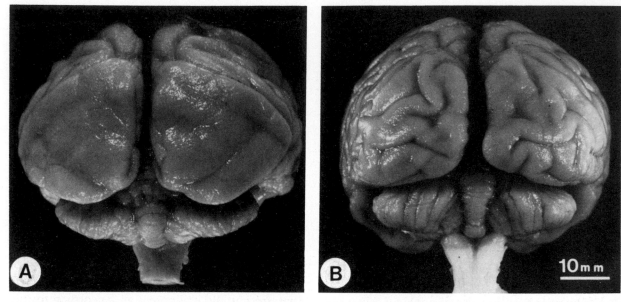

Fig. 4 Photomicrograph of the occipital lobe in a normal monkey (A) and in the age-matched animal subjected to binocular enucleation at the end of the second month of gestation (B). Both photographs are reproduced at the same magnification.

visual cortex. The occipital lobe in enucleates displays dramatic changes in the pattern of convolutions (Fig. 4), but has topographically well defined residual connections with the diminished lateral geniculate nucleus.

The primary visual cortex (area 17) of the occipital lobe in enucleates was well defined by a sharp border with the adjacent areas, indicating that a morphological distinction between them develops in the absence of any information via chains of neurons from the retina (Fig. 5). Most unexpectedly, the thickness of area 17 and its characteristic complement of layers and sublayers was within the normal range (Rakic, 1988; Rakic and Williams, 1986). However, the surface of area 17 in enucleates was less than half the size it is in the age-matched controls. Thus, despite the absence of retinal input to the lateral geniculate

nucleus and the severely reduced number of geniculo-cortical afferents, area 17 had the normal number of neurons per each layer and per each ontogenetic column. In contrast, the total number of neurons in the entire area and total surface of the area was diminished in proportion to the loss of geniculate neurons (Rakic and Williams, 1986; Rakic, 1988; and unpublished data).

The results obtained from our experiments are in harmony with several relevant findings observed in the post-mortem human brain. For example, individuals with a larger auditory cortex in the left cerebral hemisphere have a larger medial geniculate nucleus on the same side (Eidelberg and Galaburda, 1982). Also, it has been found that human anophthalmic brains have a smaller lateral geniculate nucleus and smaller surface of area 17 (Bolton, 1900). The

Fig. 5 A. Photomicrograph of the Nissl-stained occipital lobe at the border between area 17 (left) and area 18 (right) in the ▶ normal rhesus monkey. B. Corresponding photomicrograph taken from the age-matched animal subjected to binocular enucleation at the second month of gestation. Both photographs are reproduced at the same magnification.

27

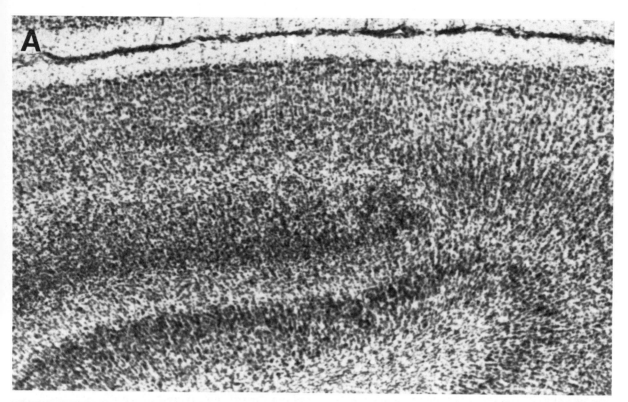

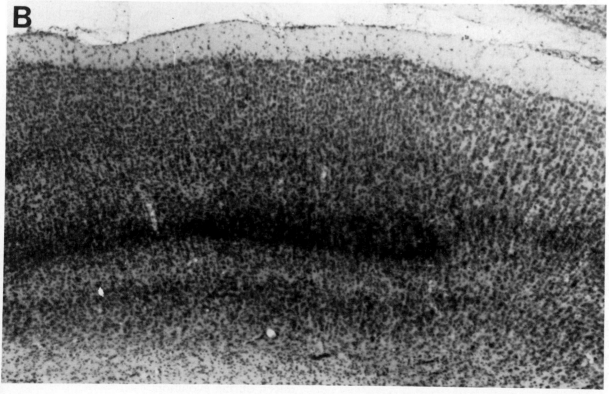

visual cortex in this case, nevertheless, had its normal laminar pattern. It may also be relevant to mention that the major neurotransmitter receptors within area 17 in early enucleated monkeys also retain their characteristic basic pattern of laminar distribution in spite of some modifications in the details and intensity (Rakic et al., 1987). Finally, synaptic density within each layer in the visual cortex, as revealed by quantitative electron microscopy, develops within the normal range (Bourgeois and Rakic, 1987). Thus, our experimental data and the pertinent literature on human anatomy reveal a correspondence between the number of specific thalamic afferents and the surface of corresponding cortical area. In the context of the radial unit hypothesis, these findings can be extrapolated to suggest that the final number of ontogenetic columns in the corresponding cortical area can be affected without altering either the number of neurons within each ontogenetic column or their differentiation into basic phenotypes (Rakic, 1988).

It should be emphasized that regulation by thalamic afferents is only part of a more complex interactive process that occurs during development and parcellation of the neocortex. As illustrated schematically in Fig. 3, the subplate zone contains numerous cortico-cortical (CC) connections in addition to thalamic radiation (TR). Prenatal resection of the fetal cortex, which eliminates or decreases the volume of specific cortico-cortical input to the subplate at early embryonic stages, also has a profound effect on the subsequent gyral pattern and connections of the other, unoperated areas in both hemispheres (Goldman-Rakic, 1981; Goldman-Rakic and Rakic, 1984; Rakic, 1988). On the basis of experiments in other systems, one can predict that multiple inputs to a given cytoarchitectonic area could have an effect on its final size (Rakic, 1986). For example, we found that monkey embryos during midgestation have about 3 million axons, which originate from each eye and terminate in an overlapping manner in the lateral geniculate nucleus (Rakic, 1976). However, this number

declines rapidly during the second half of segregation, slowing afterward until it reaches a level of about 1.2 million in adults (Rakic and Riley, 1983a). If one eye is removed at the stage of 'overshoot' or overlap of retino-geniculate projections, the remaining eye retains a larger number of ganglion cells in the retina and their axons in the optic nerve than it otherwise would (Rakic and Riley, 1983b).

Our working hypothesis is that the same general principle of competitive elimination may be at play during formation of neocortical areas that share some common synaptic targets during development. So far, this hypothesis is supported by evidence from the experimental ablation of selected areas of the cortex by prenatal neurosurgery (Goldman-Rakic, 1980; Rakic and Goldman-Rakic, 1985). For example, unilateral resection of the occipital cortex at midgestational periods results in an enlarged inferior parietal lobule on the side of lesion (Goldman-Rakic and Rakic, 1984, and unpublished data). One explanation of this dramatic result is that supernumerary cells in the parietal lobe survive in the absence of competition with projections from the occipital lobe in the subcortical structures or in the other cortical areas with which they share common synaptic targets. Another possibility is that input from the remaining areas spreads to the territories that are normally occupied by input from the removed region. In experiments with cortical ablation and experiments that reduce the size of specific thalamic nuclei (described above), ontogenetic columns initially specified for one area may receive afferents normally destined for another area. As a result, we may have created experimentally a new type of cytoarchitectonic area that has uncommon neuronal and synaptic relationships. We are currently studying the synaptoarchitecture and distribution of receptors in the zone adjacent to area 17 in early enucleates. This is an important goal of our future research, since the results may hold the key to understanding consequences of prenatal lesions as well as how new cytoarchitectonic areas may be introduced during evolution.

Radial unit model and pattern of human cortical malformations

The radial unit hypothesis has several implications for both understanding and classifying major cortical malformation in man. Among abnormalities of the cortical mantle that may be caused by defective proliferation and/or migration of cortical neurons, lissencephaly, pachygyria and polymicrogyria are perhaps the most prominent (Friede, 1975; Volpe, 1987). There are several variations of these basic types of cortical malformations but, in general, lissencephalic brains have a smoother cerebral surface, diminished total area, and usually the thickness of the cortex is approximately normal or even enlarged (Stewart et al., 1975; Richman et al., 1973). In contrast, polymicrogyria is characterized by a highly convoluted cerebrum with nearly normal surface area, and a cortex which is thinner than normal (Caviness and Williams, 1985; Volpe, 1987). Since the etiology of most cortical malformations is still a mystery, their classification in the past has been based on the appearance of the cortex at the time of death. These types of cortical malformation can now be classified into two major categories on the basis of developmental mechanisms that are outlined by the radial unit hypothesis.

The first category of cortical malformations, according to this classification scheme, consists of those cases in which the number of ontogenetic columns in the cortex is diminished while the number of neurons within each ontogenetic column remains relatively normal. The second category consists of malformations in which the number of ontogenetic columns in the cortex remains normal while the number of neurons within each column is diminished. Although malformations may predominantly display features of one or the other of these two categories, many are a mixture of both types. The picture is further complicated by subsequent transneuronal degeneration, so that a pure example of each category may be rare.

On the basis of the radial unit hypothesis, it can be expected that the first category is the result of an early defect that occurs at the time when proliferative units are being formed within the cerebral ventricular zone. The defect in this case should precede the onset of neurogenesis and therefore, in humans, it probably occurs within the first 7 weeks of gestation. Once the number of proliferative units in the ventricular zone has been established, each unit can produce the usual number of neurons that form ontogenetic columns of normal height. Neurons may or may not reach their final destinations and, as a result, a large contingent of ectopic neurons may remain in the white matter. In many of these cases, nevertheless, the cortex has nearly normal thickness but, as a rule, a considerably smaller surface.

The defect in the second category of malformations begins after the normal number of proliferative units have been established. This defect should, therefore, occur after the 7th week of gestation and it should not greatly affect the number of ontogenetic columns. However, it can be expected that it affects the number of neurons produced within each proliferative unit. As a result, ontogenetic columns should have fewer neurons and consequently a thinner cortex. It should be emphasized that a smaller number of neurons in the ontogenetic columns could be the result of low production in the proliferative unit, subsequent cell death or a failure of their migration. In the latter case, some cortical neurons may survive in ectopic positions within the white matter, as frequently occurs in polymicrogyric brains (Friede, 1975; Volpe, 1987). Although the proposed classification of cortical malformations does not address the issue of their primary etiology, it suggests possible developmental mechanisms and delineates the timing and sequence of cellular events. The pattern of cortical malformations, on the other hand, supports the radial unit hypothesis by exposing the possible consequences of defects that occur during the stages when proliferative units or columns are being formed.

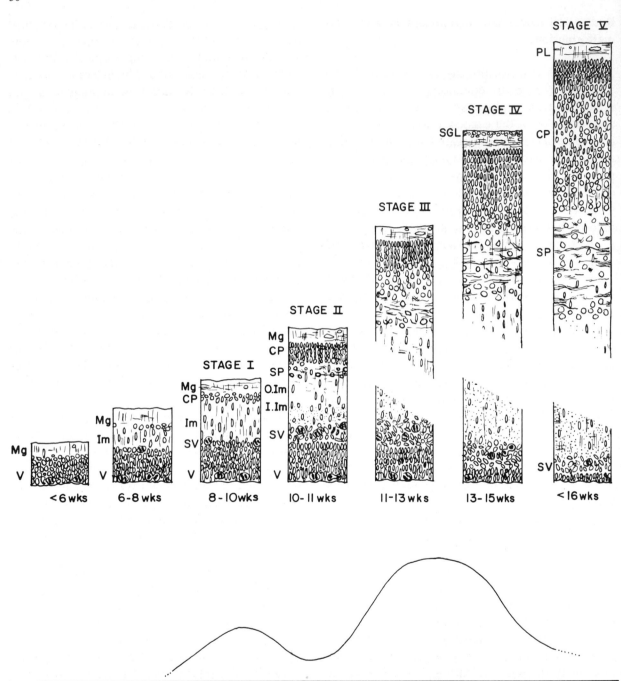

Fig. 6 Semi-diagrammatic drawings of the human cerebral wall at various gestational ages listed in fetal weeks below each column. The stages refer specifically to an arbitrarily chosen area midway along the lateral surface of the hemisphere (detailed in Sidman and Rakic, 1982). In addition, the subplate zone of Kostovic and Molliver (1974), situated below the cortical plate, is introduced in the last three stages. Because there is a gradient of maturation, as many as three of the five stages of cortical development may be observed in different regions of the neocortex in the same fetal brain. In the three columns on the right, the intermediate zone is not drawn in full because the thickness of the cerebral wall has increased markedly compared to earlier

Radial unit model and pathogenesis of cortical malformation

The radial unit hypothesis and new developmental data about the timing, pattern, and molecular mechanisms of neuronal migration provide the basis for understanding the pathogenesis of various genetic and acquired disorders of cortical development. Corticogenesis in the human fetus proceeds according to some general principles, as described for the macaque (Rakic, 1978; Sidman and Rakic, 1982). Migration in the human begins around the 6th fetal week and tapers down by midgestation (Fig. 6). The defects of migration that occur during this period can be divided into three broad categories (Rakic, 1975b): (a) complete failure of neuronal migration; (b) detention of some migratory cells along the migratory pathway; and (c) aberrant placement of postmitotic neurons within their target structure. This simple classification scheme is useful because each type of defect may have a different pathogenetic mechanism. For example, an inability of cells to dissociate from the ventricular surface or the absence of a signal to initiate movement may be involved in the first category, but do not play a role in the other two. Changes in surface molecules on the guiding substrate cells or the breakdown of machinery to propel the soma of a migrating neuron to the next position may cause the second type of migratory defect. On the other hand, an inability to recognize the target site or absence of the molecules on the target to be recognized, is significant for the third category, but not for the first two. Unfortunately, it is difficult to make the distinction between these types of cortical defects by examination of autopsy material. First, the original form of the anomaly is, by the time of death, usually obscured by secondary tissue changes. Second, malformations seemingly of the same type may be caused by a variety of factors. Conversely, the same etiological factors may cause different disorders, depending on local conditions and the timing of their action.

In the case of complete failure of migration, postmitotic cells remain close to the site of their last division. Although this type of disorder may be relatively common, it remains wholly undetected since most ectopic cells subsequently degenerate and leave no trace (Rakic, 1975b, 1988). Instructive examples of the dynamic cellular interactions during abnormal development are the studies of neurological mutant mice (Caviness and Rakic, 1978; Rakic and Sidman, 1973a,b; Sidman and Rakic, 1982; Caviness, 1982). Prior existence of this type of defect in human can be manifested by the total loss of or a significant decrease in the number of certain neuron classes observed in autopsy material. However, even when neuronal loss is evident, it is difficult to determine if the deficit was caused by a migratory defect or by cell death that occurred prior, during, or after migration was completed.

In some cases, however, ectopic neurons survive for a long time near, or at the very site of their genesis. Survival of the cells in an ectopic position is presumably dependent on formation of synapses. This type of malformation may occur as a consequence of fetal exposure to a variety of physiochemical agents including ionizing irradiation (e.g., Dekaban, 1969; Hicks et al., 1959; Jensen and Killackey, 1984). An instructive example may be the consequence of irradiation of human embryos caused by the atomic blasts at Hiroshima and Nagasaki in 1945, although so far only a few victims have died and their brain examined histologically. It is clear, however, that

stages and cannot fit into the drawing. The curve below the drawings schematically indicates waves of cell migration to the neocortex assessed by the density of migrating neurons in the intermediate zone. Abbreviations: CP, cortical plate; Im, intermediate zone; I.Im and O.Im, inner and outer intermediate zones, respectively; Mg, marginal zone, PL, plexiform layer; SGL, subpial granular layer; SP, subplate zone; SV, subventricular zone; V, ventricular zone; wks, age in fetal weeks. Modified from Rakic (1978) with permission.

many individuals who survived the initial insult (fetal at that time) were born with a smaller head size and various neurological and psychiatric disorders. Furthermore, recent psychological and psychiatric reevaluation of this population revealed a significantly higher incidence of mental retardation in individuals irradiated between 8 and 15 weeks of gestation (Otake and Schull, 1984). This period corresponds remarkably well to the time of the second wave of neuronal migration (Fig. 6). This wave in humans mostly supplies neurons to the superficial layers of the neocortex (Rakic, 1978; Sidman and Rakic, 1973) and I think it is possible that irradiation interferes with both cell proliferation and migration of these neurons. This type of radiation insult may be more widespread but difficult to detect except in extreme cases. For example, mental retardation in children exposed prenatally to multiple X-irradiation for various medical reasons (e.g., Goldstein and Murphy, 1929; Murphy et al., 1942) was reported only because it was obvious. In retrospect, the basic insult in these cases may have been caused by defective neuronal migration.

The possible effects of irradiation on the migration of cortical neurons in some victims of gamma irradiation are illustrated in a case that was exposed during the second fetal month in Hiroshima and survived for 16 years (Yokota et al., 1961; Neriishi and Matsumura, 1983). At the time of death, the brain of this individual weighed less than 1000 g, the neocortex was attenuated, missing cells of the more superficial layers, and there was a massive neuronal ectopia in the subcortical white matter near the cerebral ventricle. Obviously, a large number of neurons did not move far from the place of their origin around the lateral cerebral ventricle. Instead, they remained in the white matter, forming a large mass of ectopic gray matter that was visible even at the gross morphological level. Although only a few cases have been examined at autopsy, the application of magnetic resonance on living victims shows a band of abnormal gray matter near

the cerebral ventricle in two Hiroshima victims. Both are female and were exposed to radiation during the 12–13 weeks after fertilization (W. Shull, personal communication). The autopsy material and magnetic resonance pictures correspond remarkably well. It appears that in all three cases, cells belonging to the second migratory wave survived in abnormal positions near the lateral ventricle. Although we do not have any date in humans on the pattern of connectivity of these cells, it is reasonable to assume that they survived in this abnormal position by forming aberrant synaptic connections, as has been demonstrated with ectopic cells in experimentally irradiated animals (Jensen and Killackey, 1984).

In terms of the possible cellular and molecular mechanisms involved in migration defects caused by irradiation, the main problem is how a single dose of gamma rays, which destroys a single generation of proliferating cells, affects the migration of several generations of subsequently produced neurons. For example, if radial glia are a cell population that is selectively killed by irradiation, they could not be easily replenished. We have evidence from [^{3}H]thymidine autoradiography that the majority of radial glial cells in the monkey fetus are a stable population as they stop dividing during the midgestational period, when they serve as guides for migrating neurons (Schmechel and Rakic, 1979). Their elimination during this period may prove to be devastating, as the substrate for neuronal movement is missing. On the other hand, the loss of neural progenitor cells due to a single dose of radiation could be replenished by the regulation of subsequent cell proliferation, as observed in experimental animals (Webster et al., 1973). However, although the production of neurons can continue following irradiation, later generated cells fail to move from the proliferation zone. One possible reason for this failure is the absence of the appropriate substrate for their movement. Alternatively, radiation may prevent migration of only a single generation of cells by interference with interacting membranes. In this case, even the retention of glial guides would not help, since the affected cells of one generation may physically clog the pathway and thus preclude subsequently produced, healthy neurons from bypassing this point.

Many radiation experts believe that gamma rays interfere exclusively with nucleic acids during cell division. They state that a single dose should not permanently change the composition of cell surface membranes (e.g., Kriegel et al., 1987). However, we should not exclude an outside possibility that irradiation can also change the membrane properties of either migrating neurons or glial fibers and, thus, interfere more directly with cell movement. A migratory defect which results in ectopic neurons has been observed regularly in rats irradiated as embryos (Hicks et al., 1959). In irradiated animals, both the migration and the production of neurons seems to be diminished. However, many cells that do not move nevertheless survive. Recent studies show that in such cases, ectopic cells situated near the cerebral ventricle project to the appropriate levels of the spinal cord despite their grossly aberrant position (Jensen and Killackey, 1984). Irradiation, therefore, could produce an anomaly that can be used to study the problem of abnormal migration experimentally. Another useful approach is to directly examine the effect of irradiation on the migration of neurons in vitro using the dissociated tissue culture system of Hatten and her colleagues (Hatten and Liem, 1981; Hatten et al., 1984). Likewise, the population of atomic bomb victims should be monitored and their brains examined after death by the most advanced technology including computer-aided quantitative analysis.

The final position of a neuron and its synaptic relationships after its arrival at the cortex can also be disturbed by changing the amount and/or pattern of cortical afferents, e.g. reducing the number of monoamine neurons in the embryo by exposure to a specific neurotoxin, 6-hydroxydopamine (6-OHDA). This illustrates how external agents can play an indirect role in corticogenesis. Although reports conflict in regard to the type of morphological changes which occur in the neo-cortex of adult animals that have been exposed to 6-OHDA, there is little disagreement that the effect can be functionally devastating. Among effects that have been observed are alterations in cortical cell number, branching of dendrites, density and shape of dendritic spines, and synaptic density (Maeda et al., 1974; Wendlandt et al., 1977; Ebersole et al., 1981; Felton et al., 1982). The findings most relevant to the present topic are the observations of neuronal malposition and the presence of ectopic neurons in layer I, indicating that even moderate destruction of distant but synaptically related groups of neurons may affect the settling pattern of cells in the developing cortex.

Concluding remarks

Conceptual and factual advances in understanding neuronal migration in the past two decades have provided new insight into the pathogenesis of human brain malformations at the cellular, molecular, and functional levels. Some of these results may have direct implications for understanding the consequences of exposure to toxic substances or ionizing radiation on the fetal central nervous system in utero. The reviewed material indicates that cortical malformations can be caused by the death of a specific neuronal class or by a breakdown in cell-to-cell interactions. Although in recent years we have learned an enormous amount of information concerning differentiation of individual nerve cells, their organelles, and synaptic contacts, we are still ignorant when it comes to understanding the meaning of these events in terms of building a complex cellular assembly such as the neocortex. At least in part, this can be attributed to the failure in recognizing that a complex system such as the cerebral cortex cannot be understood by simple extrapolation of properties of elementary components without taking into account competitive interaction and the impact of the external environment. As important as competitive cell interactions are for shaping the final structure of any organ of multicellular organisms, they may be even more crucial for the development of the central nervous system. Thus, to understand either normal or abnormal development, one must take into account the entire community of interconnected nerve cells.

Logistical problems in the analysis of the development of the vertebrate brain in general and the human neocortex in particular seem insurmountable. Yet, new information that has accumulated in recent years has opened new perspectives on normal and abnormal brain development. At the moment, the significance of the research on embryonic competitive interactions is primarily in its relevance to understanding normal development. However, it has considerable implication for understanding brain malformations that occur due to exposure to a variety of environmental factors. At this point in our industrial society, we have to worry more about new man-made agents as well as natural forces that played a relatively minor role in the past. In particular, I refer here to exposure to new types of neuroactive drugs, large amounts of toxic chemicals from industrial waste, and ionizing radiation. Understanding of developmental principles is essential if we are to prevent serious damage to a large population. It is, however, still very difficult to relate new concepts from developmental neurobiology to the genesis of an abnormal human brain and even more to translate these findings into a useful explanation of abnormal behavior. Nevertheless, methodological and conceptual advances made in recent years open new possibilities for understanding the effect of the environment on synaptic connectivity in the human brain at the molecular, cellular and functional levels.

References

Angevine, J.B., Jr. and Sidman, R.L. (1961) Autoradiographic study of cell migration during histogenesis of cerebral cortex in the mouse. *Nature*, 192: 766–768.

Antomicek, H., Persohn, E. and Schachner, M. (1987) Biochemical and functional characterization of a novel neuron-glia adhesion molecule that is involved in neuronal migration. *Cell Biol.*, 104: 1587–1595.

Ariëns Kappers, C.U. (1929) *The Evolution of the Nervous System*, E.F. Bohn, Haarlem.

Ariëns Kappers, C.U., Huber, G.C. and Crosby, E.C. (1936) *The Comparative Anatomy of the Nervous System of Vertebrates Including Man*, Hafner, New York.

Bolton, J.S. (1900) The exact histological localization of the visual area of the human cerebral cortex. *Phil. Trans. R. Soc. Lond. B.*, 193: 165–205.

Bourgeois, J.-P. and Rakic, P. (1987) Distribution, density and ultrastructure of synapses in the visual cortex in monkeys devoid of retinal input from early embryonic stages. *Soc. Neurosci. Abstr.*, 13: 1044.

Bray, D. (1973) Model for membrane movements in the neural growth cone. *Nature*, 244: 93–96.

Bretscher, M.S. (1984) Endocytosis: relation to capping and cell locomotion. *Science*, 224: 681–686.

Brodmann, K. (1909) *Vergleichende Lokalisationslehre der Grosshirninde*, Brath, Leipzig.

Caviness, V.S., Jr. (1982) Development of neocortical afferent systems: studies in the reeler mouse. *Neurosci. Res. Program Bull.*, 20: 560–566.

Caviness, V.S., Jr. and Rakic, P. (1978) Mechanisms of cortical development: a view from mutations in mice. *Ann. Rev. Neurosci.*, 1: 297–326.

Caviness, V.S., Jr. and Williams, R.S. (1985) Cellular patterns in developmental malformations of neocortex: Neuronal-glial interactions. In *The Developing Brain and Its Disorders*, Karger, Basel, pp. 43–67.

Creutzfeldt, O.D. (1977) Generality of the functional structure of the neocortex. *Naturwissenschaften*, 64: 507–517.

Dekaban, A.S. (1969) Differential vulnerability to irradiation of various cerebral structures during prenatal development. In *Radiation Biology of the Fetal and Juvenile Mammal*, U.S. Atomic Energy Commission, Oak Ridge, TN, pp. 769–777.

Ebersole, P., Parnavelas, J.G. and Blue, M.E. (1981) Development of visual cortex of rats treated with 6-hydroxydopamine in early life. *Anat. Embryol.*, 162: 489–492.

Eccles, J.C. (1984) The cerebral neocortex. A theory of its operation. In E.G. Jones and A. Peters (Eds.), *Cerebral Cortex*, Vol. 2, Plenum, New York, pp. 1–36.

Eckenhoff, M.F. and Rakic, P. (1984) Radial organization of the hippocampal dentate gyrus: A Golgi, ultrastructural and immunohistochemical analysis in the developing rhesus monkey. *J. Comp. Neurol.*, 223: 1–21.

Edelman, G.M. (1983) Cell adhesion molecules. *Science*, 219: 450–457.

Eidelberg, D. and Galaburda, A.M. (1982) Symmetry and asymmetry in the human posterior thalamus. *Arch. Neurol.*, 39: 325–332.

Felton, D.L., Hallman, H. and Jonsson, G. (1982) Evidence for a neurotrophic role of noradrenalin neurons in the postnatal development of rat cerebral cortex. *J. Neurocytol.*, 11: 119–135.

Freytag, E. and Lindenberg, R. (1967) Neuropathologic findings in patients of a hospital for the mentally deficient: A survey of 359 cases. *Johns Hopkins Med. J.*, 121: 379–392.

Friede, R.L. (1975) *Developmental Neuropathology*, Springer, New York, Wien.

Goldberg, D.J. (1982) Actin and myosin in nerve cells. In D.G. Weiss (Ed.), *Axoplasmic Transport*, Springer, Berlin, pp. 73–80.

Goldman, P.S. and Nauta, W.J.H. (1977) Columnar organization of association and motor cortex: Autoradiographic evidence for cortico-cortical and commissural columns in the frontal lobe of the newborn rhesus monkey. *Brain Res.*, 122: 369–385.

Goldman-Rakic, P.S. (1980) Morphological consequences of prenatal injury to the primate brain. *Prog. Brain Res.*, 53: 3–19.

Goldman-Rakic, P.S. (1981) Development and plasticity of primate frontal association cortex. In F.O. Schmitt, F.G. Worden, S.G. Dennis and G. Adelman (Eds.), *Organization of the Cerebral Cortex*, The MIT Press, Cambridge, MA, pp. 69–97.

Goldman-Rakic, P.S. and Rakic, P. (1984) Experimental modification of gyral patterns. In N. Geschwind and A.M. Galaburda (Eds.), *Cerebral Dominance: The Biological Foundation*, Harvard Univ. Press, Cambridge, MA, pp. 179–192.

Goldstein, L. and Murphy, D.P. (1929) Etiology of the ill-health in children born after maternal pelvic irradiation. Part II. Defective children born after postconception pelvic irradiation. *Am. J. Roentgenol.*, 22: 322–331.

Hatten, M.E. and Liem, R.K.H. (1981) Astroglia provide a template for the positioning of cerebellar neurons in vitro. *J. Cell Biol.*, 90: 622–630.

Hatten, M.E. and Liem, R.K.H. and Mason, C.A. (1984) Defects in specific associations between astroglia and neurons occur in microcultures of weaver mouse cerebellar cells. *J. Neurosci.*, 4: 1163–1172.

Hatten, M.E. and Mason, C.A. (1986) Neuron-astroglia interactions in vitro and in vivo. *Trends Neurosci.* 9: 168–174.

Hemendinger, L.M. and Caviness, V.S. (1988) Cellular migration in developing cerebral wall explants in vitro. *Dev. Brain Res.*, 38: 290–295.

Hicks, S.P., D'Amato, C.J. and Lowe, M.J. (1959) The development of the mammalian nervous system. I. Malformations of the brain, especially the cerebral cortex, induced in rats by radiation. II. Some mechanisms of the malformations of the cortex. *J. Comp. Neurol.*, 113: 435–470.

Hubel, D.H. and Wiesel, T.N. (1977) Ferrier lecture. Functional architecture of macaque monkey visual cortex. *Proc. R. Soc. Lond. B.*, 198: 1–59.

Jensen, K.F. and Killackey, H.P. (1984) Subcortical projections from ectopic neocortical neurons. *Proc. Natl. Acad. Sci. USA*, 81: 964–968.

Johnston, R. and Wessells, N. (1980) Regulation of the elongating nerve fiber. *Curr. Top. Dev. Biol.*, 16: 165–206.

Kostovic, I. and Molliver, M.E. (1974) A new interpretation of the laminar development of cerebral cortex: Synaptogenesis in different layers of neopalium in the human fetus. *Anat. Rec.*, 178: 395.

Kriegel, H., Schmahl, W., Gerber, G.B. and Stieve, F.E. (1987) *Radiation Risks on the Developing Nervous System*, Fisher, Stuttgart.

Letourneau, P.C. (1975) Cell-to-substratum adhesion and guidance of axonal elongation. *Dev. Biol.*, 44: 92–101.

Levitt, P. and Rakic, P. (1980) Immunoperoxidase localization of glial fibrillary acid protein in radial glial cells and astrocytes of the developing rhesus monkey brain. *J. Comp. Neurol.*, 193: 815–840.

Levitt, P., Cooper, M.L. and Rakic, P. (1981) Coexistence of neuronal and glial precursor cells in the cerebral ventricular zone of the fetal monkey: An ultrastructural immunoperoxidase analysis. *J. Neurosci.*, 1: 27–39.

Levitt, P., Cooper, M.L. and Rakic, P. (1983) Early divergence and changing proportions of neuronal and glial precursor cells in the primate cerebral ventricular zone. *Dev. Biol.*, 96: 472–484.

Lidov, H.G.W. and Mollier, M.E. (1982) The structure of cerebral cortex in the rat following prenatal administration of 6-hydroxydopamine. *Dev. Brain Res.*, 3: 81–108.

Lindner, J., Zinser, G., Werz, W., Goridis, C., Bizzini, B. and Schachner, M. (1986) Experimental modification of postnatal cerebellar granule cell migration in vitro. *Brain Res.*, 377: 298–304.

Luskin, M.B. and Shatz, C.J. (1985) Studies of the earliest generated cells of the cat's visual cortex: cogeneration of subplate and marginal zones. *J. Neurosci.*, 5: 1062–1075.

Maeda, T., Tohyama, M. and Shimizu, N. (1974) Modification of postnatal development of neocortex in rat brain with deprivation of locus coeruleus. *Brain Res.*, 70: 515–520.

McClain, D.A. and Edelman, G.M. (1982) A neuronal cell adhesion molecule from human brain. *Proc. Natl. Acad. Sci. USA*, 79: 6380–6384.

Molgard, K., Balslev, Y., Lauritzen, B. and Norman, R. (1987) Cell junctions and membrane specializations in the ventricular zone (germinal matrix) of the developing sheep brain: a CSF-brain barrier. *J. Neurocytol.*, 16: 433–444.

Moonen, G., Grau-Wagemans, M.P. and Selak, I. (1982) Plasminogen activator – plasmin system and neuronal migration. *Nature*, 298: 753–755.

Mountcastle, V.B. (1979) An organizing principle for cerebral function: the unit module and the distributed system. In F.O. Schmitt and F.G. Worden (Eds.), *The Neurosciences: Fourth Study Program*, MIT Press, Cambridge, MA, pp. 21–42.

Murphy, D.P., Schirlock, M.E. and Doll, E.A. (1942) Micro cephaly following maternal pelvic irradiation for inter ruption of pregnancy. *Am. J. Roentgenol.*, 48: 356–359.

Neriishi, F. and Matsumura, H. (1983) Morphological observations of the central nervous system in an in-utero exposed autopsy case. *J. Radiat. Res.*, 24: 18.

Nowakowski, R.S. and Rakic, P. (1979) The mode of migration of neurons to the hippocampus: a Golgi and electron microscopic analysis in fetal rhesus monkey. *J. Neurocytol.*, 8: 697–718.

Otake, M. and Schull, W.J. (1984) In utero exposure of A-bomb radiation and mental retardation: a reassessment. *Br. J. Radiol.*, 57: 409–414.

Peters, A. and Jones, E.G. (1984) *Cerebral Cortex. Volume 1. Cellular Components of the Cerebral Cortex*, Plenum Press, New York.

Pinto-Lord, C.M., Evrard, E. and Caviness, V.S., Jr. (1982) Obstructed neuronal migration along radial glial fibers in the neocortex of the reeler mouse: a Golgi-EM analysis. *Dev. Brain Res.*, 4: 379–393.

Rakic, P. (1972) Mode of cell migration to the superficial layers of fetal monkey neocortex. *J. Comp. Neurol.*, 145: 61–84.

Rakic, P. (1974) Neurons in rhesus monkey visual cortex: systematic relation between time of origin and eventual disposition. *Science*, 183: 425–427.

Rakic, P. (1975a) Timing of major ontogenetic events in the visual cortex of the rhesus monkey. In N.A. Buckwald and M. Brazier (Eds.), *Brain Mechanisms in Mental Retardation*, Academic Press, New York, pp. 3–40.

Rakic, P. (1975b) Cell migration and neuronal ectopias in the brain. In D. Bergsma (Ed.), *Morphogenesis and Malformation of the Face and Brain (Birth Defects: Original Series)*, Alan R. Liss, New York, pp. 95–129.

Rakic, P. (1976) Prenatal genesis of connections subserving ocular dominance in the rhesus monkey. *Nature*, 261: 467–471.

Rakic, P. (1978) Neuronal migration and contact guidance in primate telencephalon. *Postgrad. Med. J.*, 54: 25–40.

Rakic, P. (1981a) Development of visual centers in primate brain depends on binocular competition before birth. *Science*, 214: 928–931.

Rakic, P. (1981b) Neuronal-glial interactions during brain development. *Trends Neurosci.*, 4: 184–187.

Rakic, P. (1981c) Developmental events leading to areal organization of the neocortex. In F.O. Schmitt, S.G. Dennis and F.G. Worden (Eds.), *The Cerebral Cortex*, MIT Press, Cambridge, MA, pp. 7–28.

Rakic, P. (1985) Contact regulation of neuronal migration. In G.M. Edelman and J.-P. Thiery (Eds.), *The Cell in Contact: Adhesions and Junctions as Morphogenetic Determinants*, Wiley and Sons, New York, pp. 67–91.

Rakic, P. (1986) Mechanisms of ocular dominance segrega- tion in this lateral geniculate nucleus: Competitive elimination hypothesis. *Trends Neurosci.*, 9: 11–15.

Rakic, P. (1987) Neuronal migration. In G. Adelman (Ed.), *Encyclopedia of Neuroscience*, Birkhauser, Boston, MA, pp. 825–827.

Rakic, P. (1988) Specification of cerebral cortical areas: the radial unit hypothesis. *Science* (submitted).

Rakic, P. and Goldman-Rakic, P.S. (1982) Development and modifiability of the cerebral cortex. *Neurosci. Res. Program Bull.*, 20: 429–611.

Rakic, P. and Goldman-Rakic, P.S. (1985) Use of fetal neurosurgery for experimental studies of structural and function brain development in nonhuman primates. In R.A. Thompson, J.R. Green and S.D. Johnson (Eds.), *Prenatal Neurology and Neurosurgery*, Spectrum Press, New York, pp. 1–15.

Rakic, P. and Riley, K.P. (1983a) Regulation of axon number in primate optic nerve by binocular competition. *Nature*, 305: 135–137.

Rakic, P. and Riley, K.P. (1983b) Overproduction and elimination of retinal axons in the fetal rhesus monkey. *Science*, 219: 1441–1444.

Rakic, P. and Sidman, R.L. (1973a) Sequence of developmental abnormalities leading to granule cell deficit in cerebellar cortex of weaver mutant mice. *J. Comp. Neurol.*, 152: 103–132.

Rakic, P. and Sidman, R.L. (1973b) Organization of cerebellar cortex secondary to deficit of granule cells in weaver mutant mice. *J. Comp. Neurol.*, 152: 133–162.

Rakic, P. and Singer, W. (1988) *Neurobiology of Neocortex*, Wiley and Sons, New York.

Rakic, P. and Williams, R.W. (1986) Thalamic regulation of cortical parcellation: an experimental perturbation of the striate cortex in rhesus monkeys. *Soc. Neurosci. Abstr.*, 12: 1499.

Rakic, P., Kritzer, M. and Gallager, D. (1987) Distribution of major neurotransmitter receptors in the visual cortex of monkeys devoid of retinal input from early embryonic stages. *Soc. Neurosci. Abstr.*, 13: 358.

Rakic, P., Stensaas, L.J., Sayre, E.P. and Sidman, R.L. (1974) Computer aided three-dimensional reconstruction and quantitative analysis of cells from serial electron microscopic montages of fetal monkey brain. *Nature*, 250: 31–34.

Richman, D.P., Stewart, R.M. and Caviness, V.S., Jr. (1973) Microgyria, lissencephaly, and neuron migration to the cerebral cortex: an architectonic approach. *Neurology*, 23: 413.

Rouslahti, E. and Pierschbacher, M.D. (1987) New perspective in cell adhesion: RGD and integrens. *Science*, 238: 491–497.

Schmechel, D.E. and Rakic, P. (1979) A Golgi study of radial glial cells in developing monkey telencephalon: morphogenesis and transformation into astrocytes. *Anat. Embryol.*, 156: 115–152.

idman, R. L. and Rakic, P. (1973) Neuronal migration, with special reference to developing human brain: a review. *Brain Res.*, 62: 1–35.

idman, R. L. and Rakic, P. (1982) Development of the human central nervous system. In W. Haymaker and R. D. Adams (Eds.), *Cytology and Cellular Neuropathology*, Charles C. Thomas, Springfield, IL, pp. 3–145.

tewart, M. R., Richman, D. P. and Caviness, V. S., Jr. (1975) Lissencephaly and pachygyria. An architectonic and topological analysis. *Acta Neuropath.*, 31: 1–12.

zenthagothai, J. (1983) The modular architectonic principle of neural centers. *Rev. Physiol. Biochem. Pharmacol.*, 98: 11–61.

renkner, E., Smith, D. and Segil, N. (1984) Is cerebellar granule cell migration regulated by an internal clock? *J. Neurosci.*, 4: 2850–2855.

Volpe, J.J. (1987) *Neurology of the Newborn*, 2nd edn., Saunders, Philadelphia.

Webster, W., Shimada, M. and Langman, J. (1973) Effect of fluorodeoxyuridine, colcemid, and bromodeoxyuridine on developing neocortex of the mouse. *Am. J. Anat.*, 137: 67–86.

Wendlandt, S., Crow, T.J. and Sterling, R.V. (1977) The involvement of the noradrenergic system arising from the locus coeruleus in the postnatal development of the neocortex in rat brain. *Brain Res.*, 125: 1–9.

Yokota, S., Tagowa, D., Tsura, S.O., Nakayama, K., Neriishi, S., Namiki, H. and Hirose K. (1961) Microcephaly in an in vitro survivor: An autopsy case. *Nagasaki Tgaku Zushi*, 38: 92–95.

G.J. Boer, M.G.P. Feenstra, M. Mirmiran, D.F. Swaab and F. Van Haaren
Progress in Brain Research, Vol. 73
© 1988 Elsevier Science Publishers B.V. (Biomedical Division)

CHAPTER 3

Implications of behavioral teratology for assessing the risks posed by environmental and therapeutic chemicals

Bernard Weiss

Environmental Health Sciences Center and Department of Biophysics, University of Rochester School of Medicine and Dentistry, Rochester, NY 14642, USA

Introduction

Ten years ago, behavioral toxicology and teratology could be described as emerging sciences. They are now well past the stage of metamorphosis. Not only have meetings and conferences multiplied to such a degree that almost any week chosen at random provides an opportunity to attend one, but legislation and regulations reflect the concern of both governments and their publics. Such acknowledgements reflect the status of a mature and influential discipline.

Toxicological background

To understand how toxicological findings are translated into policy decisions, consider the implications of terms such as the No Observable Effect Level (NOEL). This value is inferred from a dose–response function and is usually defined as that exposure level exhibiting no statistically reliable elevation in either incidence or magnitude of effect compared to control data. Typically, the NOEL based on experimental animal data gathered from chronic treatment is multiplied by a safety or uncertainty factor to provide an adequate margin of protection for humans. A common safety factor under these conditions is 100; it represents the combination of a 10-fold factor designed to

yield an adequate margin of protection and a 10-fold factor to account for species differences. A safety factor of 10 might be used when epidemiological data are believed firm enough so that a species extrapolation factor is not pertinent.

The discussion above may seem rather remote from the mechanistic themes that direct most research on neurobehavioral teratology. But consider the problems stemming from much of what is termed research on mechanisms. Often, experimental treatment consists of only a single dose value, typically administered acutely. The investigator then performs a statistical analysis to determine whether the treatment produced significant differences from control conditions in some selected endpoint. Especially if the experiment was performed to discover whether the developing organism is uniquely sensitive to the treatment, its more transparent conclusions may prove misleading from a toxicological perspective.

In Fig. 1, I have sketched the kinds of information that may be required to support research in behavioral toxicology and teratology. If behavioral measures are to serve as more than isolated curiosities to toxicology, they should be supplemented by, or be offered in the context of, other relevant measures. Dose is central, in the form of either a dose–response (for quantal measures) or a dose–effect (for continuous

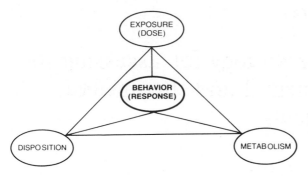

Fig. 1. Sources of coordinated data typically required to fully grasp significance of behavioral observations.

measures) function. A single point on that function is not sufficient to confirm a postulated mechanism because of the other nodes joined to behavior. Disposition refers to the distribution of the chemical in the body. Differences between effects observed at different stages of the life-cycle may arise, not from any inherent differences in sensitivity to a chemical treatment, but simply in where the chemical tends to lodge. The fetus may be more vulnerable to a specific agent than the adult only because the fetal brain-to-body weight ratio is higher than in the adult. Tracing the routes of metabolism is at least equally important. Many chemicals undergo bioactivation; that is, only after they have been transformed by the body do they become toxic. Most chemical carcinogens possess this property. The neurotoxicants, n-hexane and methyl n-butyl ketone, which produce a central-peripheral distal axonopathy, are metabolized to the compound 2,5-hexanedione, the proximate poison. Other poisons are detoxified by metabolic processes.

If a specific dose of an agent is selected which, in the developing organism, (a) produces a different pattern of distribution from that obtained in the adult, or (b) overwhelms immature mechanisms of detoxification by exceeding the capacity of rate-limited enzymes, or (c) is bioactivated at a higher rate, an experimenter could easily be misled to a faulty conclusion. This is the junction at which the abstract concept of risk joins the concrete one of mechanism. Mechanisms postulated in the absence of dose variation and dispositional and metabolic data are not especially cogent in toxicology. They lose further cogency if they are based on high doses, because another confusing feature of high-dose toxicology is the breadth of systems such doses may affect. If an agent which modifies nervous system function is administered at a dose high enough to also impair renal function, the organism's inability to excrete the agent or its metabolites could alter the agent's gamut of activity and provoke faulty conclusions. The low dose range from which the most convincing risk estimates would be drawn is also the range from which the best clues to mechanisms can be extracted.

Metal neurotoxicity

Metals offer several cogent examples of these issues and problems. Fig. 2 is a compilation of

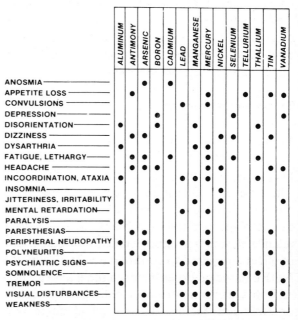

SYMPTOMS ASCRIBED TO METAL TOXICITY

Fig. 2. Signs and symptoms of behavioral toxicity associated with exposure to various metals.

various metals and their reported behavioral toxicity. This chart does not take account of the differences in toxic potency between various forms of species of a metal, but they can be enormous. Organic forms are often much more neurotoxic than inorganic forms (cf Weiss, 1983, for details). Even with this abbreviated detail, however, it is easy to see the great variety of effects that have been ascribed to excessive metal exposure. Excessive is a significant word, because many metals are also essential elements. Manganese, for example, is required for proper skeletal and connective tissue development. In fact, attempts to induce manganese toxicity in neonatal rats or mice have been reported to enhance growth. In the adult, manganese can produce a syndrome marked by both neurological and psychological aberrations (Table 1). Most of the reported victims were miners or workers exposed through inhalation to dust from manganese ore or fumes arising from ferromanganese production. This feature emphasizes the critical role of route of exposure in toxicology. Manganese consumed as part of the diet is closely regulated, and excessive amounts are excreted.

Table 1 illustrates a central problem for behavioral toxicology: the plethora of possible endpoints. Which should be chosen as a criterion for toxicity? The more overtly neurological indices are easier to measure, at least by the usual clinical

TABLE 1

Manganese neurotoxicity

Major signs	Major symptoms
Abnormal gait	Weakness
Retropulsion, propulsion	Difficulty walking
Diminished leg power	Somnolence
Impaired coordination	Clumsiness
Abnormal laughter	Bradykinesia
Expressionless face	Lack of balance
Dysarthria	Muscle pains

standards. But the subjective, psychological indices may appear earlier in the course of intoxication, although the sequence is not uniform. Some observers have reported that the psychological disturbances precede the neurological disorders; others have observed them to erupt concurrently. In some of the manganese mining communities of South America, the constellation of odd behaviors is known as 'locura manganica,' or manganese madness, and is assumed to herald the onset of the neurological component. Should we be willing to trade the possibly more sensitive but less easily measured psychological variables for the possibly more robust neurological signs in calculating safe exposure standards? Studies by Roels et al. (1987) indicate that we need not. By relying on a battery of tests which measured both types of variables more precisely and in greater depth than clinical judgment, these investigators showed that workers exposed to manganese fumes performed differently from controls on several components of the battery, although no worker provided an overt hint of toxicity. Psychological test results now offer a quantitative scale for decisions about safe exposure levels for manganese.

Lead toxicity

The metal evoking the greatest concern and debate about exposure standards is lead, and most of that concern stems from reports linking lead to reduced scores on intelligence and allied tests by children. Needleman et al. (1979) generated a radical swing in the terms of the debate. Their study of nearly 3000 children in the Boston area, based on lead in deciduous teeth, demonstrated clear differences in intelligence test scores between children with moderate and low lead levels and even showed a convincing dose–response relationship on items from an inventory of classroom behavior. The report by Needleman et al. provoked comparable studies elsewhere, although not of the same magnitude. These subsequent studies (Needleman, 1985) all confirmed the 1979 study.

Some aspects of the debate lingered, however,

because no epidemiological study can be entirely free of flaws. But prospective studies can eliminate many objections inherent in the kind of cross-sectional design adopted by Needleman et al. These are now coming to publication. The original Needleman group recently presented the results of a massive study based on over 11 000 births (Bellinger et al., 1987). From that original population, designed to provide reliable measures of prenatal lead exposure by analyses of cord blood, a sample of 249 children was chosen for intensive study. About one-third were assigned to a low-lead group (mean Pb blood levels of 1.8 μg/dl), one-third to a medium-lead group (mean of 6.6 μg/dl) and one-third to a high-lead group (mean of 14.6 μg/dl). The U.S. Centers for Disease Control define a blood level of 25 μg/dl as the upper limit of safety. When tested at two years of age by the Bayley Scales of Infant Development, the children in the high-lead group scored about eight percent less on the Bayley Mental Development Index than the children in the other two groups.

This striking difference at two years of age amplified earlier assessments at 6, 12 and 18 months of age (Bellinger and Needleman, 1985). Moreover, the statistical analyses and assignment of children to groups took account of a long list of potentially confounding variables. It included demographic variables such as maternal age and family social class, reproductive history, smoking and drinking habits, pregnancy and labor history, neonatal status, and the child's home environment. Moreover, lead exposure after birth, as measured by blood lead, seemed minimal, yielding group means for the low, medium and high children of 5.4, 7.2 and 7.7 μg/dl, respectively, at the age of two years. A unique feature of this study was its population. The parents could be characterized as mostly white, from the upper social levels, college graduates, and offering intact home environments.

The implications of such findings pose serious policy problems, because they leave no room for complacency about the reduced incidence of overt lead poisoning in developed countries. The question has shifted leftward, so to speak, on the dose–response function, and entails a much broader view even of risk. Risk typically is defined in individual terms; for example, the risk of developing cancer arising from exposure to a specific chemical at a particular level. Framing policies on substances such as lead poses another kind of challenge – one that might be termed societal risk analysis. It can be viewed from the following vantage point. Assume that modest lead exposure reduces scores on standard intelligence tests by five percent (Bellinger et al. reported a reduction of eight percent). Most such tests are arranged to yield a mean I.Q. of 100; a child with such a score is average for its age. For widely used tests such as the Stanford-Binet, the standard deviation is 15 points. Simple calculation shows that, in a population of 100 million, 2.3 million persons will score above 130 (2 standard deviations). If the mean of the population is lowered by five percent, the number of persons scoring above 130 drops to 990 thousand. Any society experiencing such a loss confronts a serious threat to its future.

The mechanisms at the source of these recent findings about prenatal sensitivity to lead are not clear because most mechanistic explanations of lead's behavioral effects, besides their dependence on biological processes studied at relatively high levels of lead exposure, must contend with the absence of a solid experimental literature (Bornshein et al., 1980). Much of the earlier research adopted crude behavioral endpoints, which, combined with inadequate measures of lead in tissue and inadequate control of variables such as food intake and body weight, virtually guaranteed an indigestible porridge of findings. The newer experimental literature displays a much greater degree of sensitivity to these variables. Rice and her colleagues (reviewed in Rice, 1983) focused their skills on primates. *Macaca fascicularis* infants were assigned immediately after birth either to control treatments or to lead administration at different dose levels ranging from 25 to 500 μg/kg daily. At 100 days of age, lead treatment produced blood levels ranging from a mean of about 55 μg/dl in the high-dose group to about 10 μg/dl in the low-dose group. After weaning from infant formula, blood levels decreased, attaining values in the high- and low-dose groups, respectively, of about 33 and 10 μg/dl. Several kinds of behavioral measures distinguished the treated from the control monkeys. Schedule-controlled performance, for example, revealed sharp differences. Similar effects are apparent in rats, a species assumed to be relatively resistant to lead toxicity. Cory-Slechta et al. (1985) have demonstrated such findings in several studies, the most recent of which (Fig. 3) confirmed significant performance effects at blood levels of 10–20 μg/dl. There seems little point any more in pursuing mechanisms of gross toxicity.

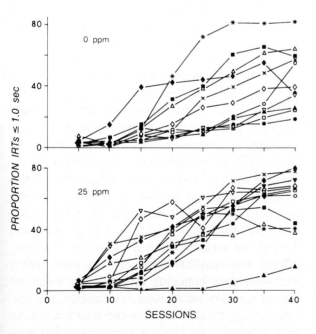

Fig. 3. Short interresponse times in rats drinking control solution (25 ppm sodium acetate) and rats drinking 25 ppm lead acetate solution. Each symbol represents an individual rat maintained on a fixed interval 1-min schedule of food reinforcement (Cory-Slechta et al., 1985).

Inorganic mercury

Mercury is also a toxic metal, and offers lessons and models of its own for behavioral teratology. Inorganic mercury compounds are usually regarded as renal poisons. In children, however, they may induce a different pattern of toxicity, one that includes a liberal nervous system component. Pink Disease, also known as acrodynia ('painful limbs'), drew its name from the signs and symptoms listed in Table 2. Speculations about its etiology abounded in the medical literature for perhaps 150 years (Weiss and Clarkson, 1982). Probably the most popular explanation was some form of infectious disease. Not until about 40 years ago, stemming from a search by Warkany and Hubbard (1951) which originally sought a possible source in arsenic poisoning, was the actual source verified: mercury. Children with Pink Disease excreted enormous amounts of mercury in urine. Probing by these investigators revealed the source to be mercurous chloride, or calomel, usually from teething powders, and sometimes from other medications such as those used to treat skin disorders.

Why was calomel added to teething powders? The most likely explanation seems to be the mystical powers with which mercury was invested by ancient and medieval physicians. Recall that the

TABLE 2

Pink disease (acrodynia)

Neurotoxic features	General features
Pain in extremities	Cold blue fingertips, toes
Numbness, tingling	Reddening of cheeks, nose
Loss of muscle tone	Sloughing of skin
Muscle twitching	Loss or loosening of teeth
Photophobia	Excessive perspiration
Tremor	Elevated blood pressure
Itching, burning sensation	Rash
Diminished reflexes	Loss of appetite

alchemists sought to transmute mercury into gold, and that mercury compounds persisted as therapy for syphilis (without success) well into the twentieth century (Goldwater, 1972). Why was mercury not uncovered earlier as the source of Pink Disease? One element of the answer is surely that only a small proportion of the children treated with teething powders and other preparations, perhaps as low as one in a thousand, displayed the full syndrome. It would have been easy to confuse an incomplete syndrome with the usual galaxy of childhood afflictions, including the pain of teething itself. The number of children exhibiting just a few of the manifestations of Pink Disease and labelled with the incorrect diagnosis must have been substantial. A recent outbreak of mercury poisoning in Argentina (Gotelli et al., 1985), arising from the addition of a phenyl mercury fungicide to a diaper cleaning process, also provoked several clear instances of Pink Disease although the renal effects were predominant.

Methylmercury

The form of mercury most closely associated with postnatal functional disturbances is methyl-

TABLE 3

Indices of methylmercury toxicity

Sensory
  Paresthesia
  Pain in limbs
  Visual disturbances (constriction)
  Hearing disturbances
  Astereognosis

Motor
  Disturbances in gait
  Weakness, unsteadiness of legs; falling
  Thick, slurred speech (dysarthria)
  Tremor

Other
  Headaches
  Rashes
  'Mental disturbance'

---

mercury, and the site where that association took form was Minamata, Japan. In the 1950s, a factory engaged in the production of acetaldehyde began to discharge an effluent into Minamata Bay which was contaminated with methylmercury. Another form of mercury had been used as a catalyst in the production process, but was converted into the deadly methyl form. Fishermen and their families who subsisted on seafood from the bay became examples of how Japan's rush to become an industrial power absorbed human suffering into the inevitable costs. The famed photographer Eugene Smith documented those costs in a searing book (Smith and Smith, 1975).

The signs and symptoms of methylmercury poisoning appear in Table 3. They reflect damage throughout the nervous system. In humans and other primates, the damage is most extensive deep in the folds of the cerebral cortex. Such localization is the reason why impairment of vision, expressed as constriction of the visual field, is such a prominent feature of the syndrome. The peripheral areas of the visual field are represented in the calcarine fissure, which is buried in the medial surface of the occipital cortex.

The original action levels determined by the FDA derived from epidemiological data gathered in Japan, Sweden and elsewhere, and were based on the appearance of paresthesias in adults. But a mass chemical disaster in the winter of 1971–1972 shifted the focus to the fetus. In the summer of 1971, drought ruined the wheat crop in Iraq, an event that led the government to order nearly 80 000 tons of seed wheat, the robust variety called Mexipak, from Mexico. But, apparently through an error in placing the order, the Iraqi officials specified that the wheat be treated with a methylmercury fungicide instead of a less dangerous mercury compound. Ordinarily, the methylmercury would be dissipated into the soil. In Iraq, however, the farmers were unfamiliar with the precautions needed to handle treated grain, and, in many areas, it arrived after the planting season. Faced with a wheat shortage, the families ground the wheat into flour and baked it into bread. Warnings on the sacks, printed in Spanish, and the skull and crossbones symbol communicated nothing to Iraqi farmers.

The long latency to signs of illness, because of the length of time it takes for methylmercury to accumulate in the brain and to damage enough nervous tissue to induce neurotoxic signs, helped produce the greatest mass chemical disaster in history (Bakir et al., 1973). By the time adverse effects had begun to appear, about Christmas of 1971, and had been traced to the treated grain, 5000 people had consumed enough methylmercury to die, and ten times that many had suffered severe damage. This acute phase, however, lasted only about three months. Adult hospital admissions had nearly ceased by March, 1972. But the most disquieting aftershocks were yet to emerge.

University of Rochester investigators, led by Thomas W. Clarkson, became involved in Iraq because Clarkson had presented a report to an international meeting about a complexing agent that accelerated the excretion of methylmercury from the body. After equipping a laboratory in Bagdhad, the investigators designed a program to help establish the extent of poisoning, its consequences, and the efficacy of various treatments. The crucial component of the strategy was to identify the exposed population so that individual members could be traced, and to establish an index of exposure, because dose was the essential variable in the total effort. Polaroid photographs, by maintaining verifiable identification of members of the study sample, helped achieve the first aim. Hair analyses helped achieve the second aim. Scalp hair was found to reflect blood concentrations of methylmercury at the time of hair formation. Since hair grows at the fairly constant rate of about one centimeter per month, exposure history could be traced by slicing hair into segments and measuring the concentration in each segment.

From this effort, one cardinal principle, suggested but not quantified at Minamata, began to predominate: the fetal brain is exceedingly sensitive to methylmercury. Women who were pregnant at the time of the Iraq disaster, although their exposure level had induced no more than minor signs of toxicity, gave birth to offspring who might manifest severe deficiencies. Those children most seriously damaged were diagnosed with cerebral palsy. But even those who superficially seemed normal showed defects when examined by pediatric neurologists (Fig. 4). Developmental milestones, such as language acquisition, appeared beyond the expected time. Seizures and abnormal reflexes might be exhibited. Subtle deficits in coordination could be detected. Collating and analysing this mass of data indicated that the fetus may be ten times more sensitive than the mature organism (Clarkson et al., 1981).

The experimental literature supports this conclusion and expands it. In one of the most influential contributions to the rise of behavioral teratology, Spyker (1975) demonstrated that mice exposed prenatally to methylmercury might appear normal to a casual observer but exhibit peculiar

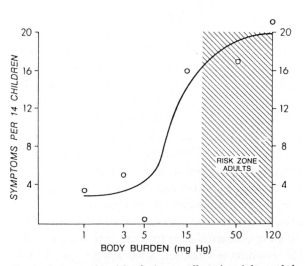

Fig. 4. Comparative risk of adverse effects in adults and the fetus, based on the episode of methylmercury poisoning in Iraq. Symptoms of poisoning (paresthesias) occur in adults at body burdens of about 25 mg. Evidence of central nervous system damage, ranging in severity from cerebral palsy to slowed language acquisition, are associated with prenatal maternal body burdens of about 2.5 mg.

behaviors under test conditions. For example, some of the treated mice walked backwards in an open field; some adopted peculiar postures while swimming. Subsequent studies by other investigators have shown even more subtle differences between treated and control offspring at doses far lower than those administered by Spyker.

Aging and neurotoxicity

In a meeting devoted to developmental phenomena it seems natural to focus on the earliest stages of the life-cycle. But development is not a process that comes to an abrupt end at maturity, and effects observed in young organisms do not convey the whole story. More subtle consequences of toxic exposure may not be observable until much later in the life-cycle, perhaps not even until senescence. The research by Spyker (1975) found that mice treated prenatally might not show any adverse effects until middle age or later. Signs such as postural deformities, excessive weight gain, hind limb weakness, and even paralysis might not appear until the mice reached 18 months of age or more.

Consider the implications for human populations. On the whole, the brain loses capacity with age as measured by indices such as nerve cell density, neurotransmitter levels, glucose utilization and oxygen consumption. The rates are different for different brain areas; some show little decline, while others show a marked reduction in various indices of function. Moreover, many compensatory processes, such as dendritic growth, are now known to occur. Still, functional declines across the population are recognized. Ponder the following question: what could be the impact of an environmental contaminant which accelerated the erosion of function with aging? Fig. 5 compares the hypothesized normal rate of brain aging (Kety, 1956) with that promoted by hypothetical increments in rate attributable to such a contaminant (Weiss and Simon, 1975). Even an increment of 0.1 percent annually exerts a pronounced effect on the relative age of the brain if compound-

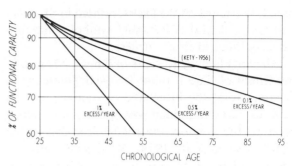

Fig. 5. Comparison of normal loss of brain function in aging (Kety, 1956) with the loss at hypothetical increments of accelerated rates of cell loss (Weiss and Simon, 1975).

ed in this way; moreover, advanced morphometrics could not discriminate such a rate of loss.

Aspects of risk assessment

Such questions must eventually become a part of risk assessment, the process by which toxicity data are transformed into conclusions about the health effects of exposure. Four components constitute this process: hazard identification, dose-response assessment, exposure assessment, and risk characterization. The last is the product of the three earlier steps, and is defined as 'The description of the nature and often the magnitude of human risk, including attendant uncertainty.' Cancer remains the focus of risk assessment, and nearly all of the efforts to devise models for quantifying risk are based on cancer. If functional endpoints such as behavior are to achieve parity, we will have to modify our efforts and devote more of them to questions bearing on risk. This does not mean a massive restructuring of the research enterprise. But it does imply a different approach to research. The most critical element is a shift from excessively high dose levels to a fuller exploration of the dose-response function and more attention to low dose levels. Such a shift would allow not only more useful estimates of human risks, but also more reasonable mechanistic explanations. A second element is a wider appreciation of all af the differences between developing and mature organisms, not simply those based on brain structure and function. Fetal and neonatal mechanisms for handling toxic chemicals are also immature: drug-metabolizing processes are less efficient, and toxic metals observe different kinetic parameters.

One of the most neglected attributes of experimental data that is significant for risk assessment if the distribution of observations. Investigators who otherwise perform acceptable statistical analyses and present measures of variability often fail to examine their data carefully for unusual patterns, and often remain unaware of the implications. If only a minority of a population consists of responders to a particular agent, conventional statistical approaches, based on group designs, will usually fail to detect an effect. Even data based on a presumably homogeneous sample of rats (for example, Cory-Slechta et al., 1985) indicate that individual differences may be enormous, and that conventional statistical analyses can be misleading. Instead of studying large groups superficially, which may be useful at the stage of hazard identification, a more direct strategy, especially during the later stages of the risk-assessment process, would study smaller groups more intensively and precisely and examine the distributions of individual responses in greater detail. Such a strategy has yielded important information about human individual differences in response to inhaled toxicants (Admur, 1980).

Summary

Neurobehavioral teratology is a discipline which has now attained a crucial role in predicting the health risks of drugs and environmental chemicals. For its findings to be translated into reasonable policies, investigators must be sensitive to the ways in which toxicological data become embodied into risk assessment. High experimental doses, although useful for preliminary work, may turn out to be misleading guides to actual risks in practice because of metabolic and dispositional variables. Crude behavioral assays, typically joined with high-dose toxicology, also blunt the usefulness of experimental observations. The joint contribution of aging and toxic exposure is a further factor that needs to be incorporated into risk evaluations. The impact of even small differences, such as changes in psychological test performance correlated with low-level lead exposure, can be seen when risk is viewed in societal rather than individual terms.

Acknowledgements

This work was supported in part by grants ES-01247, ES-01248 and ES-03054 from the National Institute of Environmental Health Sciences and in part by DOE grant DE-FG02-85ER60281 with the U.S. Department of Energy at the University of Rochester Department of Biophysics and has been assigned report No. DOE/EV/03490-2536. Such support does not constitute an endorsement by DOE of the views expressed in this article.

References

Amdur, M.O.(1980) Air pollutants. In J. Doull, C.W. Klaassen, and M.O. Amdur (Eds.), Casarett and Doull's Toxicology: *The Basic Science of Poisons*, Macmillan, New York, pp. 608–631.

Bakir, F., Damluji, S.F., Amin-Zaki, L., Murtadba, M., Kahlide, A., Al-Rawi, N.Y., Smith, J.C. and Doherty, R.A. (1973) Methylmercury poisoning in Iraq. *Science*, 181: 230–241.

Bellinger, D.C. and Needleman, H.L. (1985) Prenatal and early postnatal exposure to lead: developmental effects, correlates, and implications. *Int. J. Ment. Health*, 14: 78–111.

Bellinger, D., Leviton, A., Waternaux, C., Needleman, H. and Rabinowitz, M. (1987) Longitudinal analysis of prenatal and postnatal lead exposure and early cognitive development. *N. Engl. J. Med.*, 316: 1037–1043.

Bornshein, R., Pearson, D. and Reiter, L. (1980) Behavioral effects of moderate lead exposure in children and animal models: 2. animal studies. *CRC Crit. Rev. Toxicol.*, 7: 101–152.

Clarkson, T.W., Cox, C., Marsh, D.O., Myers, G.J., Al-Tikriti, S.K., Amin-Zaki, L. and Dabbagh, A.R. (1981) Dose–response relationships for adult and prenatal exposures to methylmercury. In G.C. Berg and H.W. Maillie (Eds.), *Measurement of Risk*, Plenum, New York, pp. 111–130.

48

Cory-Slechta, D.A., Weiss, B. and Cox, C. (1985) Performance and exposure indices of rats exposed to low concentrations of lead. *Toxicol. Appl. Pharmacol.*, 78: 291–299.

Goldwater, L.J. (1972) *Mercury. A History of Quicksilver*, York
Press, Baltimore.

Gotelli, C.A., Astolfi, E., Cox, C., Cernichiari, E. and Clarkson, T.W. (1985) Early biochemical effects of an organic
mercury fungicide on infants. 'Dose makes the poison.'
Science, 227: 638–640.

Kety, S.S. (1956) Human cerebral blood flow and oxygen
consumption as related to aging. *Res. Publ. Assoc. Nerv.
Ment. Dis.*, 35: 31–45.

Needleman, H.L. (1985) The neurobehavioral effects of low
level exposure to lead in childhood. *Int. J. Ment. Health*, 14:
64–77.

Needleman, H.L., Gunnoe, C., Leviton, A., Reed, R., Peresie,
H., Maker, C. and Barrett, P. (1979) Deficits in psycholog-
ic and classroom performance of children with elevated
dentine lead levels. *N. Engl. J. Med.*, 300: 689–695.

Rice, D.C. (1983) Central nervous effects of perinatal exposure to lead on methylmercury in the monkey. In T.W.
Clarkson, G.F. Nordberg and P.R. Sager (Eds.), *Reproductive and Developmental Toxicity of Metals*, Plenum Press,
New York, pp. 517–539.

Roels, H., Lauwerys, R., Buchet, J.P., Genet, P., Sarhan,
M.J., Hanotian, J., De Fays, M., Bernard, A. and Stane-
scu, D. (1987) Epidemiological survey among workers exposed to manganese: effects on lung, central nervous system, and some biological indices. *Am. J. Indust. Med.*, 11:
307–327.

Smith, W.E. and Smith, A.M. (1985) *Minamata*, Holt, Rine-
hart and Winston, New York.

Spyker, J.M. (1975) Behavioral teratology and toxicology. In
B. Weiss and V.G. Laties (Eds.), *Behavioral Toxicology*,
Plenum, New York, pp. 311–344.

Warkany, J. and Hubbard, D.M. (1951) Adverse mercurial
reactions in the forms of acrodynia and related conditions.
Am. J. Dis. Child., 81: 335–373.

Weiss, B. (1983) Behavioral toxicology of heavy metals. In I.
Dreosti and R. Smith (Eds.), *Neurobiology of the Trace
Elements*, The Humana Press, Clifton, NJ, pp. 1–50.

Weiss, B. and Clarkson, T.W. (1982) Mercury toxicity in
children. In *Chemical and Radiation Hazards to Children*,
Ross Laboratories, Columbus, OH, pp. 52–59.

Weiss, B. and Simon, W. (1975) Quantitative perspectives on
the long-term toxicity of methylmercury and similar
poisons. In B. Weiss and V.G. Laties (Eds.), *Behavioral
Toxicology*, Plenum, New York, pp. 429–437.

Discussion

G.J. Boer: When you were speaking about the chemical soup
around us, I got the impression that you only meant the
chemicals of industries. But don't you agree that 'natural'
chemicals of the environment (e.g. people in the inlands of
New Guinea) may also cause behavioral teratology?

B. Weiss: I did not intend to give the impression that only
synthetic chemicals pose health risks, which is one of the
reasons I chose to feature metals in my lecture. The pace of
new chemical production, however, means that an enormous
number of agents are introduced into the environment
without many accompanying data about their toxicity. Your
reference to the Western Pacific area, which I assume involves locations with an elevated prevalence of amyotrophic
lateral sclerosis (accompanied in Guam by Parkinsonism
dementia), emphasizes the difficulties presented even by a
clear clinical syndrome in places where the contaminants
seen in advanced industrial societies are largely absent. Consider how much more of a puzzle might be posed by an even
more complex chemical environment in company with more
subtle endpoints such as conduct disorders.

D.F. Swaab: Why is the developing brain so extremely sensitive to methylmercury?

B. Weiss: Several toxic mechanisms seem to be at work.
Methylmercury can interfere with developmental processes
such as neuronal migration (Choi, 1983) and cell proliferation
(Sager et al., 1982). It also inhibits protein synthesis, an
action that is more likely to kill small cells than large ones
(Syversen, 1982). Also, methylmercury half-time is longer in
the neonate than in the adult (Rowland et al., 1983). All these
factors conspire to enhance risk.

W. Lichtensteiger: Many of these agents are at subthreshold
levels in our environment, but they are probably additive in
their action. How could risk assessment of combined intake
be improved?

B. Weiss: The question of how to evaluate complex mixtures
is provoking considerable effort in the United States. The
National Academy of Sciences, with support from the
National Institute of Environmental Health Sciences, recently completed a report on complex mixtures that is scheduled
for publication in the near future. The primary source of
concern about environmental mixtures is the possibility of
unexpected synergism, or mutual enhancement exceeding a
simple model such as algebraic additivity. The report discusses current knowledge of the biological action of mixtures,
experimental strategies for estimating the toxic potency of
mixtures, and statistical modeling of outcomes. For risk assessments based on the multistage model of carcinogenesis,
additivity is a reasonable upper bound for very low exposure
levels. At higher levels, such as the interaction of cigarette
smoking and asbestos, simple additivity underestimates risk.
Unfortunately, nearly all of the current risk models are based

on cancer. Only recently have modelers turned their attention to systemic toxicants such as those acting on nervous tissue.

References

Choi, B. H. (1983) Effects of prenatal methylmercury poisoning upon growth and development of fetal nervous system. In T. W. Clarkson, G. F. Nordberg and P. R. Sager (Eds.), *Reproductive and Developmental Toxicity of Metals*, Plenum, New York, pp. 473–495.

Rowland, I. R., Robinson, R. D., Doherty, R. A. and Landry, T. D. (1983) Are developmental changes in methylmercury metabolism and excretion mediated by the intestinal microflora? In T. W. Clarkson, G. F. Nordberg and P. R. Sager (Eds.), *Reproductive and Developmental Toxicity of Metals*, Plenum, New York, pp. 745–758.

Sager, P., Doherty, R. A. and Rodier, P. M. (1982) Effects of methylmercury on developing mouse cerebellar cortex. *Exp. Neurol.*, 77: 179–193.

Syversen, T. L. M. (1982) Effects of repeated dosing of methylmercury on in vivo protein synthesis in isolated neurones. *Acta Pharmacol. Toxicol.*, 50: 391–397.

G.J. Boer, M.G.P. Feenstra, M. Mirmiran, D.F. Swaab and F. Van Haaren
Progress in Brain Research, Vol. 73
© 1988 Elsevier Science Publishers B.V. (Biomedical Division)

CHAPTER 4

Problems in studying functional teratogenicity in man

Hendrik J. Huisjes

Department of Obstetrics and Gynaecology, University Hospital Groningen, Oostersingel 59, 9713 EZ Groningen, The Netherlands

Behavioural or functional teratology has been and still is in the process of being extensively studied in experimental animals, in particular the rat. In contrast to the clinical situation, in an experimental setting most of the variables can, within limits, be manipulated and among the outcome variables not only behaviour but also morphological substrates in the brain can be studied. Since obviously the results of animal experiments cannot readily be extrapolated to the human, clinical studies have to be done. This paper highlights some important problems specific to functional teratologic studies in the human.

Development of functional teratology in the human

Teratology was mainly structural – i.e. dealing with gross morphological defects – until the early seventies, but after the sixties studies began to appear on functional teratology, first in relation to hormones (see Reinisch and Karow, 1977). There is, of course, no sharp demarcation line between structural and functional effects of chemical compounds. 'Drugs can produce biochemical or histological damage in the developing nervous system. These appear to be associated with behavioural effects' (Hutchings, 1978). Nevertheless, there are important differences. First of all, most structural defects in man can be recognized within one year after birth, whereas behavioural abnormalities may sometimes come to light when the subject is 10 or more years old. Perhaps even

more problematic is the nature of the abnormalities. Structural defects may be difficult to classify because some of them are so common (e.g. naevi and other skin 'abnormalities'). Functional defects may not only be common, they can also be subtle and difficult to recognize, e.g. a shorter attention span, lower intelligence, hyperactivity (Kolata, 1978). A third important difference is that, whereas a normal morphology can usually be defined, a description of what constitutes normal behaviour or function in an individual cannot always be given.

Clinical studies related to functional teratology in the human being less than 25 years old are still rare. Short-term functional effects, in particular withdrawal symptoms, are relatively well-known, e.g. those involving barbiturates, alcohol and narcotics (Zuspan and Zuspan, 1982). But Reinisch and Sanders, in 1982, could not find one report in the literature on the behavioural teratogenic effects of barbiturates in man, in spite of the fact that barbiturates were, and sometimes still are, extensively prescribed to pregnant women. Moreover, from animal experiments it could be suspected that prenatal exposure to barbiturates may lead to learning disabilities, decreased IQ, performance deficits, psychological maladjustment, and demasculinization of gender identity and sex role behaviour in males.

There are several other drugs which are functional teratogens in experimental animals that have not been tested in the human as yet. Sometimes functional effects of drugs are found unexpectedly. Vessey et al. (1983) detected twice as many psychiatric disorders, especially depression and anxiety, in their well-known follow-up study of over 500 offspring of women who had, when pregnant in the early fifties, taken part in a controlled study of stilboestrol treatment versus placebo. Usually, however, the search for functional effects of drugs used in pregnancy has to be an intentional undertaking.

Reasons for clinical studies

When should one test a substance for functional teratogenicity in humans? Only when there is a reasonable suspicion, based on experimental data, that there might be such an effect. Testing for functional abnormalities in general is too expensive, and too much of a burden for the subjects, not least because of the time it takes, to undertake it lightly. It is also hardly possible: one text reports the existence of over one thousand behavioural tests (Gal and Sharpless, 1984). Only when one has a rough idea of the effects to look for is it possible to devise a testing scheme which can be worked out without overloading the programme. Only then can a hypothesis be tested. At least, that seems a logical approach to a clinician. Ideally, the choice should be made on the basis of animal experiments. However, the usefulness of such experiments has also been criticized. Dobbing, for instance, in a letter to the Lancet (1982), stated: 'The evaluation of long-term behavioural outcome in rats is a most inexact, interpretive art, which is a continuing source of vigorous scientific discussion amongst those whose profession it is'. That may be true, but nevertheless one needs a basis on which clinical studies can be designed.

In The Netherlands, haloperidol is considered not dangerous to the fetus, at least not in low doses. Among the effects of perinatal administration in rats were impaired sex behaviour in male offspring (Hull et al., 1984), and delayed onset of sexual maturation in female offspring (Bhanot and Wilkinson, 1982). Other neuroleptics may have similar effects (Dukes, 1986). Whatever the significance of the rat experiments, a clinical teratological study of neuroleptics has still not been carried out and therefore is urgently needed. Even very late sequelae may be found now that neuroleptics have been in use for about 40 years.

Study design and methodological problems

How should a clinical study of functional teratology be designed? The purely experimental approach of giving a chemical substance just for the purpose of the experiment is, of course, unacceptable in man. The next-best design is to prospectively collect a group of pregnant women receiving a drug on prescription, or taking a drug or a chemical substance without prescription, and a matched control group, and follow them up for 10 or 20 years. For financial and other obvious reasons this is not often done. A third and probably in this specific field the most appropriate way is to retrospectively collect a group of pregnant women whose fetuses were exposed to a certain compound, to devise a control group of women who did not take the drug, and to try and find the children. This is not easy, even in a small country like The Netherlands. What is needed is a skilled and devoted technical staff; skilled not only in tracing the children, but also in contacting their parents and explaining to them the reason for the contact – this being the possibility of developmental damage in their child caused by a drug taken during the pregnancy several years ago.

Apart from this cumbersome problem there are a number of methodological pitfalls. Was the drug under investigation the only one used? This is improbable, since a staggering percentage of pregnant women are still using all kinds of drugs, still smoke and drink or are addicted (Krauer et al., 1984). In this respect another important question concerns the phase of gestation in which developmental disturbance resulting in functional defects is most likely to occur. If this is after the first trimester of pregnancy, when brain growth begins to accelerate, then drug use in the second and third trimester is the issue in functional teratological studies. It is often very difficult, however, to collect a sizeable sample of women who used a certain drug within a limited period of time during their pregnancy. It may, therefore, be necessary to accept the ingestion during a relatively short period of additional drugs which are not suspected of having effects on the developing brain. For instance, in a study we did on clonidine (Huisjes et al., 1986) we had to accept the use of antibiotics in some cases, because otherwise we would have had hardly any cases left. If possible, smoking – a habit of somewhat less than half of all pregnant women (Krauer et al., 1984) – should be matched for, even though it would be preferable to enrol only women who did not smoke or drink.

A second problem is matching for obstetrical and other variables. Obviously some obstetrical variables should be matched for. The most common of them are parity, sex of the baby, gestational age at birth, birthweight and social background and, last but not least, the disease for which the medication was given. There are some pitfalls here, however. It is an interesting question whether birthweight, or rather weight-for-dates, should be matched for. The answer is yes only if the contention that any deleterious effect on brain function is associated with growth retardation can be dismissed with certainty. This is not the case. It is known that in several if not most developmental abnormalities functional disturbances are associated with growth retardation (e.g. chromosomal errors). It should be realized that those variables associated with the effect to be studied are not to be considered as confounders. When matching for disease the severity of the illness is important: it may be that those treated have the disease in a more serious degree than those not treated. It may even be impossible to find patients with the same disease who have not been treated with the same drug. In that case one should decide beforehand whether the disease should be considered as a confounder, in other words, whether it may in itself have an effect on brain development.

Clearly factors other than drugs may play an important role in behaviour disturbances. Hadders-Algra et al. (1985) in our department found that, even though the neurological condition of a child influenced behaviour, in the sense that mild neurological dysfunction made the child more vulnerable to the environment, it was the environment itself together with the sex of the child that played the most important part in affecting behaviour.

A follow-up study by Hadders-Algra et al. (1988) from our department showed how some perinatal factors contribute to several behavioural outcome variables (Table 1). Male sex, for instance, roughly doubled the risk of the child being distractable, troublesome, clumsy and a poor speller. Birth in the 33rd week of gestation, or before, quadrupled the risk of the child being bad at arithmetic and troublesome in school. Other significant factors were interval complications, presence and severity of minor neurological dys-

TABLE 1

Odds ratios (comparable with relative risk ratios) of 4 selected risk variables for behaviour and cognitive factors in 9-year-old children (adapted from Hadders-Algra et al., 1988)

Outcome factors	Sex		g.a. ≤ 33 wk	Lower social class[a]	Family adversity
	♂	♀			
Distractable, P	2.7				1.8
Distractable, T				2.7	
Troublesome, P	2.2			2.0	
Troublesome, T	2.0		4.1		
Timid, P					4.5
Timid, T		2.2			2.5
Clumsy, P	1.8				
Clumsy, T	2.2			1.5	
School failure				3.0	
Poor reading				3.3	
Poor spelling	1.6			4.5	1.6
Poor arithmetic		4.5		4.5	

g.a. = gestational age; P = according to parents; T = according to teachers.
[a] Lower social class = low and lower-middle class.

function, social class and adverse family circumstances. These effects have to be taken into account in clinical teratology studies. Since randomization is not feasible, the only way to do so is by matching for factors occurring frequently, or by eliminating subjects with rare confounders, such as early preterm birth or neurological abnormality. Elimination, however, will reduce the numbers, which are often limited anyway.

Multiple interrelationships of variables

It is obvious that there is an enormous interplay between various classes of causes and effects, e.g. preterm birth and intra-uterine growth retardation, the disease for which the drug was given, damage to the nervous system due to nonchemical factors, intercurrent disease, social and other environmental variables and behaviour. In Table 2, from the same study by Hadders-Algra et al. (1988), the frequency of behaviour problems is shown in relationship with the children's neurological classification in the newborn period. Except for cognitive variables there are no significant differences between children who were neurologically normal, suspect or abnormal in the newborn period. If a direct relationship between neurological abnormality of the newborn, a direct indicator of functional impairment of the nervous system, and behaviour at nine years cannot be proved, it might be extremely difficult to do the same for relatively small doses of drugs given to the mother during pregnancy.

An additional problem is the effect of time. A gross anatomical abnormality will remain essentially the same over the years. A functional expression of damage to the nervous system is subject to the wear and tear of time. The effect of the environment has already been mentioned. In addition, there is the probability of recovery. Overt neurological dysfunction in the early neonatal period can no longer be recognized at 18 months in about 80% of the cases (Bierman-van Eendenburg et al., 1981). Even though part of the damage diagnosed shortly after birth will be the consequence of transient mechanical or chemical damage inflicted during the process of birth, no doubt later recovery may occur as well, be it through adaptation or training. And finally, everyone involved in follow-up studies should realize that the law of regression to the mean implies that severely damaged children will tend to recover rather than to deteriorate, whereas children in optimal condition can only get worse.

It seems very difficult to demonstrate behavioural consequences of teratological effects in man. There are simply too many variables, time and environment are too powerful, and the effects looked for too subtle. Nevertheless, it should be tried, if only to rule out the presence of gross functional abnormalities. If nothing is found in a well-designed study, any existing teratologic effect on development can hardly be disastrous.

TABLE 2

Percentage of 9-year-old children with behavioral problems in relation to their neonatal neurological classification (from Hadders-Algra et al., 1987)

	Normal ($n = 230$)	Mildly abnormal ($n = 207$)	Abnormal ($n = 133$)
Distractable, P	9	11	14
Distractable, T	8	8	4
Troublesome, P	13	13	17
Troublesome, T	8	7	14
Timid, P	1	1	5
Timid, T	7	10	10
Clumsy, P	13	14	20
Clumsy, T	18	20	23
School failure	16[a]	10[a]	29
Poor reading	13	7[a]	20
Poor spelling	22	17[a]	26
Poor arithmetic	10	6[a]	15

[a] $P < 0.05$ as compared with neonatally abnormal.

Two follow-up studies

Some of the above-mentioned problems can be illustrated by data from our study on the effect of clonidine (Huisjes et al., 1986). The study was undertaken because Mirmiran et al. (1983) had demonstrated hyperactivity in the open field test, a deficient sexual response in males, and a much higher incidence of large myoclonic jerks during active sleep in adult rats after neonatal exposure to clonidine. We were able to find 22 women treated for hypertension during pregnancy with clonidine only. Duration of treatment and dosage varied, but the minimum duration was 5 weeks and the minimum dosage was 150 μg per day. A

control group of 22 non-treated hypertensive gravidae was selected, matched for diastolic blood pressure during pregnancy, and sex, birthweight and gestational age of the children (Table 3). At 3–9 years of age no differences were found in head circumference or neurological findings, school performance, or behavioural characteristics as reported by parents or teachers. The only difference found was in sleeping behaviour: seven children in the study group against one in the control group scored positive in two or more of seven aspects of abnormal sleeping behaviour. Night terrors and somnambulism occurred in the study group only.

On the basis of this study alone, one cannot

TABLE 3

Matching criteria and additional variables in clonidine-treated and control groups used for behavioural teratological evaluation

	Clonidine (n = 22)	Control (n = 22)
Sex ratio (male/female)	11/11	11/11
Mean diastolic blood pressure during pregnancy (mmHg)		
range	91–108	93–110
mean $\pm$ SD	101 $\pm$ 5.2	100 $\pm$ 4.2
Number of preterm infants (34–36 wk)	4	4
Birthweight of preterm infants (g): range	1450–1930	1480–1940
Birthweight of fullterm infants (g): mean $\pm$ SD	3129 $\pm$ 478	3096 $\pm$ 455
pH umb. ven. known	19	19
<7.20	3	3
Apgar 1 min < 7	3	4
3 min < 7	0	0
Primiparae	12	11
Parturition vaginally	18	18
Caesarean section	4	4
Mothers' age (mean $\pm$ SD) in years	29.0 $\pm$ 6.4	27.1 $\pm$ 4.9
Social class		
lower/lower-middle	14	13
upper-middle/upper	8	9
Head circumference (cm)	52.5 $\pm$ 2.0	52.4 $\pm$ 1.6
Neurological examination		
normal	16	15
minimal neurological dysfunction	6	7
abnormal	–	–

TABLE 4

Means and standard deviations or distributions of matching variables in a study group of ritodrine-exposed children and in two non-exposed control groups (from Hadders-Algra et al., 1986)

	Study group	Control group A	Control group B
Sex ratio (male/female)	44/34	44/34	44/34
No. of nulliparous women	39	39	39
No. of infants of birthweight < 10th centile	10	9	9
Week of delivery	39.4 (1.1)[a]	39.4 (1.1)	39.4 (1.1)
Birthweight (g)	3159 (478)	3177 (424)	3186 (397)
Maternal age (years)	25.6 (4.7)	25.3 (4.2)	25.4 (4.6)
Social class			
1	2	4	5
2	25	25	21
3	36	43	44
4	8	4	4
Unknown	7	2	4

[a] Indicates average (SEM).

conclude that sleep disturbances are due to prenatal clonidine exposure. We feel, however, that the study was carried out sufficiently carefully to at least raise the suspicion that clonidine may have just that effect in man. The study should be repeated. Since the children were 3–9 years old at the time of the examination, we will have to wait another 10–20 years to see whether the sexual abnormalities found in rats might be present in man as well.

In another study we compared a group of 78 6-year-old children prenatally exposed to ritodrine, a widely used tocolytic agent, with two equally sized control groups of non-exposed children (Hadders-Algra et al., 1986). All children had been born at term. In the study group mothers had received ritodrine for an average of 28 ± 27 days, median 17 days. Again the groups were fairly similar for several relevant variables (Table 4). There were no differences in physical, neurological or behavioural development in the data collected, but there was one peculiar finding when functioning at school was compared

(Table 5). The proportion of children considered by their teachers as belonging to the group of best pupils was significantly smaller in the ritodrine group than in both control groups. Suprisingly there was no excess of very weak pupils in the

TABLE 5

School performance at 6 years in a study group of prenatally ritodrine-exposed children and in two non-exposed control-groups: numbers indicate percentages of 'best pupils', i.e. pupils who were classified by their teachers as belonging to the best 25% of pupils (from Hadders-Algra et al., 1986)

	Study group (n = 76)	Control group A (n = 77)	Control group B (n = 77)
Motor skills	5.3	19.5	18.2
Social skills	7.9	19.5	16.9
Emotional development	3.9	13.0	10.4
Cognitive development	7.9	19.5	15.6

study group. It is difficult to ascribe this un-expected finding to methodological flaws. All children had been born at term and therefore teachers would not have known of the adminis-tration of ritodrine, so this can hardly have caused bias. On the other hand it is striking that the deficit of bright pupils concerned all four of the aspects judged. It is difficult to interpret these findings: final judgement must await further evi-dence.

Clinical consequences

A final question is what should be the con-sequences for clinical practice? Should the use of clonidine and ritodrine be suspended until the finding of a relationship of clonidine and ritodrine with excess of sleep disturbances and lack of bright children respectively has been refuted? Replacement of the drugs by others might make matters worse instead of improving them, because nothing is known of the late sequelae of alterna-tive drugs. Not using any antihypertensive or tocolytic drug at all is clearly not the 'therapy of choice'. The only possible conclusion is that doctors should be wary of prescribing drugs to pregnant women. This is not something clinicians were not aware of. It is another question whether they act accordingly. Follow-up studies may, by showing the type and severity of effects drugs may have, stress the point and increase compliance, this time not in patients but in doctors.

Acknowledgement

Critical remarks by Mijna Hadders-Algra are gratefully acknowledged.

References

Bhanot, R. and Wilkinson, M. (1982) Treatment of pregnant rats with haloperidol delays the onset of sexual maturation in female offspring. *Experienta*, 38: 137.

Bierman-van Eendenburg, M.E.C., Jurgens-van der Zee, A.D., Olinga, A.A., Huisjes, H.J. and Touwen, B.C.L. (1981) Predictive value of neonatal neurological exami-nation: a follow-up study at 18 months. *Dev. Med. Child Neurol.*, 23: 296–305.

Dobbing, J. (1982) Teratogenicity tests and behaviour. *Lancet*, ii: 604–605.

Dukes MNG (1986) Neuroleptics. In *Side Effects of Drugs Annual*, Vol. 10, Elsevier, New York.

Gal, P. and Sharpless, M.K. (1984) Fetal drug exposure – behavioral teratogenesis. *Drug Intell. Clin. Pharm.*, 18: 186–201.

Hadders-Algra, M., Touwen, B.C.L., Olinga, A.A. and Huisjes, H.J. (1985) Minor neurological dysfunction and behavioural development. A report from the Groningen Perinatal Project. *Early Human. Dev.*, 11: 221–229.

Hadders-Algra, M., Touwen, B.C.L. and Huisjes, H.J. (1986) Long-term follow-up of children prenatally exposed to ritodrine. *Br. J. Obstet. Gynaecol.*, 93: 156–161.

Hadders-Algra, M., Huisjes, H.J. and Touwen, B.C.L. (1988) The significance of perinatal risk factors and minor neurological dysfunction for behaviour and school achievement at nine years. *Dev. Med. Child Neurol.*, in press.

Huisjes, H.J., Hadders-Algra, M. and Touwen, B.C.L. (1986) Is clonidine a behavioural teratogen in the human? *Early Hum. Dev.*, 14: 43–48.

Hull, E.M., Nishita, J.K., Bitran, D. and Dalterio, S. (1984) Perinatal dopamine-related drugs demasculinize rats. *Science*, 224: 1011.

Hutchings, D.E. (1987) *Behavioral Teratology: Embryopathic and Behavioral Effects of Drugs During Pregnancy*, Academic press, New York, pp. 7–34.

Kolata, G.B. (1978) Behavioral teratology: birth defects of the mind. *Science*, 202: 732–734.

Krauer, B., Krauer, F. and Hytten, F. (1984) *Drug Prescribing in Pregnancy*, Churchill Livingstone, Edinburgh. pp. 14–16.

Mirmiran, M., Scholtens, J., Van de Poll, N.E., et al. (1983) Effects of experimental suppression of active (REM) sleep during early dement upon adult brain and behaviour. *Dev. Brain. Res.*, 7: 277–286.

Reinisch, J.M. and Karow, W.G. (1977) Prenatal exposure to synthetic progestins and estrogens: effects on human development. *Arch. Sex. Behav.*, 6: 257–288.

Reinisch, J.M. and Sanders, S.A. (1982) Early barbiturate exposure: the brain, sexually dimorphic behavior and learning. *Neurosci. Biobehav. Rev.*, 6: 311–319.

Vessey, M.P., Fairweather, D.V.I., Norman-Smith, B. and Buckley, J. (1983) A randomized double-blind controlled trial of the value of stilboestrol therapy in pregnancy: long-term follow-up of mothers and their offspring. *Br. J. Obstet. Gynaecol.*, 90: 1007–1017.

Zuspan, F.P. and Zuspan, K.J. (1982) Drug addiction in pregnancy. In: W.F. Rayburn and F.P. Zuspan (Eds.), *Drug therapy in Obstetrics and Gynecology*, Appleton-Century-Crofts, Norwalk, p. 40.

Discussion

D.F. Swaab: You proposed to match for gestational age. However, should we not consider gestational age as a possible expression of functional teratology instead of as a confounding factor? The fetal brain influences gestational age, in both human beings and experimental animals (Swaab et al., 1977), and chemical compounds may thus influence gestational age by their action on the developing fetal brain.

H.J. Huisjes: This is an interesting suggestion which, as far as I know, has never been studied. Drugs could possibly be causative in less than one-third of preterm labours, the other two-thirds being the consequence of fetal abnormalities, fetal or maternal disease, multiple pregnancy or elective delivery. It is now accepted that some of the unexplained preterm labours are due to subclinical ascending infection. This leaves us with roughly one percent of all pregnancies, where drugs could have caused disturbed brain development resulting in spontaneous preterm labour. This is a hypothesis that could be tested by a case-control study.

Z. Annau (comment): Data on human populations could be much clearer if precise quantitative measurements used in animal studies were used, instead of clinical measurements and/or teacher/parent observations. I am not sure that this would resolve the question of difficulty of studying human populations.

H.J. Huisjes: It is certainly true that the available instruments for the assessment of functional damage in children are insufficient, and more precise measurements would be welcome. There are two problems. One is the cooperation of parents, especially in the control subjects, when time-consuming tests in an experimental setting are imposed upon their children. The other difficulty is the relevance of the findings. Deficient achievement in school may be a rather imprecise indicator; it is, however, undoubtedly a relevant one.

B.D. Perry: Have you examined sleep architecture in the offspring with sleep disturbances attributed to prenatal clonidine use?

H.J. Huisjes: No, we have not.

F. Rosa: Is weight-for-dates a key effect indicator for neurofunctional development? It is affected by many prenatal exposures and other congenital factors.

H.J. Huisjes: You are right. There are probably few developmental disturbances not associated with growth retardation. The problem is that growth retardation is a grossly defined nosological entity, in fact it is not a nosological entity at all. The only definition of growth retardation is a low body weight for dates. The etiology is far more variable than has usually been thought. Causes may be smoking and other intoxications, congenital anomalies, genetic factors, malnutrition, infections and an inadequate vascular supply, e.g. in pregnancy-induced hypertension. Thus, low weight for dates is an indicator of possible drug-induced damage in a minority of cases only.

J.F. Orlebeke: Is there an increase in the frequency of 'abnormal' children *at birth* during the last couple of decades?

H.J. Huisjes: No, if 'abnormal' means structural deformities.

Reference

Swaab, D.F., Boer, K. and Honnebier, W.J. (1977) The influence of the fetal hypothalamus and pituitary on the onset and course of parturition. In: J. Knight and M. O'Connor (Eds.), *The Fetus and Birth*, Ciba Foundation Symposium 47, Elsevier, Amsterdam, pp. 379–400.

G.J. Boer, M.G.P. Feenstra, M. Mirmiran, D.F. Swaab and F. Van Haaren
Progress in Brain Research, Vol. 73
© 1988 Elsevier Science Publishers B.V. (Biomedical Division)

CHAPTER 5

Behavioural teratology of exogenous substances: regulation aspects

Herman B.W.M. Koëter

Department of Biological Toxicology, TNO-CIVO Toxicology and Nutrition Institute, Zeist, The Netherlands

Introduction

It is a basic principle of teratology that a system is especially vulnerable during the period of differentiation. This implies in particular to the central nervous system (CNS), which consists of a number of different parts and cell types, each with its own developmental program. The susceptibility of the CNS to teratogens became evident as exposure to a number of exogenous substances during development resulted in structural central nervous defects. However, it took until the early seventies before it was understood that the same sorts of factors that had long been known to disturb the development of structures are also able, not infrequently at much lower dose levels, to disturb functional development and thus behaviour (Butcher, 1985).

One of the reasons that behavioural teratology gained acceptance in the 1970s was that the investigators of this period related their research to the principles and concepts of toxicology. Thus, several principles of behavioural teratology are framed in a toxicological perspective (Vorhees and Butcher, 1982).

Firstly, behavioural teratogenicity is expressed as delayed behavioural maturation and impaired or abnormal behaviour. This first principle is analogous to the principle in developmental toxicology that developmental disorders are expressed as retarded development, embryo- and feto-toxicity and anomalies and malformations. Although the behavioural manifestations mentioned in this first principle are thus clearly appropriate, other indices may be added in the future.

The second principle is that the period of susceptibility to behavioural teratogenesis is isomorphic with the period of CNS development. This principle refers to the biological basis of behaviour and indicates that all behaviour arises from structural and functional interactions residing within the CNS. It also indicates that the severity as well as the type of behavioural effects correlate with the period of CNS development during which exposure took place. This relationship has clearly been demonstrated by Rodier and co-workers with exposures to 5-azacytidine (Rodier 1976, 1977; Rodier et al., 1979).

The third principle is that the type and magnitude of the response are a function of (a) the type of agent administered, (b) the dose of the agent, (c) the time and duration of exposure, (d) the environment of the target organism, and (e) the genetic background of the target organism. This principle is not unique to behavioural teratology but originates from pharmacology and toxicology (Vorhees and Butcher, 1982): the unique characteristics of the chemical compound determines its biological activity and consequently its toxicity. The principle that the type and magnitude of the response are a function of the dose suggests that, as in toxicology and teratology, a no-adverse-effect level might be established.

In behavioural teratology, as in developmental toxicology, time and duration of exposure are extremely important, since the susceptibility of the developing organism to exogenous substances varies considerably with the stage of development of the CNS. The environment and the genetic background of the fetus or neonate evidently play an important role in the type and magnitude of the behavioural effect.

Although behavioural teratology gained wide acceptance since most of the research was based on these principles, there were still a number of problems to be solved. These were, among others: (a) how is 'behavioural teratology' defined, (b) should behavioural teratogenicity studies be requested upon safety evaluation of (new) substances and, if so, for which types of substance, (c) what type of behavioural functions should be assessed, (d) what is the relevance of the results of animal tests to the human situation?

Definition of behavioural teratology

The World Health Organisation (WHO) proposed the following definition: 'Behaviour teratology refers to the study of effects on behaviour which result from damage to the conceptus at any time during its development' (WHO, 1986). The most important aspect of this definition is that it says 'at any time during its development', indicating that the induction of behavioural teratogenic effects is not at all restricted to the period of gestation but could also occur after birth (Health Council of the Netherlands, 1985). Another interesting aspect of this definition is that it does not make any restrictions regarding maternal toxicity. Unfortunately, 'damage to the conceptus' is not specified and implies that, according to the definition, the study of behavioural alternations resulting from structural damage of organs other than the CNS may also be considered as behavioural teratology! In practice, however, behavioural indices will merely be used as fine

tools for the detection of CNS damage that would otherwise not have been observed in (classical) teratology studies. An alternative approach is to use the term 'functional neuroteratology', indicating that one should not regard behaviour as the sole endpoint of non-morphological anomalies but one should include all other physiological aspects subject to central regulation.

Regulations involved

The next question was: 'Should behavioural teratogenicity studies be requested upon safety evaluation of new substances'. It should be emphasized that upon safety evaluation of a compound, reproduction toxicity data and data on behavioural teratogenicity are only one aspect among many others. Therefore it was considered, especially by industry, a drastic measure when in 1974/1975 the British and Japanese authorities incorporated behavioural assessments in their guidelines for reproduction studies of pharmaceuticals. Moreover, at that time behavioural teratology was still very much in its infancy and nobody knew exactly how to tackle the problem of routine screening. The U.K. was the first to introduce a requirement. The guideline specifies that 'late effects on the progeny in terms of auditory, visual and behavioural function should be assessed'. The guidance note was deliberately designed not to be restrictive and, although auditory, visual and behavioural development are specifically mentioned in order to give some idea of the types of test which could be done, a wide range of postnatal tests have in practice been accepted in drug submissions (Barlow, 1985). At present, these rather arbitrary British guidelines are still effective. The early Japanese guideline for the testing of drugs stating that 'as to behavioural studies, appropriate tests for locomotion, learning, sensory functions or emotionality shall be done' were updated in 1984. The specifications as to which behavioural functions should be assessed have been replaced by a more general and open-ended guidenote, reading: 'for observations of growth and development, morphological, functional and behavioural examinations should be made' (Ministry of Health and Welfare Japan, 1984). Although this new guideline leaves sufficient room for the investigator to design the most appropriate test battery for a particular drug, the industry is now more than ever uncertain whether the chosen test approach is acceptable to the registration authorities. Although scientists in industry are generally in favour of the new, more liberal guidelines, their colleagues in the financial department and management may not be. For them, it is easier to live with very strict and well-defined requirements, so diminishing the chance of refusal or delay upon notification of their new drug. Moreover, strict requirements usually do not lead to unexpected and unpleasant surprises with respect to the budget of the safety assessment studies.

Apart from the U.K. and Japan, today only

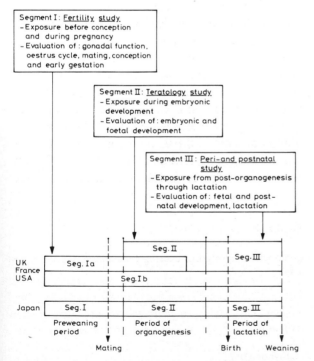

Fig. 1 Phases of testing drugs for their developmental toxicological potential and exposure periods as recommended in guidelines for developmental toxicity testing of drugs.

France has included behavioural aspects in their guidelines for the testing of drugs. Since their guidelines are essentially similar to the British ones, at present there are really only two sets.

Apart from the differences between the two sets in detailing specific behavioural functions, the Japanese and British/French guidelines also differ in another important aspect: they require behavioural evaluations in different phases of the reproductive assessment process.

Three phases of testing drugs for their developmental toxicological potential are currently distinguishable (Fig. 1).

In Segment I studies, test compounds are administered to animals prior to and during the mating period. Japanese guidelines recommend administration to females throughout early gestation, whereas European and U.S.A. guidelines suggest doing so throughout a substantial part of the period of organogenesis (Segment Ia, Fig. 1), even throughout weaning of the offspring. Apart from the evaluation of gonadal function, oestrus cycle, mating and implantation, the British/French guideline requires behavioural testing in this study, whereas the Japanese guideline does not.

In the Segment II study, the test compound is administered to pregnant females during the period of organogenesis. This test has traditionally been applied for the assessment of morphological developmental anomalies. The Japanese guideline, however, also expects the assessment of functional developmental disorders in this test.

In Segment III studies the occurrence of malformations which become apparent in the postnatal period is studied. In these studies, animals are dosed from late pregnancy throughout parturition and lactation until weaning. During lactation and after weaning the offspring are examined for structural and functional developmental disorders. Both the Japanese and the British/French guidelines include behavioural testing in this type of study.

Overlap of exposure periods is required by the

British/French guideline and the U.S.A. guideline. It is difficult to determine which phase of testing is optimal for the detection of behavioural deficits, but one working principle that has emerged from behavioural teratology does provide some insight, namely that the period of greatest vulnerability to malformations of the central nervous system is also the period of greatest vulnerability to behavioural abnormalities (Vorhees et al., 1978). This principle leads to the conclusion that applying behavioural testing in Segment I studies as required by the British/French guideline is only feasible when dosing is continued during organogenesis, since during this period the CNS is most susceptible to adverse effects. As can be seen in the diagram, this is indeed the case in the U.K. guideline. Since the Segment III study covers more of the final development of the CNS, when not only are neurotransmitter and other factors of functional organization presumably predominant (Vorhees, 1982) but also the cerebellum is still in an important stage of structural development (Rodier, 1980), it seems appropriate to include behavioural testing in this type of study as well.

Summarizing, at present the regulatory involvement in behavioural teratology is such that Japanese and British/French guidelines include some general requirements for behavioural testing which differ with respect to specification of behavioural indices that should be measured as well as to the type of study in which behaviour testing on offspring should be conducted. It may be added here that behavioural teratological testing is only required for pharmaceuticals.

In order to decide whether behavioural teratogenicity studies are necessary upon safety evaluation, and as a consequence should be incorporated in guidelines, the sensitivity and reliability of the methods used should be defined. Although the differences between the existing guidelines show that an international consensus on the methods used has not yet been reached, a number of compounds have positively been identified as behavioural teratogens.

TABLE 1

Compounds reported and confirmed as experimental behavioural teratogens

Class	Agent
Alcoholic beverages	Ethanol
Anesthetics	Halothane, nitrous oxide
Drugs	Anticonvulsants, antimitotics, antineurotics, antipsychotics
Food additives	Antioxidants, MSG
Metals	Lead, methylmercury
Narcotics	Methadone, morphine
Stimulants	Amphetamines, caffeine
Vitamins	Vitamin A excess

(Source: Vorhees and Butcher, 1982)

In Table 1 some examples of compounds reported as being experimental behavioural teratogens are listed. For each of the agents mentioned in this table behavioural teratogenicity has been observed by several investigators in different laboratories (Vorhees and Butcher, 1982). Although internationally most attention is paid to drugs, it is interesting to learn from this table that several compounds other than drugs have also been shown to be behavioural teratogens. It becomes even more interesting when compounds reported as causing behavioural deficits in humans are tabulated (Table 2). For each compound, behavioural teratogenic findings have been confirmed by a number of investigators. It is surprising to see

TABLE 2

Compounds reported as causing behavioural deficits in humans

Alcohol
Hydantoin
Lead
Methylmercury
Tobacco

(Source: Tanimura, 1980; WHO, 1986)

that almost all compounds are substances other than drugs! Therefore, the requirement for including tests of behavioural teratogenicity in guidelines for the safety assessment of drugs only does not accurately reflect the available data and should therefore be reconsidered. On the other hand, it would probably be unrealistic to recommend that behavioural teratology screening should be included as part of the screening procedure for all chemicals. To date, there is a consensus amongst the majority of scientists active in the field of (behavioural) teratology that behavioural teratology testing is a valid approach for assessing the presence of nervous system anomalies in the developing organism (Adams and Buelke-Sam, 1981; Sobotka and Vorhees, 1985, Kimmel et al., 1985). Consequently, some behavioural screening should indeed be required for drugs where it is considered essential to learn as much as possible about effects on development. With regard to other types of chemical, such as food additives, agrochemicals, industrial chemicals and toiletries and cosmetics, there was consensus among experts during the 1985 workshop on the collaborative behavioural teratology study of the National Center for Toxicological Research (NCTR) that 'behavioural teratology testing in some fashion should be carried out but that the selection of chemicals for testing should be based on certain criteria which generally indicate a potential nervous system involvement' (Sobotka and Vorhees, 1985). During the same workshop it was agreed that all compounds that are suspected of interference with the CNS should at least be subjected to some sort of behavioural teratology testing. It should be emphasized that this approach implies that for most of the novel chemicals it cannot be decided beforehand whether behavioural teratology screening is appropriate.

In The Netherlands, the Health Council has recommended that a decision on reproduction toxicity testing of novel chemicals should depend on the results of a pilot study (Health Council, 1985). Such a pilot study should be designed so that, in addition to information with respect to

gametogenesis, mating, fertility and general reproductive performance, some indication of possible (functional) developmental toxicity can be obtained (Koëter, 1983). Apart from the decision as to further testing for general reproduction toxicity, the results of such a pilot screening could also serve as a basis for decision-making with respect to behavioural teratology testing. In addition to this, priorities for such testing could also be set on the basis of other criteria. For the testing of current, insufficiently tested chemicals, the Health Council of The Netherlands has proposed the following criteria, which could also be used for setting further priorities with respect to behavioural testing (Health Council, 1985): (a) bioactivity of the agent, (b) number of men, women and children likely to be exposed either voluntarily or involuntarily, (c) available biological data such as suspected human teratogenicity, teratogenic effects in domestic animals or wildlife and toxicity in the adult at low doses, and (d) available information on ecotoxicity such as biodegradation and bioaccumulation.

Summarizing, some behavioural teratogenicity studies should indeed be included in safety evaluation for a greater number of substances. However, guidelines should not be rigid in this respect and the decision as to whether behavioural teratology screening is necessary should depend on a variety of factors and criteria, most of which are related to toxicity data derived from other studies. But also the type of application and the environmental conditions should be taken into account. The best approach for industry would be to discuss proposals for toxicity study programmes with the relevant registration authorities, prior to the start of these programmes. Of course, the authorities responsible should be willing to advise in this matter.

Behavioural functions to be assessed

When it is thus recommended that for certain substances behavioural teratology screening should be considered for safety evaluation, the next problem is how to make a choice with respect to type of behavioural functions that should be assessed. At present, no single approach or behavioural test battery has been identified as the most reliable, sensitive and economical means of detecting behavioural dysfunction following developmental insult. Moreover, the current state of knowledge is such that although various approaches and test batteries have been described (Adams, 1986; Adams and Buelke-Sam, 1981; Kimmel et al., 1985; Rodier, 1978; Spijper Cranmer and Goad, 1983). Mechanisms underlying behavioural deficits are not fully understood (WHO, 1984, 1986). Therefore, at present the majority of scientists in the field are of the opinion that fixed protocols should not yet be included in routine experimental animal studies. There is, however, much agreement with respect to the strategy of testing. A well-accepted strategy is that behavioral teratology tests should be performed at two levels of sensitivity and complexity.

Initial testing of chemicals should ensure that behavioural effects are not missed. It should be broad and comprehensive with regard to the types of function assessed. This is necessary because many types of function, including fertility, may be adversely affected by an agent and these effects cannot be reliably predicted (WHO, 1984).

Secondary testing should be performed if behavioural alterations are observed in initial testing. More sophisticated and selective behavioural techniques, perhaps also in other species, should be used to help delineate the type(s) and extent of effects produced and the possible mechanisms involved. Also, at this stage, more selective exposure regimens and testing schedules should be employed. Secondary behavioural evaluations should be flexibly designed with agent specificity in mind (Adams and Buelke-Sam, 1981).

With respect to initial testing, two different concepts are distinguishable. Firstly, the so-called 'apical test strategy' (Grant, 1976; Butcher, 1976). In essence, this strategy is based on the assumption that successful completion of a multi-behavioural test by an animal implies that all contributory functions are normal. On the other hand, it is assumed that if one or more of the component functions is deficient, then the overall performance of the animal will be impaired. This approach, however, is not widely recommended, since there is insufficient knowledge of the extent to which experimental animals are able to compensate for specific deficiencies in such a way that the overall performance remains satisfactory. It is also unclear to what degree a particular function need be affected in order to produce a specific behavioural effect (Vorhees and Butcher, 1982).

The second concept, and at present still the most adequate strategy for initial testing, is to employ a test system that combines a wide exposure period with a series of developmental tests which sample a broad range of CNS functions (Adams and Buelke-Sam, 1981). For each category of behavioural functions separate tests should be conducted. In general, measures of both early neurological, physical and behavioural development and behaviour at adulthood should be included. With respect to the categories of function to be assessed in the initial phase of testing the consensus opinion of experts in the field is that the following should receive sufficient attention (WHO, 1984; Kimmel et al., 1985):

(a) *Physical growth and maturation.* Although these parameters are not really behavioural indices, they are essential for evaluation of behavioural test results and as such are used as co-variables in statistical analyses.

(b) *Reflexive behaviour.* As a measure of neurological development reflexes are very important and this category should include both reflexes that develop early and those that develop late during the postnatal period.

(c) *Sensory-motor evaluation.* Tests of this category are based on the localization or orientation responsiveness to stimuli. Although preferably sensory functions should be assessed separately from motor functions, in practice this appears to be very difficult as the response to stimuli is usually expressed by some sort of motor activity.

(d) *Emotionality or motivational state*. These states of the animal, which are difficult to define, are usually measured as spontaneous activity, reactivity, habituation and exploratory behaviour. In addition, sleep testing is occasionally applied.
(e) *Learning evaluations*. Learning tests include habituation as an example of non-associative learning. This category further includes relatively simple associative learning (Pavlovian conditioning) as well as complex forms of learning.

For each of these categories a number of tests are available and well-documented (Health Council of The Netherlands, 1985; WHO, 1984). The selection should be made by the investigator and will depend on practical aspects, knowledge and experience with certain tests and the nature of the agent to be tested. However, upon selection it is strongly recommended to consider the so-called 'roofing-tile principle'. This implies that tests should have a certain overlap, through which it is possible to confirm a positive finding with respect to a certain behaviour in a different test, conducted under different conditions. Consequently, a positive finding should only be considered of toxicological significance when the finding is confirmed in another test.

Depending on the results of the initial testing phase and on the (social) importance of the substance tested, it could be decided whether or not secondary testing is appropriate. As mentioned earlier, secondary testing should be performed in a 'tailor-made fashion', based on earlier findings and application of the agent.

Relevance of behavioural effects in animals to man

The number of examples in which there is a correspondence between developmental behavioural defects observed in humans and effects seen in animal studies is limited to a few agents such as methylmercury, lead and some psychoactive drugs (Lorente, 1981; Needleman et al., 1984; Vorhees and Butcher, 1982). As developmental neurobehavioural toxicology is a recently developed field of research, only limited evidence has so far accumulated to convincingly demonstrate parallel effects in animals and humans. In addition, there is considerable disagreement concerning the importance or meaning of behavioural teratology data. In particular, the importance of transient changes in behaviour and accelerated or delayed maturation of reflexes is sometimes considered questionable. A better understanding can only be achieved when more information from animal and human data has been accumulated. Further, more research with respect to possible correlations between behavioural changes and structural or biochemical CNS alterations is urgently needed. In this respect, the research of Rodier and colleagues (Rodier, 1977; Koëter and Rodier, 1985; Rodier et al., 1986) on cell proliferation in the developing brain after exposure to behavioural teratogens as well as that of others (see other chapters in this volume) significantly contribute to a better understanding of the importance of developmental behavioural effects.

It should be clear from the above that there is still a lot to learn before deviant behaviours are really understood and before behavioural effects in (young) animals can be extrapolated to the human situation with sufficient confidence.

Summary

It has been shown that the same factors that have long been known to disturb the structural development are also able to disturb functional development and thus behaviour.

At present, behavioural teratogenicity studies are only required by registration authorities for drugs. Although it is generally accepted that at least some data on behavioural teratogenicity should be available for all new drugs, the majority of compounds known as being experimental, behavioural teratogens are chemicals other than drugs. Therefore, the rationale for including behavioural teratogenicity testing in guidelines for the safety assessment of drugs only is unclear.

As it would probably be unrealistic to recommend that behavioural teratogenicity screening should be included as part of the reproduction toxicity study programme for all chemicals, a procedure for the selection of priority chemicals needs to be developed. Criteria for such a selection procedure are proposed: (a) indications of a potential nervous system involvement, (b) positive results from a pilot reproduction study, (c) bioactivity of the chemical, (d) expected human exposures and (e) available information on ecotoxicity.

When behavioural testing is considered relevant, a well-accepted strategy is to perform tests at two levels of sensitivity and complexity. The most adequate approach for initial testing is to employ a test system that combines a wide exposure period with a series of tests, sampling a broad range of CNS functions.

Furthermore, tests should overlap. This should facilitate confirmation of a positive finding by a different test, conducted under different conditions. Depending on the results of the initial testing phase it can be decided whether secondary testing, to be performed in a 'tailor-made fashion', is appropriate.

References

Adams, J. (1986) Methods in behavioral teratology. In E.P. Riley and C.V. Vorhees (Eds.), *Handbook of Behavioral Teratology*, Plenum Press, New York.

Adams, J. and Buelke-Sam, J. (1981) Behavioural assessment of the postnatal animal: testing and methods development. In C.A. Kimmel and J. Buelke-Sam (Eds.), *Developmental Toxicology*, Raven Press, New York, pp. 233–258.

Barlow, S.M. (1985) United Kingdom: Regulatory attitudes towards behavioural teratology testing. *Neurobehav. Toxicol. Teratol.*, 7: 643–646.

Butcher, R.E. (1976) Behavioural testing as a method for assessing risk. *Environm. Health Perspect.*, 18: 75–78.

Butcher, R.E. (1985) A historical perspective on behavioural teratology. *Neurobehav. Toxicol. Teratol.*, 7: 537–540.

Grant, L.D. (1976) Research strategies for behavioural teratology studies. *Environm. Health Perspect.*, 18: 85–94.

Health Council of The Netherlands (1985) The evaluation of the teratogenicity of chemical substances. Report No. 1985/6E.

Kimmel, C.A., Buelke-Sam, J. and Adams, J. (1985) Collaborative Behavioural Teratology Study: implications, current applications and future directions. *Neurobehav. Toxicol. Teratol.*, 7: 669–673.

Koëter, H.B.W.M. (1983) Relevance of parameters related to fertility and reproduction in toxicity testing. *Am. J. Ind. Med.*, 4: 81–86.

Koëter, H.B.W.M. and Rodier, P.M. (1985) Behavioural effects in rats and morphologic and behavioural effects in mice after exposure to inhalant anesthetics during early development. *Neurobehav. Toxicol. Teratol.*, 7: 676.

Lorente, C.A., Tassinari, M.S. and Keith, D.A. (1981) The effects of phenytoin on rat development: an animal model system for fetal hydantoin syndrome. *Teratology*, 24: 169–180.

Ministry of Health and Welfare, Japan (1984) Information on the guidelines of toxicity studies required for application for approval to manufacture (import) drugs. Notification No. 118 of the Pharmaceutical Affairs Bureau, Ministry of Health and Welfare.

Needleman, H.L., Rabinowitz, M., Leviton, A., Luin, S. and Schoenbaum, S. (1984) The relationship between prenatal exposure to lead and congenital anomalies. *J. Am. Med. Assoc.*, 251: 2956–2959.

Rodier, P.M. (1976) Critical periods for behavioural anomalies in mice. *Environm. Health Perspect.*, 18: 79–83.

Rodier, P.M. (1977) Correlations between prenatally induced alternations in CNS cell populations and postnatal function. *Teratology*, 16: 235–246.

Rodier, P.M. (1978) Behavioral teratology. In Wilson and Frazier (Eds.), *Handbook of Teratology, Vol. 4*, Plenum Press, New York.

Rodier, P.M. (1980) Chronology of neuron development: animal studies and their clinical implications. *Dev. Med. Child Neurol.*, 22: 525–545.

Rodier, P.M., Reynolds, S.S. and Roberts, W.N. (1979) Behavioural consequences of interference with CNS development in the early fetal period. *Teratology*, 19: 327–336.

Rodier, P.M., Aschner, M., Lewis, L.S. and Koëter, H.B.W.M. (1986) Cell proliferation in developing brain after brief exposure to nitrous oxide or halothane. *Anesthesiology*, 64: 680–687.

Sobotka, T.J. and Vorhees, C.V. (1985) Application of behavioural teratology testing procedures. *Neurobehav. Toxicol. Teratol.*, 7: 665.

Spijper Cranmer, J. and Goad, P.T. (1983) Validation of selected behavioral tests for evaluating low-level toxicity. In G. Zbinden (Ed.), *Application of Behavioural Pharmacology in Toxicology*, Raven Press, New York.

Suter, K.E. and Schön, H. (1985) Possibilities and limitations of current methods in behavioural teratology screening: an industrial view-point. In Proceedings of the symposium: 'Aktuelle Probleme der Biomedizin', Salzburg, September 18–20, 1985.

Tanimura, T. (1984) Prospects of the reproductive toxicology with special reference to the developmental hazards due to the treatment at the stages from prefertilization to implantation. *Congenital Anomalies*, 24: 319–328.

Vorhees, C. V., Brunner, R. L., MacDaniel, C. R. and Butcher, R. E. (1978) The relationship of gestational age to vitamin A induced postnatal dysfunction. *Teratology*, 17: 271–276.

Vorhees, C. V. and Butcher, R. E. (1982) Behavioural teratogenicity. In K. Snell (Ed.), *Developmental Toxicology*, Croom Helm, London, pp. 247–298.

W. H. O. (1984) Principles for evaluating health risks to progeny associated with exposure to chemicals during pregnancy. *Environm. Health Criteria*, 30.

W. H. O. (1986) Draft Guidelines for the assessment of drugs and other chemicals for behavioural teratogenicity, WHO Regional Office for Europe, Copenhagen.

Discussion

A. J. Friedhoff: We know that very many non-psychotropes as well as all psychotropic drugs enter the brain, and it is likely that many of both types of drug affect brain development in ways we do not yet know. As we find out more about behavioral teratogenicity of drugs that enter the brain it is going to be necessary to learn now to differentiate among positive, negative and neutral effects, or we will probably have to ban very many drugs, because they have some effect on development.

H. B. W. M. Koëter: Behavioral effects should never be extrapolated from the period of development to the adult situation. Since behavioral teratogenicity studies are only part of the developmental toxicity study program for the compound, and, moreover, even reproductive toxicity is only one aspect of the toxicology profile, there is always more information needed and often available. Only on the basis of this full toxicity profile should a compound be evaluated.

T. D. Yih: A number of drug classes were mentioned that should be submitted to behavioral teratological testing, among which are CNS-active drugs. Do you mean drugs developed for treatment of CNS disorders or drugs which affect CNS physiology (e.g. neurotransmitter levels)? The majority of newly developed drugs have to some extent such side effects. Should they all be tested?

H. B. W. M. Koëter: In my opinion all drugs intended to be active at the CNS level should indeed be tested. It should be emphasized, however, that results of behavioral tests should only be evaluated within the context of the full toxicological profile.

P. M. Rodier: Where guidelines are flexible, will regulators emphasize the use of positive controls and soforth, to ensure that tests have some validity?

H. B. W. M. Koëter: To date, not so many compounds have been evaluated by regulatory authorities. To my knowledge, there are no requirements as to positive controls or other means to ensure the validity of the tests applied. Authorities should be encouraged to implement such controls.

C. V. Vorhees: I agree that more information is needed on the relevance of animal to human behavioral change. However, I would not like to have your comments leave the impression that this problem is any more difficult than with malformations, or cancer, where also one cannot precisely extrapolate specific effects from animals to human.

H. B. W. M. Koëter: Although your argument is valid, I feel that upon the introduction of any new discipline in toxicology the same mistake (made some 25 years ago when the majority of toxicity test methods were introduced) of being merely descriptive should not be made again. As in pharmacology, one should strive after understanding mechanisms rather than describe gross findings only.

SECTION II

Lasting Effects of Early Hormone Imbalance

G.J. Boer, M.G.P. Feenstra, M. Mirmiran, D.F. Swaab and F. Van Haaren
Progress in Brain Research, Vol. 73
© 1988 Elsevier Science Publishers B.V. (Biomedical Division)

CHAPTER 6

Teratogenic mechanisms of dysthyroidism in the central nervous system

Andrea Vaccari

Department of Neurosciences, Chair of Medical Toxicology, Via Porcell 4, 09124 Cagliari, Italy

Introduction

The regulatory influence of hormones on the development of the Central Nervous System (CNS) is manifest both pre- and postnatally. Consequently, alterations in hormone homeostasis may affect a number of biochemical and morphologic events involved in functional and behavioral maturation (see Timiras, 1972). Thyroid hormones, thyroxine (T_4) and triiodothyronine (T_3) are well-known growth-promoting factors for the CNS, their effects being at a peak when the cell ceases to divide and begins to differentiate. In humans a decrease in or lack of thyroid influences, whatever the cause may be, in late fetal or early postnatal periods, when the brain is more plastic and its growth more accelerated, may result in developmental abnormalities such as stunted body growth and skeletal maldevelopment, spastic displegia, ataxic gait, abnormal hearing, strabismus and, most importantly, in various levels of mental deficiency (cretinism) (Whybrow and Ferrell, 1974; Jubiz, 1979). One must recall that the placental transport of thyroid hormones is minimal (Fisher et al., 1977; Varma et al., 1978), which, from the beginning of the second trimester of gestation onwards, makes the brain development of the human fetus dependent on the activity of its own thyroid gland.

Causes of thyroid deficiency may be: (1) congenital agenesis or maldevelopment of the fetal or neonatal gland, (2) impaired mechanisms for making or secreting thyroid hormones, or (3) resistance to thyroid hormones perhaps due to a decreased number of their specific binding sites (Sawin, 1985). Thus, thyroid deficiency in humans, during the sensitive period of brain development (from about the 19th gestational week until the 2nd or 3rd year after birth) may represent a strong teratogen the effects of which can be reversed or prevented only when adequate doses of thyroid hormones and iodine (Vanderpas et al., 1986) are administered as soon as the diagnosis is made postnatally. Although one cannot precisely state whether the deadline for starting the therapy lies at 3, 6 or 9 weeks after birth (Glorieux et al., 1983; New England Congenital Hypothyroidism Collaborative, 1984), thyroid hormone supplementation should preferentially be initiated during the first 30 days of life in order to prevent irreversible brain damage (Wolter et al., 1980), and continued up to the 4th year of life (Klein, 1986). In other words, the critical period for brain development seems to extend well beyond the very first weeks after birth, although clinical evidence shows that hypothyroidism starting after the 2nd year of life allows the achievement of a relatively good level of mental performance. Of course it is to be expected that if an adequate treatment of neonatal thyroid hypofunction leads to a return of the normal situation, this is obtained by repairing structural abnormalities and by a normalization of the CNS developmental schedule, which would be highly retarded otherwise (Brasel and Boyd, 1975).

Thyroid hyperfunction is a rare pediatric pathology which may lead to psychomotoric and behavioral perturbances (Grave's disease) or represent a true teratogenic factor as it occurs in neonatal thyrotoxicosis, when underweight, skull malformations and, most frequently, mental retardation may occur (Hollingsworth et al., 1980).

During the last 15 years a great number of experimental studies have dealt with morphological (Legrand, 1984), biochemical (Vaccari, 1983; Puymirat, 1985) and molecular (Nunez, 1985) mechanisms which probably do underlie the dysthyroidism-related abnormal development of the CNS, and may eventually lead to cretinism-associated neurological and mental abnormalities. This effort has been almost entirely based upon experimental models of congenital or acquired adult hypothyroidism, the rat being the most widely used animal (Döhler et al., 1979). The popularity of rodents in the 'market' of experimental dysthyroidism is justified by a well-stated similarity in the general scheme of neurodevelopmental events in humans and several mammalian species. The newborn rat 'may be compared with a human fetus in the second trimester of pregnancy, and the newborn human baby to a 6–10-day-old rat' (Fisher et al., 1977; Legrand, 1984). Of course, similarity of human and animal brain development does not mean that information obtained from experimentally provoked dysthyroidism, when the causative agent is well-known, may entirely reflect spontaneously occurring thyroid disease in humans, where pathogenesis may be complex and of unknown origin.

In this survey I shall briefly describe the mechanisms of action of thyroid hormones in the brain, their effects on the establishment of neuronal networks, and dysthyroidism-associated abnormalities of central monoaminergic neurotransmission as an index for altered number of interneuronal interactions.

Molecular mechanisms of dysthyroidism-related CNS teratogenesis

Teratogenic influences of early thyroid insufficiency may result from impaired DNA transcription or depressed synthesis of active proteins in the immature brain. Since thyroid hormones do normally have a regulatory (inductive, repressive) role in the expression of the genetic program of nerve cells, protein perturbance may result in a retarded differentiation and proliferation, and in a defective establishment of the neuronal network in the immature brain. Protein depression is just the last of several events where T_3 (5,5,3'-triiodothyronine), the active 5'-deiodination product of T_4 (3,5,3',5'-tetraiodothyronine), after having been taken up by the neuropile and nerve endings (Dratman et al., 1982), binds to nuclear, chromatin-associated receptor proteins (Schwartz and Oppenheimer, 1978a). The T_3-nuclear receptor complex may then trigger the production of messenger RNAs to be translated to specific proteins (see Menezes-Ferreira and Torresani, 1983), thus influencing the thyroid-dependent gene expression in specific neuronal cells of different brain regions.

Thyroid hormone-binding proteins have been also identified in the cytosol or plasma membranes and cytoplasmic reticulum of brain cells (Dillman et al., 1974; Geel, 1977), where they would regulate the retention and supply of T_3 to the various cell compartments, primarily nuclei and mitochondria (Dozin-Van Roye and De Nayer, 1978; Menezes-Ferreira and Torresani, 1983).

The discovery that reverse $T_3(rT_3)$ (3,3',5'-triiodothyronine), the alternative extrathyroidal 5-deiodination metabolite of T_4, also binds to nuclear receptors where it can competitively inhibit all of the T_3 binding (Latham et al., 1976) is of great interest. Since the levels of rT_3 may be high in fetal circulation (and are more than 10-fold the T_3 levels, as is the case in the human amniotic fluid before 30 weeks; Chopra et al., 1978), rT_3 might conceivably result in a significant occupation of T_3 receptors, thus influencing fetal thyroid hormone-regulated functions. Furthermore, rT_3 would inhibit the conversion of T_4 to T_3. Information is lacking about hypothyroidism-associated increases in the levels of rT_3 which would hinder T_3 from triggering its action in humans. Certainly the antithyroid drug propylthiouracyl (PTU), which is widely used to induce experimental hypothyroidism in rats, is a potent producer of rT_3 (Jubiz, 1979).

The presence of thyroid hormone receptors in the CNS has stimulated investigators to study whether there are receptor alterations in the developing hypothyroid brain (Fig. 1). At first it was stated that the density of nuclear T_3 receptors is at a peak either in cerebral hemispheres (Valcana and Timiras, 1978) or in the whole brain and cerebellum (Schwartz and Oppenheimer, 1978b) of rats during the first 2 days of postnatal life, and that it declines to adult levels by the 2nd week, thus correlating with the critical dependence of the brain on thyroid hormones. Hypothyroidism is known to affect cerebellar development markedly, in spite of the low T_3 binding capacity in this region (Ruel et al., 1985), and it has been shown to increase the density of nuclear T_3 receptors in the brain consistently, as early as

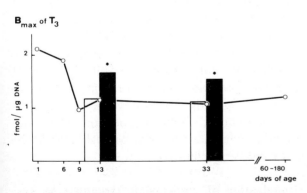

Fig. 1. Postnatal development of triiodothyronine (T_3) binding to nuclear receptors in rat cerebral hemispheres ($\bigcirc$), and effects of neonatal radiothyroidectomy on T_3 binding (open column = euthyroids; solid column = hypothyroids). * $P < 0.05$ vs. euthyroids. Results are from Valcana and Timiras (1978).

13 days after neonatal radiothyroidectomy (Fig. 1), compared to euthyroid rats (Valcana and Timiras, 1978). Neonatal hyperthyroidism does not affect binding characteristics of T_3 (Timiras, 1979). Therefore the developing hypothyroid brain would react to a smaller availability of the T_3 ligand, with an adaptive, greater binding capacity for thyroid hormones. Similarly, in synaptic transmission, excess of neurotransmitters decreases, and a deficit increases the number of pertinent receptors. In contrast, researchers have also observed a decreased binding of T_3 due to a lower than normal affinity for the hormone of nuclear receptors in human lymphocytes or fibroblasts from a hypothyroid subject suffering from familial peripheral tissue resistance to thyroid hormones (Bernal et al., 1978). Beyond all these considerations and the need for additional studies aimed at ascertaining whether alterations in T_3 binding capacity are long-lasting (even lifetime), little doubt exists that thyroid hormones in health and disease have a regulatory role on their nuclear receptors (Valcana and Timiras, 1978).

Morphogenetic alterations in dysthyroidism

The stuctural consequences of altered thyroid states during the neonatal age have been thoroughly considered in an excellent review (Legrand, 1984). Here I will only summarize some of most relevant findings.

The most important maturational steps in the CNS are (a) cell proliferation, which occurs prenatally in the rat cortex, starts from birth and continues up to approximately the 15th day of life in the cerebellum, and continues after birth in cortical glial cells, the hippocampus and olfactory bulbs (Patel et al., 1976); and (b) neuronal differentiation, a process that is mostly postnatal in the rat, begins with a change in cell shape, followed by neurite outgrowth, leading to the establishment of interneuronal contacts (synaptogenesis). T_4 administration has been shown to increase the synaptic density and the number and size of nerve processes in the cerebellum of neonatal rats

74

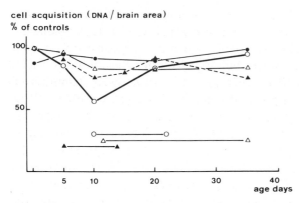

cell acquisition (DNA / brain area)
% of controls

Fig. 2. Effects of propylthiouracyl (PTU)-provoked hypothyroidism on postnatal cell acquisition (cell number) in the
forebrain (●), cerebellum (○), olfactory bulbs (▲) and
hippocampus (△) of newborn rats. Results are expressed as
the percent content of DNA (μg P/brain region) with respect
to euthyroid counterparts. The horizontal bars indicate the
period when the differences between hypothyroid and
euthyroid rats were significant. Results are from Patel et al.
(1976) and Rabié et al. (1979).

(Legrand, 1979). Conversely, thyroid hormone
deficiency does dramatically affect the neuronal
cell differentiation and to a smaller extent the
region-specific cell acquisition (Fig. 2) (Patel
et al., 1976; Legrand, 1984; Nunez, 1984). This
statement is based upon a number of experimental
studies where attention was focused on the rat
cortex and cerebellum. The latter region proved to
be particularly useful for studying dysthyroidism-
related alterations (Lauder, 1977), thanks to its
simple and homogeneous structure and its almost
entirely postnatal development. A number of observations are noteworthy. First of all, the density
of cortical axonal terminals in layer IV and the
dendritic branching of pyramidal neurons are decreased to the point that a deficit in dendro-
axonal processes may lead to a 50% decrease in
synaptic numbers in the neonatal hypothyroid
brain (Eayrs, 1971). Disturbances in synaptogenesis have also been demonstrated in rat visual
and auditory cortex, and in the caudate nucleus
(see Legrand, 1984), a region where the postnatal
density of neurons is lower, compared to

euthyroid counterparts. There is also a marked
reduction in the size and density of hippocampal
cells (Rabié et al, 1979). Secondly, the migration
of cerebellar, external granular cells towards the
molecular or the inner granular layer is delayed,
and there is a compensatory prolongation of proliferative activity, as compared to the euthyroid
cerebellum. The final result is a normal total number of cells in the hypothyroid cerebellum (Patel
et al., 1976), while similar disturbances in the cell
migration from the germinal ventricular layer in
the hippocampus and olfactory bulbs do not
coincide with compensatory mechanisms. The
number of Purkinje cells is not affected in hypothyroidism, though their histological maturation is
delayed and the density and branching of their
dendritic spines is markedly diminished (Rebière
and Legrand, 1972). Thirdly, there is increased
death of newly formed and differentiating cells in
the internal granular layer, perhaps a consequence
of a lower availability of synaptic sites in the hypothyroid cerebellum (Rabié et al., 1977; see Rami
et al., 1986). As a matter of fact, the most relevant
effect of neonatal hypothyroidism seems to be a
deficient synaptogenesis along with alterations in
the qualitative distribution and specification of
available synapses (Nunez, 1984), which might
help in explaining the electrical, neurotransmitter
and behavioral alterations which are associated
with both experimental and spontaneous hypothyroidisms. Finally, the myelination process is
retarded and myelin content is decreased in the
hypothyroid brain, which is partially the result of
a delayed formation and maturation of oligodendrocytes (Legrand, 1980). Conversely, in neonatal
hyperthyroidism, both oligodendrocytes and
myelin accumulate more precociously than in the
euthyroid cerebellum.

Organization of cytoplasmic structures in dys-
thyroidism

Changes in cell shape and neurite outgrowth, i.e.
dendritic branching, axonal sprouting and synapse formation, thus all those differentiation

processes which are under thyroid control, strictly depend on the massive assembly of cell microtubules and neurofilaments (Yamada et al., 1970; Nunez, 1985). Microtubules are linear, polymeric structures composed of tubulin and microtubule-associated proteins (MAPs and TAU) which work as assembly-promoting factors of the microtubule itself. Neurofilaments also have a protein matrix, including actin and several actin-binding proteins (ABP). All groups of proteins share the build-up of the nerve cell structure, axons and dendrites included. The finding that the efficiency of microtubule assembly depends on the stage of brain development is of great relevance to the understanding of dysthyroidism effects at this level (Lennon et al., 1980). Thus, the rate of tubulin polymerization steeply increases from the fetal period up to peak levels at approximately 1 month after birth in rat and mouse brain supernatants. Furthermore, prenatally caused hypothyroidism proved to slow down the rate of assembly during the first 15 days of life, though this effect was transient in the rat. Replacement therapy with thyroid hormones brought the rates of microtubule assembly back to normal (see Nunez, 1985).

Finally, the composition of MAPs changes with age and is thyroid-dependent. More precisely, among the three major types of MAPs, the HMW_1 (350 kDa), the HMW_2 (300 kDa) and TAU (65 kDa), the TAU fraction is heterogeneous and displays neonatal- and adult-specific components which are probably regulated by different genes (Nunez, 1984). The TAU_3 protein is almost missing in microtubules from hypothyroid brains (Nunez, 1985).

If one assumes that different kinds of MAPs underlie the expression of specific types of microtubules which, in their turn, trigger the differentiation of specific neuronal cells, it is easy to suspect the importance of any dysthyrodism-associated impairment of the microtubule machinery.

Effects of dysthyroidism on central neurotransmission

Thyroid deficiency during brain development leads to a dramatic reduction in the number and specificity of synaptic junctions (Legrand, 1984). Therefore, it is no wonder that both pre- and postsynaptically-located neurotransmitter functions in neonatal dysthyroidism are extensively impaired (see Vaccari, 1983; Puymirat, 1985). Such alterations involve levels and turnover of neurotransmitters, their release and uptake processes, the activities of pertinent synthesizing and catabolic enzymes, and their specific receptors.

Although consistent evidence shows that disruptions of biogenic amine homeostasis may be of importance to neuropsychiatric disorders (Barchas et al., 1977), neurotransmitter alterations in dysthyroidism often display conflicting trends. This makes it difficult to correlate them with neurobehavioral aberrations. There may be several reasons for such inconsistency. (1) The age- and brain region-specific sensitivity of mammalians to dysthyroid procedures, and the time schedule of brain development in different species. (2) The experimental model chosen to provoke hypothyroidism. Thus, surgical thyroidectomy cannot be performed neatly soon after birth in rats, and in any case it involves parathyroid ablation. Radiothyroidectomy at birth can only be accomplished by using huge amounts of ^{131}I, about one hundred times (on a body weight basis) the quantity applied in the treatment of human hyperthyroidism. Therefore the involvement of extrathyroidal tissues in the response to radioactivity cannot be excluded. The sulphydryl goitrogens methimazole (MMI) and propylthiouracil (PTU) have membrane-perturbing effects (Biassoni and Vaccari, 1985) which may superimpose on those of the thyroid deprivation they provoke (Fig. 3). (3) The time-lag between the last administration of antithyroid drugs and the death of the animal may be important in order to avoid any direct influence of MMI or PTU on neurotransmitter parameters studied. (4) The

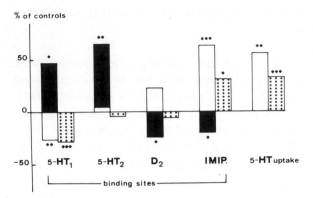

Fig. 3. Effects of methimazole (MMI)-provoked hypothyroidism (solid column) and in vitro influences of $1 \cdot 10^{-4}$ M MMI (open column) or PTU (dotted column) on 5-HT$_1$, 5-HT$_2$, D$_2$ and imipramine binding sites of rat brain membranes, and on the synaptosomal uptake of 5-HT. Rats were given MMI, 5–20 mg/kg/day s.c. form birth to day 30 of age. $*P < 0.05$; $**P < 0.02$; $***P < 0.005$ or 0.001 vs. controls. Results are from Vaccari and Timiras (1981), Vaccari et al. (1983b), Vaccari (1985) and Biassoni and Vaccari (1985).

effects of malnutrition, which are often associated with both experimental hypo- (Strupp and Levitsky, 1983) and hyperthyroidism (Pascual-Leone et al., 1985), may partially mask dysthyroidism-specific alterations. (5) Last but not least, thyroid disease is known to influence corticosteroid metabolism, hypo- and hyperthyroidism being associated with decreased or increased catabolism of corticosteroids in humans, respectively (Pittman, 1971; Linquette et al., 1976). Furthermore, there are adrenal changes in genetically hypothyroid mice (Shire and Beamer, 1984). Inasmuch as corticosteroids may influence the developing neurotransmission and act as teratogen agents by themselves (see Meyer, 1985; Biegon et al., 1985), the effects of adrenal dysfunction may become confused with those of dysthyroidism.

In the final analysis, the fact that similar experimental schedules lead to contrasting results may just indicate that it is normal to have physiological fluctuations within a certain range. It is always difficult, indeed, to determine when an alteration of neurotransmitter homeostasis is statistically significant, in order to provoke neurobehavioral impairment.

Presynaptic alterations

At the time that these considerations were reviewed for the first time (Vaccari, 1983), the overall picture of dysthyroidism-associated presynaptic alterations in neurotransmitter pathways was rather confusing. Now, in spite of a degree of uncertainty, mostly related to the status of monoamine levels (see Savard et al., 1983), little doubt exists that both neonatal and adult hypothyroidism depress synthesis and turnover rates of 5-HT, thus suggesting a serotonergic hypoactivity in the CNS (Vaccari, 1982). In addition, the existence of a depression of the dopaminergic system is supported by several studies showing decreased steady-state levels of dopamine (DA) in the whole brain, the diencephalon, or in striatal, hypothalamic and brain stem tissues of newborn hypothyroid rats (Rastogi et al., 1976; Puymirat, 1985; Leret and Fraile, 1986), along with a consistent decrease of hypothalamic DOPAC content (Puymirat, 1985). According to the available literature, a depression of norepinephrine (NE) pathways in the neonatal or adult hypothyroid brain also seems likely to occur. Finally, some evidence indicates that neonatal and adult hyperthyroidisms increase the synthesis and turnover rates of 5-HT and catecholamines (see Vaccari, 1983; Puymirat, 1985).

Neurotransmitter-linked enzyme activities have been shown to respond differently to thyroid manipulations. Thus, tyrosine hydroxylase and monoamine oxidase (MAO) activities may be either increased or decreased in the hypothyroid brain (Rastogi et al., 1976; Vaccari et al., 1977 and 1983a) depending on the experimental variables previously discussed in the text.

In summary, it is sufficiently proven that neonatal and, to a lesser extent, adult hypothyroidism depress the monoaminergic tone, while the opposite occurs in hyperthyroidism.

TABLE 1

Receptor alterations in the dysthyroid CNS

Receptor[a]	Dysthyroidism	Brain region	Age of onset of dysthyroidism	Effect[b]		References
Dopamine (D_2)	Hypo-	Striatum	Newborn	Decrease	(c)	Vaccari and Timiras (1981); Kalaria and Prince (1985)
			Newborn	No change	(Tx)	Del Cerro et al. (1986)
			Weaned	Increase	(d)	Overstreet et al. (1984)
			Adult	Decrease	(c)	Kalaria and Prince (1986)
			Adult	No change	(c)	Crocker and Overstreet (1984)
			Adult	Increase	(d)	Crocker et al. (1986)
	Hyper-	Striatum	Newborn	Decrease		Vaccari and Timiras (1981)
			Adult	No change		Atterwill (1981)
Serotonin						
5-HT$_1$	Hypo-	Brain	Newborn	Increase	(c)	Vaccari et al. (1983b)
			Newborn	No change	(HI)	Vaccari et al. (1983b)
5-HT$_2$	Hypo-	Brain	Newborn	Increase	(c)	Vaccari et al. (1983b)
			Newborn	No change	(HI)	Vaccari et al. (1983b)
5-HT$_1$	Hyper-	Brain	Newborn	No change		Vaccari et al. (1983b)
5-HT$_2$	Hyper-	Brain	Newborn	No change		Vaccari et al. (1983b)
Imipramine	Hypo-	Cortex	Newborn	Decrease	(c)	Vaccari (1985)
		Striatum	Newborn	No change	(c)	Vaccari (1985)
		Cortex, striatum	Adult	No change	(c)	Vaccari (1985)
Adrenergic						
Alpha$_1$	Hypo-	Cortex	Adult	Decrease	(c)	Gross et al. (1981); Kalaria and Prince (1986)
	Hyper-	Cortex	Adult	Increase		Gross et al. (1981)
		Spinal cord	Newborn	No change		Lau et al. (1985)
Alpha$_2$	Hypo-	Cortex	Adult	Decrease	(c)	Gross and Schümann (1981)
	Hyper-	Cortex	Adult	No change		Gross and Schümann (1981)
Beta	Hypo-	Forebrain, cerebellum	Newborn	Decrease	(c)	Smith et al. (1980)
		Cortex, striatum, hypothalamus	Adult	Decrease	(c)	Gross et al. (1980b); Atterwill et al. (1984)
		Lymphocytes (human)	Adult	Increase		Fantozzi et al. (1983)
	Hyper-	Cortex, hypothalamus	Newborn	No change		Atterwill et al. (1984)
		Striatum	Newborn	Increase		Atterwill et al. (1984)
		Forebrain, cerebellum	Newborn	Increase		Smith et al. (1980)
		Spinal cord	Newborn	Increase		Lau et al. (1985)
		Cortex	Adult	Decrease		Schmidt and Schultz (1985)
		Striatum, hypothalamus	Adult	Increase		Atterwill et al. (1984)
Histamine (H_1)	Hypo-	Brain	Newborn	Decrease	(c)	Codolà and Garcia (1985)
		Brain	Adult	Decrease	(c)	Codolà and Garcia (1985)
	Hyper-	Brain	Newborn	Increase		Codolà and Garcia (1985)
		Brain	Adult	No change		Codolà and Garcia (1985)
Cholinergic (Muscarinic)	Hypo-	Forebrain, cortex, striatum	Newborn	No change	(c)	Patel et al. (1980); Kalaria et al. (1981)
		Cerebellum	Newborn	Increase	(c)	Patel et al. (1980)
		Brain, cortex, striatum	Adult	No change	(c)	Kastrup and Christensen (1984); Kalaria and Prince (1986)

TABLE 1 (continued)

Receptor[a]	Dysthyroidism	Brain region	Age of onset of dysthyroidism	Effect[b]	References
	Hyper-	Forebrain	Newborn	No change	Patel et al. (1980)
		Cerebellum	Newborn	Decrease	Patel et al. (1980)
		Brain	Adult	No change	Kastrup and Christensen (1984)
GABA	Hypo-	Cerebellum	Newborn	Decrease (c)	Patel et al. (1980)
		Forebrain, striatum	Newborn	No change (c)	Patel et al. (1980); Kalaria and Prince (1985)
		Cerebellum, striatum	Newborn	Increase (Tx)	Del Cerro et al. (1986)
		Cortex	Adult	Decrease (c)	Kalaria and Prince (1986)
		Striatum	Adult	No change (c)	Kalaria and Prince (1986)
	Hyper-	Forebrain	Newborn	No change	Patel et al. (1980)
		Cerebellum	Newborn	Increase	Patel et al. (1980)
Glutamate	Hypo-	Striatum	Newborn	Decrease (c)	Kalaria and Prince (1985)
Benzodiazepine	Hypo-	Cortex	Adult	Increase (Tx)	Medina et al. (1984)
	Hyper-	Cortex	Adult	Decrease	Medina et al. (1984)
			Adult	Increase	Gavish et al. (1986)

[a] The ligands used were: [^{3}H]spiperone (D_2; 5-HT$_2$); [^{3}H]5-HT (5-HT$_1$); [^{3}H]WB4101 or [^{3}H]prazosin (alpha$_1$); [^{3}H]clonidine (alpha$_2$); [^{3}H]dihydroalprenolol (beta); [^{3}H]GABA or [^{3}H]muscimol (GABA); [^{3}H]glutamate (glutamate); [^{3}H]QNB (muscarinic); [^{3}H]mepyramine (histamine); [^{3}H]flunitrazepam (benzodiazepine); [^{3}H]imipramine (imipramine/5-HT uptake).
[b] The methods used to induce hypothyroidism in rats are indicated in brackets: (c) = methimazole or propylthiouracyl; (Tx) = surgical ablation; (r) = ^{131}I; (d) = iodine-deficient diet; (HI) = high-iodine diet.

Of particular relevance to the central effects of dysthyroidism is the possibility that iodothyronine hormones enter into a neurotransmitter pathway, serving as substrates for biogenic amine-forming enzymes (Dratman et al., 1984). A neurotransmitter-precursor role for thyroid hormones is strongly suggested by the structural similarity of T_4 and tyrosine (Dratman, 1974).

Receptors and their functions in dysthyroidism

Since thyroid hormones regulate the synthesis or degradation of specific proteins at the transcriptional or translational level, every receptor protein in central neurotransmission may be a putative target for thyroid influences in health and disease. Such a primary, direct effect of dysthyroidism may be either amplified or counteracted by subsequent receptor alterations (increased or decreased density of receptors, modifications in their affinity for ligands) secondary to the synaptic availability of pertinent transmitters (Reisine, 1981). Of course, the mere description of any receptor alteration is not very informative, unless they are correlated with modifications of receptor-mediated functions.

The study of receptor functions is usually based upon the behavioral or biochemical effects of receptor-specific agonists or antagonists. Correlating receptors to functional aberrations is a difficult task. This is particularly true in dysthyroidism studies, where there is already disagreement about the behavioral effects intrinsic to hormone dysfunction (see Table 2), and where the use of receptor-specific drugs to assess receptor functions may introduce an additional variable in the system. Thus, all of us who are familiar with thyroid studies know that neonatal and adult hyperthyroid rats are hyperactive and hyperreactive,

TABLE 2

Putative receptor functions in dysthyroidism

Receptor system	Dysthy-roidism[a]	Age of onset of dysthyroidism	Effect[b]		References
Intrinsic	Hypo-	Newborn	Spontaneous locomotion	Decrease (c)	Rastogi et al. (1976); Tamasy et al. (1986)
		Newborn	Spontaneous locomotion	Increase (c)	Schalock et al. (1977)
		Newborn	Spontaneous locomotion	No change (c, d)	Overstreet et al. (1984); Comer and Norton (1985)
		Newborn	Learning ability	Decrease (c, d, Tx)	Schalock et al. (1977); Hendrich et al. (1984); Overstreet et al. (1984)
		Newborn	Learning ability	No change (c)	Tamasy et al. (1986)
		Adult	Spontaneous locomotion	Decrease (c, Tx)	Ito et al. (1977); Fundarò et al. (1985)
		Adult	Learning ability	Decrease (c)	Fundarò et al. (1985)
	Hyper-	Newborn	Spontaneous locomotion	Increase	Rastogi et al. (1981)
		Newborn (mice)	Spontaneous locomotion	No change	Forster et al. (1981)
		Adult	Spontaneous locomotion	Increase	Ito et al. (1977); Kulcsàr et al. (1980)
		Adult	Learning ability	No change	Fundarò et al. (1985)
Serotonin	Hypo-	Newborn	5-HT syndrome	Decrease (c)	Vaccari (1982)
		Adult	5-HT syndrome	Decrease (Tx)	Heal et al. (1983)
	Hyper-	Adult	5-HT syndrome	Increase	Atterwill (1981); Brochet et al. (1985)
		Adult (human)	L-Tryptophan effect	Increase	Coppen et al. (1972)
Dopamine	Hypo-	Newborn	Apomorphine behavior	Increase (d)	Overstreet et al. (1984)
		Adult	Apomorphine behavior	Increase (r)	Crocker et al. (1986)
		Adult	Haloperidol catalepsy	Decrease (c, r)	Crocker and Overstreet (1984); Crocker et al. (1986)
	Hyper-	Newborn	Apomorphine behavior	Decrease	Atterwill (1981)
		Newborn	Apomorphine behavior	Increase	Rastogi et al. (1981)
		Newborn (mice)	Amphetamine behavior	Increase	Forster et al. (1981)
		Adult	Apomorphine behavior	Decrease	Atterwill (1981)
		Adult	Apomorphine behavior	No change	Strömbom et al. (1977)
		Adult	Apomorphine behavior	Increase	Heal and Atterwill (1982)
		Adult	Haloperidol catalepsy	Increase	Atterwill (1981); Crocker and Overstreet (1984)
		Adult	Dopamine behavior	Increase	Engström et al. (1974); Atterwill (1981); Heal and Atterwill (1982)
		Adult	Dopamine behavior	No change	Strömbom et al. (1977)
Adrenergic Alpha$_2$	Hypo-	Newborn	Clonidine activity	Increase (c)	Heal et al. (1984)
		Adult	Clonidine activity	Decrease (c)	Atterwill et al. (1984)
		Adult	Clonidine activity	Increase (Tx)	Heal et al. (1983)
		Adult	NE release	No change (c)	Gross et al. (1980a)
	Hyper-	Newborn	Clonidine activity	Increase	Heal et al. (1984)
		Adult	Clonidine activity	Increase	Strömbom et al. (1977); Atterwill et al. (1984)
Beta	Hypo-	Adult	cAMP accumulation	Decrease (c)	Gross et al. (1980a)
		Adult	Firing of Purkinje cells	Decrease (c)	Marwaha and Prasad (1981)
	Hyper-	Adult	cAMP accumulation	Decrease	Schmidt and Schultz (1985)
Benzodiazepine	Hyper-	Adult	Anticonvulsant thresholds	No change	Atterwill and Nutt (1983)

[a] The methods used to induce hypothyroidism in rats are indicated in brackets: (c) = methimazole or propylthiouracyl; (Tx) = surgical ablation; (r) = ^{131}I; (d) = iodine-deficient diet.
[b] Apomorphine behavior = stereotypy, spontaneous locomotion etc.; amphetamine behavior = hyperactivity; 5-HT syndrome = shaking behavior, side-to-side head movements, stereotypy; clonidine activity = sedation or hyperactivity, depending on the dose.

80

they bite, and that hypothyroids are calm and can be easily manipulated. Nonetheless, spontaneous activity and reactivity in hypothyroid rats have been described as either decreased, or increased, or fluctuating in different studies (see Table 2). Avoidance learning, curiosity and 'memory', however, appear to be consistently decreased in experimental hypothyroidism, thus mimicking some aspects of the human cretinoid syndrome.

The up-to-date status of dysthyroidism-associated receptor alterations is summarized in Table 1. The density of dopaminergic D_2-type receptors is consistently decreased in striatal membranes from newborn and adult rats given goitrogenic drugs (Vaccari and Timiras, 1981; Kalaria and Prince, 1985, 1986), whereas an iodine-deficient diet given to weaned pups (i.e. late in development) (Overstreet et al., 1984) or ^{131}I to adult rats (Crocker et al., 1986) increases the number of D_2 receptors. The hyperthyroidism-associated D_2-receptor deficit we have found (Vaccari and Timiras, 1981) might either be due to T_3 toxicity, or represent the adaptive response towards an increased dopaminergic tone. As a matter of fact, the DA system is overactive in neonatal and adult hyperthyroids, as may be inferred from a number of studies showing enhanced behavioral responses to the stimulation of DA neurons as obtained with directly or indirectly acting DA-agonists such as apomorphine, L-DOPA, DA itself, or amphetamine (Table 2). However, no precise statement can be made concerning the status of DA transmission in hypothyroidism (Table 2). For this purpose it will be important to characterize the complex behavioral components of DA stimulation, e.g. locomotor activity, stereotypy, catalepsy, etc., more thoroughly. Such behaviours might be triggered by different types of DA receptors, or co-mediated by additional transmitters, and may respond differently to thyroid dysfunctions.

Hypothyroid newborn and adult rats undergo a clear-cut serotonergic hypoactivity (Vaccari, 1982; Heal et al., 1983), while the opposite occurs in adult hyperthyroid rats and mice (Atterwill,

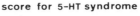

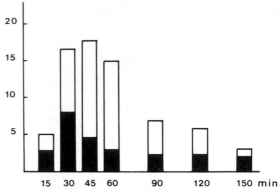

Fig. 4. Time-course of the serotonergic behavioral syndrome (tremors, wet dog shakes, side-to-side head movements etc.) induced by an i.p. injection of 220 mg/kg L-5-hydroxytryptophan to 32–34-day-old, euthyroid (open column) and MMI-hypothyroid (solid column) rats. Results are from Vaccari (1982).

1981; Brochet et al., 1985) as assessed by the behavioral syndrome which is believed to reflect activation of central 5-HT neurons, after treatment of dysthyroid animals with 5-HT precursors (Fig. 4). It is interesting that the antidepressant activity of the 5-HT precursor L-tryptophan or of imipramine (a marker for the 5-HT reuptake system) is potentiated in human hyperthyroids (Coppen et al., 1972). The maximum number of both 5-HT$_1$- and 5-HT$_2$-type receptors has been found to increase in the brain of MMI-treated newborn rats, and to be unchanged in T_3- treated hyperthyroids (Vaccari et al., 1983b). The greater density of 5-HT receptors might be an additional adaptive reaction to the hypothyroidism-related depression of the 5-HT pathways.

It is generally agreed that neonatal and adult hypothyroidisms decrease the number of α_1-, α_2- and β-adrenoceptors in cortical, striatal, hypothalamic and brain membranes (Table 1). The effects of hyperthyroidism are less obvious. Moreover, it is noteworthy that the number of membrane β-adrenoceptors of lymphocytes from human hypothyroids is increased (Fantozzi et al., 1983).

The dysthyroidism-provoked alterations of adrenoceptors do not fit well with the impairments of functions they probably mediate. For example, clonidine has been widely used as a ligand or as an agonist of α_2-receptors. The density of clonidine binding sites decreases or remains the same in cortical membranes of adult hypo- and hyperthyroid rats, respectively (Gross and Schümann, 1981). In contrast, clonidine-induced sedation, an index for stimulation of presynaptic α_2-receptors which regulate the feedback inhibition of NE release (Westfall, 1984), is enhanced in both hypo- and hyperthyroid newborn rats (Heal et al., 1984), and diminished in adult hypothyroids (Atterwill et al., 1984). An explanation for these discrepancies might be that receptor binding assays almost exclusively reveal postsynaptic α_2-adrenoceptors (U'Prichard et al., 1980), which might not react to dysthyroid insults in the same way as presynaptically located α_2-autoreceptors (Heal et al., 1984). In addition, age-related differences in the ratio of pre- and postsynaptic α_2-receptor numbers may be an important variable between studies (Dausse et al., 1982). Thus, one might cautiously conclude that in the CNS of hypothyroid newborn rats only, or in hyperthyroidism, there is a greater α_2-mediated inhibition of NE release than in euthyroidism.

As far as β-adrenoceptors are concerned, their hypothyroidism-associated decreased density in cortical, striatal and cerebellar membranes (Smith et al., 1980; Gross et al., 1980b; Atterwill et al., 1984) agrees well with the decrease of NE- or isoprenaline-stimulated cAMP accumulation in cortical slices of hypothyroid rats (Gross et al., 1980a) and with the depressed firing responses of Purkinje neurons to NE (Marwaha and Prasad, 1981), as indices of β-mediated central adrenergic activity. A receptor-to-function correlation is less easily stated in hyperthyroidism, due to inconsistency of the available results (see Tables 1 and 2). A similar conclusion can be drawn for benzodiazepine receptors: in fact, hyperthyroidism has been found to either increase or decrease the density of flunitrazepam binding sites in cortical

membranes of adult rats (Medina et al., 1984; Gavish et al., 1986). Furthermore, hyperthyroidism does not affect the flurazepam-induced increase or the FG 7142-provoked decrease in pentetrazol seizure thresholds, as an index of benzodiazepine receptor function (Atterwill and Nutt, 1983).

Cerebellar GABAergic and cholinergic muscarinic receptors seem to be sensitive targets for dysthyroidism-related influences as well (Table 1). Finally, the density of histamine H_1-type receptors and of imipramine binding sites decreases in the brain and cortex of newborn and adult hypothyroid rats (Vaccari, 1985; Codolà and Garcia, 1985).

Conclusions

Experimentally provoked thyroid dysfunctions during the fetal and early postnatal period in mammalians induce a morphologic and biochemical cascade of events underlying abnormal brain development, and ending with behavioral aberrations which are in some aspects similar to the neuropsychiatric disturbances of human dysthyroidism. A lack or deficiency of thyroid hormones results in an abnormal regulation of the synthesis or degradation of specific proteins such as nuclear or cytosol T_3 receptors, microtubules and neurofilaments, enzymes and receptors involved in neurotransmitter pathways. Alterations in the kinetics of microtubule assembly may affect the build-up of the nerve cytostructure and lead to a deficient synaptogenesis. Abnormalities in the synaptic network would then, as expected, result in a widespread malfunction of the neurotransmitter machinery. The receptor alterations that are primarily due to protein abnormalities might be further complicated by compensatory adaptations of their number or affinity, a consequence of dysthyroidism-associated excessive or deficient availability of pertinent transmitters.

Consistent with the hypothesis of a monoamine imbalance in the origin of mental disorders, a central serotonergic, noradrenergic and, probably, dopaminergic hypofunction in neonatal hypothyroidism would underlie behavioral teratogenesis.

Such conclusions are necessarily inferred from animal studies; a promising approach to a better understanding of the mechanisms underlying central teratogenic consequences of human dysthyroidism will be based on the use of blood platelets as a model of peripheral neurons.

References

Atterwill, C.K. (1981) Effects of acute and chronic triiodothyronine (T_3) administration to rats on central 5-HT and dopamine-mediated behavioral responses and related brain biochemistry. *Neuropharmacology*, 20: 131–144.

Atterwill, C.K. and Nutt, D.J. (1983) Thyroid hormones do not alter brain benzodiazepine receptor function in-vivo. *J. Pharm. Pharmacol.*, 35: 767–768.

Atterwill, C.K., Bunn, S.J., Atkinson, D.J., Smith, S.L. and Heal, D.J. (1984) Effects of thyroid status on presynaptic alpha$_2$-adrenoceptor function and beta-adrenoceptor binding in the rat brain. *J. Neural Transm.*, 59: 43–55.

Barchas, J.D., Elliott, G.R. and Berger, P.A. (1977) Biogenic amine hypotheses of schizophrenia. In J.D. Barchas, P.A. Berger, R.D. Ciaranello and G.R. Elliott (Eds.), *Psychopharmacology*, Oxford University Press, New York, pp. 100–120.

Bernal, J., Refetoff, S. and De Groot, L.J. (1978) Abnormalities of triiodothyronine binding to lymphocyte and fibroblast nuclei from a patient with peripheral tissue resistance to thyroid hormone action. *J. Clin. Endocrinol. Metab.*, 47: 1266–1272.

Biassoni, R. and Vaccari, A. (1985) Selective effects of thiol reagents on the binding sites for imipramine and neurotransmitter amines in the rat brain. *Br. J. Pharmacol.*, 85: 447–456.

Biegon, A., Rainbow, T.C. and McEwen, B.S. (1985) Corticosterone modulation of neurotransmitter receptors in rat hippocampus: a quantitative autoradiographic study. *Brain Res.*, 332: 309–314.

Brasel, J.A. and Boyd, B. (1975) Influence of thyroid hormone on fetal brain growth and development. In D.A. Fisher and G.B. Burrow (Eds.), *Perinatal Thyroid Physiology and Disease*, Raven Press, New York, pp. 59–71.

Brochet, D., Martin, P., Soubrie, P. and Simon, P. (1985) Effects of triiodothyronine on the 5-hydroxytryptophan-induced head twitch and its potentiation by antidepressants in mice. *Eur. J. Pharmacol.*, 112: 411–414.

Chopra, I.J., Solomon, D.H., Chopra, U., Wu, S.Y., Fisher, D.A. and Nakamura, H. (1978) Pathways of metabolism of thyroid hormones. *Rec. Progr. Horm. Res.*, 34: 521–567.

Codolà, R. and Garcia, A. (1985) Effect of thyroid state on histamine H$_1$ receptors in adult and developing rat brain. *Biochem. Pharmacol.*, 34: 4131–4136.

Comer, C.P. and Norton, S. (1985) Behavioral consequences of perinatal hypothyroidism in postnatal and adult rats. *Pharmacol. Biochem. Behav.*, 22: 605–611.

Coppen, A., Whybrow, P.C., Noguera, R., Maggs, R. and Prange, A.J. (1972) The comparative antidepressant value of L-tryptophan and imipramine with and without attempted potentiation by triiodothyronine. *Arch. Gen. Psychiatry*, 26: 234–241.

Crocker, A.D. and Overstreet, D.H. (1984) Modification of the behavioural effect of haloperidol and of dopamine receptor regulation by altered thyroid status. *Psychopharmacology*, 82: 102–106.

Crocker, A.D., Overstreet, D.H. and Crocker, J.M. (1986) Hypothyroidism leads to increased dopamine receptor sensitivity and concentration. *Pharmacol. Biochem. Behav.*, 24: 1593–1597.

Dausse, J.P., Le Quan-Bui, K.H., Gallagher, D.W. and Agajanian, G.K. (1982) Alpha$_1$- and alpha$_2$-adrenoceptors in rat cerebral cortex: effects of neonatal treatment with 6-hydroxydopamine. *Eur. J. Pharmacol.* 78: 15–20.

Del Cerro, M.R., Somoza, G., Segovia, S. and Guillamòn, A. (1986) Effects of neonatal thyroidectomy on neurotransmitter receptors in several regions of the rat brain. *IRCS Med. Sci.*, 14: 92–93.

Dillman, W., Surks, M.I. and Oppenheimer, J.H. (1974) Quantitative aspects of iodothyronine binding by cytosol proteins of rat liver and kidney. *Endocrinology*, 95: 492–498.

Döhler, K.D., Wong, C.C. and Von Zur Mühlen, A. (1979) The rat as a model for the study of drug effects on thyroid function: consideration of methodological problems. *Pharmac. Ther.*, 5: 305–318.

Dozin-Van Roye, B. and De Nayer, P. (1978) Triiodothyronine binding to brain cytosol receptors during maturation. *FEBS Lett.*, 96: 152–154.

Dratman, M.B. (1974) On the mechanism of action of thyroxin, an amino acid analog of tyrosine. *J. Theor. Biol.*, 46: 255–270.

Dratman, M.B., Crutchfield, F.L. and Gordon, J.T. (1984) Thyroid hormones and adrenergic neurotransmitters. In E. Usdin, A. Carlsson, A. Dahlström and J. Engel (Eds.), *Catecholamines: Neuropharmacology and Central Nervous System–Theoretical Aspects*, A.R. Liss, New York, pp. 425–439.

Dratman, M.B., Futaesaka, Y., Crutchfield, F.L., Berman, N., Payne, B., Sar, M. and Stumpf, W.E. (1982) Iodine-125-labeled triiodothyronine in rat brain: evidence for localization in discrete neural systems. *Science*, 215: 309–312.

Eayrs, J.T. (1971) Thyroid and developing brain: anatomical and behavioral effects. In M. Hamburgh and E.J. Barrington (Eds.), *Hormones in Development*, Appleton Century Crofts, New York, pp. 345–355.

Engström, G. Svensson, T.H. and Waldeck, B. (1974) Thyroxine and brain catecholamines: increased transmitter synthesis and increased receptor sensitivity. *Brain Res.*, 77: 471–483.

Fantozzi, R., Brunelleschi, S., Cuomo, S., Defeo, L., Maggi, M., Mannelli, M., Serio, M. and Ledda, F. (1983) Changes in the density of human lymphocyte beta adrenergic receptors in hypothyroidism. *Acta Pharmacol. Toxicol.*, 53: Suppl.1, 120.

Fisher, D.A., Dussault, J.H., Sack, J.H. and Chopra, I.J. (1977) Ontogenesis of hypothalamic-pituitary-thyroid function and metabolism in man, sheep and rat. *Rec. Progr. Horm. Res.*, 33: 59–116.

Forster, M.J., Nagy, Z.M. and Murphy, J.M. (1981) Potentiation of amphetamine-induced hyperactivity in the adult mouse following neonatal thyroxine administration. *Bull. Psychonomic Soc.*, 18: 337–339.

Fundarò, A., Molinengo, L. and Cassone, M.C. (1985) The transition from a fixed ratio to a fixed interval schedule of reinforcement in hypo and hyperthyroid rats. *Pharmacol. Res. Commun.*, 17: 463–470.

Gavish, M., Weizman, A., Okun, F. and Youdim, M.B. (1986) Modulatory effects of thyroxine treatment on central and peripheral benzodiazepine receptors in the rat. *J. Neurochem.*, 47: 1106–1110.

Geel, S.E. (1977) Development-related changes of triiodothyronine binding to brain cytosol receptors. *Nature*, 269: 428–430.

Glorieux, J., Dussault, J.H., Letarte, J., Guyda, H. and Morissette, J. (1983) Preliminary results on the mental development of hypothyroid infants detected by the Quebec screening program. *J. Pediatr.*, 102: 19–22.

Gross, G., Brodde, O.E. and Schümann, H.J. (1980a) Effects of thyroid hormone deficiency on pre- and postsynaptic noradrenergic mechanisms in the rat cerebral cortex. *Arch. Int. Pharmacodyn. Thér.*, 244: 219–230.

Gross, G., Brodde, O.E. and Schümann, H.J. (1980b) Decreased number of beta-adrenoceptors in cerebral cortex of hypothyroid rats. *Eur. J. Pharmacol.*, 61: 191–194.

Gross, G. and Schümann, H.J. (1981) Reduced number of alpha$_2$-adrenoceptors in cortical brain membranes of hypothyroid rats. *J. Pharm. Pharmacol.*, 33: 552–554.

Gross, G., Brodde, O.E. and Schümann, H.J. (1981) Regulation of alpha$_1$-adrenoceptors in the cerebral cortex of the rat by thyroid hormones. *Naunyn-Schmied. Arch. Pharmacol.* 316: 45–50.

Heal, D.J. and Atterwill, C.K. (1982) Repeated administration of triiodothyronine (T_3) to rats enhances nigrostriatal and mesolimbic dopaminergic behavioural responses. *Neuropharmacology*, 21: 159–162.

Heal, D.J., O'Shaughnessy, K.M., Smith, S.L. and Nutt, D.J. (1983) Hypophysectomy alters both 5- hydroxytryptamine- and alpha$_2$-adrenoceptor-mediated behavioural changes in the rat. *Eur. J. Pharmacol.*, 89: 167–171.

Heal, D.J., Smith, S.L. and Atterwill, C.K. (1984) Effects of thyroid status on clonidine-induced hypoactivity responses in the developing rat. *J. Neural Transm.*, 60: 295–302.

Hendrich, C.E., Jackson, W.J. and Porterfield, S.P. (1984) Behavioral testing of progenies of Tx (hypothyroid) and growth hormone-treated Tx rats: an animal model for mental retardation. *Neuroendocrinology*, 38: 429–437.

Hollingsworth, D.R., Mabry, C.C. and Reid, M.C. (1980) Congenital Grave's disease. In C. La Cauza and A.W. Root (Eds.), *Problems in Pediatric Endocrinology*, Academic Press, New York, P. 169.

Ito, J.M., Valcana, T. and Timiras, P.S. (1977) Effects of hypo- and hyperthyroidism on regional monoamine metabolism in the adult rat brain. *Neuroendocrinology*, 24: 55–64.

Jubiz, W. (1979) *Endocrinology – A Logical Approach for Clinicians*, McGraw-Hill, New York, pp. 45–79.

Kalaria, R.N., Kotas, A.M., Prince, A.K. and Reynolds, R. (1981) Neuronal development in discrete areas of rat brain during neonatal thyroid deficiency. *Br. J. Pharmacol.*, 77: 103P.

Kalaria, R.N. and Prince, A.K. (1985) Effect of thyroid deficiency on the development of cholinergic, GABA, dopaminergic and glutamate neuron markers and DNA concentrations in the rat corpus striatum. *Int. J. Dev. Neurosci.*, 3: 655–666.

Kalaria, R.N. and Prince, A.K. (1986) Decreased neurotransmitter receptor binding in striatum and cortex from adult hypothyroid rats. *Brain Res.*, 364: 268–274.

Kastrup, J. and Christensen, N.J. (1984) Lack of effects of thyroid hormones on muscarine cholinergic receptors in rat brain and heart. *Scand. J. Clin. Lab. Invest.*, 44: 33–38.

Klein, R. (1986) Screening for congenital hypothyroidism. *Lancet*, 8503: 403.

Kulcsàr, A., Kulcsàr-Gergely, J. and Kulcsàr, L. (1980) A hyperthyreosis model experiment in rats. *Arzneim.-Forsch.*, 30: 44–47.

Latham, K.R., Ring, J.C. and Baxter, J.D. (1976) Solubilized nuclear 'receptors' for thyroid hormones. Physical characteristics and binding properties, evidence for multiple forms. *J. Biol. Chem.*, 251: 7388–7397.

Lau, C., Pylypiw, A. and Ross, L.L. (1985) Development of serotonergic and adrenergic receptors in the rat spinal cord: effects of neonatal chemical lesions and hyperthyroidism. *Dev. Brain Res.*, 19: 57–66.

Lauder, J. (1977) The effects of early hypo- and hyperthyroidism on the development of rat cerebellar cortex. III. Kinetics of cell proliferation in the external granular layer. *Brain Res.*, 126: 31–51.

Legrand, J. (1979) Morphogenetic actions of thyroid hormones. *Trends Neurosci.*, 2: 234–236.

Legrand, J. (1980) Effects of thyroid hormones on brain development, with particular emphasis on glial cells and myelination. In C. Di Benedetta, R. Balàsz, G. Gombos and G. Porcellati (Eds.), *Multidisciplinary Approach to Brain Development*, Elsevier, Amsterdam, pp. 279–292.

Legrand, J. (1984) Effects of thyroid hormones on central nervous system development. In J. Yanay (Ed.), *Neurobehavioral Teratology*, Elsevier, Amsterdam, pp. 331–363.

Lennon, A. M., Francon, J., Fellous, A. and Nunez, J. (1980) Rat, mouse and guinea pig brain development and microtubule assembly. *J. Neurochem.*, 35: 804–813.

Leret, M. L. and Fraile, A. (1986) Influence of thyroidectomy on brain catecholamines during the postnatal period. *Comp. Biochem. Physiol.*, 83: 117–121.

Linquette, M., Lefebvre, J., Racadot, A., Cappoen, J. P. and Fontaine-Delort, S. (1976) Taux de production et concentration plasmatique moyenne du cortisol dans l'hyperthyroïdie. *Ann. Endocrinol. (Paris)*, 37: 331–345.

Marwaha, J. and Prasad, K. N. (1981) Hypothyroidism elicits electrophysiological noradrenergic subsensitivity in rat cerebellum. *Science*, 214: 675–677.

Medina, J. H., Tumilasci, O. and De Robertis, E. (1984) Thyroid hormones regulate benzodiazepine receptors in rat cerebral cortex. *IRCS Med. Sci.*, 12: 158–159.

Menezes-Ferreira, M. M. and Torresani, J. (1983) Mécanismes d'action des hormones thyroïdiennes au niveau cellulaire. *Ann. Endocrinol. (Paris)*, 44: 205–216.

Meyer, J. S. (1985) Biochemical effects of corticosteroids on neural tissues. *Physiol. Rev.*, 65: 946–1020.

New England Congenital Hypothyroidism Collaborative (1984) Characteristics of infantile hypothyroidism discovered on neonatal screening. *J. Pediatr.*, 104: 539–544.

Nunez, J. (1984) Effects of thyroid hormones during brain differentiation. *Mol. Cell. Endocrinol.*, 37: 125–132.

Nunez, J. (1985) Microtubules and brain development: the effects of thyroid hormones. *Neurochem. Int.*, 7: 959–968.

Overstreeet, D. H., Crocker, A. D., Lawson, C. A., McIntosh, G. H. and Crocker, J. M. (1984) Alterations in the dopaminergic system and behaviour in rats reared on iodine-deficient diets. *Pharmacol. Biochem. Behav.*, 21: 561–565.

Pascual-Leone, A. M., Escrivà, F., Alvarez, C., Goya, L. and Rodriguez, C. (1985) Influence of hormones and undernutrition on brain development in newborn rats. *Biol. Neonate*, 48: 228–236.

Patel, A. J., Rabié, A., Lewis, P. D. and Balàsz, R. (1976) Effects of thyroid deficiency on postnatal cell formation in the rat brain. A biochemical investigation. *Brain Res.*, 104: 33–48.

Patel, A. J., Smith, R. M., Kingsbury, A. E., Hunt, A. and Balàsz, R. (1980) Effects of thyroid state on brain development: muscarinic acetylcholine and GABA receptors. *Brain Res.*, 198: 389–402.

Pittman, J. A. (1971) *The Thyroid*, Harper and Row, New York, pp. 644–655.

Puymirat, J. (1985) Effects of dysthyroidism on central catecholaminergic neurons. *Neurochem. Int.*, 7: 969–977.

Rabié, A., Favre, C., Clavel, M. C. and Legrand, J. (1977) Effect of thyroid dysfunction on the development of the rat cerebellum, with special reference to cell death within the internal granular layer. *Brain Res.*, 120: 521–531.

Rabié, A., Patel, A. J., Clavel, M. C. and Legrand, J. (1979) Effect of thyroid deficiency on the growth of the hippocampus in the rat. A combined biochemical and morphological study. *Dev. Neurosci.*, 2: 183–194.

Rami, A., Rabié, A. and Patel, A. J. (1986) Thyroid hormone and development of the rat hippocampus: cell acquisition in the dentate gyrus. *Neuroscience*, 19: 1207–1216.

Rastogi, R. B., LaPierre, Y. and Singhal, R. L. (1976) Evidence for the role of brain biogenic amines in depressed motor activity seen in chemically thyroidectomized rats. *J. Neurochem.*, 26: 443–449.

Rastogi, R. B., Singhal, R. L. and LaPierre, Y. D. (1981) Effects of apomorphine on behavioural activity and brain catecholamine synthesis in normal and L-triiodothyronine-treated rats. *J. Neural Transm.*, 50: 139–148.

Rebière, A. and Legrand, J. (1972) Données quantitatives sur la synaptogenèse dans le cervelet du rat normal et rendu hypothyroïdien par le propylthiouracile. *C. R. Acad. Sci. (Paris)*, 274: 3581–3584.

Reisine, T. (1981) Adaptive changes in catecholamine receptors in the central nervous system. *Neuroscience*, 6: 1471–1502.

Ruel, J., Faure, R. and Dussault, J. H. (1985) Regional distribution of nuclear T_3 receptors in rat brain and evidence for preferential localization in neurons. *J. Endocrinol. Invest.*, 8: 343–348.

Savard, P., Mérand, Y., Di Paolo, T. and Dupont, A. (1983) Effects of thyroid state on serotonin, 5-hydroxyindole acetic acid and substance P contents in discrete brain nuclei of adult rats. *Neuroscience*, 10: 1399–1404.

Sawin, C. T. (1985) Hypothyroidism. *Med. Clin. N. Am.*, 69: 989–1004.

Schalock, R. L., Brown, N. J. and Smith, R. L. (1977) Neonatal hypothyroidism: behavioral, thyroid hormonal and neuroanatomical effects. *Physiol. Behav.*, 19: 489–491.

Schmidt, B. H. and Schultz, J. E. (1985) Chronic thyroxine treatment of rats down-regulates the noradrenergic cyclic AMP generating system in cerebral cortex. *J. Pharmacol. Exp. Ther.*, 233: 466–472.

Schwartz, H. L. and Oppenheimer, J. H. (1978a) Nuclear triiodothyronine receptor sites in brain: probable identity with hepatic receptors and regional distribution. *Endocrinology*, 103: 267–273.

Schwartz, H. L. and Oppenheimer, J. H. (1978b) Ontogenesis of 3,5,3'-triiodothyronine receptors in neonatal rat brain: dissociation between receptor concentration and stimulation of oxygen consumption by 3,5,3'-triiodothyronine. *Endocrinology*, 103: 943–948.

Shire, J.G. and Beamer, W.G. (1984) Adrenal changes in genetically hypothyroid mice. *J. Endocrinol.*, 102: 277–280.

Smith, R.M., Patel, A.J., Kingsbury, A.E., Hunt, A. and Balász, R. (1980) Effects of thyroid state on brain development: beta-adrenergic receptors and 5'-nucleotidase activity. *Brain Res.*, 198: 375–387.

Strömbom, U., Svensson, T.H., Jackson, D.M. and Engström, G. (1977) Hyperthyroidism, specifically increased response to central NA-(alpha)-receptor stimulation and generally increased monoamine turnover in brain. *J. Neural Transm.*, 41: 73–92.

Strupp, B.J. and Levitsky, D.A. (1983) Early brain insult and cognition: a comparison of malnutrition and hypothyroidism. *Dev. Psychobiol.*, 16: 535–549.

Tamasy, V., Meisami, E., Vallerga, A. and Timiras, P.S. (1986) Rehabilitation from neonatal hypothyroidism: spontaneous motor activity, exploratory behavior, avoidance learning and responses of pituitary-thyroid axis to stress in male rats. *Psychoneuroendocrinology*, 11: 91–103.

Timiras, P.S. (1972) *Developmental Physiology and Aging*, MacMillan Co., New York, pp. 129–165.

Timiras, P.S. (1979) Distribution, development and function of thyroid hormone receptors in the brain. *Proc. West. Pharmacol. Soc.*, 22: 371–374.

U'Prichard, D.C., Reisine, T.D., Mason, S.T., Fibiger, H.C. and Yamamura, H.I. (1980) Modulation of rat brain alpha- and beta-adrenergic receptor populations by lesion of the dorsal noradrenergic bundle. *Brain Res.*, 180: 143–154.

Vaccari, A., Valcana, T. and Timiras, P.S. (1977) Effects of hypothyroidism on the enzymes for biogenic amines in the developing rat brain. *Pharmacol. Res. Commun.*, 9: 763–780.

Vaccari, A. and Timiras, P.S. (1981) Alterations in brain dopaminergic receptors in developing hypo- and hyperthyroid rats. *Neurochem. Int.*, 3: 149–153.

Vaccari, A. (1982) Decreased central serotonin function in hypothyroidism. *Eur. J. Pharmacol.*, 82: 93–95.

Vaccari, A., Biassoni, R. and Timiras, P.S. (1983a) Selective effects of neonatal hypothyroidism on monoamine oxidase activities in the rat brain. *J. Neurochem.*, 40: 1016–1025.

Vaccari, A., Biassoni, R. and Timiras, P.S. (1983b) Effects of neonatal dysthyroidism on serotonin type 1 and type 2 receptors in rat brain. *Eur. J. Pharmacol.*, 95: 53–63.

Vaccari, A. (1983) Effects of dysthyroidism on central monoaminergic neurotransmission. In M. Schlumpf and W. Lichtensteiger (Eds.), *Drugs and Hormones in Brain Development*, Karger, Basel, pp. 78–90.

Vaccari, A. (1985) Effects of neonatal antithyroid treatment on brain ^{3}H-imipramine binding sites. *Br. J. Pharmacol.*, 84: 773–778.

Valcana, T. and Timiras, P.S. (1978) Nuclear triiodothyronine receptors in the developing rat brain. *Mol. Cell. Endocrinol.*, 11: 31–41.

Vanderpas, J.B., Rivera-Vanderpas, M.T., Bourdoux, P., Luvivila, K., Lagasse, R., Perlmutter-Cremer, N., Delange, F., Lanoie, L., Ermans, A.M. and Thilly, C.H. (1986) Reversibility of severe hypothyroidism with supplementary iodine in patients with endemic cretinism. *N. Eng. J. Med.*, 315: 791–795.

Varma, S.K., Murray, R. and Stanbury, J.B. (1978) Effects of maternal hypothyroidism and triiodothyronine on the fetus and newborn in rats. *Endocrinology*, 102: 24–30.

Westfall, T.C. (1984) Evidence that noradrenergic transmitter release is regulated by presynaptic receptors. *FASEB Proc.*, 43: 1352–1357.

Whybrow, P. and Ferrell, R. (1974) Thyroid state and human behaviour: contributions from a clinical perspective. In A.J. Prange (Ed.), *The Thyroid Axis, Drugs and Behaviour*, Raven Press, New York, pp. 5–28.

Wolter, R., Noël, P., De Cock, P., Craen, M., Ernould, C.H., Malvaux, P., Verstraeten, F., Simons, J., Mertens, S., Van Broek, N. and Vanderschueren-Lodewyckx, M. (1980) Neuropsychological study in treated thyroid dysgenesis. *Acta Pediatr. Scand.*, 277: 41–46.

Yamada, K.M., Spooner, B.S. and Wessels, N.K. (1970) Axon growth: role of microfilaments and microtubules. *Proc. Natl. Acad. Sci. USA*, 66: 1206–1212.

Discussion

R. Balazs: I would take issue with your proposal that all the effects of thyroid disorders are the result of a single influence followed by a cascade of alterations.

A. Vaccari: Of course, simplifying the intimate mechanisms of any pathological event like dysthyroidism is a difficult task. There is no doubt that the very first *single* influence of thyroid disorders is an alteration in the synthesis or turnover of specific proteins. For example, Lemarchand-Béraud et al. (1987) have shown that the modulation of pituitary nuclear T_3-receptors in hypothyroid rats is impaired by the protein synthesis inhibitor cycloheximide. From then onwards, all the different steps in the cascade sequence that I have suggested may occur either at the same time, or follow each other, or may even be absent, depending on variables such as the stage of brain development and the severity of thyroid insults. I have focused attention on the putative role of established neurotransmitters in the etiogenesis of behavioral disorders. It will be also necessary to consider the role of trophic factors and neurotransmitter peptides in the origin of dysthyroidism-related central teratogenesis.

A.J. Patel (comment): In your talk you proposed a direct relationship between modification in the composition of microtubule-associated protein reduction and the reduction in the number of synaptic junctions in hypothyroid animals. In this context, another possibility to be considered is the alterations in specific cell surface molecules that are believed to be involved in cell-to-cell interaction and recognition (see Edelman, 1984). A severe reduction in the ontogenesis of neural cell adhesion molecule (N-CAM)-like glycoprotein (D_2) and changes in its molecular forms on the one hand, and in the number of synapses per nerve on the other has been observed in the cerebellum of young hypothyroid or hyperthyroid rats (Patel et al., 1985).

References

Edelman, G.M. (1984) Modulation of cell adhesion during induction, histogenesis and perinatal development of the nervous system. *Annu. Rev. Neurosci.*, 7: 339–377.

Lemarchand-Béraud, T., Von Overbeck, K. and Rognoni, J.B. (1987) The modulation by 3,5,3'-triiodothyronine (T_3) of pituitary T_3 nuclear receptors in hypothyroid rats is inhibited by cycloheximide. *Endocrinology*, 121: 677–683.

Patel, A.J., Hunt, A. and Meier, E. (1985) Effects of undernutrition and thyroid state on the ontogenetic changes of D_1, D_2 and D_3 brain-specific proteins in rat cerebellum. *J. Neurochem.*, 44: 1581–1587.

G.J. Boer, M.G.P. Feenstra, M. Mirmiran, D.F. Swaab and F. Van Haaren
Progress in Brain Research, Vol. 73
© 1988 Elsevier Science Publishers B.V. (Biomedical Division)

CHAPTER 7

The role of the insulin-like growth factors in the regulation of brain development

Vicki R. Sara and Christine Carlsson-Skwirut

Karolinska Institute's Department of Psychiatry, St. Göran's Hospital, Box 12500, 112 81 Stockholm, Sweden

Introduction

In simple terms, cellular growth occurs initially as the rapid proliferation of undifferentiated cells. This is followed by the period of differentiation until finally the mature cell has emerged. These two stages are common to the growth of all cells. Their uniqueness lies in the timing and the rate of their growth. During their most rapid growth phase, cells are especially vulnerable and therefore this is referred to as their critical period. In man, for example, the critical period of cell proliferation in the brain is during fetal and neonatal life, whereas this occurs around puberty in the gonads. Life-span and renewal ability are also characteristic features of a cell. For example, blood cells such as erythrocytes have a short life-span and are constantly renewed from their stem cells, whereas the fully differentiated neurone does not normally divide during its long life-span. Fibroblasts and hepatocytes maintain proliferative potential which can be evoked as a repair response. Growth is thus a continual process of anabolism throughout life. Hormones which regulate this anabolic process may thus evoke different responses according to the genetic program of the target cell. Nutrition provides the substrates and energy source for growth, and hormones regulate the rate of growth. The term hormone refers not only to regulatory substances which act distal to their site of origin (endocrine

hormone) but also to those which are locally produced to act on neighbouring cells (paracrine hormone) or even the cell of origin (autocrine hormone).

In all species, the critical period of brain growth occurs during the early stages of development. The hormones which regulate the growth of the brain are gradually being identified. In this review, the role of the somatomedins or insulin-like growth factors (IGFs) in the regulation of brain growth will be discussed. These growth promoting peptide hormones have recently been characterized in the brain, where they are produced as paracrine hormones and regulate cell proliferation and hypertrophic growth. The IGFs were first implicated in the regulation of brain growth with the hypothesis of a brain growth factor whose production could be stimulated by growth hormone (Sara et al., 1974). During purification attempts it became clear that this brain growth factor belonged to the IGF family of, at that time, as yet incompletely characterized hormones. In recent years, the brain growth factor has been isolated and its chemical structure determined. This has established the IGFs as brain growth-promoting hormones.

Since the IGFs regulate brain growth during normal development, abnormalities in their production or the sensitivity of their target cells will result in growth disturbances, and even possibly malformations in the brain. The means whereby

88

teratogenic agents, such as chemicals and other environmental factors, produce abnormalities in brain development are largely unknown. However, one mechanism may involve interference in normal IGF regulation, which may mediate the influence of teratogenic agents on the developing brain.

Chemical structure

The somatomedins or insulin-like growth factors are a family of growth-promoting peptide hormones (Hall and Sara, 1983). Depending on the methods employed to assay for their presence, these peptides were initially termed sulfation factor activity (SFA), non-suppressible insulin-like activity (NSILA) and multiplication-stimulating activity (MSA). The first insulin-like growth factors to be characterized were insulin-like growth factors 1 (IGF-1) and 2 (IGF-2) isolated from adult human plasma (Rinderknecht and Humbel, 1978a,b). Somatomedins A (SMA) and C (SMC) were subsequently shown to be identical to IGF-1, disregarding possible deamidation differences (Svoboda et al., 1980; Engberg et al., 1984). MSA, purified from conditioned medium of fetal rat liver cells, is the rat homologue to human IGF-2 (Marquardt et al., 1981).

IGF-1 and IGF-2 are structurally related to proinsulin, relaxin and β-nerve growth factor, suggesting that these peptides diverged from a com-

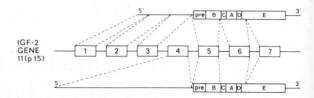

Fig. 2. Schematic representation of the IGF-2 gene and protein product. Alternative splicing of the 7 gene exons (□) results in different 5'-untranslated regions.

mon ancestor during evolution (Blundell and Humbel, 1980). Like proinsulin, IGF-1 and IGF-2 are single-chain molecules composed of an amino-terminal B region, a connecting C-region and an A-region (Figs. 1 and 2). In addition, the IGFs also contain a carboxyl-terminal D-region not present in proinsulin. IGF-1 and IGF-2 consist of 70 and 67 amino acids, respectively. Several variant forms of both IGF-1 and IGF-2 have been identified (Zumstein et al., 1985), although the IGFs, and especially IGF-1, are well conserved between different species (Marquardt et al., 1981; Honegger and Humbel, 1986). Although only small structural alterations exist between the IGFs from various species and their variant forms, they result in different immunological and biological properties.

The IGFs in the human brain have been isolated and characterized (Sara et al., 1986a; Carlsson-Skwirut et al., 1986). Two forms of IGFs were purified from human fetal and adult brain. Structural analysis identified these peptides as a variant of IGF-1 with a truncated amino terminal region and IGF-2. The amino-terminal amino acid threonine of the truncated IGF-1 variant aligns with the amino acid in position 4 of IGF-1. With this alignment, the amino acid sequences of variant IGF-1 from human fetal and adult brain, i.e. positions 1–29 and 1–19 respectively, are identical to the sequence of IGF-1 between positions 4–32 and 4–22 respectively. The carboxyl-terminal amino acid of the truncated IGF-1 variant from human fetal brain has been shown to be identical to that of IGF-1. Thus

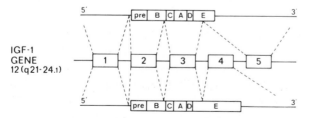

Fig. 1. Schematic representation of the IGF-1 gene and its protein products. Alternative splicing of the 5 gene exons (□) results in two prepro IGF-1s which both contain intact IGF-1 (B, C, A, D domains) but differ in the length and structure of their E domains.

the amino-terminus truncation is likely to be the only structural difference between brain IGF-1 and circulating IGF-1.

Biosynthesis

Gene protein

The genes for human IGF-1 and IGF-2 have been identified and mapped to the long arm of chromosome 12 (q 22 – q 24.1) and the short arm of chromosome 11 (p 15) respectively (Bell et al., 1985). The IGF-1 gene contains at least 5 exons, which can be spliced to result in alternative IGF-1 mRNAs (Fig. 1). Two IGF-1 cDNAs have been described (IGF-1a and IGF-1b) which result from exons 1, 2, 3 and 5 or 1, 2, 3 and 4 respectively (Rotwein et al., 1986). These different IGF-1 mRNAs result from alternative RNA splicing from a single gene transcript. They encode two IGF-1 precursor proteins of either 153 and 195 amino acids which differ in the length and sequence of their carboxyl-terminal extensions. The biological role of the two IGF-1 precursors has yet to be clarified. The IGF-2 gene contains 7 exons of which the first 4 are 5′-nontranslated exons and exons 5–7 encode the IGF-2 precusor (de Pagter-Holthuizen et al., 1986, 1987) (Fig. 2). Two alternative transcripts containing either exons 4–7 or 1–3 together with 5–7 have

been identified in human hepatoma cells or adult liver respectively (de Pagter-Holthuizen et al., 1987).

The genes for IGF-1 and IGF-2 are expressed in the central nervous system. An IGF-1 mRNA of approximately 1.1 kb has been identified in the human brain. Expression of the IGF-2 gene has been reported only in the adult and not the fetal human brain (Scott et al., 1985). In the rat, both IGF-1 and IGF-2 mRNAs are present in the fetal brain, whereas only IGF-2 mRNA has been consistently detected in the adult brain (Table 1). Expression of both IGF genes appears to be tissue- and development-specific. Several mRNA species have been identified and their relative abundance varies during development in different tissues. IGF-2 gene expression in the rat brain is developmentally regulated, with a greater abundance of mRNA occurring in the fetus compared to the adult. This is presumably regulated by the distinct promotor regions of the IGF-2 gene, whose appearance is developmentally specific (Soares et al., 1986; de Pagter-Holthuizen et al., 1987). Tissue-specific IGF gene expression was first suggested by Soares et al. (1985), who demonstrated that the size and abundance of rat IGF-2 transcripts varied in different organs. It is necessary, however, to determine the functional activity of these transcripts, whose size differences could represent incomplete RNA processing or polyadenylation.

Identification of variant IGF-1 as the final protein product indicates CNS-specific processing from the IGF-1 gene. This can occur at either the mRNA or precursor protein level. Variant IGF-1 most probably arises from CNS-specific proteolytic processing of the precursor protein (Sara, in press) since the amino-terminus of IGF-1 is not an intron/exon hinge region (Jansen et al., 1983). As the variant IGF-1 has increased neurotrophic potency (Sara et al., 1986a), the amino-terminus truncation of IGF-1 in the human brain is proposed to be a neurospecific regulatory mechanism to enhance the neuroactivity of the peptide (Sara, in press). Thus

TABLE 1

IGF mRNA in rat brain

Fetal/neonatal	Adult	Reference
IGF-1	Not detectable	Lund et al., 1986
IGF-2	IGF-2	Soares et al., 1985, 1986
Cortex, brain stem, hypothalamus, spinal cord	Cortex, cerebellum, hippocampus, hypothalamus, medulla, striatum, spinal cord	Brown et al., 1986; Lund et al., 1986

through differential RNA and precursor hormone processing, a single gene can express a multitude of alternative protein products with differing biological activity and whose appearance can be regulated at multiple sites in the biosynthetic pathway.

Localization and regulation

The IGFs are produced as paracrine or autocrine hormones within the CNS. As yet, however, the cellular site of synthesis remains to be identified. A glial cell origin is suggested by studies showing the majority of IGF activity in the conditioned media of glial rather than neuronal cells in culture. It is now well established that IGF biosynthesis occurs throughout the CNS as well as the peripheral and autonomic nervous systems. No area appears as the specific site of production. In earlier studies in the cat, IGF activity was detected in all CNS areas as well as sympathetic ganglia, vagus and sciatic nerves (Sara et al., 1982a). Similarly, immunoreactive IGF-2 is distributed throughout the human brain (Haselbacher et al., 1985). Immunoreactive IGF-1 has been identified in neurones and Schwann cells in the rat autonomic and peripheral nervous system (Hansson et al., 1986). Interestingly, these authors reported an increase in immunoreactive IGF-1 in Schwann cells surrounding the rat sciatic nerve following its transection. This finding suggests a role for IGF in neural regeneration and repair after injury. The above studies of IGF localization cannot distinguish whether the peptide is produced or merely transported. The site of biosynthesis can only be identified by studies of gene expression. Unfortunately no in situ hybridization studies have yet been reported. However, as shown in Table 1, several studies have recently reported the presence of IGF mRNA in several CNS areas (Soares et al. 1985, 1986; Brown et al., 1986; Lund et al., 1986). Soares et al. (1986), for example, found IGF-2 mRNA in all regions of the rat brain, thus supporting the earlier evidence of widespread peptide localization.

The mechanisms which regulate IGF biosynthesis and secretion in the nervous system are still unknown. In contrast to other tissues, GH does not appear to influence IGF production of the CNS (D'Ercole et al., 1984). Whilst triiodothyronine stimulates IGF production by fetal hypothalamic cells, this effect may be secondary to that of maturation (Binoux et al., 1985). Instead, nutrition has been proposed to be the primary regulator of IGF production in the brain (Sara, in press). IGF synthesis may simply depend upon the availability of substrates to the cell.

Although release mechanisms in the CNS are unknown, it was previously observed that electrical stimulation led to a rapid release of IGF from cat brachial and sciatic nerves, suggesting neural release after depolarization (Sara et al., 1982a). Recent studies also indicate rapid axoplasmic transport of IGF-1 in rat sciatic nerve (Hansson et al., 1987).

After release, the IGFs are bound to carrier proteins. In cerebrospinal fluid or in glial and neuronal conditioned media, IGF appears as a higher molecular weight complex of around 40 kDa consisting of IGF bound to a carrier protein. The predominant binding protein in CSF is approximately 35 kDa and preferentially binds IGF-2 (Binoux et al., 1986). Similar specificity has not been observed in the binding proteins from brain cytosol or glial and neuronal conditioned media. The functional importance of the binding proteins presumably resides in regulating the transport and availability of the IGFs to their target cells, by both transport through the microcirculation and protection from enzymic degradation. The release of IGFs from the carrier proteins may depend upon the equilibrium between binding affinity to the carrier protein and that to the target cell. During periods of rapid growth, cells display an increased IGF receptor affinity and thus may be capable of stripping IGF from its binding protein. This mechanism would provide for transport to selective cells.

Biological action

Receptors

The biological action of a hormone depends upon the ability of the target cell to respond to the level of hormone in its extracellular milieu. This is a function of the sensitivity of the cell receptors for the hormone and of the ability of the intracellular machinery to respond to the hormonal signal. Receptor sensitivity thus provides one of the mechanisms for regulating cellular responsiveness. Two distinct IGF receptors have been characterized (Rechler and Nissley, 1986). As shown in Fig. 3, these proteins are transmembranally located in the plasma membrane. The Type 1 or IGF-1 receptor is a glycoprotein with molecular weight of approximately 350 kDa which consists of 2 extracellular α-subunits (approx. 130 kDa) and 2 transmembranal β-subunits (approx. 95 kDa). The primary structure of the IGF-1 receptor has recently been identified from its cDNA sequence, and its gene mapped to chromosomal locus 15 q 25–26 (Ullrich et al., 1986). This receptor preferentially binds IGF-1

but the homologous IGF-2 also crossreacts to a lesser degree. At high concentrations insulin crossreacts weakly in the IGF-1 receptor, which is structurally related to the insulin receptor. IGF-1 binds to the extracellular α-subunit and the hormonal signal is transmitted intracellularly by the consequent stimulation of β-subunit tyrosine kinase activity and autophosphorylation. The Type II or IGF-2 receptor is an approximately 250 kDa protein whose primary structure has recently been determined (Morgan et al., 1987). The receptor preferentially binds IGF-2 and less potently its homologue IGF-1; however, the mechanism of intracellular signal transduction is unclear.

Both IGF-1 and IGF-2 receptors have been identified in the central nervous system. The ontogenesis of these receptors has been followed in the human brain (Sara et al., 1983b). During early fetal life, crossreaction studies suggest the presence of an immature form of membrane receptor displaying the unique characteristics of neither an IGF-1 nor an IGF-2 receptor. Around midgestation, however, a distinct IGF-1 receptor can be identified. This receptor preferentially recognizes the truncated variant IGF-1. The concentration of this IGF-1 receptor is greatest during the intrauterine growth spurt of the human brain. The emergence of a distinct IGF-1 receptor around 18 weeks of gestation which remains unchanged throughout life suggested that this receptor may be located on neurones. This is supported by studies using primary neuronal or glial cell cultures, which have demonstrated a much greater abundance of IGF-1 receptors on neurones rather than glia (Burgess et al., 1987). Moreover, the neuronal IGF-1 receptor shows structural differences from the Type 1 receptor in other tissues, having a smaller α-subunit of around 115 kDa. This may be due to differences in glycosylation (Heidenreich et al., 1986). Such modification in the carbohydrate domain of the α-subunit of the receptor may have functional significance by affecting the orientation of the hormone binding site. In contrast to the neuronal

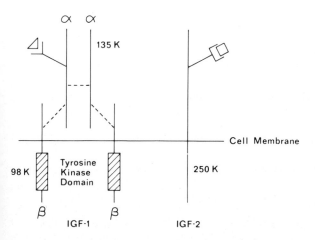

Fig. 3. Schematic representation of IGF-1 and IGF-2 receptors. The extracellular hormone binding sites are shown as well as the intracellular tyrosine kinase domain of the IGF-1 receptor subunit. The approximate molecular weights of the receptors are given. The α and β subunits of the IGF-1 receptor are joined by disulphide bonds.

receptor, rat astroglial cells display an IGF-1 receptor with an α-subunit of approximately 130 kDa which is identical to that found in other tissues (Han et al., 1987). These findings suggest a specific subtype of IGF-1 receptor in neurones which emerges with their differentiation. The specificity of the neuronal receptor may reside in modification of the hormone binding domain to accommodate the truncated IGF-1 variant synthesized in the brain.

The IGF-1 receptors are widely distributed throughout the adult human brain (Sara et al., 1982b). In accordance with their proposed neuronal location, the greatest concentration is found in neuronal-rich regions such as cerebral cortex and various nuclei, with few receptors being found in predominantly fibre-rich areas such as the corpus callosum. Receptors for IGF-2 are also distributed throughout the brain. This

receptor is similar to the IGF-2 receptor found in other tissues and has a molecular weight of approximately 240 kDa. The IGF-2 receptor has been identified on rat astroglial cells together with the IGF-1 receptor (Han et al., 1987). It remains to be determined whether the IGF-2 receptor is also present on neurones. In general, the biological role of the IGF-2 receptor is at present undefined, especially since many of the growth-promoting actions of IGF-2 can be attributed to its crossreaction in the IGF-1 receptor.

In vitro action

Serum has long been recognized as an essential ingredient in culture medium for growing neuronal and glial cells. Artificial media require high concentrations of insulin to replace serum. It is now established that one of the major growth-promoting ingredients of serum, and that replaced by the

TABLE 2

Neurobiological action of IGFs

Peptide	Target	Action	Reference
IGF	Fetal rat brain cells	DNA synthesis	Sara et al., 1979
IGF-1	Fetal rat brain cells	DNA synthesis, cell proliferation, GAD, CAT, ACE, CNP	Lenoir and Honneger, 1983
IGF-1/IGF-2	Fetal rat brain cells	DNA synthesis	Enberg et al., 1985
IGF-1	Neonatal rat brain cells	Oligodendrocyte proliferation	McMorris et al., 1986
IGF-1	Fetal rat neuronal cells	RNA synthesis	Burgess et al., 1987
IGF-1/IGF-2	Neonatal rat astroglial cells	DNA synthesis	Han et al., 1987
IGF-2	Human neuroblastoma SH-SY5Y cells	Neurite formation, NGF binding	Recio-Pinto et al., 1984
IGF-2	Human neuroblastoma SH-SY5Y cells	Neurite outgrowth	Recio-Pinto and Ishii, 1984
IGF-2	Human neuroblastoma SH-SY5Y cells	Neurite formation, tubulin mRNA	Mill et al., 1985
IGF-1/IGF-2	Human neuroblastoma SH-SY5Y cells	DNA synthesis, ODC	Mattsson et al., 1986
IGF-2	Chick sympathetic and sensory neurons	Neurite formation, survival	Recio-Pinto et al., 1986
IGF	Hypox rat in vivo	Incorporation of labelled amino acid into brain protein	Sara et al., 1981
IGF-1	Neonatal rat brain in vivo	Brain weight	Philipps et al., 1987

high doses of insulin, is the IGFs. The IGFs have a direct biological action on neural and glial cells in vitro. This biological response is mediated by interaction with IGF receptors. Table 2 summarizes the findings of studies which have investigated the biological effects of purified IGFs on the nervous system. These studies initially used primary cell suspensions of rat fetal or neonatal brain cells. Later studies have used relatively pure preparations of either neuronal or glial cells. Several studies have also used human neuroblastoma cell lines. Both IGF-1 and IGF-2 elicit a mitogenic response when added to the incubation medium in physiological concentrations (approx. 10^{-9} M). No consistent significant difference in potency between IGF-1 and IGF-2 has been reported. The truncated IGF-1 variant, however, displays increased neurotrophic activity. Fig. 4 illustrates the influence of truncated variant IGF-1, IGF-1 and IGF-2 on fetal rat brain cell DNA synthesis. Insulin elicits a similar mitogenic response only when added in supraphysiological concentrations of at least 100-fold greater molar concentration that IGFs. This corresponds to the concentration of insulin required to interact in the IGF-1 receptor. Thus the growth-promoting

effect of insulin on neural tissue is undoubtedly mediated by its crossreaction in the IGF receptor. As summarized in Table 2, the IGFs have been reported to have a wide variety of growth-promoting effects on neural and glial cells. The IGFs stimulate DNA synthesis and cell proliferation, neurite formation and outgrowth, neuronal and glial enzyme activity and oligodendrocyte development (Table 2). These studies not only show a potent IGF action on the growth of both neurones and glial cells, but also suggest a possible role in differentiation. For example, McMorris et al. (1986) demonstrated a selective induction of oligodendrocyte development and suggested that IGF-1 may be involved in the regulation of myelination.

Studies of neuronal and neuroblastoma cells in culture have suggested an interaction between the IGFs and NGF. Recio-Pinto et al. (1984) reported that the loss of NGF binding and biological response observed in neuroblastoma cells in a serum-free medium could be restored by IGF-2. These results suggested that the IGFs may potentiate NGF action by receptor induction. Recently, Burgess et al. (1987) reported that the 7 S NGF complex, which is thought to be the storage form of the peptide, crossreacted in the neuronal IGF-1 receptor, whereas the biologically active β-NGF did not. This interesting observation requires further investigation to clarify a possible functional relationship between the IGFs and NGF.

In vivo action

Until the development of recombinant DNA technology, it was impossible to study IGF action in vivo. Since only small amounts of these peptides could be purified, only in vitro studies could be performed. Using a partially purified preparation containing both IGF-1 and IGF-2, however, a potent stimulation of labelled amino acid uptake and incorporation into brain protein could be demonstrated after administration to hypophysectomized rats (Sara et al., 1981). The recent availability of recombinant IGF-1 has provided

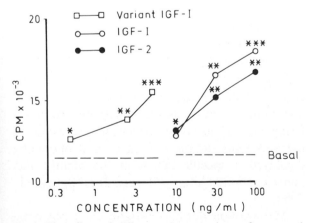

Fig. 4. The effect of different concentrations of truncated IGF-1, IGF-1 and IGF-2 on the uptake of [³H]thymidine into DNA of rat fetal brain cells in primary suspension culture. The method is described in detail in Enberg et al. (1985) * $P < 0.05$, ** $P < 0.01$, *** $P < 0.001$.

opportunities for in vivo studies of biological action. Philipps et al. (1987) have examined the effect of recombinant IGF-1 on the growth of neonatal rats. Administration of 2 nmoles recombinant IGF-1 twice daily from day 3 to day 15 of postnatal growth significantly increased body weight and length. The growth of several organs, particularly the brain, was also stimulated. Earlier eye-opening time was also observed, suggesting enhanced maturation in IGF-1-treated animals. Equimolar GH administration during this early developmental period had no such significant effect. Significantly, the effects of IGF-1 on neonatal growth were dependent upon nutritional status, as little growth stimulation could be observed in poorly nourished growth-retarded animals. Undernutrition was suggested to induce changes in receptor sensitivity so that cell responsiveness to IGF-1 was impaired.

These studies of biological action both in vitro and in vivo support the hypothesis that the IGFs regulate the growth and development of the nervous system.

Role of IGFs in disorders of brain development and mental retardation

A disturbance in IGF production has been suggested to be involved in disorders of brain development arising from both genetic and environmental factors. In Down's syndrome, for example, although the primary defect is trisomy on chromosome 21, one of the secondary effects appears to involve a disorder of IGF biosynthesis throughout development (Sara et al., 1983a). It has been suggested that there is a delay in the onset of IGF production during early fetal life resulting in an IGF deficit during the critical period of neuronal proliferation and migration. After birth, IGF-1 levels in serum fail to rise during childhood, remaining at low values throughout life. This IGF-1 deficit undoubtedly accounts for the postnatal somatic growth retardation observed in many patients with Down's syndrome. Normal IGF receptors are present in

Down's syndrome, suggesting an ability to respond to exogenous hormone (Sara et al., 1984). IGF-1 production is regulated after birth by GH (Hall and Sara, 1983). Although endogenous GH appears normal in growth-retarded Down's syndrome patients, GH administration stimulates their IGF production and growth velocity (Annerén et al., 1986). These findings may suggest a subsensitivity of GH regulation of IGF-1 biosynthesis in growth-retarded Down's syndrome children. A change in receptor sensitivity may have resulted from the delayed maturation of IGF synthesis during fetal life. If there exists a critical period for establishment of the 'hormostat' for GH-IGF-1 regulation, then an out-of-phase development may bring about a change in the critical threshold level. It is important to be clear, however, that GH stimulation of IGF-1 production is only a postnatal phenomenon and any effect elicited by this treatment can only influence postnatal growth. Furthermore, CNS production of IGF appears to be independent of GH regulation throughout postnatal life (Bäckström et al., 1984) and thus GH administration is unlikely to influence CNS development.

It is not yet clear whether disturbances in IGF are specific to Down's syndrome or may reflect general disorders in brain development. The latter possibility may be more likely, since altered serum levels have been observed in children with unclassified mental retardation (Sara et al., 1981) as well as minimal brain dysfunction (Rasmussen et al., 1983). Disturbances may also occur in membrane receptor development, thereby interfering with cellular responsiveness. For example, the only fetus examined with fetal alcoholpathy displayed a specific deficit in the affinity and concentration of brain IGF receptors (Sara et al., 1984).

Malnutrition during fetal and early postnatal life is frequently associated with impaired brain development and mental retardation. Nutrition is believed to be the primary regulator of paracrine IGF biosynthesis during this time (Sara and Hall,

1984). The growth retardation resulting from malnutrition is invariably accompanied by reduced IGF levels in serum (Maes et al., 1984; Philipps, 1986: Soliman et al., 1986). In the growing rat, both caloric and especially protein intake are important in maintaining IGF biosynthesis (Prewitt et al., 1982). The marked association between serum IGF levels and growth impairment suggests that the deleterious effects of malnutrition are mediated by the IGFs. In the rat, for example, preweaning malnutrition which results in brain growth retardation is accompanied by IGF deficiency (Sara et al., 1979b). However, animal studies using recombinant IGF-1 make it clear that IGF-1 alone is insufficient to restore growth impairment when administered during undernutrition (Philipps et al., 1987). These findings suggest an accompanying alteration in receptor sensitivity to IGF. An increase in the threshold of cellular responsiveness to IGF may be part of an adaptive mechanism to regulate cellular growth according to nutrient availability. During early development there appears to be a critical period for imprinting of the IGF 'hormonostat'. In rats, for example, malnutrition during the preweaning period induces a permanent reduction in IGF biosynthesis which is accompanied by growth retardation throughout life (Sara et al., 1986b). Thus teratogenic agents during early development may induce permanent alterations in the setting of the IGF 'hormonostat'. This could have important implications for later brain function. IGFs are synthesized in the mature brain, where they are believed to have an anabolic action as maintenance hormones (Sara et al., 1981). Any permanent alteration in their biosynthesis may thus impair neuronal and glial cell metabolism throughout life.

Conclusion

The IGFs are paracrine hormones produced in the nervous system throughout life. The chemical structure of these neuropeptides has been established as truncated variant IGF-1 and IGF-2. The genes for both these peptides are expressed in neural tissues and the biosynthesis of the peptide appears to involve neural-specific RNA and precursor hormone processing. IGF receptors have been identified throughout the nervous system, where structural alteration in the IGF-1 receptor similarly indicates neural-specific receptor biosynthesis. The IGFs have a potent growth-promoting action on neural tissues and are proposed to be major growth-regulating hormones for the central nervous system. This is supported by clinical studies, where a disturbance in IGF biosynthesis and action is found in disorders of brain development and mental retardation.

Acknowledgements

This work was supported by the Swedish Medical Research Council, Sävstaholmsföreningen, Expressens Prenatal Research Fund, Loo and Hans Osterman Fund and Nordic Insulin Fund.

References

Annerén, G., Sara, V.R., Hall, K. and Tuvemo, T. (1986) Growth and somatomedin responses to growth hormone in children with Down's syndrome. *Arch. Dis. Child.*, 61: 48–52.

Bell, G.I., Gerhard, D.S., Fong, N.M., Sanchez-Pescador, R. and Rall, L.B. (1985) Isolation of the human insulin-like growth factor genes: insulin-like growth factor II and insulin genes are contiguous. *Proc. Natl. Acad. Sci. USA*, 82: 6450–6454.

Binoux, M., Faivre-Bauman, A., Lassarre, C., Barret, A. and Tixier-Vidal, A. (1985) Triiodothyronine stimulates the production of insulin-like growth factor (IGF) by fetal hypothalamus cells cultured in serum-free medium. *Dev. Brain Res.*, 21: 319–321.

Binoux, M., Lassarre, C. and Gourmelen, M. (1986) Specific assay for insulin-like growth factor (IGF) II using the IGF binding proteins extracted from human cerebrospinal fluid. *J. Clin. Endocrinol. Metab.*, 63: 1151–1155.

Blundell, T.L. and Humbel, R.E. (1980) Hormone families: pancreatic hormones and homologous growth factors. *Nature*, 287: 781–787.

Brown, A. L., Graham, D. E., Nissley, S. P., Hill, D. J., Strain, A. J. and Rechler, M. M. (1986) Developmental regulation of insulin-like growth factor II mRNA in different rat tissues. *J. Biol. Chem.*, 261: 3144–3150.

Burgess, S. K., Jacobs, S., Cuatrecasas, P. and Sahyoun, N. (1987) Characterization of a neuronal subtype of insulin-like growth factor I receptor. *J. Biol. Chem.*, 262: 1618–1622.

Bäckström, M., Hall, K. and Sara, V. R. (1984) Somatomedin levels in cerebrospinal fluid from adults with pituitary disorders. *Acta Endocrinol.*, 107: 171–178.

Carlsson-Skwirut, C., Jörnvall, H., Holmgren, A., Andersson, C., Bergman, T., Lundquist, G., Sjögren, B. and Sara, V. R. (1986) Isolation and characterization of variant IGF-1 as well as IGF-2 from adult human brain. *FEBS Lett.*, 201: 46–50.

de Pagter-Holthuizen, P., van Schaik, F. M. A., Verduijn, G. M., van Ommen, G. J. B., Bouma, B. N., Jansen, M. and Sussenbach, J. S. (1986) Organization of the human genes for insulin-like growth factors I and II. *FEBS Lett.*, 195: 179–184.

de Pagter-Holthuizen, P., Jansen, M., van Schaik, F. M. A., van der Kammen, R., Oosterwijk, C., Van den Brande, J. L. and Sussenbach, J. S. (1987) The human insulin-like growth factor II gene contains two development-specific promoters. *FEBS Lett.*, 214: 259–264.

D'Ercole, A. J., Stiles, A. D. and Underwood, L. E. (1984) Tissue concentrations of somatomedin C: further evidence for multiple sites of synthesis and paracrine or autocrine mechanisms of action. *Proc. Natl. Acad. Sci. USA*, 81: 935–939.

Enberg, G., Carlquist, M., Jörnvall, H. and Hall, K. (1984) The characterization of somatomedin A, isolated by microcomputer-controlled chromatography, reveals an apparent identity to insulin-like growth factor I. *Eur. J. Biochem.*, 43: 117–124.

Enberg, G., Tham, A. and Sara, V. R. (1985) The influence of purified somatomedins and insulin on fetal brain DNA synthesis in vitro. *Acta Physiol. Scand.*, 125: 305–308.

Francis, G. L., Read, L. C., Ballard, F. J., Bagley, C. J., Upton, F. M., Gravestock, P. M. and Wallace, J. C. (1986) Purification and partial sequence analysis of insulin-like growth factor I from bovine colostrum. *Biochem. J.*, 233: 207–213.

Hall, K. and Sara, V. R. (1983) Growth and somatomedins. *Vitam. Horm.*, 40: 175–233.

Han, V. K. M., Lauder, J. M. and D'Ercole, A. J. (1987) Characterization of somatomedin/insulin-like growth factor receptors and correlation with biologic action in cultured neonatal rat astroglial cells. *J. Neurosci.*, 7: 501–511.

Hansson, H. A., Dahlin, L. B., Danielsen, N., Fryklund, L., Nachemson, A. K., Polleryd, P., Rozell, B. Skottner, A., Stemme, S. and Lundborg, G. (1986) Evidence indicating trophic importance of IGF-1 in regenerating peripheral nerves. *Acta Physiol. Scand.*, 126: 609–614.

Hansson, H.-A., Rozell, B. and Skottner, A. (1987) Rapid axoplasmic transport of insulin-like growth factor I in the sciatic nerve of adult rats. *Cell Tissue Res.*, 247: 241–247.

Haselbacher, G. K., Schwab, M. E., Pasi, A. and Humbel, R. E. (1985) Insulin-like growth factor II (IGF-II) in human brain: regional distribution of IGF-II and of higher molecular mass forms. *Proc. Natl. Acad. Sci. USA*, 82: 2153–2157.

Heidenreich, K. A., Freidenberg, G. R., Figlewicz, D. P. and Gilmore, P. R. (1986) Evidence for a subtype of insulin-like growth factor I receptor in brain. *Regul. Pept.*, 15: 301–310.

Honegger, A. and Humbel, R. E. (1986) Insulin-like growth factors I and II in fetal and adult bovine serum. *J. Biol. Chem.*, 261: 569–575.

Jansen, M., van Schaik, F. M. A., Ricker, A. T., Bullock, B., Woods, D. E., Gabbay, K. H., Nussbaum, A. L., Sussenbach, J. S. and Van den Brande, J. L. (1983) Sequence of cDNA encoding human insulin-like growth factor I precursor. *Nature*, 306: 609–611.

Jansen, M., van Schaik, F. M. A., van Tol, H., Van den Brande, J. L. and Sussenbach, J. S. (1985) Nucleotide sequences of cDNAs encoding precursors of human insulin-like growth factor II (IGF-II) and an IGF-II variant. *FEBS Lett.*, 179: 243–246.

Lenoir, D. and Honegger, P. (1983) Insulin-like growth factor I (IGF-I) stimulates DNA synthesis in fetal rat brain cell cultures. *Dev. Brain Res.*, 7: 205–213.

Lund, P. K., Moats-Staats, B. M., Hynes, M. A., Simmons, J. G., Jansen, M., D'Ercole, A. J. and Van Wyk, J. J. (1986) Somatomedin-C/insulin-like growth factor I and insulin-like growth factor II mRNAs in rat fetal and adult tissues. *J. Biol. Chem.*, 261: 14539–14544.

McMorris, F. A., Smith, T. M., DeSalvo, S. and Furlanetto, R. W. (1986) Insulin-like growth factor I/somatomedin C: a potent inducer of oligodendrocyte development. *Proc. Natl. Acad. Sci. USA*, 83: 822–826.

Maes, M., Underwood, L. E., Gérard, G. and Ketelslegers, J.-M. (1984) Relationship between plasma somatomedin-C and liver somatogenic binding sites in neonatal rats during malnutrition and after short and long term refeeding. *Endocrinology*, 115: 786–792.

Marquardt, H., Todaro, G. J., Henderson, L. E. and Oroszlan, S. (1981) Purification and primary structure of a polypeptide with multiplication-stimulating activity from rat liver cell cultures. *J. Biol. Chem.*, 256: 6859–6865.

Mattsson, M. E. K., Enberg, G., Ruusala, A.-I., Hall, K. and Pahlman, S. (1986) Mitogenic response of human SH-SY5Y neuroblastoma cells to insulin-like growth factor I and II is dependent on the stage of differentiation. *J. Cell Biol.*, 102: 1949–1954.

Mill, J. F., Chao, M. V. and Ishii, D. N. (1985) Insulin, insulin-like growth factor II, and nerve growth factor effects on tubulin mRNA levels and neurite formation. *Proc. Natl. Acad. Sci. USA*, 82: 7126–7130.

Morgan, D.O., Edman, J.C., Standring, D.N., Fried, V.A., Smith, M.C., Roth, R.A. and Rutter, W.J. (1987) Insulin-like growth factor II receptor as a multifunctional binding protein. *Nature*, 329: 301–307.

Philipps, A.F., Persson, B., Hall, K., Lake, M., Skottner, A., Sanengen, T. and Sara, V.R. (1987) The effects of biosynthetic insulin-like growth factor I. Supplementation on somatic growth, maturation and erythropoiesis on the neonatal rat. *Pediatr. Res.*, in press.

Philipps, L.S. (1986) Nutrition, somatomedins, and the brain. *Metabolism*, 35: 78–87.

Prewitt, T.E., D'Ercole, A.J., Switzer, B.R. and Van Wyk, J.J. (1982) Relationship of serum immunoreactive somatomedin-C to dietary protein and energy in growing rats. *J. Nutr.*, 112: 144–150.

Rasmussen, F., Sara, V.R. and Gustavson, K.-H. (1983) Serum levels of radioreceptor-assayable somatomedins in children with minor neurodevelopmental disorder. *Uppsala J. Med. Sci.*, 88: 121–126.

Rechler, M.M. and Nissley, S.P. (1986) Insulin-like growth factor (IGF)/somatomedin receptor subtypes: structure, function, and relationships to insulin receptors and IGF carrier proteins. *Horm. Res.*, 24: 152–159.

Recio-Pinto, E. and Ishii, D.N. (1984) Effects of insulin, insulin-like growth factor II and nerve growth factor on neurite outgrowth in cultured human neuroblastoma cells. *Brain Res.*, 302: 323–334.

Recio-Pinto, E., Lang, F.F. and Ishii, D.N. (1984) Insulin and insulin-like growth factor II permit nerve growth factor binding and the neurite formation response in cultured human neuroblastoma cells. *Proc. Natl. Acad. Sci. USA*, 81: 2562–2566.

Recio-Pinto, E., Rechler, M.M. and Ishii, D.N. (1986) Effects of insulin, insulin-like growth factor II, and nerve growth factor on neurite formation and survival in cultured sympathetic and sensory neurons. *J. Neurosci.*, 6: 1211–1219.

Rinderknecht, E. and Humbel, R.E. (1978a) The amino acid sequence of human insulin-like growth factor I and its structural homology with proinsulin. *J. Biol. Chem.*, 253: 2769–2776.

Rinderknecht, E. and Humbel, R. (1978b) Primary structure of human insulin-like growth factor II. *FEBS Lett.*, 89: 283–286.

Rotwein, P., Pollock, K.M., Didier, D.K. and Krivi, G.G. (1986) Organization and sequence of the human insulin-like growth factor I gene. *J. Biol. Chem.*, 261: 4828–4832.

Rubin, J.S., Mariz, I., Jacobs, J.W., Daughaday, W.-H. and Bradshaw, R.A. (1982) Isolation and partial sequence analysis of rat basic somatomedin. *Endocrinology*, 110: 734–740.

Sara, V.R. Insulin-like growth factors in the nervous system: characterization, biosynthesis and biological role. In M. Preece and J. Tanner (Eds.), *Annals of Human Biology*, Oxford University Press, London; in press.

Sara, V.R. and Hall, K. (1984) The biosynthesis and regulation of fetal somatomedin. In P. Gluckman and F. Ellendorf (Eds.), *Fetal Neuroendocrinology*, Perinatal Press, New York, p. 213.

Sara, V.R., Lazarus, L., Stuart, M.C. and King, T. (1974) Fetal brain growth; selective action by growth hormone. *Science*, 186: 446–447.

Sara, V.R., Hall, K., Wetterberg, L., Fryklund, L., Sjögren, B. and Skottner, A. (1979a) Fetal growth: the role of the somatomedins and other growth-promoting peptides. In G. Giordano, J.J. Van Wyk and F. Minuto (Eds.), *Somatomedins and Growth*, Academic Press, London, pp. 225–230.

Sara, V.R., Hall, K., Sjögren, B., Finnson, K. and Wetterberg, L. (1979b) The influence of early nutrition on growth and circulating levels of immunoreactive somatomedin A. *J. Dev. Physiol.*, 1: 343–350.

Sara, V.R., Hall, K. and Wetterberg, L. (1981) Fetal brain growth: proposed model for regulation by embryonic somatomedin. In M. Ritzén, A. Apéria, K. Hall, A. Larsson and R. Zetterström (Eds.), *The Biology of Normal Human Growth*, Raven Press, London, p. 241.

Sara, V.R., Uvnäs-Moberg, K., Uvnäs, B., Hall, K., Wetterberg, L., Poslonec, B. and Goiny, M. (1982a) The distribution of somatomedins in the nervous system of the cat and their release following neural stimulation. *Acta Physiol. Scand.*, 115: 467–470.

Sara, V.R., Hall, K., von Holtz, H., Humbel, R., Sjögren, B. and Wetterberg, L. (1982b) Evidence for the presence of specific receptors for insulin-like growth factors I (IGF-1) and II (IGF-2) and insulin throughout the adult human brain. *Neurosci. Lett.*, 34: 39–44.

Sara, V.R., Gustavson, K.-H., Annerén, G., Hall, K. and Wetterberg, L. (1983a) Somatomedins in Down's syndrome. *Biol. Psychiatry*, 18: 803–811.

Sara, V.R., Hall, K., Mizaki, M., Fryklund, L., Christensen, N. and Wetterberg, L. (1983b) The ontogenesis of somatomedin and insulin receptors on the human fetus. *J. Clin. Invest.*, 71: 1084–1094.

Sara, V.R., Sjögren, B., Annerén, G., Gustavson, K.-H., Forsman, A., Hall, K. and Wetterberg, L. (1984) The presence of normal receptors for somatomedin and insulin in fetuses with Down's sydrome. *Biol. Psychiatry*, 19: 591–598.

Sara, V.R., Carlsson-Skwirut, C., Andersson, C., Hall, E., Sjögren, B., Holmgren, A. and Jörnvall, H. (1986a) Characterization of somatomedins from human fetal brain: identification of a variant form of insulin-like growth factor I. *Proc. Natl. Acad. Sci. USA*, 83: 4904–4907.

Sara, V.R., Hall, K., Menolascino, S., Sjögren, B., Wetterberg, L., Müntzing, K., Oldfors, A. and Sourander, P. (1986b) The influence of maternal protein deprivation on the developmental pattern of serum immunoreactive insulin-like growth factor I (IGF-1) levels. *Acta Physiol. Scand.*, 126: 391–395.

Scott, J., Cowell, J., Robertson, M. E., Priesley, L. M., Wadey, R., Hopkins, B. Pritchard, J., Bell, G. I., Rall, L. B., Graham, C. F. and Knott, T. J. (1985) Insulin-like growth factor II gene expression in Wilms' tumor and embryonic tissues. *Nature*, 317: 260–262.

Soares, M. B., Ishii, D. N. and Efstratiadis, A. (1985) Developmental and tissue-specific expression of a family of transcripts related to rat insulin-like growth factor II mRNA. *Nucleic Acids Res.*, 13: 1119–1134.

Soares, M. B., Turken, A., Ishii, D., Mills, L., Episkopou, V., Cotter, S., Zeitlin, S. and Efstratiadis, A. (1986) Rat insulin-like growth factor II gene. A single gene with two promoters expressing a multitranscript family. *J. Mol. Biol.*, 192: 737–752.

Soliman, A. T., Hassan, A. E. H. I., Aref, M. K., Hintz, R. L., Rosenfeld, R. G. and Rogol, A. D. (1986) Serum insulin-like growth factors I and II concentrations and growth hormone and insulin responses to arginine infusion in children with protein-energy malnutrition before and after nutritional rehabilitation. *Pediatr. Res.*, 20: 1122–1130.

Svoboda, M. E., Van Wyk, J. J., Klapper, D. G., Fellows, R. E., Grissom, F. E. and Schlueter, R. J. (1980) Purification of somatomedin-C from human plasma: chemical and biological properties, partial sequence analysis, and relationship to other somatomedins. *Biochemistry*, 19: 790–797.

Ullrich, A., Gray, A., Tam, A. W., Yang-Feng, T., Tsubokawa, M., Collins, C., Henzel, W., Le Bon, T., Kathuria, S., Chen, E., Jacobs, S., Francke, U., Ramachandran, J. and Fujita-Yamaguchi, Y. (1986) Insulin-like growth factor I receptor primary structure: comparison with insulin receptor suggests structural determinants that define functional specificity. *EMBO J.*, 5: 2503–2512.

Zumstein, P. P., Lüthi, C. and Humbel, R. E. (1985) Amino acid sequence of a variant pro-form of insulin-like growth factor II. *Proc. Natl. Acad. Sci. USA*, 82: 3169–3172.

Discussion

A. Dekker: Given that insulin-like growth factor I (IGF-1) levels remain high, whereas cell number degenerates, is there any evidence for a change in IGF-1 receptors with aging?

V. Sara: During aging, serum levels of IGF-1 fall and also there is a decline in the sensitivity of the IGF receptors. It is therefore not difficult to consider that the IGFs may be involved in cell aging and could be therapeutically used in degenerative disorders. Studies in rat by Hansson et al. (1986) suggest that IGF-1 is elicited as a repair response after sciatic nerve transsection and that it stimulates neural regeneration.

G. J. Boer: You provided evidence for the synthesis of IGFs in the brain. Has the production site been further localized? And are glial or nerve cells, or both, synthesizing the IGFs?

V. Sara: The cell of origin for IGF synthesis in the CNS has yet to be determined. Using in situ hybridization with synthetic oligonuleotide probes, Han et al. (1987) localized IGF mRNA in the human fetus in connective tissues or cells of mesenchymal origin. They suggested mesenchymal cells as the primary site of biosynthesis. The authors were unable to identify IGF mRNA in the cerebral cortex. Using cDNA probes, we have identified IGF-1 mRNA in the human fetal cortex but as yet have no results on localization. However, I suspect a glial origin, since astrocytoma cells provide a rich source of IGF activity (Prisell et al., 1987).

J. M. Lauder: In response to G. J. Boer's question regarding sites of IGF synthesis in brain, Hynes et al. (1988) have shown with in situ hybridization using an oligonucleotide probe to IGF-2 that only the choroid plexus has mRNA for IGF-2. Would you comment on this?

V. Sara: These results are in accordance with unpublished findings of Meister showing IGF-2 immunoreactivity around the choroid plexus in the developing rat brain. The in situ hybridization findings do not rule out other cells as sites of production. Several studies demonstrate that both IGF-1 and 2 mRNAs are widely distributed within the CNS. However, it has been difficult to define their cellular localization with present techniques.

A. J. Patel: It has been shown by Recio-Pinto et al (1984) that treatment with insulin and with IGF-2 increases specific and saturable nerve growth factor (NGF) binding sites in cultured human neuroblastoma cells. Would you comment on these results in the light of your observations? In addition, do you know of similar interactions between IGFs and other hormones of neurohumoural agent receptors?

V. Sara: The relationship between NGF and the IGFs remains to be clarified. In addition, Burgess et al. (1987) reported that the high molecular weight 7 S complex, which is the stable storage form of the NGF dimer, but not the biologically active NGF, crossreacted with the IGF-1 receptor. It seems clear, however, that growth results from an interaction between several growth factors. For example, IGFs act as progression factors for cellular growth after cells have been committed to DNA synthesis by other growth factors such as platelet-derived growth factor (PDGF) or fibroblast growth factor (FGF), in this respect called competence factors (Stiles et al. 1979). Interestingly, PDGF also stimulates IGF production in fibroblasts (Clemmons and Shaw, 1983).

D. F. Swaab: You showed that IGF is normal in anencephalic blood and mentioned that their growth is normal. The latter is only true for anecephalics younger than 20 weeks (Honnebier and Swaab, 1974). Are your data indeed from early anencephalics, and, if so, do you also have data on late gestation in anencephalics?

V. Sara: The anencephalics we have been able to examine were all less than 21 weeks gestational age. We have not examined late gestation anenecephalics. It is clear, however, that in man IGF-1 production does not become regulated by GH until after birth (Sara and Hall, 1984). In the rat, this occurs around the time of weaning (Sara and Hall, 1984). The influence of other hypothalamic or pituitary hormones on IGF synthesis during intrauterine life has yet to be elucidated.

References

Burgess, S. K., Jacobs, S., Cuatrecasas, P. and Sahyoun, N. (1987) Characterization of a neuronal subtype of insulin-like growth factor I receptor. *J. Biol. Chem.*, 262: 1618–1622.

Clemmons, D. R. and Shaw, D S. (1983) Variables controlling somatomedin production by cultured human fibroblasts. *J. Cell. Physiol.*, 115: 137–142.

Han, V. K. M., D'Ercole, A. J. and Lund, P. K. (1987) Cellular localization of somatomedin (insulin-like growth factor) messenger RNA in the human fetus. *Science*, 236: 193–197.

Hansson, H. A., Dahlin, L. B., Danielsen, N., Fryklund, L., Nachemson, A. K., Polleryd, P., Rozell, B., Skottner, A., Stemme, S. and Lundborg, G. (1986) Evidence indicating trophic importance of IGF-I in regenerating peripheral nerves. *Acta Physiol. Scand.*, 126: 609–614.

Honnebier, W. J. and Swaab, D. F. (1974) Influence of alpha-melanocyte-stimulating hormone (alpha-MSH), growth hormone (GH) and fetal brain extracts on intrauterine growth of fetus and placenta in the rat. *J. Obstet. Gynaecol. Br. Commonw.*, 81: 439–447.

Hynes, H..A., Brooks, P.J., Van Wyck, J.J. and Lund, P.K. (1988) Insulin-like GF II messenger RNAs are expressed in choroid plexus of rat brain. *Mol. Endocrinol.*, in press.

Prisell et al. (1987) Somatomedins in tumor cyst fluid; cerebrospinal fluid and tumor cytosol in patients with glial tumours. *Acta Neurochirur.*, 89: 48–52.

Recio-Pinto, E., Lang, F. F. and Ishii, D. M. (1984) Insulin and insulin-like growth factor II permit nerve growth factor binding and the neurite formation response in controlled human neuroblastoma cells. *Proc. Natl. Acad. Sci. USA*, 81: 2562–2566.

Sara, V. R. and Hall, K. (1984) The biosynthesis and regulation of fetal somatomedin. In P. Gluckman and F. Ellendorf (Eds.), *Fetal Neuroendocrinology*, Perinatal Press, New York, p.213.

Stiles, C. D., Capone, G. T., Scher, C. D., Antoniades, H. N., Van Wyk, J. J. and Pledger, W. J. (1979) Dual control of cell growth by somatomedins and platelet-derived growth factor. *Proc. Natl. Acad. Sci. USA*, 76: 1279–1284.

G.J. Boer, M.G.P. Feenstra, M. Mirmiran, D.F. Swaab and F. Van Haaren
Progress in Brain Research, Vol. 73
© 1988 Elsevier Science Publishers B.V. (Biomedical Division)

CHAPTER 8

Stress, glucocorticoids and development

E. Ronald De Kloet[1], Patricia Rosenfeld[2], J. Anke M. Van Eekelen[1], Winardi Sutanto[1] and Seymour Levine[2]

[1]*Rudolf Magnus Institute for Pharmacology, University of Utrecht, Vondellaan 6, 3521 GD Utrecht, The Netherlands, and* [2]*Department of Psychiatry, Stanford University, Stanford, CA 94305, USA*

Introduction

In the adult organism, glucocorticoids (GCs) serve a wide variety of regulatory and permissive functions, aimed basically at controlling the organism's responses to stress, and at regulating circadian-driven activities. Most of these GC effects are readily reversible. During development, however, GCs have also been shown to produce, in experimental animals, permanent effects on growth and differentiation of a number of systems, including the central nervous system. In rats, for example, high doses of GCs administered neonatally cause a decrease in mitosis and myelination, as well as altered neural morphogenesis. Animals thus treated show reduced DNA content and brain size as well as impaired neuroendocrine responsiveness as adults. Long-lasting or permanent behavioral abnormalities have also been extensively documented. Although high doses administered postnatally impair brain development, low, constant levels of GCs seem to be indispensable for normal maturation. In support of this notion, it has been shown that plasma GC levels are low and the hypothalamus-pituitary-adrenal (HPA) axis is hyporesponsive to stressful stimuli during the first weeks of life in the rat, while circadian fluctuations in plasma GC concentrations do not develop fully until approximately 3 weeks after birth. This would ensure low and relatively unperturbed levels of circulating GCs during this critical period of development.

In this chapter first an overview of the current understanding of the dynamics of the HPA system in the adult rat is given, placing particular emphasis on the role of glucocorticoid receptors in this process. In the following sections the ontogeny of this system is described, after which we elaborate on the functional implications of some of its more salient features. Since most of the work in this area has been carried out in the rat, attention will be focussed on this species. In the final section of the chapter, we shall briefly review some of the relevant human literature and consider the implications of animal studies for the field of human functional teratology.

The mature hypothalamic-pituitary-adrenal axis

The principal GC synthesized by the rat adrenal cortex is corticosterone (CORT). CORT levels display a pronounced circadian rhythmicity: they are highest immediately preceding the animal's active period, and lowest at the end of this period. In addition to these daily fluctuations in concentration, GC plasma levels may show dramatic increases as a result of stress-induced secretion. GCs evoke a wide range of cellular and metabolic effects with profound consequences for the organism. The hypothesis developed by Munck et al. (1984), and in germinal form presented as early as 1951 by Tausk, states that these GC effects all have in common the protection of the organism from its own rapid responses to stress-induced disturbances of homeostasis. A large body of evidence supports this notion. GCs have been shown, for example, to block synthesis,

release and action of intercellular mediators involved in inflammation (prostaglandins, leukotrienes, histamine), immune responses (lymphokines), water resorption (vasopressin), glucose utilization (insulin) and the responses of the central nervous system to stress, all of which constitute primary defense reactions. GCs act, moreover, in a delayed fashion. In this way they allow the appropriate defense mechanisms sufficient time to exert their effects while at the same time preventing them from overshooting and thus constituting, themselves, a threat to homeostasis. The secretion of GCs is under the control of the central nervous system. The steroids are in fact the last chain in a cascade of neurohumoral events that is organized in the HPA system (Fig. 1).

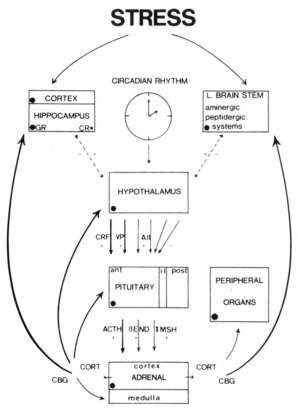

Fig. 1. The hypothalamo-pituitary-adrenocortical (HPA) axis in the rat. Corticotrophin-releasing factor (CRF) released from the paraventricular nucleus (PVN) in the hypothalamus stimulates the pituitary pro-opiomelanocortin (POMC) gene, leading to enhanced release of adrenocorticotrophin (ACTH), which subsequently triggers the secretion of adrenocortical steroids. The system has two modes of operation: mediator of the animal's ability to cope with stress, and coordinator of daily activity and sleep-related events. VP = arginine vasopressin; AII = angiotensin II; β-END = beta-endorphin (predominantly from the intermediate lobe); Ant = anterior pituitary; il = intermediate lobe; post = posterior lobe; CORT = corticosterone; CBG = corticosteroid binding globulin; GR = Type 2 glucocorticoid receptor; CR = Type 1 corticosterone-preferring receptor.

Peptides released from brain and pituitary

The hypothalamus is of critical importance in the integration and coordination of endocrine, behavioral and autonomic responses. Within the hypothalamus, the neurons of the paraventricular nucleus (PVN) play a key role in the organization of the stress response. The parvocellular neurons of the PVN synthesize corticotrophin-releasing factor (CRF), which reaches the anterior pituitary via the hypothalamo-hypophyseal tract and the portal vasculature. Here it activates the pro-opiomelanocortin (POMC) cells. Vasopressin appears to be co-localized with CRF in these PVN neurons and has been found to potentiate CRF action on the pituitary POMC cells (Kiss et al., 1984). Recently, a number of other neuropeptides were also found to co-localize under certain experimental conditions with CRF (e.g. angiotensin II, enkephalin, cholecystokinin, neurotensin) (Swanson et al., 1986). All these peptides, together with circulating adrenomedullary hormones (amines, dynorphins), are thought to converge as multifactorial signals on the pituitary cell membrane and assist CRF in stimulating second-messenger systems, thus leading to an integrated response of the POMC cell (Kordon et al., 1987). The CRF-containing neurons, in turn, are influenced by a number of sources.

Visceral sensory information is conveyed to them via highly differentiated pathways from the lower brain stem. These have been identified as adrenergic C_{1-3} and noradrenergic A_{1-2} neurons (Swanson et al., 1986; Mezey et al., 1987). Information from the limbic system is provided by an input arising from the bed nucleus of the stria terminalis. This nucleus receives massive neural inputs from the amygdala and the hippocampal formation. The function of this limbic circuitry is to integrate sensory information and neocortical influences. Accordingly, the bed nucleus may be thought of as the end of a limbic pathway transducing cognitive influences on CRF release (Swanson et al., 1986). The hippocampus is thought to exert an inhibitory influence on CRF release which depends on the 'state' of the animal (Bohus et al., 1987). Direct inputs to the CRF neurons arise from all of the preoptic and hypothalamic nuclei, as well as from the periventricular region (Palkovits, 1987). Small intrinsic CRF-containing neuronal networks are present throughout the brain. The peptide is thought, in this case, to stimulate sympathetic outflow. Vasopressin, on the other hand, is synthesized only in a few neuronal cell groups in the hypothalamus and extrahypothalamic brain regions which are involved in regulation of autonomic and motor responses (Buys, 1983).

POMC genes are expressed in cells in the anterior and intermediate lobes of the pituitary, as well as in a few hundred cells in the periarcuate region of the medial-basal hypothalamus. These three sources of POMC are in close vascular and neural contact and their wide distribution suggests a system with great integrative capacity (De Kloet et al., 1986). Proteolytic cleavage of the POMC molecule provides a number of end-products, predominantly the various peptides related to the endorphins and adrenocorticotrophin (ACTH) with distinct and often opposite biological activity, both in the periphery and in the CNS. The opiate activity displayed by β-endorphin is in general inhibitory, in contrast to ACTH, which has overall excitatory and arousing effects. The POMC system, therefore, may be considered as a homeostatic control system in its own right, which controls brain function in a way similar to that in which the autonomic system controls organ function (De Wied, 1987).

Corticosteroid receptors in brain and pituitary

The main effect of ACTH in the periphery is to stimulate GC secretion by the adrenal cortex. These GCs, in addition to their previously mentioned effects on the immune system, glucose metabolism, etc., also feed information back to the brain and pituitary to prevent the higher components of the HPA system from over-reacting and to restore homeostasis (McEwen et al., 1986). The feedback action of GC is mediated by receptors (Fig. 2). GC receptors are found in abundance in the POMC cells of the anterior pituitary, as well as in the hypothalamic CRF neurons, where they mediate the GC-dependent suppression of the stress-induced activity of the HPA system (Jones et al., 1982; Keller-Wood and Dallman, 1984).

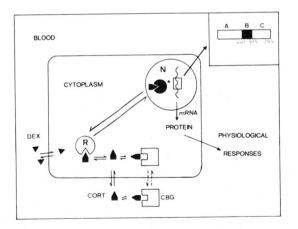

Fig. 2. Mechanism of action of corticosteroids in the anterior pituitary. Corticosterone (CORT) is taken up by cell and binds to receptor (R). Upon binding of CORT the receptor complex displays enhanced affinity for DNA in the cell nucleus (N), where it alters transcription and leads to altered synthesis of proteins underlying the appropriate physiological response. Inset represents three functional domains of receptor. A = immunoreactive domain; B = DNA binding domain; C = steroid binding domain.

104

Recent research has shown that there are actually two types of corticoid receptor in the central nervous system: Type 1 and Type 2 (Reul and De Kloet, 1985; Funder and Sheppard, 1987). The Type 1 receptors are the same in their primary amino-acid sequence as the kidney mineralocorticoid receptor. They are localized principally in the hippocampal CA_1 and CA_2 neurons and in the neurons of the dentate gyrus and in the septum (Gerlach and McEwen, 1972), and they are the receptors originally discovered by McEwen et al. (1968). In the rat, CORT (in other

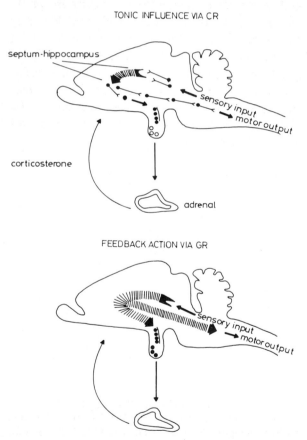

TONIC INFLUENCE VIA CR

septum-hippocampus

sensory input
motor output

corticosterone

adrenal

FEEDBACK ACTION VIA GR

sensory input
motor output

Fig. 3. Tonic and feedback action of corticosterone (CORT) via CR (Type 1 corticosterone-preferring receptor) in neurons of the septum-hippocampus. Feedback action on stress-activated brain circuits takes place via GR (Type 2 gluco-corticoid receptors). (From De Kloet and Reul (1987) Psychoneuroendocrinology, 12: 83–105, with permission.)

species, cortisol) and aldosterone are bound with high affinity. A peculiar property of the Type 1 receptors in the brain is that they mediate with stringent specificity the action of CORT, while aldosterone often acts as an antagonist. In our view (Fig. 3), Type 1 regulates on-going behavior and thus is involved in synchronization and co-ordination of circadian activities (food-seeking behavior, exploration, sleep-related events), and in the subtle adjustments of the HPA system during its basal state of activity (De Kloet and Reul, 1987; Dallman, 1987). Its almost exclusive hippocampal localization suggests a role in appropriate interpretation of environmental stimuli and expression of proper behavioral and neuroendocrine responses. The Type 2 receptor is the classical GC receptor which displays highest affinity for potent synthetic GCs. Its affinity to the natural ligand, CORT, however, is 6–10-times lower than that shown by Type 1 receptors. Radioligand binding studies and immunocyto-chemistry using monoclonal antibodies have shown a widespread localization in glial cells and neurons, especially in those neurons involved in the regulation of the autonomic, behavioral and neuroendocrine responses to stress. Thus, high concentrations of Type 2 glucocorticoid receptors are found in the CRF neurons and in the β-endorphin and neuropeptide Y immunoreactive neurons of the arcuate nucleus, as well as in the ascending monoaminergic neurons, i.e. the adrenergic neurons C_{1-3}, the noradrenergic neurons A_{1-7} and the serotonergic neurons B_{1-9} (Fuxe et al., 1985; Van Eekelen et al., 1987). Via Type 2 receptor-mediated feedback, the steroid blocks the stress-induced ACTH synthesis and CRF/AVP release, facilitates extinction of stress-induced behavioral responses and exerts a long-term effect on brain functions serving adaptive processes (De Kloet and Reul, 1987).

CORT circulates partly bound to cortico-steroid-binding globulin (CBG, transcortin). The free fraction is assumed to be available for inter-action with the receptors. Dallman (1987) has shown that the percentage of free corticosterone increases dramatically after small changes in total plasma CORT level; linear increases in total plasma CORT level appeared to result in nearly logarithmic increases in non-CBG bound CORT. At morning base levels of plasma CORT in rat, the non-CBG bound steroid could be expected to saturate the Type 1 sites and result in about 10–20% occupation of Type 2 (Reul and De Kloet, 1985; Dallman, 1987). The pituitary corticotropes have been found to contain intracellular CBG-like proteins (De Kloet et al., 1977). Occupation of the Type 2 receptors in such tissues would be even lower due to competition with CBG for CORT (Fig. 2). Accordingly, tissue-localized CBG-like binders are thought to diminish the feedback signal of corticosterone at the level of pituitary (Koch et al. 1978; De Kloet et al., 1977, 1984). As will be pointed out in the next section, CBG and CBG-like binders in the pituitary are lacking during the second week of postnatal development in the rat. This appears to be an important consideration when attempting to understand corticosteroid action during that time.

The immature hypothalamic-pituitary-adrenal axis

In the developing organism, GCs display a wide variety of functions, above and beyond those described for the adult. During ontogeny, GCs have, besides those regulatory and permissive functions already mentioned, a number of critical, and permanent, organizational effects.

The components of the HPA system show a characteristic pattern of development (Fig. 4). During the final days of gestation and immediately after birth, basal levels of CORT in the rat are extremely high. Within the first two days of life, however, concentrations decrease dramatically. They remain at this very low level until approximately day 12. Beginning near the end of the second postnatal week concentrations once again start to rise, reaching a peak at about day 24 (Henning, 1978; Sapolsky and Meaney, 1986). Given the crucial role of GCs in the adult, this

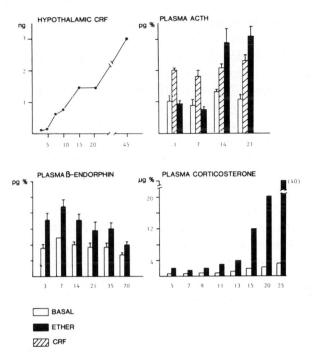

Fig. 4. Ontogeny of the HPA axis. Hypothalamic CRF content (Walker et al., 1986); basal, ether and CRF-induced plasma ACTH level (Guillet and Michaelson, 1978); basal and ether-induced plasma β-endorphin level (Iny et al., 1987); basal and ether-induced plasma corticosterone level (Schoenfield et al., 1980). Values are given at various postnatal ages of the rat.

'vanishing act' is unexpected and, at first instance, counterintuitive. Even more surprising, however, is the fact that during this period of low circulating CORT, the entire HPA system seems to be hyporesponsive to stressful stimuli. In other words, stimuli which in adult organisms reliably elicit a large increase in circulating GCs fail to do so (or do so only minimally) in the infant. This period, which extends, roughly, over the first two weeks of life, has become known in the literature as the 'stress hyporesponsive period' (SHRP). The SHRP has been extensively documented by a number of investigators using a variety of physiological and psychological challenges. These have included exposure of the rats to electric shock, ether, histamine, heat and cold or novel environment (Ader and Grota, 1973; Sapolsky and Meaney, 1986).

It is important to note that, although the HPA axis may function 'as a whole', this certainly does not imply that the different components of the system follow similar ontogenetic patterns. Thus, for example, circadian rhythmicity in CORT secretion is fully developed by day 25 (Ader and Grota, 1973) whereas the characteristic sex differences in plasma CORT and CBG levels are apparent by 2 months of age (Ramaley, 1976) and pituitary ACTH content continues increasing up to two months of age (Levine, 1970; Walker et al., 1986a,b). By about 4 weeks of age, the capacity to respond to challenges with a large increase in GC secretion is comparable to that found in adults. However, although stress-responsiveness has reached adult levels by this age, the feedback action of corticosteroids has not yet developed fully. One-month-old animals, for example, show prolonged elevated plasma CORT levels following stress and are less responsive to blockade of stress-induced HPA activity by exogenous dexamethasone (Goldman et al., 1973).

Peptides released from brain and pituitary

Considerable insight has been obtained in recent years regarding the anatomical and physiological details of the maturation of the HPA axis (Fig. 4). In the following sections we shall review the development of the components of this system, placing particular emphasis on their capacity (or lack thereof) to respond to stress during the SHRP. At the hypothalamic level, CRF immunostaining is detectable by fetal day 18 (Bugnon et al., 1982). In the first few hours after birth, CRF-like immunoreactivity decreases substantially and remains low (about 20% of day 21 levels) during the first week of life. The hypothalamic-hypophyseal portal vessel system, though, is not fully developed until 2 weeks after birth (Glydon, 1957). This may contribute to attenuating the CRF signal which reaches the pituitary. However, in spite of this, CRF is apparently released in response at least to certain

stressors and does act on the pituitary during the SHRP. This can be deduced from the fact that ACTH output in response to a potent stressor (urethane) diminishes after CRF immunoneutralization (Walker et al., 1986). Finally, neural inputs to the CRF neurons may not be fully developed during the SHRP. This would result in a diminished CRF response to stress. Within the pituitary, a substantial amount of CRF receptors has been reported to be present on cell membranes during the first week of life. These receptors respond to CRF both in vivo and in vitro, although with a diminished sensitivity (Walker et al., 1986). POMC is present in pituitary corticotrophs and brain of prenatal (f17) and neonatal rat (Chatelaine and Dupouy, 1985). Processing of the molecule to its biologically active endproducts has also been reported. As is the case with CRF, immunoreactive and bioactive ACTH levels are low the first week after birth and only achieve adult concentrations some six weeks later (Walker et al., 1986a). Despite these low levels, exposure of the one-week-old animals to certain stressors is capable of eliciting an ACTH response, although this response is relatively small. The adrenal cortex of the neonatal rat is capable of both synthesizing and secreting CORT in response to ACTH stimulation. However, during the SHRP, a certain degree of refractoriness seems to be evident (Levine and Mullins, 1966). Most interestingly, the β-endorphin levels are high during the SHRP and they respond to stress (Iny et al., 1987). Apparently during this period a POMC precursor outside the anterior pituitary (probably in the intermediate lobe cells) is responsible for these increased endorphin levels (see below).

Up to this point we have seen that the hypothalamus, pituitary and adrenal cortex are capable of synthesizing and secreting their respective hormones, albeit in an attenuated manner. The relative immaturity of these components, therefore, could partially, but not totally, account for the SHRP. As we will attempt to show below, further insight into the nature and development of the SHRP may be gained by looking at the particular features of the CORT binding systems in the pituitary and brain.

Corticosteroid receptors in brain and pituitary

The three corticosteroid binding systems in the pituitary display a remarkably divergent pattern of development. The Type 2 GC receptor is present from birth and changes very little in concentration and affinity during development. The receptor in the pituitary is capable of retaining in vivo administered tracer doses of radio-labelled steroids and is biologically active (i.e. blocks the expression of the POMC gene). The mineralo-corticoid (Type 1) receptor in the anterior pituitary only becomes detectable in in vitro cytosol binding assays from the sixth day on. Concentrations then increase rapidly and reach adult levels approximately one month after birth (Sakly and Koch, unpublished observation). Finally, the CBG-like binding system is present at high levels around the time of birth but then decreases rapidly and is undetectable between days 6 and 10. Levels then rise gradually, reaching adult concentrations at about four weeks of age. In this respect, the CBG-like binding system closely parallels the changes in concentration of circulating plasma CBG (Sakly and Koch, 1981, 1983). During the CBG-devoid period, in consequence, endogenous CORT is circulating mostly in the unbound form and can interact freely with the receptors in the pituitary. Since in the adult rat CBG-like molecules in the pituitary are thought to diminish the corticosterone feedback signal, it has been argued that during this period the CORT signal to the pituitary is greatly amplified, with the consequent failure of the pituitary gland to secrete ACTH. In favour of this line of reasoning, it has been shown recently that in adrenalectomized neonatal animals, pituitary ACTH synthesis and release is increased and does show an enhanced response to stress and to exogenous CRF (Walker et al., 1986b). Thus, the SHRP seems to be largely due to the inability of most stressors to evoke a sufficiently large CRF signal to overcome the GC

feedback at the pituitary level (Fig. 5). In this respect, it is important to note that the diminished CRF signal may not necessarily be due to immaturity of the appropriate neural inputs. A large body of evidence points to specific maternal cues as being responsible for the inhibition of the stress-induced HPA response during the SHRP. Thus, during this period, mother-deprived pups show a small adrenocortical response both to novelty and to ACTH administration, in contrast to non-deprived pups, which show no response. The critical variable seemed to be thermotactile contact with a lactating dam. It remains to be established how this maternal signal is transduced into a diminished responsivity in the infant.

Regarding the ontogenetic pattern of brain corticosteroid receptors, it is important to note that previous studies have either measured the total (i.e. Type 1 + Type 2) pool of corticosteroid receptors, or have detected with in vivo tracer

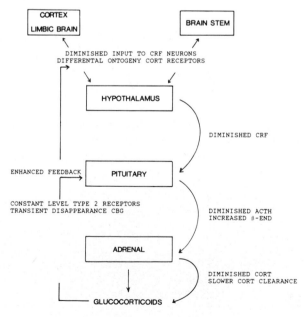

Fig. 5. HPA axis during development of the rat: Overview of different components. The axis in general is rather quiescent in responses which evoke a response in the adult animal. Note that levels of β-endorphin (and α-MSH) in plasma and brain are still highly responsive to challenging stimuli.

techniques (autoradiography and cell-nuclear uptake studies) solely the Type 1 receptor system (Olpe and McEwen, 1976; Clayton et al., 1977; Turner, 1978; Meaney et al., 1985a,b). Since both methodologies in this early work were invariably regarded to yield measurements of a single 'glucocorticoid receptor type' involved in feedback action, it is thus essential to update the interpretation of some parts of these studies.

Using high-resolution autoradiography after administration of tracer doses of [^{3}H]CORT, Turner (1978) showed a high density of GC receptors in the hippocampal CA_2 and CA_1 pyramidal cells, as well as in parts of the cingular cortex, at the end of the first postnatal week. Given the tracer amounts of [^{3}H]CORT administered, it can be expected that mainly Type 1 receptors were labelled. As late as day 9 the CA_3 and CA_4 cell fields were largely devoid of Type 1 receptors. In the dentate gyrus, the most heavily labelled cells were the oldest granular neurons, while newly arrived neurons did not appear to have Type 1 receptors (Turner, 1978). Thus, Type 1 receptors are present in the hippocampus

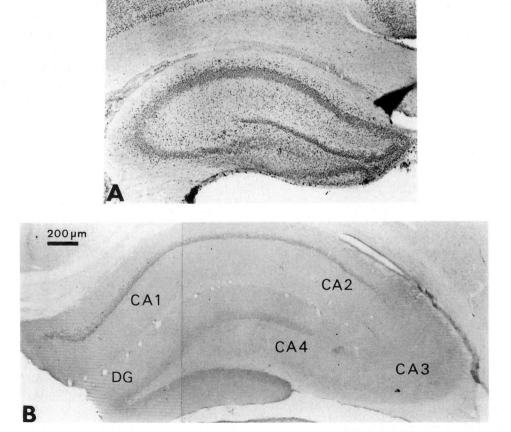

Fig. 6. Immunocytochemistry of the Type 2 glucocorticoid receptor in the rat hippocampus. A, post-natal day 2; B, 3-month-old (adult). Immunostaining was obtained by using a monoclonal antibody raised against the activated rat liver glucocorticoid receptor. The antibody was kindly provided by Dr. H. M. Westphal, Marburg, FRG. Note the disappearance of immunostaining from the CA_3 and CA_4 cell field, as well as the more densely packed stained cell in the CA_1 and CA_2 region of the adult rat. Magnification × 40.

but their density and topography seem largely to depend on the pattern of post-natal neurogenesis (Turner, 1978).

Using a monoclonal antibody to the Type 2 receptor, we have recently been able to follow the ontogenetic pattern of the Type 2 antigen in the brain of the intact neonatal rat (Van Eekelen et al., 1987; Rosenfeld et al., 1988). The monoclonal antibody was raised against the rat liver gluco-corticoid receptor and allows visualization of the Type 2 receptor conformation in its DNA binding state (Fig. 2). The intensity of nuclear immuno-reactive staining in the hippocampal CA_1 and CA_2 pyramidal cell fields and in the dentate gyrus was high in 2-day-old animals, moderate in 4- and 8-day-old animals and low in the 12-day-olds. Staining then increased gradually until achieving adult intensity at approximately 20 days of age (Fig. 6). Within the hypothalamus, nuclear staining in animals 8 days of age or older was mostly confined to those nuclei which also show Type 2 immunoreactivity in the adult (PVN, supraoptic nucleus, arcuate nucleus). Finally, in the perinatal rat, a high intensity of Type 2 immunoreactivity was detectable in the CA_3 and CA_4 pyramidal cell regions of the hippocampus (Fig. 6) as well as in the suprachiasmatic nucleus of the hypothalamus. These regions have less receptor in the adult (Van Eekelen et al., 1987).

In order to determine the ontogeny of the binding constants of Type 1 and Type 2 receptors we employed an in vitro cytosol binding assay of neonatal rat hippocampal tissue (Rosenfeld et al., 1988). Type 1 receptors are absent in both 2- and 4-day-old rats. In animals 8 days old or older, the receptors resemble those found in adult tissue in both affinity and capacity ($K_d \approx 1$ nM, $B_{max} \approx 40$ fmol/mg protein). The Type 2 receptor capacity is about 30.0 fmol/mg protein at day 2 and then increases slowly 5-fold during the next three weeks. However, this is still half the adult values.

These data from immunocytochemistry and radioligand binding suggest that the corticoid receptors show dramatic alteration during a critical period of developmental changes in the functional regulation of the HPA axis.

Environmental effects on brain development

The first two weeks of life in the rat are characterized by low basal levels of GCs and an HPA axis which, though capable of responding to stimulation, does so in a dramatically reduced way. As pointed out in the previous section, this appears to be due to a number of factors. Maternal cues seem to be important in the inhibition of the stress response. At the same time, many of the peripheral and central components of the system are still immature. At the pituitary level, an enhanced negative-feedback system seems to be operating to reduce CRF-induced ACTH release. Finally the biological half-life of CORT is prolonged to about three times that observed in adult rats (Burnstein and Westort, 1967). The outcome is a period of relatively unperturbed HPA activity and constant CORT levels, which is apparently necessary for normal development. A number of questions immediately come to mind. Does the hyporesponsiveness of the HPA system to stress imply that the organism, as a whole, is somehow shielded against the effects of stress? Do stimuli, which in adult organisms evoke an HPA response, have the ability to alter brain development? If so, through which mechanisms are they acting? Can the HPA system be manipulated during the SHRP? What would happen if GC levels were not 'low and constant'? The answers to these questions are not yet clear. However, intensive research in this area has yielded some clues as to what those answers may be. Exhaustive reviews on these subjects have been published by Ader and Grota (1973), Ader (1975), Ballard (1979), Doupe and Patterson (1982), Bohn (1984, 1986), Meyer (1985) and Sapolsky and Meaney (1986).

Two general approaches have been used to throw light on these questions. In the first, 'environmental' challenges (cold, heat, electric shock, handling, exposure to novelty, etc.) are used as independent variables, and the short- and long-term effects on morphological, physiological and/or behavioral (assumed) dependent variables are then assessed. This approach is likely to yield data of physiological relevance, but may lead to difficulty in identifying the chain of events linking cause with effect. In the second approach, the system is altered directly by adding known (usually, large) doses of steroids and looking, again, at their short- and long-term effects. In this case, the cause-effect relationship is easier to distinguish; however, the physiological relevance of the data is not always clear. This latter type of experimental paradigm is well suited to detecting comparatively gross teratological effects; the former type is better suited to illustrating the more subtle (though not, for that, less important) effects which GCs (and other hormones of the HPA axis) may have during ontogeny. It should be emphasized that neither 'approach' is more or less valid. In fact, some of the more interesting findings, as we shall see, have arisen from a 'multiple-approach' kind of strategy. In this section we shall evaluate the results proceeding from some of this research, especially those which have (or potentially may have) teratological implications.

'Handling' and brain development

With regard to the first question posed, i.e., whether the animal, during the SHRP, is shielded from the effects of stress, recent findings seem to point to a qualified yes as an answer. This 'protection' seems to proceed from at least two different sources. On the one hand, as we have seen, the HPA axis shows at this time a marked refractoriness. On the other hand, however, the endorphin system is far from quiescent during this period. Basal β-endorphin plasma levels in the neonatal rat are higher than those observed in the adult, and stress evokes a pronounced increase in their release (Iny et al., 1987). This is somewhat surprising, when we consider that this same stimulus does not produce an increase in the levels of ACTH, the other main end-product of the POMC molecule. The precise source of β-endorphin is not known. Both pituitary and brain contain high quantities of β-endorphin and α-MSH (Bayon, 1979). It is generally accepted

that β-endorphins have an inhibitory and depressant activity on neural activity, while the effects of α-MSH-related peptides are trophic and excitatory (De Wied, 1987). Thus, it would appear that an exquisite set of mechanisms is operating during this period to maintain the relatively constant internal milieu necessary for normal growth to occur. This leads us on to the next questions: can stimuli, which in adults provoke a vigorous HPA response (though not in infants, or only to a minimal degree), alter brain development? If so, how? Once again, the answer seems to be yes, at least in the case of certain stimuli. Electric shock, heat stress, exposure to novelty and handling of the neonate, to name a few, have been shown to produce long-lasting or permanent physiological, morphological and/or behavioral effects (Levine and Mullins, 1966; Ader, 1975; and Chapter 21 of this volume). In most of these cases it is hard to establish the intermediary chain of events linking the initial procedure with the final outcome. Although the CORT increase produced as a result of these manipulations would appear to be too small to be of any significance, there is as yet insufficient evidence to rule it out as a possible mediating mechanism. Exposure of the developing animal to environmental stimuli has been shown to advance maturation of circadian rhythmicity (Ader and Grota, 1973). Similarly, even presumably innocuous procedures such as handling of the neonate will cause a reduction in both the duration and the magnitude of the SHRP. In a 1966 review, Levine and Mullins showed that daily handling of the animals during the first week of life primed the HPA system to the effect of electric shock. Handled animals showed a small but significant increase in GC secretion in response to shock when tested during their second week; non-handled control showed none. Whether or not the actual mechanisms have been elucidated, the indisputable fact still stands: the neonatal brain, even during (or, perhaps, especially during) the SHRP, is highly sensitive to, and modifiable by, environmental stimuli. In this respect, the 'early handling' paradigm constitutes a particularly interesting model. It can be used both to demonstrate the above-mentioned statement and as a starting point from which to investigate the underlying causative mechanisms. In the following paragraphs, we shall proceed to elaborate further on this subject, especially on those aspects more closely related to the HPA axis.

Neonatal handling has long been known to produce less emotional and seemingly 'better adapted' rats. Animals that have been handled during infancy, for example, show a greater initial corticosteroid response to electric shock than that displayed by untreated animals when tested as adults. Non-handled animals respond more slowly to stress but the adrenocortical secretion appears to persist over a much longer period. Apparently, such animals are less capable of terminating stress–induced HPA activity either by a neurally mediated mechanism or by GC feedback action (Levine and Mullins, 1966). Based on animal studies, it is possible to state that rapid production of GCs is consistent with good adjustment to the environment – so long as efficient termination of GC secretion can also occur. The brain Type 1 and Type 2 corticosteroid receptor systems are an important consideration in the turning on and off of the HPA activity, respectively (De Kloet and Reul, 1987; McEwen and Brinton, 1987). Higher brain and pituitary CORT receptor levels have been shown, for example, to correlate with a more efficient feedback mechanism and better performance of conditioned behaviors (Sapolsky et al., 1985; Angelucci et al., 1983). Does handling (or, more in general, environmental stimuli) modify CORT receptor ontogeny? If so, which are the underlying mechanisms?

Corticosteroid receptors and brain development

From recent studies carried out on rats, it seems that neonatal handling does indeed result in a persistently elevated level of hippocampal corticosteroid receptor capacity (Meaney et al., 1985c). A number of factors are known to be involved in regulation of receptor number in the adult rat. Among these are certain neuropeptides (related to ACTH and vasopressin), neurotransmitters and the homologous hormone (De Kloet et al., 1986, 1987). The few studies to date devoted to this subject in the neonatal rat show that the ability of CORT receptors to adjust to changing circulating CORT levels appears slowly during the 2nd to 3rd week of life (Sapolsky et al., 1985). Administration of high doses of thyroid hormone during development has been reported to increase the number of GC receptors during adulthood. Furthermore, a large amount of propylthiouracil (a thyroid hormone synthesis inhibitor) interfered with the normal development, including that of the GC receptors (Meaney et al., 1987). Thus thyroid hormone might also be involved in GC receptor maturation. It was thought that handling causes hypothermia with consequent release of thyroid hormones. Although this proposal is both ingenious and challenging, data on the physiological stimulation of the thyroid gland during ontogeny are still lacking.

GC receptors display a considerable degree of plasticity during development. The immunocytochemical studies have clearly pointed to migration of GC receptor immunopositive cells in the brain and dramatic changes in GC receptor density. Type 2 immunoreactivity (Type 2-ir) localization showed a distinctive developmental trend towards greater compactness within the cell fields, with a greater restriction of immunostaining to the cell fields and exclusion of adjoining areas. This migration of Type 2-ir cells was particularly evident in the hippocampus and hypothalamus. Moreover, in the hippocampal CA_3 and CA_4 cell fields, as well as in the suprachiasmatic nucleus, Type 2-ir density is high perinatally and disappears during the second week of life. Finally, while in the adult animal GC receptor agonists easily induce a conformational change in the receptor, this activation of the Type 2 receptor seems impaired transiently during the second week of life as judged from the inability of GR receptor agonist to enhance immunostaining in the brain (Van Eekelen et al., 1987; Rosenfeld et al., 1988). Studies in the adult rat have shown that GC receptor expression is sensitive to presynaptic activity. Thus, an increase in Type 2 receptor number is observed following lesioning of the commissural-associational fibers of the hippocampus (De Ronde et al., 1986) and denervation of the intermediate lobe of the pituitary (Seger et al., 1987). In the hippocampus, at least, this receptor increase is transient, correlating with the re-innervation of the receptor-containing neurons. This would suggest that the formation of a functional neural input suppresses Type 2 gene expression. It is of general interest that the disappearance of the Type 2 receptor from the suprachiasmatic nucleus and the hippocampal CA_3 and CA_4 region during development coincides with a period of intense synaptogenesis. The neonatal brain, therefore, may in a way constitute a natural 'lesion and recovery' model and it is tempting to speculate that in the neonate, suppression of functional Type 2 receptors may also occur as a result of the formation of synaptic contacts. The similarity between the neonate brain and the denervation of nerve cells may be taken one step further with respect to the functional consequence. Our recent observations in the intermediate lobe show that in the denervated cell, the newly generated GC receptor molecules seem to mediate GC action on POMC gene expression. However, while in the anterior lobe GC suppresses POMC gene expression, it stimulates POMC in the denervated cell (Seger et al., 1987). Could it be that a similar mechanism explains the high circulating endorphin levels in the neonate? Taken together, the presently available evidence indicates that steroid hormones, including the corticosteroids, have an important influence on the permanent structural organization of the brain. It is likely that most of these corticosteroid effects are exerted via receptors. Transynaptic modulation of Type 2 receptor expression during ontogeny may thus contribute to the pattern of GR-ir. The remarkable changes in Type 2 receptor localization and density could thus account for the great variety in corticosteroid effects observed at different postnatal ages: areas containing at that time large amounts of functionally active receptors would constitute the 'windows of vulnerability'.

Glucocorticoid effects on brain development

During the SHRP, the HPA axis is sensitive to very subtle manipulations. The question can now be raised as to whether these (relatively) small increases in GC secretion could be involved in the organization of neural circuitry during development. There is an extensive literature dealing with the effects of perinatal GC administration on the development of the CNS in general. Unfortunately, most studies have used pharmacological doses of GCs in their experimental paradigms. In consequence, the ensuing results are not necessarily relevant from a physiological point of view and the question posed above must, for now, remain open. Nevertheless, the relevance of these studies to the field of functional neuroteratology is obvious. In the remainder of this contribution we shall briefly review some of the more salient effects of GC administration during ontogeny. Table I gives an overview of the effects of neonatal GC administration on brain morphology, chemistry and function.

Effects on cell acquisition

GCs are predominantly catabolic. They inhibit cell division, protein synthesis, and amino acid and glucose uptake in both the adult and the immature organism (Munck, 1984). In addition to these general, widespread effects, there is evidence for a specific action of CORT on the developing nervous system. High levels of GCs have profound effects on neurogenesis and gliogenesis (for review see Bohn, 1984). They have been shown to inhibit the rate of cell proliferation, alter the time course over which various types of microneurons are generated ('neuronal birthdays') as well as cause a precocious cessation of cell division in some stem cells. In cells that have

TABLE 1A

Summary of effects after treatment of neonatal rats with high and low doses of glucocorticoids. A: Short-term and long-term damaging effects of high doses of glucocorticoids (data taken from Angelucci et al., 1983; Nyakas et al., 1983; Bohn et al., 1984). B: Glucocorticoid requirement for brain development (data taken from Doupe and Patterson, 1982; Meyer, 1985; Bohn et al., 1986). TH = tyrosine hydroxylase; PNMT = phenylethanolamine N-methyl-transferase.

Effects of high (milligram) doses of glucocorticoids on brain development

---

Short term:
    Inhibits neurogenesis and gliogenesis
    Alters neuronal birthdays
    Causes precocious cessation of cell division
    Retards myelination, formation of dendritic spikes, axonal growth and synaptic genesis
    Delays maturation of evoked potentials
    Delays appearance of HPA circadian rhythmicity
    Affects stress hyporesponsive period
    Delays spontaneous alternating behavior

Long term:
    Causes permanent reduction of brain weight, size and shape, DNA content and myelination
    Produces deficit in passive and active avoidance behavior
    Produces deficit in problem solving
    Increases general motor activity
    Increases novelty-induced ambulation

TABLE 1B

Examples of glucocorticoid requirement for brain development

Determination of cellular and neurotransmitter phenotype
    Chromaffin cells vs. sympathetic neurons
    Adrenergic vs. cholinergic sympathetic neurons
Acceleration of differentiation and maturation of a previously determined phenotype
    Increases TH in sympathetic neurons
    Increases PNMT in chromaffin cells
Stimulation of expression of glial enzymes
    Glycerolphosphate dehydrogenase
    Glutamine synthetase

---

ceased division, GCs retard myelination, the formation of dendritic spines, axonal growth and synaptogenesis. Depending upon the time of GC treatment, these effects may be irreversible (Bohn, 1984). GC treatment in the late developmental period, for instance, has permanent effects on neurogenesis and gliogenesis. The effects are more pronounced in those areas undergoing active growth and differentiation at the moment of treatment. Extensive postnatal neurogenesis, for example, occurs in the cerebellum and hippocampus. Forty-five percent of the granular neurons in the dentate gyrus of the hippocampus are formed during the first postnatal week. These are small round microneurons which make contact with the prenatally formed axonal processes that innervate the hippocampus. GCs severely inhibit neurogenesis in this area. However, if treatment is discontinued sufficiently early, cell proliferation may compensate for the prior inhibition, leading to a normal-sized tissue in the adult (Bohn, 1984). In contrast, in the cerebellum, size and weight remain reduced throughout development and in the adult, irrespective of when treatment is terminated. It should be noted, however, that qualitative as well as quantitative effects have also been described. Thus, the deficit in the number of cells present in the adult may not accurately reflect the extent of the damage caused. This can be clearly seen in the cerebellum: while early GC treatment results in a much smaller deficit in the final number of cells when compared to animals treated late in development, the early treatment has a far more dramatic effect than the late treatment on the shape of the cerebellum, resulting in grossly malformed lobules in the adult (Bohn, 1984). It would be preposterous to assume that these morphological aberrations have no pathophysiological and/or behavioral consequences. Glial cell proliferation is also depressed by GC administration. This results in a, possibly permanent, reduction in myelination (Bohn, 1984).

Effects on differentiation, proliferation and enzymes
    In vitro experiments have shown that GCs play

an important role in the choice between several cellular and neurotransmitter phenotypes. They permit preferentially the development of chromaffin cells over sympathetic neurons from a precursor cell, i.e. the small intensely fluorescent cells, and prevent adrenergic sympathetic neurons of the superior cervical ganglion (SCG) from developing cholinergic properties (MacLennan et al., 1980). In both these cases, GCs apparently act by modulating the influence of other developmental signals. Thus, the chromaffin cell phenotype may result from GC suppression of NGF-induced neuronal differentiation. At the same time, by inhibiting the release of cholinergic inducing factor from the non-neuronal tissue surrounding the sympathetic neurons, GCs prevent the sympathetic SCG neurons from changing to the cholinergic phenotype (Fukuda, 1980; Hendry et al., 1987).

GCs accelerate both the differentiation and the maturation of a previously determined phenotype. Thus, they increase tyrosine hydroxylase (TH) levels in sympathetic neurons both directly and via a transsynaptic mechanism. In the adrenomedullary chromaffin cells GCs cause an increase in the levels of phenylethanolamine N-methyltransferase (PNMT), the enzyme which catalyses the methylation of norepinephrine to epinephrine (Bohn et al., 1986). Thus, in the absence of GC norepinephrine predominates and after administration of GC the epinephrine levels rise. GCs appear to exert this effect via a CORT-dependent endogenous stabilizing factor, S-adenosylmethionine, which protects PNMT against denaturation (Ciaranello, 1978; Doupe and Patterson, 1982). GCs are also required for the expression of certain glial enzymes during development (Meyer, 1985). Glycerol-phosphate dehydrogenase, a glial cell-specific enzyme important in myelination, apparently requires the continuous presence of GCs for both its induction and developmental increase. Another GC-induced glial enzyme is glutamine synthetase. This enzyme catalyses the formation of glutamine from glutamate and ammonia. It may serve a role in the reduction of glutamate and ammonia levels in the brain. This function may be particularly important after stress, when levels of both substrates are high: glutamate is a well-known excitatory transmitter, while ammonia is a toxic metabolite (Munck et al., 1984).

Effects on physiology

GCs also delay the maturation of a number of endogenous features of the CNS. Electrophysiological studies have demonstrated a pronounced effect of neonatal GC administration on the maturation of evoked potentials (Salas and Schapiro, 1970) and electro-shock seizure threshold (Vernadakis and Woodbury, 1963). High doses of GCs administered neonatally have profound effects on the development of the HPA system. Thus, for example, they have been found to delay the appearance of the circadian rhythm in HPA activity as well as the HPA response to stressful stimuli (Krieger, 1972). Finally, at a behavioral level, GCs have been shown to delay the manifestation of spontaneous alternating behavior, assumed to be under the control of the hippocampus (Nyakas, 1983), and, in much lower doses (approx. 1 μg), to impair approach and following behavior in one-day-old chicks. This latter effect is reversed by prior administration of GC antiserum. This would seem to indicate that GCs (or ACTH-related peptide fragments) are needed for imprinting to occur (Martin, 1978).

Numerous long-term behavioral and physiological effects of perinatal GC manipulation have been documented. Either GCs were administered directly into the new-born, or studies were performed with GC-nursed neonatal rats which received the steroids via the mother. The great variety in dosage (mg range) and timing schedule of GC administration does not allow a uniform inference of the effects. Commonly, general motor activity and novelty-induced ambulatory activity, for example, appear to be increased in adults treated with GCs during postnatal days 1–5, but hyperactivity and deficient motor performance are observed with GCs administered during postnatal day 7. Several aspects of learning and memory functions are impaired: deficits in passive and active avoidance behavior and problem-solving paradigms have been found. Reproductive functions also appear to be impaired (Angelucci et al., 1983; Nyakas, 1983; Bohn, 1984; Pavlik et al., 1985). Other studies have used prenatal GC manipulation by treating the pregnant mothers with steroids or with compounds such as metopirone which interfere with mother and fetal corticosteroidogenesis. As in the case with postnatal GC treatment, prenatal GC administration results in reduced adrenocortical reactivity and behavioral impairments of the adult rats (Naumenko and Dygalo, 1980; Bohn, 1984; Peruzovic and Milkovic, 1986). In addition to the (presumably) central effects described, the primary-induced GC defect in all species studied (except, apparently, in humans) is cleft palate (Schardein, 1981).

Surprisingly few human neuroteratological effects have been described in the clinical literature. Marton and Szondy (1982) found a slowing of psychomotor development in prematurely born children who had been exposed in utero to high doses of GC. This deficit still persisted at 2 years of age (Marton and Szondy, 1982; Swaab and Mirmiran, 1986). EEG alteration, pituitary-adrenal depression and immunosuppression in these same children were also reported. GCs are the major cause of drug-induced growth retardation in childhood; dosages only slightly above physiological level cause a slowing or complete cessation of statural growth (Marton, 1982). It is not known, though, whether these early childhood GC effects persist until and during adulthood.

Concluding remarks

In rats, postnatal GCs reduce cell number in the developing brain and regulate the phenotypic expression of certain cell types. At the same time, GCs have a pronounced influence on growth and differentiation of monoaminergic neurotransmitter systems in brain and periphery. In addition, they may affect other hormonal systems also involved in developmental processes. Thus,

whereas high levels of GCs are damaging for postnatal maturation, low levels seem to be an absolute requirement for this maturation to progress normally.

Our recent immunocytochemical studies in the rat indicate that CORT receptors have considerable plasticity during development. Receptors are expressed in certain brain regions during the first postnatal days but disappear at the time neural contacts are established. Examples of such temporary expression can be found in the suprachiasmatic nucleus and the CA_3 region of the hippocampus of the rat; these areas contain an abundance of GC receptors only during the first postnatal days. This apparent dependency of expression of steroid receptors on functional neural input is reminiscent of the effects of neurotransmitters on steroid-receptor expression in brain of the adult animal. As mentioned previously, selective lesioning of neurotransmitter input induces the appearance of GC receptors in target cells which previously did not contain detectable levels of receptor. Therefore, it is not unlikely that at least some of the regulatory processes operating in the adult animal during recovery from brain damage may be similar to those taking place during the neonatal period.

The importance of GC receptors for growth and differentiation processes is highlighted by the studies showing receptor-dependent induction of cleft palate (Goldman, 1984). Similarly, the lungs of premature babies suffering from myeline membrane disease or idiopathic respiratory distress syndrome have been shown to lack the normal large concentrations of GC receptor (Ballard and Ballard, 1974), suggesting that this lack may be one of the causes of the disease. Given the critical role the receptor plays within the HPA axis, it would be of interest to know the extent to which these early experiences and developmental events affect receptor ontogeny in particular, and HPA reactivity in general. Although at this stage mostly circumstantial, there are some data linking early experience, HPA reactivity, personality types and ability to cope with environmental challenges – a matter of obvious relevance for the fields of medicine and psychiatry.

Little is known about transplacental effects on fetal neural development following GC treatment. The data available show that there are wide differences among species in metabolism and transplacental transport of steroid hormones, and, in particular, in the timing and vulnerability of fetal development (Bohn, 1984). The rat, however, is an altricious species. Studies of GC effects on brain development in the perinatal rat are therefore of possible significance in estimating potential teratological hazards in human prenatal care.

As has been pointed out in this chapter, GCs are potent teratogens in laboratory animals. They produce an extensive array of effects, ranging from subtle changes in 'emotionality' to overt physical aberrations such as cleft palate. However, and probably due to the fact that most GC effects are hard to identify, particularly in humans (which does not mean, of course, that they do not exist), little attention has been paid, in the clinical setting, to this compelling body of evidence. GCs are commonly employed as treatment for a variety of childhood diseases, either as anti-inflammatory agents or in the prevention of respiratory distress syndrome in premature infants. In view of this widespread use of GC, a more in-depth evaluation of the possible complications of corticosteroid therapy and the potential toxicity of GC prophylaxis in the neonatal human has become a matter of critical urgency.

References

Ader, R. and Grota L.J. (1973) Adrenocortical mediation of the effects of early life experiences. In E. Zimmermann, W.H. Gispen, B.H. Marks and D. De Wied (Eds.), *Drug Effects on Neuroendocrine Regulation, Progress in Brain Research, Vol. 39*, Elsevier, Amsterdam, pp. 396–406.

Ader, R. (1975) Neonatal stimulation and maturation of the 24–hour adrenocortical rhythm. In W.H. Gispen, T.B. Van Wimersma-Greidanus and D. De Wied (Eds.), *Hormones, Homeostasis and the Brain, Progress in Brain Research, Vol. 42*, Elsevier, Amsterdam, pp. 333–341.

Angelucci, L., Patacchioli, F.R., Chierichetti, C. and Laureti, S. (1983) Changes in behavior and brain glucocorticoid receptor detected in adult life of corticosterone-nursed rats. In G. Zbinden, V. Cuomo, G. Racagni and B. Weiss (Eds.), *Application of Behavioral Pharmacology in Toxicology*, Raven Press, New York, pp. 277–291.

Balazs, R. and Cotterrell, M. (1972) Effect of hormonal state on cell number and functional maturation of the brain. *Nature (London)*, 236: 348–350.

Ballard, P.L. and Ballard, R.A. (1974) Cytoplasmic receptor for glucocorticoids in lungs of the human fetus and neonate. *J. Clin. Invest.*, 53: 477–486.

Ballard, P.L. (1979) Glucocorticoids and glucocorticoid hormone action. In J.D. Baxter and G.G. Rousseau (Eds.), *Monographs in Endocrinology, Vol. 12*, Springer-Verlag, Berlin, pp. 495–515.

Bayon, A., Shoemaker, W.E., Bloom, F.E., Mauss, A. and Guillemin, R. (1979) Perinatal development of the endorphin- and enkephalin-containing systems in the rat. *Brain Res.*, 179: 93–101.

Boer, G.J. (1987) Development of vasopressin systems and their function. In D.M. Gash and G.J. Boer (Eds.), *Vasopressin, Principles and Properties*, Plenum Press, New York, in press.

Bohn, M.C. (1984) Glucocorticoid induced teratologies of the nervous system. In J. Yauci (Ed.), *Neurobehavioral Teratologies of the Nervous System*, Elsevier, Amsterdam, pp. 365–387.

Bohn, M. Goldstein, M. and Black, I.B. (1986) Expression and development of phenylethanolamine *N*-methyltransferase (PNMT) in rat brain stem: studies with glucocorticoids. *Dev. Biol.*, 114: 180–193.

Bohus, B., Benus, R.F., Fokkema, D.S., Koolhaas, J.M., Nyakas, C., Van Oortmerssen, G.A., Prins, A.J.A., De Ruiter, A.J.H., Scheurink, A.J.W. and Steffens, A.B. (1987) Neuroendocrine states and behavioural and physiological stress responses. In E.R. de Kloet, V.M. Wiegant and D. De Wied (Eds.), *Neuropeptides and Brain Function, Progress in Brain Research, Vol. 72*, Elsevier, Amsterdam, pp. 57–70.

Bugnon, C. Feldman, D. Gouget, A. and Cardot, J. (1982) Ontogeny of the corticoliberin neuroglandular system in rat brain. *Nature*, 298: 159–161.

Buys, R.M. (1983) Vasopressin and oxytocin: their role in neurotransmission. *Pharmacol. Ther.*, 22: 127–141.

Burnstein, S. and Westort, C. (1967) Developmental pattern of hepatic steroid sulfatase activity. *Endocrinology*, 92: 1120–1126.

Chatelain, A. and Dupouy, J.P. (1985) Adrenocorticotropic hormone in the anterior and neuro-intermediate lobes of the rat during the perinatal period: polymorphism, biological and immunological activities of ACTH. *Biol. Neonate*, 47: 235–248.

Clayton, C.J., Grosser, B.I. and Stevens, W. (1977) The ontogeny of corticosterone and dexamethasone receptors in the rat brain. *Brain Res.*, 134: 445–453.

Ciaranello, R.D. (1978) Regulation of phenylethanolamine-N-methyltransferase synthesis and degradation. I. Regulation by rat adrenal glucocorticoids. *Mol. Pharmacol.*, 14: 478–489.

Dallman, M.F. (1987) Regulation of ACTH secretion: variation on a theme of B. *Rec. Progr. Horm. Res.*, in press.

De Kloet, E.R., Burbach, J.P.H. and Mulder, G.H. (1977) Localization and role of transcortin-like molecules in the anterior pituitary. *Mol. Cell. Endocr.*, 7: 261–273.

De Kloet, E.R., Voorhuis, T.A.M., Leunissen, J.L.M. and Koch, B. (1984) Intracellular CBG-like molecules in the rat pituitary. *J. Steroid. Biochem.*, 20: 367–371.

De Kloet, E.R., Palkovits, M. and Mezey, E. (1986) Opioid peptides: localization, source and avenues of transport. In D. De Wied, W.H. Gispen and Tj.B. van Wimersma-Greidanus (Eds.), *Neuropeptides and Behavior, Encyclopedia of Pharmacology and Therapeutics, Vol. 1*, Pergamon Press, New York, pp. 1–41.

De Kloet, E.R., Reul, J.M.H.M., de Ronde, F.S.W., Bloemers, M. and Ratka, A. (1986) Function and plasticity of brain corticosteroid receptor system: action of neuropeptides. *J. Steroid. Biochem.*, 25: 723–731.

De Kloet, E.R. and Reul, J.M.H.M. (1987) Feedback action and tonic influence of corticosteroids on brain function: a concept arising from heterogeneity of brain receptor system. *Psychoneuroendocrinology*, 12: 83–105.

De Kloet, E.R., Ratka, A., Reul, J.M.H.M., Sutanto, W. and Eekelen, J.A.M. (1987) Corticosteroid receptor types in brain: regulation and putative function. *Annals N.Y. Acad. Sci.*, in press.

De Ronde, F.S.W., De Kloet, E.R. and Nyakas, C. (1986) Corticosteroid receptor plasticity and recovery of a deficient hippocampus associated behavior after unilateral (dorsal) hippocampectomy. *Brain Res.*, 374: 219–226.

De Wied, D. (1987) The neuropeptide concept. In E.R. De Kloet, V.M. Wiegant and D. De Wied (Eds.), *Neuropeptides and Brain Function, Progress in Brain Research, Vol. 72*, Elsevier, Amsterdam, pp. 93–108.

Doupe, A.J. and Patterson, P.H. (1982) Glucocorticoids and the developing nervous system. In D. Ganten and D. Pfaff (Eds.), *Current Topics in Neuroendocrinology, Vol. 2*, Springer-Verlag, Berlin, pp. 23–43.

Fukuda, K. (1980) Hormonal control of neurotransmitter choice in sympathetic neurone cultures. *Nature*, 287: 552–555.

Funder, J.W. and Sheppard, K. (1987) Adrenocortical steroids and the brain. *Annu. Rev. Physiol.*, 49: 397–411.

Fuxe, K., Wikstrom, A.C., Okret, S., Agnati, L.F., Harfstrand, F., Yu, Z.-Y., Granholm, L., Zoli, M., Vale, W. and Gustafsson, J.-A. (1985) Mapping of glucocorticoid receptor immunoreactive neurons in the rat tel- and diencephalon using a monoclonal antibody against liver glucocorticoid receptor. *Endocrinology*, 117: 1803–1812.

Gerlach, J.L. and McEwen, B.S. (1972) Rat brain binds adrenal steroid hormone: radioautography of hippocampus with corticosterone. *Science*, 175: 1133–1136.

Glydon, R.J. (1957) The development of blood supply of the pituitary in the albino rat with special reference to the portal vessels. *J. Anat.*, 91: 237–250.

Goldman, L., Winget, C., Hollingshead, G.W. and Levine, S. (1973) Postweaning development of the negative feedback in the pituitary adrenal system of the rat. *Neuroendocrinology*, 12: 199–211.

Goldman, A.S. (1984) Biochemical mechanism of glucocorticoid and phenytoin-induced cleft palate. *Curr. Top. Dev. Biol.*, 19: 217–224.

Guillet, R. and Michaelson, S.M. (1978) Corticotropin responsiveness in the neonatal rat. *Neuroendocrinology*, 27: 119–125.

Gustafsson, J., Carlstedt-Duke, J., Poellinger, L., Okret, S., Wikstrom, A., Bronnegard, M., Gillner, M., Dong, Y., Fuxe, K., Cintra, A., Harfstrand, A. and Agnati, L. (1987) Biochemistry, molecular biology and physiology of the glucocorticoid receptors. *Endocr. Rev.* 8: 185–234.

Hendry, I.A., Hill, C.E. and McLennan, I.S. (1987) RU38486 blocks the steroid regulation of transmitter choice in cultured rat sympathetic ganglion. *Brain Res.*, 402: 264–268.

Henning, S.J. (1978) Plasma concentrations of total and free corticosterone during development in the rat. *Am. J. Physiol.*, 235: E451–456.

Iny, L.J., Gianoulakis, C., Palmour, R.M. and Meaney, M.J. (1987) The β-endorphin response to stress during postnatal development in the rat. *Dev. Brain Res.*, 31: 177–181.

Jones, M.T., Gillham, B., Greenstein, B.D., Beckford, U. and Holmes, M.C. (1982) Feedback action of adrenal steroid hormones. In D. Ganten and D. Pfaff (Eds.), *Adrenal Action of the Brain, Current Topics in Neuroendocrinology, Vol. 2*, Springer-Verlag, Berlin, pp. 45–68.

Keller-Wood, M.E. and Dallman, M.F. (1984) Corticosteroid inhibition of ACTH-secretion. *Endocr. Rev.* 5: 1–24.

Kiss, J.Z., Mezey, E. and Skirboll, L. (1984) Corticotropin-releasing factor-immunoreactive neurons of the paraventricular nucleus become vasopressin positive after adrenalectomy. *Proc. Natl. Acad. Sci. USA* 81: 1854–1858.

Koch, B., Lutz-Bucher, B., Briaud, B. and Mialhe, C. (1978) Specific interaction of corticosteroids with binding sites in the plasma membranes of the rat anterior pituitary gland. *J. Endocrinol.* 79: 215–222.

Kordon, C., Bluet-Pajot, M.T., Clauser, H., Drouva, S., Enjalbert, A. and Epelbaum, J. (1987) New designs in neuroendocrine systems. In E.R. De Kloet, V.M. Wiegant and D. De Wied (Eds.), *Neuropeptides and Brain Function, Progress in Brain Research, Vol. 72*, Elsevier, Amsterdam, pp. 27–34.

Krieger, D.T. (1972) Corticosteroid periodicity: critical period for abolition by neonatal injection of corticosteroid. *Science*, 178: 1205–1207.

118

Levine, S. and Mullins, R.F.Jr. (1966) Hormonal influences on brain organization in infant rats. *Science*, 152: 1585–1592.

Levine, S. (1970) The pituitary-adrenal system and the developing brain. In D. De Wied and J.A.W.M. Weijnen (Eds.), *Pituitary, Adrenal and the Brain, Progress in Brain Research, Vol. 32.*, Amsterdam, pp. 79–85.

MacLennan, I.S., Hill, C.E. and Hendry, I.A. (1980) Glucocorticoids modulate neurotransmitter choice in developing superior cervical ganglion. *Nature*, 283: 206–207.

Martin, J.T. (1978) Imprinting behavior, pituitary-adrenocortical modulation of the approach response. *Science*, 200: 563–567.

Marton, I.S., Gati, I., Nemenyi, M. and Szondy, M. (1979) Psychomotor development and cord endocrine parameters of premature newborn exposed to steroid in utero. In L. Zichella and P. Pancheri (Eds.), *Psychoneuroendocrinology in Reproduction*, Elsevier, Amsterdam, pp, 509–514.

Marton, I.S. and Szondy, M. (1982) Possible neuroendocrine hazards of prenatal steroid exposure. In E. Endroczi (Ed.), *Neuropeptides, Neurotransmitters and Regulation of Endocrine Processes*, pp, 535–543.

McEwen, B.S., Weiss, J.M. and Schwartz, L.S. (1968) Selective retention of corticosterone by limbic structures in rat brain. *Nature*, 220: 911–912.

McEwen, B.S., De Kloet, E.R. and Rostene, W. (1986) Adrenal steroid receptors in the nervous system. *Physiol. Rev.*, 66: 1121–1189.

McEwen, B.S. and Brinton, R.E. (1987) Neuroendocrine aspects of adaptation. In E.R. De Kloet, V.M. Wiegant and D. De Wied (Eds.), *Neuropeptides and Brain Function, Progress in Brain Research, Vol. 72*, Elsevier, Amsterdam, pp. 11–26.

Meaney, M.J., Aitken, D.H., Bodnoff, S.R., Iny, L.J., Tatarewicz, J.E. and Sapolsky, R.M. (1985a) Early postnatal handling alters glucocorticoid receptor concentrations in selected brain regions. *Behav. Neurosci.*, 99: 765–770.

Meaney, M.J., Sapolsky, R.M. and McEwen, B.S. (1985b) The development of glucocorticoid receptor system in the rat limbic brain. I. Ontogeny and autoregulation. *Dev. Brain Res.*, 18: 159–164.

Meaney, M.J., Sapolsky, R.M. and McEwen, B.S. (1985c) The development of the glucocorticoid receptor system in the rat limbic brain. II. An autoradiographic study. *Dev. Brain Res.*, 18: 165–168.

Meaney, M.J., Aitken, D.H. and Sapolsky, R.M. (1987) Thyroid hormones influence the development of hippocampal glucocorticoid receptors in the rat: a mechanism for the effects of postnatal handling on the development of the adrenocortical stress response. *Neuroendocrinology*, 45: 278–283.

Meyer, J.S. (1985) Biochemical effects of corticosteroids on neural tissues. *Physiol. Rev.*, 65: 946–1021.

Mezey, E., Young III, W.S., Siegel, R.E. and Kovacs, K. (1987) Neuropeptides and neurotransmitters involved in regulation of corticotropin-releasing factor-containing neurons in the rat. In E.R. De Kloet, V.M. Wiegant and D. De Wied (Eds.) *Neuropeptides and Brain Function, Progress in Brain Research, Vol. 72*, Elsevier, Amsterdam, pp. 119–127.

Munck, A., Guyre, P.M. and Holbrook, N.J. (1984) Physiological functions of glucocorticoids in stress and their relation to pharmacological actions. *Endocr. Rev.* 5: 25–44.

Munck, A. and Guyre, P.M. (1986) Glucocorticoids, physiology, pharmacology and stress. In G.P. Chrousos, D.L. Loriaux and M.B. Lipsett (Eds.), *Steroid Hormone Resistance – Mechanisms and Clinical Aspects, Advances in Experimental Medicine and Biology, Vol. 196*, Plenum Press, New York, pp. 81–96.

Naumenko, E.V. and Dygalo, N.N. (1980) Noradrenergic brain mechanisms and emotional stress in adult rats after prenatal hydrocortisone treatment. In H. Parvez and S. Parvez (Eds.), *Biogenic Amines in Development*, Elsevier, Amsterdam, pp. 373–388.

Nyakas, C. (1983) Behavioral effects of infantile administration of glucocorticoid hormones. In G. Zbinden (Ed.), *Application of Behavioral Pharmacology and Toxicology*, Raven Press, New York, pp. 265–276.

Olpe, H. and McEwen, B.S. (1976) Glucocorticoid binding to receptor-like proteins in rat brain and pituitary: ontogenetic and experimentally induced changes. *Brain Res.*, 105: 121–128.

Palkovits, M. (1987) Organization of the stress response at the anatomical level. In E.R. De Kloet, V.M. Wiegant and D. De Wied (Eds.), *Neuropeptides and Brain Function, Progress in Brain Research, Vol. 72*, Elsevier, Amsterdam, pp. 47–55.

Pavlik, A., Benesova, O. and Buresova, M. (1985) Model studies of perinatal insults: a comprehensive approach to behavioral teratology. *Physiol. Bohemoslov., Suppl.* 34: 117–120.

Peruzovic, M. and Milkovic, K. (1986) Prenatal ACTH and corticosteroids, development and behavior in rat. In M.M. Cohen (Ed.), *Monographs in Neural Sciences, Vol. 12*, Karger, Basel, pp. 103–111.

Ramaley, J.A. (1976) Entrainment of the adrenal rhythm to photoperiod prior to puberty: effects of early experience in the adrenal rhythm and puberty. *Neuroendocrinology* 21: 225–235.

Reul, J.M.H.M. and De Kloet, E.R. (1985) Two receptor systems for corticosteroids in the brain: microdistribution and differential occupation. *Endocrinology*, 117: 2505–2511.

Reul, J.M.H.M., Van Den Bosch, F. and De Kloet, E.R. (1987) Differential response of type I and type II corticosteroid receptors to changes in plasma steroid level and circadian rhythmicity. *Neuroendocrinology*, 45: 407–412.

Rosenfeld, P., Van Eekelen, J.A.M., Levine, S. and De Kloet, E.R. (1988) Ontogeny of the glucocorticoid receptor: an immunocytochemical study. *Dev. Brain Res.*, in press.

Rosenfeld, P., Sutanto, W., Levine, S. and De Kloet, E.R. (1988) Ontogeny of Type 1 and Type II corticosteroid receptors in the rat hippocampus. *Dev. Brain Res.*, in press.

Sakly, M. and Koch, B. (1981) Ontogenesis of the glucocorticoid receptor in the anterior pituitary gland: transient dissociation among cytoplasmic receptor density, nuclear uptake and regulation of corticotropic activity. *Endocrinology* 108: 591–596.

Sakly, M. and Koch, B. (1983) Ontogenetical variations of transcortin modulate glucocorticoid receptor function and corticotropic activity in the pituitary gland. *Horm. Metab. Res.*, 15: 92–96.

Salas, M. and Schapiro, S. (1970) Hormonal influences upon the maturation of the rat brain's responsiveness to sensory stimuli. *Physiol. Behav.*, 5: 7–11.

Sapolsky, R.M. and Meaney, M.J. (1986) Maturation of the adrenal stress response: neuroendocrine control mechanisms and the stress hyporesponsive period. *Brain Res. Rev.*, 11: 65–76.

Sapolsky, R.M. and Meaney, M.J. and McEwen, B.S. (1985) The development of the glucocorticoid receptor system in the rat limbic brain. III. Negative feedback regulation. *Dev. Brain Res.*, 18: 169–173.

Schardein, J.L. (1986) *Chemically Induced Birth Defects*, Marcel Dekker, New York, p. 307.

Schoenfield, N.M., Leathem, J.H. and Rabii, J. (1980) Maturation of adrenal stress response in the rat. *Neuroendocrinology*, 31: 101–105.

Seger, M., Van Eekelen, J.A.M., Kiss, J.Z., Burbach, J.P.H. and De Kloet, E.R. (1988) Stimulation of pro-opiomelanocortin gene expression by glucocorticoids in the denervated rat intermediate pituitary gland. *Neuroendocrinology*, in press.

Swaab, D. and Mirmiran, M. (1986) Functional and teratogenic effects of chemicals on the developing brain. In M.M. Cohen (Ed.), *Monographs in Neural Sciences, Vol. 12*, Karger, Basel, pp. 46–57.

Swanson, L.W., Sawchenko, P.E. and Lind, R.W. (1986) Regulation of multiple peptides in CRF parvacellular neurosecretory neurons: implications for the stress response. In T. Hokfelt, K. Fuxe and and B. Pernow (Eds.), *Progress in Brain Research, Vol. 68*, Elsevier, Amsterdam, pp. 169–190.

Tausk, M. (1951) Hat die Nebenniere tatsachlich eine Verteidigungsfunktion. In *Das Hormon*, Vol. 3, Organon, The Netherlands, p. 1.

Turner, B.B. (1978) Ontogeny of glucocorticoid binding in the rodent brain. *Am. Zool.*, 18: 461–475.

Van Eckelen, J.A.M., Kiss, J.Z., Westphal, H.M. and De Kloet, E.R. (1987) Immunocytochemical study on the intracellular localization of the type 2 glucocorticoid receptor in the rat brain. *Brain Res.*, 436: 120–128.

Van Eekelen, J.A.M., Rosenfeld, P. and De Kloet, E.R. (1987) Post-natal disappearance of glucocorticoid receptors from the suprachiasmatic nucleus. *Neurosci. Res. Commun.*, 1: 129–133.

Vernadakis, A. and Woodbury, D.M. (1963) Effect of cortisol on electroshock seizure thresholds in developing rats. *J. Pharmacol. Exp. Ther.*, 139: 110–113.

Walker, C.D., Perrin, M., Vale, W.W. and Rivier, C. (1986a) Ontogeny of the stress response in the rat: role of the pituitary and the hypothalamus. *Endocrinology*, 118: 1445–1451.

Walker, C.D., Sapolsky, R.M., Meaney, M.J., Vale, W.W. and Rivier, C.L. (1986b) Increased pituitary sensitivity to glucocorticoid feedback during the stress nonresponsive period in neonatal rat. *Endocrinology*, 119: 1816–1821.

Discussion

M. Mirmiran: You observed high levels of glucocorticoid receptors in the suprachiasmatic nucleus (SCN) at 5 days of postnatal age. Does this suggest a relationship between glucocorticoids and circadian rhythm in development?

E.R. De Kloet: Yes, indeed we have recently observed a gradual disappearance of the Type 2 glucocorticoid receptor in the SCN during the first two postnatal weeks of the rat. It could therefore well be that periodicity in metabolic and electrical activity of the SCN is entrained by the circadian rhythmicity in glucocorticoid secretion by the mother, in particular during the late prenatal period.

M. Mirmiran: Is there any circadian rhythmicity in stress response or corticosteroid response to stress?

E.R. De Kloet: There is indeed a circadian rhythm in responsiveness of the hypothalamo-pituitary-adrenal (HPA) axis to stress (Jones, 1979).

G.J. Boer: Since you made clear that postnatal stress does not induce a corticosteroid response but results in a β-endorphin release, could early stress-induced changes in the brain be explained by increased levels of the latter peptide?

E.R. De Kloet: Indeed it is remarkable that β-endorphin and α-MSH release shows a stress response in the neonatal rat, while the ACTH-corticosteroid axis shows only minimal changes. It can therefore be assumed that these end-products of pro-opiomelanocortin (POMC) processing have an important function in the development of the central nervous system. On the other hand, it should be pointed out that even persisting minimal changes in the corticosteroid level may have profound effects on brain development as well.

B.S. McEwen: Meany et al (1987) have shown that thyroid activation by handling mediates increased hippocampal glucocorticoid receptors. As suggested by G.J. Boer's question, might this not also be one of the 'other factors' which mediate the effects of handling and early experience? Do you have any experience in your lab in the role of thyroid hormone?

E.R. De Kloet: We do not have any evidence on the role of thyroid hormone in corticosteroid receptor regulation during development, but I am aware of the findings of Meany et al (1987). It is unclear from their experiments which of the two corticosteroid receptor types is increased following handling, which renders these findings difficult to interpret at present. Nevertheless, these findings may be of importance. Whether thyroid hormone underlies these 'handling' effects is difficult to say. In their postulate handling causes hypothermia, which was assumed to evoke thyroid hormone release. I don't remember whether they actually showed thyroid activation. I do remember, though, that they have used rather high doses of thyroid hormone and propylthiouracil to see their long-lasting effects on receptor concentration.

M.V. Johnston: Sapolsky and Pulsinelli (1985) found that corticosteroid sensitizes the adult hippocampus to ischemic injury. Is there any evidence that, in the fetus, steroids might have a similar effect to accentuate the injury caused by other teratogens?

E.R. De Kloet: Chronically elevated corticosteroid levels in general have effects on growth and differentiation of the central nervous system. Furthermore, as is the case in the adult rat, glucocorticoids are catabolic and inhibit glucose uptake and protein synthesis in the neonate. Although there is not much evidence at present, it can be expected that Sapolsky and Pulsinelli (1985) will observe similar effects of corticoids on ischemic injury in the neonatal brain as they did before in the adult.

References

Jones, M.T. (1979) Control of adrenocortical hormone secretion. In V.H.T. James (Ed.), *The Adrenal Gland.* Raven Press, New York, pp. 93–130.

Meany, M.J., Aitken, D.H. and Sapolsky, R.M. (1987) Thyroid hormone influence on the development of hippocampal glucocorticoid receptors in the rat: a mechanism for the effects of postnatal handling on the development of the adrenocortical stress response. *Neuroendocrinology*, 45: 278–282.

Sapolsky, R.M. and Pulsinelli, W. (1985) Glucocorticoids potentiate ischemic injury to neurons: therapeutic implication. *Science*, 229: 1397–1399.

G.J. Boer, M.G.P. Feenstra, M. Mirmiran, D.F. Swaab and F. Van Haaren
Progress in Brain Research, Vol. 73
© 1988 Elsevier Science Publishers B.V. (Biomedical Division)

CHAPTER 9

Actions of sex hormones on the brain: 'organization' and 'activation' in relation to functional teratology

Bruce S. McEwen

Laboratory of Neuroendocrinology, The Rockefeller University, 1230 York Avenue, New York, NY 10021, USA

Introduction

The nervous system responds to hormones secreted by the gonads, adrenals and thyroid gland during its development and in maturity. Hormonal responsiveness is related to the presence of receptor sites which mediate actions of these hormones at the level of gene expression (McEwen, 1988). These hormone receptors are proteins with a steroid binding domain and a DNA binding domain, which regulate genomic activity through binding to specific DNA sequences called 'enhancers' (Yamamoto, 1985).

Genomic activity is not confined to development, either in the nervous system or in any other organ of the body, but is does change qualitatively and quantitatively as the life of each organism progresses (McEwen, 1987). More importantly, genomic activity of brain cells is responsive to changes in the internal and external environment through the endocrine system. As the environment and experiences of an animal change, this is reflected in altered output of gonadal, adrenal, thyroid and other hormones under control of the hypothalamus via the pituitary gland. These hormones act in turn to modify structure and neurochemistry of brain cells and modify behavior, neuroendocrine output and other aspects of neural activity (McEwen, 1988).

When hormones are secreted in abnormal amounts or at the wrong time, or when hormones or pseudohormones are ingested or absorbed from medications, foodstuffs or toxicants, the nervous system may respond in abnormal ways and functional pathology or teratological consequences may result. Such abnormal hormone actions are significant when, for example, an adult male is exposed to high levels of female hormones, but they are more serious, and more likely to be permanent, when a developing organism is exposed to the wrong hormone at the wrong time. In this article, we shall examine the impact of gonadal hormones on the nervous system which are or may be related to functional teratologies. We shall do this after first examining the basic neuroendocrinology underlying gonadal steroid actions on the developing and adult brain.

Gonadal steroid receptors and actions in the brain

Adult brain

The mature brain of males and females contains receptors for estrogens, progestins and androgens and enzymes for converting these steroids to more or less active hormone metabolites (McEwen, 1988). The most important enzymes are those which aromatize testosterone or androstenedione to estrogens and those which convert testosterone and progesterone to 5 alpha reduced metabolites. Estrogen receptors are rather discretely localized within the pituitary, hypothalamus, preoptic area and amygdala, with

122

lesser concentrations in hippocampus and midbrain central gray (Pfaff and Keiner, 1973). Androgen receptors show a similar distribution, but there are lesser differences in concentration between brain areas (Sar and Stumpf, 1977). Progestin receptors are distributed in two ways: (1) those inducible by estrogen are found in pituitary, hypothalamus and preoptic area; (2) those not induced by estrogens are found throughout the rat brain, including amygdala, where there are many estrogen receptors, and cerebral cortex, where estrogen receptor content is very low (McEwen et al., 1983). Species like the guinea pig, hamster and ferret show similar patterns of progestin receptors as the rat, but the bonnet macaque shows very low levels of the non-inducible progestin receptor throughout the brain and shares with other species the estrogen induction of progestin receptors in pituitary and hypothalamus (McEwen et al., 1983). Not only estrogens but also androgens are connected to progestin receptors, and this occurs via the aromatase enzyme system. Conversion of testosterone to estradiol is responsible for inducing progestin receptors in the male brain to levels comparable, in intact males, with those found in proestrus female rats (McEwen et al., 1983).

If males and females are endowed with similar complements of gonadal hormone receptors and steroid converting enzymes, what is responsible for the differences between male and female brain function? The answer lies at several different levels. First and most obvious is that there are differences in hormone levels: estradiol is high in females and testosterone is high in males, and thus androgen receptors are occupied in males and estrogen receptors in females. Aromatizing enzymes are not evenly distributed among estrogen-receptor-rich areas, and, in fact, are virtually absent in rat pituitary and present in high concentrations in rat amygdala (Fig. 1). Thus circulating testosterone gives a different pattern of estrogen receptor occupancy to that produced by circulating estradiol (Lieberburg and McEwen, 1977).

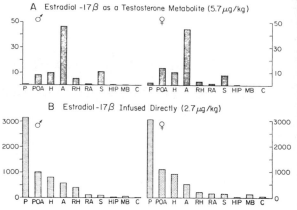

Fig. 1. (A) Levels of radioactivity identified as estradiol (E$_2$) present in brain cell nuclear fractions 2 h after [^{3}H]testosterone administration (5.7 µg/kg) to castrated-adrenalectomized adult male and female rats. (B) Levels of radioactivity present in brain cell nuclear fractions 2 h after [^{3}H]E$_2$ administration (2.7 µg/kg) to castrated-adrenalectomized adult male and female rats. Values are means of four determinations for each sex. Abbreviations: P = whole pituitary; POA = preoptic area: H = basomedial hypothalamus; A = cortico-medial amygdala; RH = rest of hypothalamus; RA = rest of amygdala; S = septum; HIP = hippocampus; MB = midbrain-central gray; C = parietal cortex. Reprinted by permission from Lieberburg and McEwen (1977).

The second level of sex differences in hormone action is in hormone responsiveness of discrete brain areas in spite of apparent similarities in content of the primary hormone receptor (McEwen, 1988). This may be illustrated by sex differences in the response of progestin receptor induction to estradiol, where male hypothalamus tends to respond less well to estrogen priming than female hypothalamus, not only in rats but also in guinea pigs and hamsters (Blaustein et al., 1980; Rainbow et al., 1982; Parsons et al., 1984; Brown et al., 1987; Fraille et al., 1987; Coirini and McEwen, 1987). Within the hypothalamus, sex differences in estrogen responsiveness are also apparent – the ventromedial nuclei, which are important for controlling feminine sexual behavior, show lesser response in males than in females compared to the neighboring arcuate nuclei (Rainbow et al., 1982: Parsons et al., 1984;

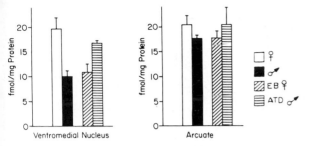

Fig. 2. The effects of hormonal manipulation during perinatal development on the induction of cytosol progestin receptors (CPR) by estradiol benzoate (EB) is shown. Analysis of variance tests revealed a significant treatment effect of perinatal EB and androstratriene-3,17-dione (ATD) administration on CPR levels in the ventromedial nucleus (VMN) ($F = 8.23$; $P < 0.001$), but not in other brain regions. Comparisons of individual means in the VMN using the Newman-Keuls test revealed that CPR induction in normal females and ATD-treated males differed significantly from those in normal males and EB-treated females ($P < 0.05$). There were no significant differences in VMN CPR levels between normal females and ATD-treated males or between normal males and EB-treated females. Student's t test revealed a sex difference (normal males vs. normal females) in CPR levels in the VMN ($P < 0.05$), but not in other brain regions. Each treatment group consisted of 24 animals; results were pooled to generate 8 independent determinations. All results are the means + S.E.M. expressed as femtomoles per mg protein. Data from Parsons et al. (1984).

Brown et al., 1987; Coirini and McEwen, 1987; See Fig. 2). Time course is important, and it even appears that the arcuate nuclei may respond more rapidly in males than in females (Coirini and McEwen, 1987). There are other examples of differential responsiveness of males and females to estrogens. These include estrogen actions to increase muscarinic receptors in basal hypothalamus, where females respond and males do not, and estrogen actions to alter serotonin-1 receptor levels, where estrogens produce different effects in male than in female brains (McEwen et al., 1987a).

How can these different estrogen actions be explained when there appear to be similar levels of estrogen receptors in male and female brains? The most general statement of an explanation is

that genomic responsiveness to the estrogen receptor differs, but how might this occur? One possibility is differential regulation of estrogen receptor function through neurotransmitter actions (De Nicola et al., 1981; Carrillo et al., 1983; Clark et al., 1985; Gietzen and Woolley, 1986; Blaustein, 1986; Blaustein et al., 1986). Additional sex differences may exist at the genomic levels in terms of which genes may be activated (McEwen, 1984). Finally, related to both possibilities, is the unknown contribution of sex differences in neuroanatomical connectivity, resulting in amounts and distributions of neurotransmitter release.

How do steroid hormones like estradiol influence cellular function in mature neurons, and what cellular changes take place? Perhaps the most careful observations to date have been made in the ventromedial (VMN) and arcuate (ARC) nuclei of the hypothalamus in response to estradiol (E). First of all, brief exposure to E for 2 h induces in VMN increased neuron soma diameter, nuclear and nucleolar size increases and increased cytoplasmic stacked rough endoplasmic reticulum; the neighboring arcuate nucleus does not respond within only 2 h but does respond after a longer time (McEwen et al., 1987b). In fact, within 6 h after E, both VMN and ARC show increased amounts of 28S ribosomal RNA, as judged by in situ hybridization (Jones et al., 1986). Brief exposure to E also evokes a pattern of change of protein synthesis, as judged from two-dimensional separation of proteins labeled in vitro with [^{35}S]methionine after in vivo hormone priming (McEwen et al., 1987b). Some proteins are induced, while synthesis of others appears to be suppressed (McEwen et al., 1987b). Different patterns of proteins are induced or repressed in VMN as opposed to medial preoptic area (McEwen et al., 1987b). Moreover, the pattern of regulated proteins changes as a function of time after E exposure is begun, suggesting that E triggers a cascade of genomic activation events over a number of hours (McEwen et al., 1987b). Progesterone exposure

124

appears to evoke its own pattern of protein synthesis, which is more pronounced in E-primed than in non-E-primed VMN and medial preoptic area (McEwen et al., 1987b).

As time passes after E exposure, various cellular features change in VMN, including increases by 24–72 h in progestin receptor levels and levels of muscarinic cholinergic (Rainbow et al., 1980; 1984) and oxytocin receptors (De Kloet et al., 1985) and decreases in type A gamma aminobutyric acid receptors (O'Connor et al., 1985) and cholecystokinin receptors (Akesson et al., 1987). Proenkephalin mRNA levels increase in VMN (Romano et al., 1986). Moreover, there is also evidence of increased synaptic density in the VMN 48 h after E treatment (Carrer and Aoki, 1982), suggesting the possibility of increased synaptic number or rearrangement of synaptic projections resulting from the hormone treatment under conditions where the effects are likely to be reversible ones.

Developing brain

The developing rat brain shows expression of receptors for estrogens, progestins and androgens within a few days or more after the time of final cell division in hypothalamus, preoptic area and amygdala (McEwen, 1985). In general, estrogen receptors are detectable earlier than progestin receptors, and progestin receptors are not inducible fully by E for a number of days after they first appear (MacLusky and McEwen, 1980: see Fig. 3). For the most part, estrogen and progestin receptors appear in the developing brain in exactly those places where they exist in the mature nervous system. However, the major exception is the cerebral cortex, which shows both estrogen and progestin receptor expression postnatally up to 2 weeks after birth, when receptor levels decline to low adult values (McEwen et al., 1982). Curiously, a left-right hemisphere sex difference in estrogen receptor level exists which may relate to sex differences in adult rat cerebral thickness (Sandhu et al., 1986). These differences in adult cerebral cortical thickness are on opposite sides

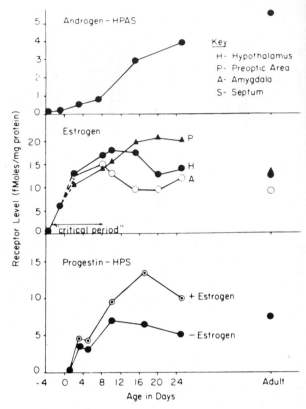

Fig. 3. Developmental time course of gonadal steroid receptors in female rat brains. Receptor levels are expressed as fmol/mg cytosol protein versus age in days post- or prenatal. Brain structures are denoted by letters (see key); note that they were studied individually (estradiol) or as tissue pools (eg., hypothalamus–preoptic area–septum–amygdala (HPAS) and hypothalamus–preoptic area–septum (HPS)). Androgen receptors were measured with [3H]testosterone and were isolated by DNA cellulose chromatography. Estrogen receptors were measured with [3H]R-2858 (moxestrol) by Sephadex LH-20 gel filtration method. Progestin receptors were measured with [3H]R-5020 by the LH-20 method. Arrows denote critical period for defeminization. Reprinted by permission from McEwen (1982).

from the elevated estrogen receptor levels and they are modified by gonadectomy early in life, leading to the hypothesis that they may be the result of a growth inhibition by gonadal steroids (Sandhu et al., 1986). In primate cerebral cortex, estrogen receptors are present perinatally and appear to be associated with aromatase activity so that testosterone (T) in males is a source of E to occupy these receptors and affect cortical development (MacLusky et al., 1986).

As in adult brain, developing rat brain shows no indications of having sex differences in levels of estrogen receptors, the only exception being the left-right cortical sex differences cited above. Aromatizing enzyme activity is high perinatally in the male and female brain (George and Ojeda, 1982) and leads to the production, in males, of high levels of E to occupy the estrogen receptors. Thus, the differential secretion of T in males perinatally is responsible for initiating sexual differentiation of brain, as well as the reproductive tract, through the differential occupation of gonadal steroid receptors that are present in both male and female brains and reproductive tract anlage.

Testosterone actions via androgen receptors are involved in the masculinization of sexual behavior and of the behavior called 'rough-and-tumble' play behavior, and these actions occur to a large extent through androgen receptors (Meaney et al., 1983). T actions via conversion to E lead to defeminization of the ability to ovulate or to show female sexual behavior (McEwen, 1983). Because males show less feminine sexual behavior than females and are particularly refractory to the actions of progesterone, we investigated whether the sex difference in progestin receptor induction by E in VMN could be reversed by blocking perinatal defeminization. As shown in Fig. 2, immediate postnatal blockade of aromatization in males by the steroidal inhibitor of this enzyme complex, androstatriene-3,17-dione (ATD), prevented defeminization of progestin receptor induction; and, although not shown in Fig. 2, it also prevented defeminization of female sexual behavior (Parsons et al., 1984). We have previously shown that ATD produces a 'chemical castration' at the level of blocking estrogen receptor occupancy in developing male hypothalamus (McEwen et al., 1982). Postnatal treatment of females with E defeminizes sexual behavior and also reduces progestin receptor inducibility to the level found in control males (Fig. 2). Further

studies must be done to determine whether some of the other sex differences in biochemical response to E treatment, described above, may also follow the same pattern of developmental hormonal influence as the progestin receptor induction in VMN.

What are the primary events associated with actions of T to produce sexual differentiation of the brain? The differential occupancy of estrogen receptors in perinatal males by E derived from T through aromatization leads to differential effects on neural development and differentiation. These actions include hormone effects on growth of neurites (Toran-Allerand, 1984) that lead to morphological (Arnold and Gorski, 1984) and biochemical (McEwen, 1983) sex differences. According to this scheme, neurite outgrowth and related neuronal differentiation initiated by hormonal signals in neurons that have expressed estrogen receptors lead to differences in neural circuitry and differences in the neurochemical properties and regulatory responses of neurons in adult male brains. In this way, some of the masculinizing and defeminizing effects of T are produced on the developing brain. As noted above, other actions of T on sexual differentiation are mediated by T acting through androgen receptors which are also expressed equally in male and female brains but are differentially occupied in males because of the testicular secretion of T during perinatal development (McEwen et al., 1982; McEwen, 1983; Meaney et al., 1983). These may also involve morphological changes (e.g., neurite outgrowth) and neuronal differentiation like those produced by E (Arnold and Gorski, 1984; Arnold and Breedlove, 1985). Paradoxically, the actions of T involving androgen receptors can be inhibited by estrogens, because estrogens have the ability to inhibit the secretion of gonadotrophins which stimulate T secretion by the testes (Greene et al., 1939).

Reactivation of developmental programs

Whereas the distinction between developmental actions of gonadal hormones and their effects in adulthood was formerly rather rigid, it now appears to be somewhat less so, due to the recognition that there may be some temporal overlap and some commonality of cellular response to hormones between development and adult life (Arnold and Breedlove, 1985). One area where this new view is particularly evident is in the response of the brain to damage in adulthood. Damaged neural tissue shows some collateral sprouting of undamaged neurons and reoccupancy of vacant synaptic sites, and treatment with estrogens, androgen and glucocorticoids has been found to enhance axon growth of new synapse formation (Matsumoto and Arai, 1979; Zhou and Azmitia, 1985; Yu and Srinivasan, 1981). This response may represent reactivation of developmental programs, called into play by the denervation and loss of nearby neurons. It remains to be seen whether the steroidal enhancement of this process is beneficial to or interferes with functional recovery.

In contradistinction to the growth-promoting actions of estrogens, androgens and glucocorticoids are actions of these same hormones which contribute to neuronal damage and loss during adult life and in aging (see also De Kloet et al., Chapter 8 of this volume). Of particular relevance to the present discussion of gonadal hormones are the observations that the ovaries contribute to drug-induced and age-related neural damage and loss of hypothalamic cyclicity in relation to ovulation (Brawer et al., 1980; Felicio et al., 1983). This type of effect, which is due to persistent and long-term secretion of ovarian steroids, is permanent, like the teratological effects of gonadal steroid during brain development which will be discussed below.

Functional teratogenicity of gonadal hormones or pseudohormones

Neural teratogens that work through endocrine mechanisms may be hormones, or substances which work like hormones (pseudohormones), or substances which alter hormone secretion. The presence of the wrong hormone at the wrong time, or abnormally high hormone levels, may induce an abnormal response in the nervous system. The consequences may be particularly serious and long-lasting when the hormone exposure occurs during development, but the actions of hormones on the adult brain may also be noteworthy. In this section, we consider both the probable and actual functional teratogenicity of gonadal hormones in adult and developing brain.

Adult brain

In the mature nervous system, functional pathological actions of hormones might be defined as effects of abnormally high levels of hormones or pseudohormones which affect adult brain function in ways which can be irreversible as well as reversible. Because the lines discriminating between developmental and adult effects of hormones are somewhat less distinct (Arnold and Breedlove, 1985), long-lasting hormone effects on the adult brain must be considered when discussing functional teratology. In the case of gonadal steroids we can point to the types of effects which one might expect to occur as a result of exposure of adults to high levels of pseudohormones in the diet. Estrogen elevation in male rats increases locomotor activity and produces a biphasic effect on amphetamine-induced hyperactivity (Menniti and Baum, 1981; West and Michael, 1986). Estrogen treatment also antagonizes apomorphine-induced yawning in male rats (Serra et al., 1984). Many of these effects are believed to involve action on the basal ganglia (Van Hartesveldt and Joyce, 1986), and biphasic changes in both acetylcholine and dopamine neurochemistry are reported to result from estrogen treatment (Euvrard et al., 1979; Piccardi et al., 1983; Van Hartesveldt and Joyce, 1986). Another action of estrogen elevation in male as well as in female rats is to increase pituitary prolactin gene transcription and prolactin levels (Shull and Gorski, 1984; Willoughby et al., 1983) and chronic hyperprolactinemia has effects of its own on neural tissue. These include effects on hypothalamic dopamine turnover (Simpkins et al., 1982) and striatal dopamine release (Chen and Ramirez, 1982), induction of grooming behavior (Drago et al., 1981), suppression of copulatory behavior (Svare et al., 1979; Doherty et al., 1985) and inhibition of luteinizing hormone release (Marchetti and Labrie, 1982).

Androgen elevation has a suppressive effect on response of the CNS serotonergic system to elevated endogenous serotonin through treatment with pargyline plus tryptophan (Fischette et al., 1984). These effects do not, however, appear to be long-lasting and tend to disappear after castration of males or over days after androgen administration to females.

Developing brain

Developmental effects of external agents related to the brain-pituitary-gonadal axis may be divided into two categories: (1) the actions of hormones and pseudohormones administered or ingested or secreted at the wrong time of development; (2) the actions or other toxic agents, such as alcohol, narcotics, nicotine, amphetamine and tetrahydrocannabinol, which can alter hormone output and produce teratological actions through this pathway. Category 2 is extensively discussed by Lichtensteiger and by others in this volume. In this section we shall consider category 1.

Synthetic progestins. Synthetic progestational steroids were administered to pregnant women to prevent threatened miscarriages or were given in the course of pregnancy testing or were ingested as oral contraceptives after fertilization had occurred. The unanticipated and deleterious side-effects of their administration appear to be due to the ability of these steroids to act as 'pseudohormones'. Specifically, they appear to act as androgens and also as glucocorticoids. Virilizing, androgen-like effects of synthetic progestins were noted on genital appearance (Wilkins et al., 1958) and they were subsequently extended to include psychosexual identity (Ehrhardt and Money, 1967), other aspects of personality (Reinisch,

1977) and potential for aggression (Reinisch, 1981). Less well-known and not as thoroughly studied are influences of synthetic progestins which may cause mental retardation, cranio-facial abnormalities and growth retardation (Lorber et al., 1978). Although the mechanism of action for these effects is not known, one possibility is that some of the synthetic progestins mimic glucocorticoids and may be acting as pseudoglucocorticoids to produce these abnormalities. One of the most prominent of these steroids, Provera, is a synthetic progestational steroid which is also a potent glucocorticoid (Camanni et al., 1963; Kimmel et al., 1979). Glucocorticoids are known to cause cranial malformations (e.g. cleft palate) (Kimmel et al., 1979; Goldman et al., 1978) and to retard neural growth and development (see De Kloet et al., Chapter 8 of this volume). Additional studies are called for in order to explore this aspect of synthetic progestin action, especially in view of the extensive use of synthetic progestins in obstetric and gynecological practice.

Actions of estrogens and pseudoestrogens. One of the most potent developmental neural teratogens is the pseudoestrogen, diethylstilbestrol (DES), to which between 0.4 and 2.6 million women and their fetuses were exposed over the past four

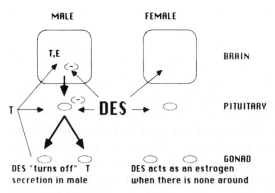

Fig. 4. Schematic summary of how DES may differentially affect sexual differentiation of the brain in male and female fetuses.

decades (Meyer-Bahlburg et al., 1984, 1985, 1987; Ehrhardt et al., 1985). Prenatal DES exposure alters general measures of personality and alters sexual behavior patterns in adolescence and adulthood by reducing the formation of heterosexual relationships (Ehrhardt et al., 1985). These effects of DES could not be explained by higher levels of sexual dysfunctions related to the genitalia, but rather appear to be due to psychosocial and neuroendocrine factors resulting from the DES exposure in utero (Ehrhardt et al., 1985; Meyer-Bahlburg et al., 1985). One way of understanding the different consequences of prenatal DES exposure in men and women is to look at the known interactions of DES with the neuroendocrine axis of the male and female fetus (Fig. 4). In males, DES suppresses the secretion of T by acting on the hypothalamus and pituitary gland and thus deprives the developing male of normal levels of T, resulting in some hypomasculinization. Although this results in some reduction in masculine gender role behavior in males, it does not result in increased levels of male homosexual or bisexual behavior (Meyer-Bahlburg et al., 1987). In females, DES acts as an estrogen when there is no circulating estrogen or testosterone and thus provides a hormone that normally is not there (Fig. 4). The consequences, as noted above, include a significant increase in bisexuality but only minimal alterations in gender role behavior, which is generally believed to depend on androgens and not on estrogens or aromatization of T (Ehrhardt et al., 1985).

DES is also reported to have a paradoxical masculinizing effect in some human infants exposed to this agent alone during gestation (Bongiovanni et al., 1959), as well as in rats (Greene et al., 1939). This is difficult to explain, since DES is not an androgen. However, some DES-exposed women show elevated T levels and thus may respond to DES with abnormal androgen production, which therefore is the immediate cause of the masculine traits (Meyer-Bahlburg et al., 1985).

Since the developing brains of both sexes re-

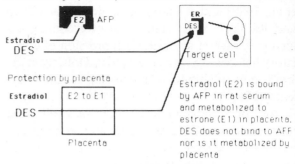

Fig. 5 Schematic summary of protection mechanisms which retard actions of estradiol in development but which do not prevent DES from acting to affect brain development.

spond to gonadal steroids, are there mechanisms to protect the fetus in utero from hormones circulating in the mother? Possible mechanisms are presented in Fig. 5. One mechanism involves the serum protein, alpha fetoprotein (AFP), which binds estradiol in rats and mice (Plapinger and McEwen, 1978). DES is much more potent than E in causing brain sexual differentiation because it does not bind to AFP (Plapinger and McEwen, 1978). AFP appears to be most important in protecting the brain postnatally from estrogens in the mother's milk, because it is during the postnatal period that the rat brain is most sensitive to defeminizing actions of estrogens that would sterilize female offspring. Why do other species like the guinea pig and human lack an estrogen binding form of AFP? Most likely this is because defeminizing actions involving estrogens take place in utero in these species and thus the estrogen binding domain of AFP may have been lost during the course of evolution since it serves no useful protective role in postnatal life.

In view of these considerations, the fetal-placental unit must be carefully scrutinized for the protection which it affords. The placenta has a selective effect on estradiol, secreting it toward the maternal circulation (Walsh and McCarthy, 1981). In addition, as schematized in Fig. 5, estradiol is converted to estrone, a less potent estrogen, and the fetus has much higher levels of estrone relative to estradiol than the mother (Walsh and MacCarthy, 1981; Slikker et al., 1982). In contrast, as shown in Fig. 5, DES is able to pass to the fetus unmetabolized and in relatively high levels where it can act potently as an estrogen (Slikker et al., 1982). The inability of the fetal-placental unit to handle DES is like the inability of AFP to bind DES, and any pseudoestrogen in the environment which is similar to DES may also gain access to the developing fetus.

Many substances in the environment have estrogenic properties, including certain natural products of plants, a number of insecticides and the stilbene derivatives, of which DES is one example (McLachlan, 1985). A phenolic ring is a common feature of all of these estrogens, and it is capable of producing estrogen receptor activation (McLachlan, 1985). What we do not know is the extent to which environmental estrogens like the insecticides, DDT and methoxychlor, or the plant estrogens, like daidzein, coumestrol or zearalenone, may be able, like DES, to bypass fetal-placental protection mechanisms.

Discussion

Gonadal steroids affect the developing and adult brain through protein receptor sites which interact directly with the genome. The effects produced through this interaction are diverse, but they can be categorized into growth-related actions and effects on neurochemistry. At first it was thought that the two actions might be strictly separated temporally, with growth-related actions occurring during the perinatal period of synaptogenesis and neurochemical effects taking place in the mature brain. Recent evidence indicates some overlap in these two manifestations of hormone action, such as the recurrence of synaptic sprouting in damaged adult brain tissue and the occurrence of neuronal growth after estrogen treatment in undamaged adult hypothalamic neurons.

Gonadal steroid effects are not confined to processes related to reproduction but have more widespread consequences for brain function. Estrogen actions in the adult rat brain increase cholinergic enzyme activity of neurons projecting to cerebral cortex and hippocampus (Luine, 1985), and estrogen treatment improves indices of cognitive function and affect in aging women, including some patients suffering from late-onset senile dementia (Fillit et al., 1986). During development, gonadal steroid actions influence cortical development as well as hypothalamic differentiation, and recent studies indicate that there are sex differences in behavioral adaptation to stress (Kennett et al., 1986) as well as in spatial memory (Williams and Barnett, 1987).

One important consequence of the developmental action of gonadal steroids is the programming of the male and female brain to respond differently to the same hormones. Recent studies indicate that male and female brain tissue differs in response to estrogens and androgens with respect to induction of cholinergic enzymes (Luine and McEwen, 1983), regulation of serotonin receptors (Fischette et al., 1983) and response of CNS serotonin receptors to elevated serotonin as a result of tryptophan and pargyline (Fischette et al., 1984). Male and female striatum also differs in the dopamine-releasing effects of prolactin (Chen and Ramirez, 1982). Sex differences are also found in the actions of dexamethasone on the hippocampal cAMP response to noradrenaline and vasoactive intestinal peptide (Harrelson and McEwen, 1987). What these sex differences may mean is that the brain will respond somewhat differently to exogenous drugs and endogenous neurotransmitters depending not only on which hormones are present at the time but also on whether the brain is in a male or a female.

What does this mean for the actions of neural teratogens? Insofar as drugs, plant products or environmental toxicants either alter secretion or mimic the actions of gonadal steroids, they may well produce some of the effects alluded to in this chapter. As noted, teratogenic actions in development may be the most serious because their consequences are potentially longer-lasting. Are such effects of major consequence in our society? With the widespread use of pesticides, DES and plant products which have estrogenic activity, we cannot exclude the possibility of subtle effects on neuronal development and behavior. Could disorders such as anorexia nervosa, dyslexia and perhaps presenile dementia be traced in part to actions of such environmental agents? It is unfortunately almost impossible to design studies which would test such a hypothesis.

Summary and concluding remarks

In this brief overview of a complex and growing field, we have seen that gonadal steroids produce multiple effects on the adult and developing nervous system. In most cases, these effects are ones which modulate genomic activity and produce long-term consequences for the structure and function of the brain. In the adult nervous system, normal effects include facilitation of sexual and aggressive behavior, whereas abnormal effects include actions that alter dopamine-dependent motor activity or elevate sexual and aggressive behavior inappropriately and artificially. Although these effects are reversible, there are also permanent changes resulting from prolonged estrogen exposure, such as the so-called 'hypothalamic disconnection syndrome' in rats (Brawer et al., 1980).

During development, testosterone is responsible for the masculinizing and defeminizing aspects of sexual differentiation. When testosterone, or estrogens like DES, are allowed to reach the developing female, teratological consequences include masculinization and defeminization of brain and behavior; when DES reaches the developing male, the consequences are understandable in terms of blockade of normal testosterone secretion and interference with normal masculinization processes. The consequences of DES exposure in humans are at least partially understandable by these types of actions and illustrate the value of animal research for studies of human psychosexual differentiation. What remains to be established in future research is the extent to which early teratological effects of agents like DES predispose the adult nervous system to show pathological responses to hormones and to drugs. In a like manner, the normal sexual differentiation of the brain, resulting in a sexually differentiated neural substrate, may also result in sex differences in the pathological actions of hormones and drugs in adulthood.

Acknowledgements

Research in the author's laboratory on this topic is supported by NIH Grant NS07080. Ms. Inna Perlin provided editorial assistance.

References

Akesson, T., Mantyh, P., Mantyh, C., Matt, D. and Micevych, P. (1987) Estrous cyclicity of ^{125}I-cholecystokinin octapeptide binding in the ventromedial hypothalamic nucleus. *Neuroendocrinology*, 45: 257–262.

Arnold, A. and Breedlove, S.M. (1985) Organizational and activational effects of sex steroids on brain and behavior: a reanalysis. *Horm. Behav.*, 19: 469–498.

Arnold, A. and Gorski, R. (1984) Gonadal steroid induction of structural sex differences in the central nervous system. *Annu. Rev. Neurosci.*, 7: 413–442.

Blaustein, J. (1986) Cell nuclear accumulation of estrogen receptors in rat brain and pituitary gland after treatment with a dopamine-β-hydroxylase inhibitor. *Neuroendocrinology*, 42: 44–50.

Blaustein, J., Ryer, H. and Feder, H. (1980) A sex difference in the progestin receptor system of guinea pig brain. *Neuroendocrinology*, 31: 403–409.

Blaustein, J., Brown, T. and Swearengen, E. (1986) Dopamine-beta-hydroxylase inhibitors modulate the concentration of functional estrogen receptors in female rat hypothalamus and pituitary gland. *Neuroendocrinology*, 43: 150–158.

Bongiovanni, A., Di George, A. and Grumbach, M. (1959) Masculinization of the female infant associated with estrogenic therapy alone during gestation. *J. Clin. Endocrinol.*, 19: 1004–1011.

Brawer, J., Schipper, H. and Naftolin, F. (1980) Ovary-dependent degeneration in the hypothalamic arcuate nucleus. *Endocrinology*, 107: 274–279.

Brown, T., Clark, A. and MacLusky, N. (1987) Regional sex differences in progestin receptor induction in the rat hypothalamus: effects of various doses of estradiol benzoate. *J. Neurosci.*, 7: 2529–2536.

Camanni, F., Massara, F. and Molinatti, G. (1963) The cortisone-like effect of 6-alpha-methyl-27-alpha-acetoxyprogesterone in the adrenalectomized man. *Acta Endocrinol.* 43: 477–483.

Carrer, H. and Aoki, A. (1982) Ultrastructural changes in the hypothalamic ventromedial nucleus of ovariectomized rats after estrogen treatment. *Brain Res.*, 240: 221–233.

Carrillo, A., Steger, R. and Chamness, G. (1983) Dopaminergic stimulation of pituitary but not hypothalamic estrogen receptors in ovariectomized rats. *Endocrinology*, 112: 1839–1846.

Chen, Y.-F. and Ramirez, V. (1982) Prolactin stimulates dopamine release from male but not female rat striatal tissue superfused in vitro. *Endocrinology*, 111: 1740–1742.

Clark, A., Nock, B., Feder, H. and Roy, E. (1985) α_1-Noradrenergic receptor blockade decreased nuclear estrogen receptor binding in guinea pig hypothalamus and preoptic area. *Brain Res.*, 330: 197–199.

Coirini, H. and McEwen, B. S. (1987) Progesterone receptor induction and sexual behavior by different estrogen treatment in male and female rats. *Abstr. Soc. Neurosci.*, 13, Abstr. 68.1.

De Kloet, E. R., Voorhuis, T. A. and Elands, J. (1985) Estradiol induces oxytocin binding sites in rat hypothalamic ventromedial nucleus. *Eur. J. Pharmacol.*, 118: 185–186.

De Nicola, A. F., Weisenberg, L., Arakelian, M. and Libertun, C. (1981) Effects of bromocriptine on ^{3}H-estradiol binding in cytosol of anterior pituitary. *Endocrinology*, 109: 83–86.

Drago, F., Bohus, B., Canonico, P. and Scapagnini, U. (1981) Prolactin induces grooming in the rat: possible involvement of nigrostriatal dopaminergic system. *Pharm. Biochem. Behav.*, 15: 61–63.

Doherty, P., Bartke, A., Smith, M. S. and Davis, S. (1985) Increased serum prolactin levels mediate the suppressive effects of ectopic pituitary grafts on copulatory behavior in male rats. *Horm. Behav.*, 19: 111–121.

Ehrhardt, A. and Money, J. (1967) Progestin-induced hermaphroditism: IQ and psychosexual identity in a study of ten girls. *J. Sex. Res.*, 3: 83–100.

Ehrhardt, A., Meyer-Bahlburg, H., Rosen, L., Feldman, J., Veridiano, N., Zimmerman, I. and McEwen, B. S. (1985) Sexual orientation after prenatal exposure to exogenous estrogen. *Arch. Sex. Behav.*, 14: 57–75.

Euvrard, C., Labrie, F. and Boissier, J. (1979) Effect of estrogen on changes in the activity of striatal cholinergic neurons induced by DA drugs. *Brain Res.*, 169: 215–220.

Felicio, L., Nelson, J., Gosden, R. and Finch, C. (1983) Restoration of ovulatory cycles by young ovarian grafts in aging mice: potentiation by long-term ovariectomy decreases with age. *Proc. Natl. Acad. Sci. USA*, 80: 6076–6080.

Fillit, H., Weinreb, H., Cholst, I., Luine, V., Amador, R.,

Zabriskie, J. and McEwen, B. S. (1986) Hormonal therapy for Alzheimer's disease. In T. Crook, R. Bartrus, S. Ferris, S. Gershon (Eds.), *Treatment Development Strategies for Alzheimer's Disease.* Mark Powley Associates, Connecticut, pp. 151–171.

Fischette, C., Biegon, A. and McEwen, B. S. (1983) Sex differences in serotonin 1 binding in rat brain. *Science*, 222: 333–335.

Fischette, C., Biegon, A. and McEwen, B. S. (1984) Sex steroid modulation of the serotonin behavioral syndrome. *Life Sci.*, 35: 1197–1206.

Fraille, I., Pfaff, D. W. and McEwen, B. S. (1987) Progestin receptors with and without estrogen and female hamster brain. *Neuroendocrinology*, 45: 487–491.

George, F. and Ojeda, S. (1982) Changes in aromatase activity in the rat brain during embryonic, neonatal and infantile development. *Endocrinology*, 111: 522–529.

Gietzen, D. and Woolley, D. (1986) Sex differences in ^{3}H-estradiol binding in brain and pituitary after acute dopaminergic treatment. *Neuroendocrinology*, 42: 334–343.

Goldman, A., Shapiro, B. and Katsumato, M. (1978) Human foetal palatal corticoid receptors and teratogens for cleft palate. *Nature*, 272: 464–466.

Greene, R., Burrill, M. and Ivy, A. (1939) Experimental intersexuality, the paradoxical effects of estrogens on the sexual development of the female rat. *Anat. Rev.*, 74: 429–438.

Harrelson, A. and McEwen, B. S. (1987) Gonadal steroid modulation of neurotransmitter-stimulated cAMP accumulation in the hippocampus of the rat. *Brain Res.*, 404: 89–94.

Jones, K., McEwen, B. S. and Pfaff, D. W. (1986) Regional specificity in estradiol effects on ^{3}H uridine incorporation in rat brain. *Mol. Cell. Endocrinol.*, 45: 57–63.

Kennett, G., Chaouloff, F., Marcou, M. and Curzon, G. (1986) Female rats are more vulnerable than males in an animal model of depression: the possible role of serotonin. *Brain Res.*, 382: 416–421.

Kimmel, G., Hartwell, B. and Andrew, F. (1979) A potential mechanism in medroxyprogesterone acetate teratogenesis. *Teratology*, 171–176.

Lieberburg, I. and McEwen, B. S. (1977) Brain cell nuclear retention of testosterone metabolites, 5alpha-dihydrotestosterone and estradiol 17beta in adult rats. *Endocrinology*, 100: 588–597.

Lorber, C., Cassidy, S. and Engfl, E. (1978) Is there an embryo-fetal exogenous sex steroid exposure syndrome (efesses)? *Fertil. Steril.*, 31: 21–24.

Luine, V. (1985) Estradiol increases choline acetyltransferase activity in specific basal forebrain nuclei and projection areas of female rats. *Exp. Neurol.*, 89: 484–490.

Luine, V. and MacEwen, B. (1983) Sex differences in cholinergic enzymes of diagonal band nuclei in the rat preoptic area. *Neuroendocrinology*, 36: 475–482.

MacLusky, N. and McEwen, B. S. (1980) Progestin receptors

132

in the developing rat brain and pituitary. *Brain Res.*, 189: 262–268.

MacLusky, N., Naftolin, F. and Goldman-Rakic, P. (1986) Estrogen formation and binding in the cerebral cortex of the developing rhesus monkey. *Proc. Natl. Acad. Sci. USA*, 83: 513–516.

Marchetti, B. and Labrie, F. (1982) Prolactin inhibits pituitary luteinizing hormone-releasing receptors in the rat. *Endocrinology*, 111: 1209–1216.

Matsumoto, A. and Arai, Y. (1979) Synaptogenic effect of estrogen on the hypothalamic arcuate nucleus of the adult female rat. *Cell. Tiss. Res.*, 198: 427–433.

McEwen, B.S. (1982) Sexual differentiation of the brain: gonadal hormone action and current concepts of neuronal differentiation. In I. Brown (Ed.), *Molecular Approaches and Neurobiology*, Academic Press, New York, pp. 199–213.

McEwen, B.S. (1983) Gonadal steroid influences on brain development and sexual differentiation. In R. Greep (Ed.), *Reproductive Physiology IV*, University Park Press, University Park, MD, Vol. 27, pp. 99–145.

McEwen, B.S. (1984) Gonadal hormone receptors in developing and adult brain: relationship to the regulatory phenotype. In F. Ellendorff, P. Gluckman and N. Parvizi (Eds.), *Fetal Neuroendocrinology*, Perinatology Press, Ithaca, pp. 149–159.

McEwen, B.S. (1985) Steroid hormone receptors and actions in the developing brain. In R. Jaffe and S. Dell'Acqua (Eds.), *The Endocrine Physiology of Pregnancy and the Peripartal Period*, Serono Symposia Publications, Raven Press, New York, pp. 183–193.

McEwen, B.S. (1987) Steroid hormones and the brain: linking 'nature' and 'nurture'. *Neurochem. Res.*, in press.

McEwen, B.S. (1988) Endocrine effects on the brain and their relationship to behavior. In G. Siegel, W. Albers, B. Agranoff, R. Katzman (Eds.) *Basic Neurochemistry*, Little Brown, Boston, in press.

McEwen, B.S., Biegon, A., Davis, P., Krey, L., Luine, V., McGinnis, M., Paden, C., Parsons, B. and Rainbow, T. (1982) Steroid hormones: humoral signals which alter brain cell properties and functions. *Rec. Prog. Horm. Res.*, 38: 41–92, Academic Press, New York.

McEwen, B.S., Davis, P., Gerlach, J., Krey, L., MacLusky, N., McGinnis, M., Parsons, B. and McEwen B.S. (1983) Progestin receptors in the brain and pituitary gland. In C. Bardin, P. Mauvais-Jarvis and Milgrom (Eds.), *Progesterone and Progestin*, Raven Press, New York, pp. 59–76.

McEwen, B.S., Luine, V. and Fischette, C. (1987a) Developmental actions of hormones: from receptors to function. In S. Easter, K. Barald and B. Carlson (Eds.), *From Message to Mind: Directions in Developmental Neurobiology*, A. Sinauer, Connecticut, in press.

McEwen, B.S., Jones, K. and Pfaff, D.W. (1987b) Hormonal control of sexual behavior in the female rat: molecular, cellular and neurochemical studies. *Biol. Reprod.*, 36: 37–45.

McLachlan, J. (Ed.) (1985) *Estrogen in the Environment. II. Influences on Development*, Elsevier, Amsterdam.

Meaney, M., Stewart, J., Poulin, P. and McEwen, B.S. (1983) Sexual differentiation of social play in rat pups is mediated by the neonatal androgen receptor system. *Neuroendocrinology*, 37: 85–90.

Menniti, F. and Baum, M. (1981) Differential effects of estrogen and androgen on locomotor activity induced in castrated male rats by amphetamine, a novel environment, or apomorphine. *Brain Res.*, 216: 89–107.

Meyer-Bahlburg, H., Ehrhardt, A., Rosen, L., Feldman, J., Veridiano, N., Zimmerman, I. and McEwen, B.S. (1984) Psychosexual milestones in women prenatally exposed to diethylstilbestrol. *Horm. Behav.*, 18: 359–366.

Meyer-Bahlburg, H., Ehrhardt, A., Feldman, J., Rosen, L., Veridiano, N. and Zimmerman, I. (1985) Sexual activity level and sexual functioning in women prenatally exposed to diethylstilbestrol. *Psychosom. Med.*, 47: 497–511.

Meyer-Bahlburg, H., Ehrhardt, A., Whitehead, D. and Felix, V. (1987) Sexuality in males with a history of prenatal exposure to diethylstilbestrol (DES). *Am. Cancer. Soc.*, Psychosexual and Reproductive Issues of Cancer Patients, in press.

O'Connor, L., Nock, B. and McEwen, B.S. (1985) Quantitative autoradiography of GABA receptors in rat forebrain: receptor distribution and effects of estradiol. *Soc. Neurosci. Abstr.* 11: 223.5.

Parsons, B., Rainbow, T.C. and McEwen, B.S. (1984) Organizational effects of testosterone via aromatization on feminine reproductive behavior and neural progestin receptors in rat brain. *Endocrinology*, 115: 1412–1417.

Pfaff, D.W. and Keiner, N. (1973) Atlas of estradiol-concentrating cells in the central nervous system of the female rat. *J. Comp. Neurol.* 151: 121–158.

Piccardi, P., Bernardi, F., Rossetti, Z. and Corsini, G. (1983) Effect of estrogens on dopamine autoreceptors in male rats. *Eur. J. Pharm.* 91: 1–9.

Plapinger, L. and McEwen, B.S. (1978) Gonadal steroid-brain interactions in sexual differentiation. In J. Hutchison (Ed.), *Biological Determinants of Sexual Behavior*, John Wiley, New York.

Rainbow, T., DeGroff, V., Luine, V. and McEwen, B.S. (1980) Estradiol-17β increases the number of muscarinic receptors in hypothalamic nuclei. *Brain Res.*, 198: 239–243.

Rainbow, T.C., Parsons, B. and McEwen, B.S. (1982) Sex differences in rat brain oestrogen and progestin receptors. *Nature*, 300: 648–649.

Rainbow, T., Snyder, L., Berck, D.J. and McEwen, B.S. (1984) Correlation of muscarinic receptor induction in the ventromedial hypothalamic nucleus with the activation of feminine sexual behavior by estradiol. *Neuroendocrinology*, 39: 476–480.

Reinisch, J. (1977) Prenatal exposure of human fetuses to synthetic progestin and oestrogen affects personality. *Nature*, 266: 561–562.

Reinisch, J. (1981) Prenatal exposure to synthetic progestins increases potential for aggression in humans. *Science*, 211: 171–173.

Romano, G., Harlan, R., Schivers, B., Howells, R. and Pfaff, D.W. (1986) Estrogen increases proenkephalin mRNA in the mediobasal hypothalamus of the rat. *Abstr. Soc. Neurosci.*, 12: 188.17.

Sandhu, S., Cook, P. and Diamond, M. (1986) Rat cerebral cortical estrogen receptors, male-female, right-left. *Exp. Neur.*, 92: 186–196.

Sar, M. and Stumpf, W.E. (1977) Distribution of androgen target cells in rat forebrain and pituitary after ^{3}H-dihydrotestosterone administration. *J. Steroid Biochem.*, 8: 1131–1135.

Serra, G., Collu, M., Serra, A. and Gessa, G. (1984) Estrogens antagonize apomorphine-induced yawning in rat. *Eur. J. Pharmacol.*, 104: 383–386.

Shull, J. and Gorski, J. (1984) Estrogen stimulates prolactin gene transcription by a mechanism independent of pituitary protein synthesis. *Endocrinology*, 114: 1550–1557.

Simpkins, J., Hodson, C., Kalra, P. and Kalra, S. (1982) Chronic hyperprolactinemia depletes hypothalamic dopamine concentrations in male rats. *Life Sci.*, 30: 1349–1353.

Slikker, W., Hill, D. and Young, J. (1982) Comparison of the transplacental pharmacokinetics of 17-beta estradiol and diethylstilbestrol in the subhuman primate. *J. Pharmacol. Exp. Ther.*, 221: 173–182.

Svare, B., Bartke, A., Doherty, P., Mason, I., Michael, S. and Smith, M. (1979) Hyperprolactinemia suppresses copulatory behavior in male rats and mice. *Biol. Reprod.*, 21: 529–535.

Toran-Allerand, C.D. (1984) On the genesis of sexual differentiation of the central nervous system: morphogenetic consequences of exposure and possible role of alpha-fetoprotein. In G. De Vries, J. De Bruin, H. Uylings and M. Corner (Eds.), *Progress in Brain Research, Vol. 61*, Elsevier, Amsterdam, pp. 63–98.

Van Hartesveldt, C. and Joyce, J. (1986) Effects of estrogen on the basal ganglia. *Neurosci. Biobehav. Rev.*, 10: 1–14.

Walsh, S. and McCarthy, M. (1981) Selective placental secretion of estrogens into fetal and maternal circulations. *Endocrinology*, 109: 2152–2159.

West, C. and Michael, R. (1986) Time-dependent modulation by estrogen of amphetamine-induced hyperactivity in male rats. *Pharmacol. Biochem. Behav.*, 25: 919–923.

Wilkins, L., Jones, H., Holman, G. and Stempel, R. (1958) Masculinization of the female infant associated with administration of oral and intramuscular progestins during gestation: non-adrenal female pseudohermaphrodism. *J. Clin. Endocrinol. Metab.*, 18: 559–585.

Williams, C. and Barnett, A. (1988) Organizational effects of early gonadal secretions on sexual differentiation in spatial memory. *Behav. Neurosci. Neurosci.*, in press.

Willoughby, J., Pederick, H., Jervois, P. and Menadue, M. (1983) Sustained oestrogen-induced hyperprolactinemia results from a pituitary defect. *J. Endocr.*, 99: 477–483.

Yamamoto, K. (1985) Steroid receptor regulated transcription of specific genes and gene networks. *Annu. Rev. Genet.*, 19: 209–252.

Yu, W.A. and Strinivasan, R. (1981) Effect of testosterone and 5-alpha-dihydrotestosterone on regeneration of the hypoglossal nerve in rats. *Exp. Neurol.*, 71: 431–435.

Zhou, F.-C. and Azmitia, E. (1985) Effects of 5,7-dihydroxytryptamine on HRP retrograde transport from hippocampus to midbrain raphe nuclei in the rat. *Brain Res. Bull.*, 10: 445–451.

Discussion

J.M. Lauder: Handa et al. (1986) have shown that serotonergic terminals in the medial preoptic area may also be important for development of sexual dimorphism in this region. This suggests that we should also consider the role of neurotransmitters and their possible interactions with sex steroids as part of the mechanism involved in the ontogeny of sexual dimorphisms. Would you comment on this?

B.S. McEwen: These results are complemented by some of our own data which show that denervating serotonergic input to ventromedial hypothalamus of adult male rat unmasks feminine sexual behavior in response to estrogen plus progesterone (Moreines et al., 1987). The response of the male to this denervation is more dramatic than that of females, suggesting that serotonin inhibition is more significant in males and that serotonin may be involved in sexual differentiation of the lordosis response.

J.W. Olney: Have studies been done to determine whether sexually dimorphic nuclei (SDN) in human homosexuals can be distinguished by cell counting, autoradiography etc. from such nuclei in heterosexuals?

Answered by D.F. Swaab: There is no difference in the size of the human SDN in the few homosexual brains studied so far (Swaab et al., 1987).

P.E. Treffers: With respect to the differences in sexual interest and orientations: is it possible to differentiate between the psychological influence of knowing that you are a DES daughter, that your vagina is abnormal, and the prenatal influence of the DES (diethylstilbestrol) itself?

B.S. McEwen: This is a possibility and one which Ehrhardt et al. (1985) are concerned about addressing. The key is an appropriate control group. Thus far controls were taken who show positive PAP smears and therefore have some similar concerns about themselves as DES subjects do, but they do not show the same characteristics.

K. Boer: The controls that you showed for the DES daughter when testing sexual behaviour might have less homosexual behaviour and less heterosexual activity because they had deviant PAP smears!

B.S. McEwen: I doubt it, because controls who had positive PAP smears and did not get DES did not show bisexuality.

M.V. Johnston: Is there evidence of differences in spatial abilities or genetic chromosomal disorders such as Turner's syndrome?

B.S. McEwen: Several ongoing studies in the USA (e.g. Resnick et al., 1986) are pursuing the question in adrenogenital syndrome, Turner's syndrome, and other disorders. Although I believe there are some positive results I do not know what they are.

R. Ravid: In which stage of development do estrogen and testosterone receptors appear? Secondly, what comes first: the hormone or its receptor and could this determine the sexual differentiation of the brain?

B.S. McEwen: In the rat brain, estrogen and androgen receptors appear equally and at the same time in males and females (McEwen, 1983). Their appearance follows the first cell divisions of the neurons which made them, and is independent of circulating gonadal and adrenal hormones. We have performed transplant experiments of 16–17-day-old fetal hypothalamus into adult female brains and shown normal development of estrogen and progestin receptors even when hosts are gonadectomized and adrenalectomized (Paden et al., 1985). Thus, circulating steroids are not required for development of estrogen and progestin receptors, and the fact that androgen and estrogen receptors are equal in male and female brains argues against a role for testosterone in their development because testosterone is produced only by males. Only a few studies were done with human fetal tissue because it is hard to obtain, and one can only say that both estrogen receptors and aromatase are present. Exactly when they appear no one knows. Androgen receptors have been difficult to detect, but this may be a technical problem. In the late stages of gestation, the rhesus monkey brain has estrogen and androgen receptors.

References

Ehrhardt, A., Meyer-Bahlburg, H., Rosen, L., Feldman, J., Veridiano, N., Zimmerman, I. and McEwen, B.S. (1985) Sexual orientation after prenatal exposure to exogenous estrogen. *Arch. Sex. Behav.*, 14: 57–77.

Handa, R.J., Hines, M., Schoonmaker, J.N., Shryne, J.E. and Gorski, R.A. (1986) Evidence that serotonin is involved in the sexually dimorphic development of the preoptic area in the rat brain. *Brain Res.*, 395: 278–282.

Paden, C., Gerlach, J. and McEwen, B.S. (1985) Estrogen and progestin receptors appear in transplanted fetal hypothalamus-preoptic area independently of the steroid environment. *J. Neurosci.*, 9: 2374–2381.

McEwen, B.S. (1983) Gonadal steroid influences on brain development and sexual differentiation. In R. Greep (Ed.), *Reproductive Physiology IV, Vol. 27*, University Park Press, University Park, pp. 99–145.

Moreines, J., Kelton, M., Luine, V., Pfaff, D.W. and McEwen, B.S. (1987) Hypothalamic serotonin lesions unmask hormone responsiveness of lordosis in adult male rats. *Neuroendocrinology*, in press.

Resnick, S., Gottesman, I., Berenbaum, S. and Bouchard, T. (1986) Early hormonal influences on cognitive functioning in congenital adrenal hyperplasia. *Dev. Physiol.*, 22: 191–198.

Swaab, D.F., Roozendaal, B., Ravid, R., Velis, D.N., Gooren, L. and Williams, R.S. (1987) Suprachiasmatic nucleus in aging, Alzheimer's disease, transsexuality and Prader-Willi syndrome. In E.R. De Kloet, V.M. Wiegant and D. De Wied (Eds.), *Neuropeptides and Brain Function, Progress in Brain Research, Vol. 72*, Elsevier, Amsterdam, pp. 301–310.

SECTION III

Neuroactive Drugs as Functional Teratogens

G.J. Boer, M.G.P. Feenstra, M. Mirmiran, D.F. Swaab and F. Van Haaren
Progress in Brain Research, Vol. 73
© 1988 Elsevier Science Publishers B.V. (Biomedical Division)

CHAPTER 10

Prenatal adverse effects of nicotine on the developing brain

Walter Lichtensteiger, Urs Ribary, Margret Schlumpf, Brigitte Odermatt and Hans Rudolf Widmer

Pharmakologisches Institut, Universität Zürich, Gloriastrasse 32, CH-8006 Zürich, Switzerland

Behavioral abnormalities in children and experimental animals

Smoking has been reported to affect fetal motor behavior, as shown by a reduction of fetal movements (Kelly et al., 1984). During childhood, several studies have revealed a statistical relationship between behavioral abnormalities and smoking in pregnancy (Davie et al., 1972; Denson et al., 1975; Dunn et al., 1977, Saxton, 1978; Rantakallio, 1983; Naeye and Peters, 1984). The part played by different components of tobacco smoke (especially nicotine and carbon monoxide) can hardly be assessed in clinical studies, but animal experiments clearly implicate nicotine as a behavioral teratogen (Martin and Becker, 1971; Hudson et al., 1973; Peters et al., 1979, Baer et al., 1980; Johns et al., 1982; Peters and Tang, 1982; Genedani et al., 1983; Lichtensteiger and Schlumpf, 1985). Nicotine readily crosses the placental barrier and is found in human fetal (cord) serum in concentrations that are at least as high as, if not higher than, the corresponding maternal serum levels (Luck et al., 1985).

Nicotine acts on many different central and peripheral processes in the adult organism; its developmental effects can thus be expected to result from an interaction of direct effects on the developing brain with actions of nutrition, metabolism and endocrine systems of both fetal and maternal organisms, including the placenta. Few of these possible effects have actually been tested so far. The behavioral abnormalities seen in children of mothers who smoked during pregnancy (see references quoted above and Landesman-Dwyer and Emanuel, 1979) resemble the symptoms of minimal brain dysfunction (attention deficit disorder): short attention span, hyperactivity, decrements in reading ability, certain sensory deficits and difficulties in social adjustment. Since alterations in central catecholamine neurons may play a role in this syndrome (Shaywitz et al., 1976; Oke and Adams, 1978; Raskin et al., 1984) and since these systems are typical targets for nicotine in the adult brain, the first part of this presentation will focus on the complex of nicotinic input, central catecholamine systems and target neurons as a model system for interactions of nicotine with the developing brain. However, we think that adaptive processes could also be found in other neurotransmitter systems. The second part of this article addresses some aspects of metabolic and endocrine actions of nicotine that might indirectly affect the developing brain. Adverse effects on developing neuroendocrine systems may represent an important factor in functional teratology (Lichtensteiger and Schlumpf, 1984).

Regional ontogeny of nicotinic receptors in relation to catecholamine neurons and other transmitter systems

In vitro receptor autoradiography reveals specific binding sites for [³H]nicotine in rat lower brain stem and spinal cord from gestational day (GD) 12 (Schlumpf and Lichtensteiger, 1987; GD 1 = 24 h after a 2 h mating period). During the following days, nicotinic sites spread rostrally to appear in the posterior diencephalon between GD 14 and 15 (Fig. 1; Lichtensteiger et al., 1987). A similar caudo-rostral developmental gradient is seen with muscarinic cholinergic and benzodiazepine binding sites (Schlumpf et al., 1983, 1984), but with considerable differences in detailed regional distribution patterns. [³H]Nicotine binding sites are very abundant in fetal brainstem; they are also found in regions with catecholaminergic and serotonergic nerve cells which develop during the same period (Fig. 2; Schlumpf et al., 1980). In some regions such as substantia nigra, catecholamine nerve cell

areas overlap with areas of high density of nicotinic binding sites (Fig. 3). Since adult nigral dopamine neurons receive a direct nicotinic input (Lichtensteiger et al., 1982), it seems probable that at least some [³H]nicotine binding sites are situated on dopamine neurons. The situation is less clear with noradrenergic neurons of the locus coeruleus, since electrophysiological experiments failed to demonstrate a direct nicotinic input even if these neurons are excited by systemic administration of nicotine (Svensson and Engberg, 1980). The main input to locus coeruleus appears to stem from two lower brainstem nuclei (Aston-Jones et al., 1986), but it is not known whether nicotinic mechanisms are present there.

The innervation of forebrain areas by catecholamine projections and the formation of dopaminergic and noradrenergic receptor sites are closely associated processes. This was already noted in biochemical investigations (Bruinink et al., 1983; Bruinink and Lichtensteiger, 1984), but has become especially evident in autoradiographic studies on beta-receptor development

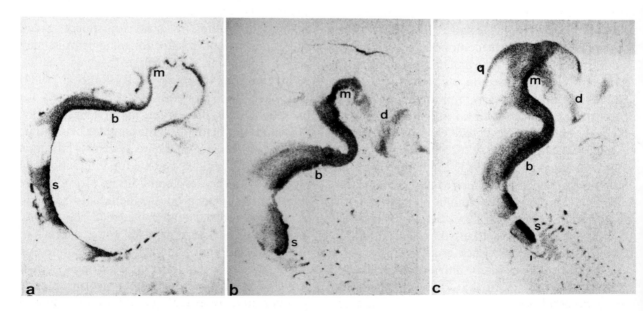

Fig. 1 Binding sites for [³H]nicotine in fetal rat brain at GD 14 (a), GD 15 (b) and GD 18 (c). In vitro autoradiography of sagittal sections. s, spinal cord; b, lower brainstem; m, mesencephalic flexure; d, diencephalon; q, quadrigeminal plate.

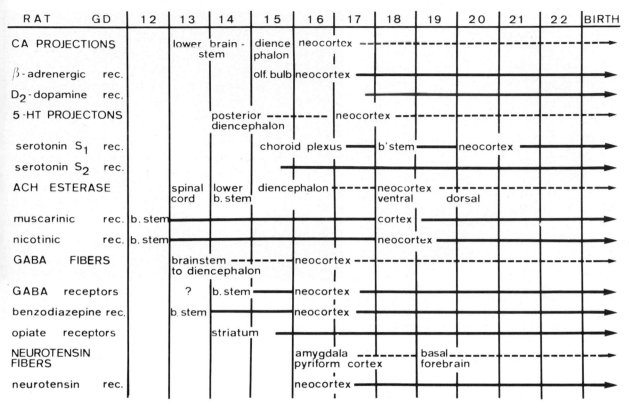

Fig. 2 Development of drug binding sites and neurotransmitter systems in fetal rat brain. Source: catecholamine (CA) projections, Schlumpf et al. (1980); beta-adrenergic receptors ([³H]dihydroalprenolol), Schlumpf et al. (1987a), Bruinink and Lichtensteiger (1984); D₂ dopamine receptors ([³H]spiperone), Bruinink et al. (1983); serotonin (5-HT) projections, Lidov and Molliver (1982), Wallace and Lauder (1983); serotonin S1 (5-HT 1) receptors ([³H]5-HT, Schlumpf et al. (1985, 1987a); serotonin S₂ receptors ([³H]spiperone), Bruinink et al. (1983); acetylcholinesterase, M. Schlumpf (unpublished observations); muscarinic-cholinergic receptors ([³H]N-methylscopolamine), Schlumpf and Lichtensteiger (1987), Schlumpf et al. (1987a); nicotinic-cholinergic receptors ([³H]nicotine), Schlumpf and Lichtensteiger (1987), Lichtensteiger et al. (1987); GABA fibers, Lauder et al. (1986); GABA receptors ([³H]GABA and [³H]muscimol), M. Schlumpf (unpublished observations); benzodiazepine receptors ([³H]flunitrazepam and [³H]Ro 15–1788), Schlumpf et al. (1983, unpublished observations); opiate receptors ([³H]naloxone), Kent et al. (1982); neurotensin fibers, Hara et al. (1982); neurotensin receptors ([³H]neurotensin), Palacios et al. (1987).

(Schlumpf et al., 1987a). While the first appearance of [³H]dihydroalprenolol binding sites, at GD 15 in olfactory bulb, may actually slightly precede catecholaminergic innervation, neocortical beta-adrenergic binding sites are first seen at GD 16, the time of catecholaminergic innervation (Fig. 2). They first occupy the marginal cortical layer and, at GD 18, the two layers situated above and below the cortical plate (anlage of the molecular layer and deep lamina bordering the intermediate zone: Schlumpf et al., 1987a), i.e., the

same layers that also receive the first ingrowing catecholamine fibers (Schlumpf et al., 1980). [³H]Nicotine binding sites are detected in deep layers of neocortex at GD 18, i.e., two days after the appearance of catecholamine fibers and receptor sites. In the first week and at least until postnatal day 14, a band of high nicotinic receptor density is observed at the level of the innermost cortical layer, which also shows the highest density of ChAT-positive nerve fibers (Widmer et al., 1986; Fig. 4). This distribution of [³H]nicotine

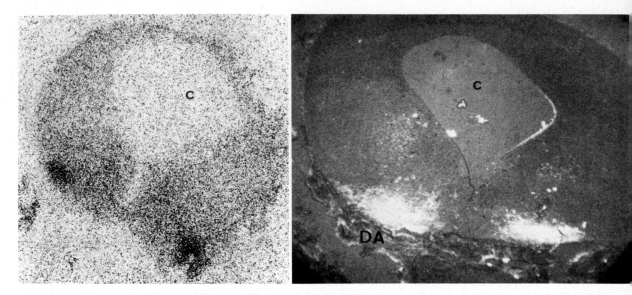

Fig. 3 Coronal sections through midbrain of rat fetuses at GD 15. Left: autoradiogram showing [³H]nicotine binding sites. Right: midbrain dopamine nerve cell groups (DA) demonstrated by formaldehyde-induced fluorescence. Note the overlap of the area of high density of [³H]nicotine binding sites with the dopamine neuron group of each side. c: central canal.

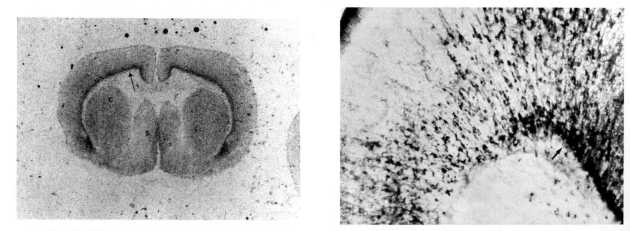

Fig. 4 Coronal sections through rat forebrain at postnatal day 6. Left: in the autoradiogram, a band of high density of [³H]nicotine binding sites is seen at the level of the innermost layer of cerebral cortex (arrow). Right: nerve fibers immuno-reactive for choline acetyltransferase (ChAT) are densely packed in the innermost layer (arrow) of parietal cortex. PAP method using a monoclonal antibody to ChAT from F. Eckenstein, Boston. Specificity was checked by absence of staining after omission of the first antibody (Widmer et al., 1986). s: septum, c: caudate-putamen.

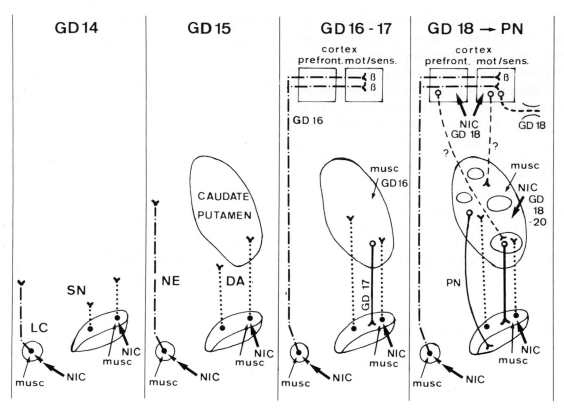

Fig. 5 Development of ascending and descending projections in rat brain from fetal to early postnatal life. Ascending catechol-amine fibers (norepinephrine = NE, dopamine = DA) from locus coeruleus (LC) and substantia nigra (SN) reach caudate-putamen at gestational day (GD) 15 and neocortex at GD 16 (Schlumpf et al., 1980, Specht et al., 1981); β-adrenergic binding sites are found in neocortex at GD 16 (Schlumpf et al., 1987a). A striatonigral projection from neurons later localized in striatal patches is established at GD 17; the descending projection from striatal matrix develops early postnatally (PN; Fishell and van der Kooy, 1987). A first population of outgrowing fibers from sensorimotor cortex reaches the corpus callosum at GD 18 and the contralateral cortex at GD 19 (Floeter and Jones, 1985). Comparable data on corticostriatal projections were not available (question marks). 'NIC' and 'musc' indicate the presence of nicotinic ([³H]nicotine) and muscarinic ([³H]N–methyl-scopolamine) binding sites, with time of appearance (Schlumpf et al., 1987a; Lichtensteiger et al., 1987; Schlumpf and Lichtensteiger, 1987).

binding sites differs completely from the adult stage, where these sites are maximally concentrated in layers I and III/IV (Clarke et al., 1985). It is interesting to note that in olfactory bulb, the postnatal rise of ChAT activity and muscarinic binding sites parallel each other, whereas no such correlation has been observed with alpha-bungarotoxin binding sites (Large et al., 1986). This apparent discrepancy with our observations can be explained by the fact that in brain, [³H]nicotine and [¹²⁵I]alpha-bungarotoxin bind to different

populations of receptor sites (Clarke et al., 1985).

A drug given during fetal life will directly or indirectly hit a number of developing transmitter systems (Fig. 2). Thereby, the neural circuitry which is affected changes continuously (Fig. 5). Thus, nicotine administered during the early fetal period will act at brainstem sites up to the meso-diencephalic junction, including catecholamine nerve cells which possess nicotinic receptor sites (Lichtensteiger et al., 1982). From the midfetal period, drug-induced changes in catecholamine

142

release may affect forebrain projection areas such as neocortex through actions on catecholamine receptor sites. In contrast, direct actions of nicotine on neocortical areas, mediated through nicotinic receptor sites, would be expected only during subsequent developmental stages (Fig. 5). At that time, nicotine might exert additional presynaptic actions on catecholamine fibers, e.g., in striatum, where a nicotinic mechanism has been observed in adult slice preparations (Giorguieff et al., 1976). Whether the newly established descending projections (Fig. 5) could already play a regulatory role is not known at the present time.

Prenatal nicotine: choice of the treatment schedule

The treatment schedule represents a critical issue especially with nicotine. Because of the short duration of action of this drug (Lichtensteiger et al., 1976, 1982; Svensson and Engberg, 1980; Taylor, 1985), the continuous exposure obtained by smoking can hardly be mimicked by individual injections. Moreover, it seems desirable to avoid effects of handling. As an alternative to injections, nicotine has been administered in the drinking water (Peters et al., 1979; Peters, 1984) or by osmotic minipump (Lichtensteiger and Schlumpf, 1985; Murrin et al., 1987; Slotkin et al., 1987b). The short ether anesthesia required for implantation of the minipump has been found not to affect the parameters studied (Lichtensteiger and Schlumpf, 1985; Murrin et al., 1987). In most of these studies, a daily dose of 6 mg/kg has been chosen, though probably on the basis of different reasoning. We have extrapolated from earlier electrophysiological experiments (Lichtensteiger et al., 1976, 1982; Svensson and Engberg, 1980), aiming at a dose that would cause a moderate activation of nigrostriatal and locus coeruleus neurons in adult animals. A recent analysis of blood levels of nicotine in rats bearing an osmotic minipump (Murrin et al., 1987) provides a basis for comparison with human data. As shown in Fig. 6, a daily dose of 6 mg/kg (= 0.25 mg/kg × h)

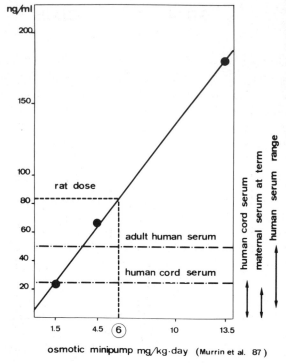

Fig. 6 Comparison between plasma nicotine levels (ordinate) in pregnant rats obtained by delivery from subcutaneously implanted osmotic minipumps at various daily doses (abscissa), and range of baseline nicotine levels in human serum (vertical arrows). Rat data are from Murrin et al., (1987), serum levels of smoking pregnant women at term and of their fetuses (cord serum) are derived from Luck et al. (1985) and the general concentration range in smokers from data by Isaac and Rand, (1972), McNabb et al. (1982), Hill et al. (1983) and Benowitz and Jacob (1984). The dose used most frequently, i.e., 6 mg/kg × day, is encircled.

administered by osmotic minipump to female Sprague Dawley rats caused blood levels of nicotine corresponding to 2–4 times the baseline or trough levels present in smokers (Isaac and Rand, 1972; McNabb et al., 1982; Hill et al., 1983; Benowitz and Jacob, 1984) and in maternal and fetal human blood at term (Luck et al., 1985). This would appear to be a reasonable dose range.

Effect of prenatal nicotine treatment on nicotinic binding sites

It seems conceivable that prenatal nicotine exposure might interfere with the regulation of nicotinic cholinergic binding sites. Observations in other transmitter systems suggest that such interactions may cause long-lasting changes in the number of receptor sites (Rosengarten and Friedhoff, 1979; Gavish et al., 1985). Chronic prenatal nicotine exposure has been found to induce an increase in the number of [^{3}H]nicotine binding sites in the brain of rat fetuses (Hagino and Lee, 1985; Slotkin et al., 1987a) and neonates (Sershen et al., 1982) and in midbrain + brainstem and cerebral cortex of early postnatal offspring (Slotkin et al., 1987a). No significant changes were seen in cerebellum, which develops later. The effect on the number of nicotinic binding sites is a transient one; control levels are again reached by postnatal day 15 (Slotkin et al., 1987a). Whether any alterations in binding sites exist in adulthood (after puberty) is not known at the present time. Also, data have not yet been analysed separately for the two sexes.

The description given above refers to the effect of prenatal treatment by osmotic minipump. Data on combined tissues from male and female offspring were obtained with a moderate daily dose of 6 mg/kg (GD 4–GD 20; Slotkin et al., 1987a), while one study on fetuses (Hagino and Lee, 1985) was based on a high daily dose of between 21 and 12 mg/kg (compare with Fig. 6; dose expressed as 0.175 mg/kg × h per Sprague Dawley rat, corresponding to 21.0–12.6 mg/kg × day with assumed body weights between 200 and 330 g). Slotkin and coworkers (1987a) noted that twice-daily injections of pregnant dams with nicotine (2 × 3 mg/kg s.c.) resulted in a different early postnatal pattern of nicotinic binding sites in midbrain + brainstem and cerebral cortex, characterized by an isolated departure from control levels at day 10 or 15, respectively. Thereafter, the number of binding sites remained at control levels until day 30, the last day studied. With this type of treatment, the cerebellum, which in the rat undergoes a major period of development after birth, was particularly affected. To what extent this might have been due to postnatal influences cannot yet be decided because the pups have not been cross-fostered.

The available data on changes in receptor sites in response to prenatal drug treatment do not yet provide a coherent picture. The increase in the number of nicotinic binding sites in fetal and neonatal rats after treatment with the agonist corresponds to what is observed in adult animals after chronic nicotine treatment (Marks et al., 1983; Schwartz and Kellar, 1983). In the adult system, the effect is explained by desensitization of the nicotinic receptor and a consequent reduction in nicotinic transmission which could result in receptor up-regulation (Marks et al., 1983). This need not be the mechanism operating in the fetal system, even if the end result is similar. Chronic exposure to high doses of another agonist, benzodiazepine, has for instance been reported to produce down-regulation of receptor sites after treatment in prenatal life (Gavish et al., 1985) as well as after treatment in adulthood (Rosenberg and Chiu, 1981). After daily application of a low dose of diazepam (1.25 mg/kg s.c.) between GD 14 and GD 20, we have also found a reduction of [^{3}H]flunitrazepam binding sites in brain areas such as neocortex and caudate-putamen of adult rat offspring (unpublished quantitative autoradiographic data by M. Schlumpf). In contrast, observations on dopaminergic binding sites suggest differences in receptor regulation of fetal and adult systems. These binding sites were diminished in rat offspring after prenatal reduction of dopaminergic transmission by a neuroleptic or by catecholamine synthesis inhibition, which suggests a facilitatory influence of this agonist on receptor formation during fetal development (Rosengarten and Friedhoff, 1979). The apparent discrepancies between different receptor types may result in part from differences between developmental stages studied. As will be shown in the following section, prenatal drug exposure appears to initiate a process that is subject to changes during subsequent development. In addition, true differences in the underlying regulatory processes should also be considered.

In spite of its preliminary nature, this set of data indicates that effects of drugs on the development of their own receptor sites represent one possible teratogenic mechanism. In terms of functional and ontogenetic consequences, it should be noted that the nicotinic receptor population affected in the rat by nicotine treatment during early and mid-fetal life is mainly situated in the brainstem up to the level of the diencephalon. A majority of telencephalic receptor locations will be directly influenced only by late fetal and postnatal treatment. The role of drug-sensitive periods in relation to receptor development in individual brain regions should be studied more thoroughly in the future.

Prenatal effects of nicotine on central catecholamine systems and their receptors

Nicotine may also affect brain development through actions on other transmitter systems; drug-induced changes in these systems may in turn influence developmental processes in their projection areas. Central catecholamine neurons, which are typical targets for nicotine in adulthood, represent an interesting example because they develop early and establish contact with certain brain regions before the appearance of nicotinic receptors, and because they have been implicated in certain behavioral abnormalities seen also after prenatal nicotine exposure.

We tested the acute effect of nicotine on central catecholamine systems of rat fetuses at GD 21 by determining catecholamines and their metabolites (Ribary et al., 1986), since the turnover approach with tyrosine hydroxylase inhibition has been found to be inappropriate for the condition of the pregnant dam. For reasons of animal protection, the acute experiments were performed using urethane-anesthesia in order to facilitate the preparation of fetuses. In adult rats, this pre-treatment

does not change the nicotine-induced metabolite pattern (Lichtensteiger et al., 1982). In fetuses of both sexes, a single injection of nicotine (1 mg/kg s.c.) given to the dam at GD 21 elicited a marked rise in fetal forebrain dopamine (DA), 3,4-dihydroxyphenylacetic acid (DOPAC) and homovanillic acid (HVA) within 30 min (Lichtensteiger et al., 1984 and in preparation).

Norepinephrine (NE) and its metabolite 3-methoxy-4-hydroxyphenylethylene glycol (MOPEG) increased significantly in Sprague Dawley fetuses, whereas Long Evans fetuses only showed an increase in the MOPEG/NE ratio (Ribary, 1985). These data demonstrate an acute responsiveness of fetal central catecholamine systems to nicotine. The biochemical pattern differs somewhat from that seen with adult systems; in particular, no increase in amine concentrations is seen after acute nicotine treatment in adulthood, and the metabolite pattern looks different, with an increase in HVA but no change in DOPAC at the same time-point after nicotine injection (Lichtensteiger et al., 1982). As the regulation of catecholamine synthesis, turnover and metabolism is not known for this developmental stage, a more detailed functional interpretation of the acute effects cannot be given.

Chronic prenatal nicotine treatment of time-pregnant Long Evans rats affects central catecholamine and metabolite levels of their offspring until adulthood. The drug-induced pattern of biochemical alterations changes during ontogeny and exhibits sex differences (Fig. 7; Lichtensteiger et al., 1984, 1987, and in preparation). Nicotine was administered from GD 12 until GD 18/19, i.e., during an important phase of development of catecholamine neurons and their projections (Fig. 2 Schlumpf et al., 1980), by an s.c. implanted osmotic minipump containing nicotine hydrogen tartrate or tartaric acid and adjusted to deliver 0.25 mg/kg × h (daily dose 6 mg/kg; see Fig. 6). The content of the pump lasted for about one week (until GD 19), i.e., beyond the time of innervation of neocortex by catecholamine fibers. In view of the short half-life of nicotine, the

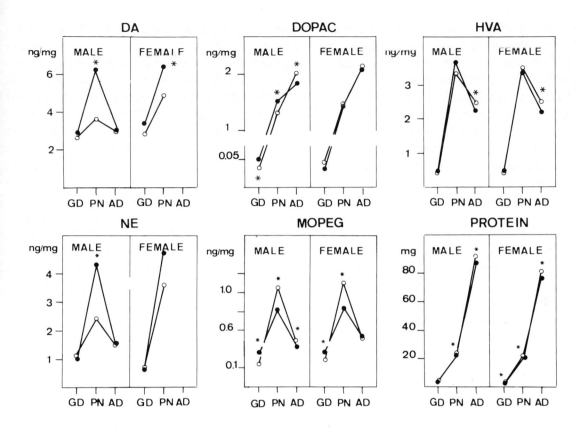

Fig. 7 Effect of prenatal nicotine exposure on catecholamines and their metabolites in fetuses and offspring. Nicotine (0.25 mg/kg × h) was delivered to time-pregnant Long Evans rats by osmotic minipump between GD 12 and GD 18/19. Controls were implanted with tartaric acid-containing osmotic minipumps. Forebrain was analysed in fetuses at gestational day 18 (= GD), in offspring at postnatal day 15 (= PN) and in adulthood (2.5 months, = AD). Control data are given in open circles and nicotine data in closed circles; * = different from control for $P < 0.05$.

pregnant dams can be expected to be drug-free before birth. This treatment does not noticeably influence the pregnant dams; it does not affect litter size or sex distribution but can cause a slight reduction of neonatal body weight which is corrected subsequently (Lichtensteiger and Schlumpf, 1985).

At GD 18, during the last phase of nicotine exposure, fetuses of both sexes show evidence for an increased turnover of NE (rise in MOPEG with NE at control level; Fig. 7) which is in keeping with data from chronically treated adult rats (Bhagat, 1970). DA metabolism is affected only in males, with an increase in DOPAC. It is interesting to note that nicotine again caused a

change in fetal DOPAC rather than HVA, quite in contrast to its effect in adult male rats (Lichtensteiger et al., 1976, 1982) and in pregnant dams, where forebrain HVA rather than DOPAC is elevated (Ribary, 1985, and in preparation).

In prenatally nicotine-exposed offspring, the metabolism of central catecholamine systems remains disturbed until adulthood (Figs. 7 and 8). The postnatal phase – which has been drug-free – is characterized by a reversal of metabolite and amine levels occurring at different developmental stages for NA and DA systems. This development is linked with the sex of the animal. Prenatally nicotine-exposed offspring of both sexes first switch from elevated forebrain MOPEG levels at

GD 18 to reduced levels at postnatal day (PN) 15; this is accompanied in males by significantly higher NE levels. These data point to a marked reduction in NE turnover. Evidence for reduced NE turnover is still found in adult male offspring at 2½ months (reduction in MOPEG in the presence of a normal NE concentration), whereas the NE system of adult female offspring (studied on diestrous day 1) appears to be normalized. These observations are consistent with a report by Peters (1984), who found an increase of adrenergic alpha-2 and beta receptor sites in cerebral cortex of adult male, but not female, offspring after prenatal exposure to a comparable dose of nicotine administered in the drinking water.

Developmental changes are also seen in DA metabolism of nicotine-exposed offspring. At the adult endpoint, either one or both DA metabolites are reduced (DOPAC + HVA in males, HVA in females; Figs. 7 and 8), indicating a reduced turnover of this amine. At the intermediary stage, PN 15, DOPAC is still elevated in males, but DOPAC/DA and HVA/DA ratios are significantly reduced in this sex because of a marked rise in DA concentration, suggesting a reduced DA turnover under conditions of elevated amine levels. No significant changes are noted in PN 15 females except for a modest rise in DA. It is interesting to note that prenatal nicotine exposure exerts significant effects on DOPAC levels throughout pre- and postnatal ontogeny but exclusively in males, whereas abnormal values of HVA are encountered only in adult offspring but are then present in both sexes.

At the present time, we can only speculate

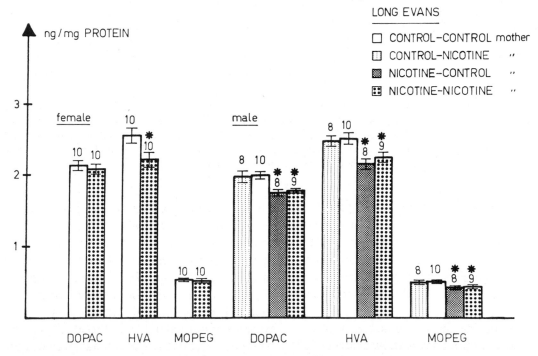

Fig. 8 Effect of prenatal nicotine exposure on forebrain catecholamine metabolites of adult Long Evans rat offspring (2.5 months), cross-fostering data (means ± S.E.M. and number of determinations; * = different from control for $P < 0.05$). Neonates were cross-fostered at birth, litter size was reduced to 8–10 pups. Control-Control: offspring of tartaric acid-treated dams raised by dams treated with tartaric acid during pregnancy. Control-Nicotine: offspring of tartaric acid-treated dams raised by fostermothers treated with nicotine during pregnancy. Nicotine-Control: Prenatally nicotine-exposed pups raised by fostermothers treated with tartaric acid during pregnancy. Nicotine-Nicotine: offspring raised by their own mother which had been treated with nicotine during pregnancy.

about the mechanisms underlying the nicotine-induced changes in central catecholamine metabolism. It is evident from the cross-fostering experiment (Fig. 8) that the alteration in adult metabolite levels was due to the prenatal drug treatment. Some changes in catecholamine metabolism may stem from variations in nicotinic input. An interesting temporal coincidence exists at PN 15 between the reduction of forebrain NE turnover of both sexes and of male DA turnover on one hand, and the normalization of the number of [^{3}H]nicotine binding sites in regions containing catecholamine cell bodies (midbrain + brainstem) and terminals (cerebral cortex; Slotkin et al., 1987a) on the other hand. For a comparison of the two data sets, it is important that at this stage at least the NE turnover change is the same in both sexes, since brain regions from male and female off-spring were pooled in the [^{3}H]nicotine binding study. A possible role of the nicotinic input in adulthood cannot be assessed before binding data on adult, prenatally nicotine-exposed offspring are available.

The functional state of catecholamine neurons could further be affected by drug-induced changes in adrenergic or dopaminergic receptors. Whether the alterations in the number of adrenergic receptor sites seen in adulthood (Peters, 1984) represent a primary phenomenon or are secondary to adult NE turnover changes cannot be decided, since data from intervening stages are lacking. The presence of normal adrenergic receptor levels in another NE projection area, i.e., cerebellum (Peters, 1984), is suggestive of an early developmental change in cerebral cortex, where beta-adrenergic receptor sites are formed during the

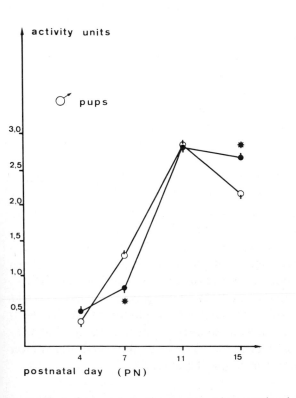
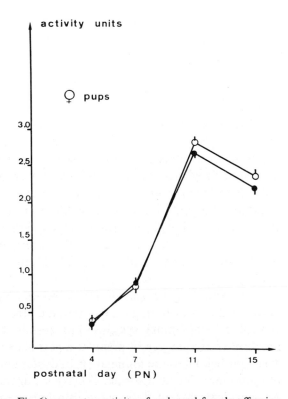

Fig. 9 Effect of prenatal nicotine treatment by osmotic minipump (see Fig. 6) on motor activity of male and female offspring at postnatal days 4 to 15. Control treatment, open circles; nicotine-exposed offspring, closed circles (means + S.D. from individual measurements on 10–16 pups, * = different from control for $P < 0.05$). Activity of individual pups was measured for 3 min on a warm platform (30 °C) by a newly designed activity meter (Schlumpf et al., 1987b).

second part of nicotine treatment (Fig. 2; Schlumpf et al., 1987a). It seems conceivable that long-term changes in receptor regulation (including receptors from additional neurotransmitter systems) play an important part.

The rise in DA and NE levels at PN 15 (and of cortical NE at PN 8 as observed by Peters, 1984) could result from various influences, including number of nerve terminals, turnover changes or transient effects on catecholamine-synthesizing enzymes. Some support for the first possibility may be seen in a report on an increase in [^{3}H]NE uptake by rat neocortex one week after 3–4 days of postnatal nicotine treatment (Jonsson and Hallman, 1980), though the condition would have to be further clarified. In rats exposed to nicotine during pregnancy and lactation, striatal tyrosine hydroxylase activity was not significantly changed at PN 10 but was reduced at PN 20 and PN 40 (Carr et al., 1985). Neonatal administration of a single high dose of nicotine (10 mg/kg) induced only an initial significant increase in adrenal tyrosine hydroxylase activity; however, adrenal dopamine-beta-hydroxylase activity was increased between PN 2 and PN 50 (Rosenthal and Slotkin, 1977). Altogether, the question of drug effects on enzymes of catecholamine synthesis and metabolism remains unsettled. A significant role of unspecific effects such as undernutrition seems unlikely in the present case, since the effect of the treatment on pup size was negligible and since quite different changes in central catecholamines have been reported to be linked with undernutrition (Shoemaker and Wurtman, 1971; Marichich et al., 1979).

It is tempting to search for a relationship between the alterations in the functional state of central catecholamine systems and certain behavioral consequences of prenatal nicotine exposure that belong to the minimal brain dysfunction (or attention deficit disorder, ADD) syndrome. An interpretation of data along this line is still difficult because the relative role of different central DA and NE systems is not yet clear. In a recent review of clinical and experimental data,

Raskin and collaborators (1984) relate neonatal lesions of DA systems to increased motor activity and decreases in performance of young rats (comparable to human ADD with hyperactivity), while selective lesions of NE systems are reported to produce learning deficits without concomitant activity change (ADD without hyperactivity). When we studied the development of motor activity in prenatally nicotine-exposed offspring, we observed a reduction of activity at PN 7 and an increase above control levels at PN 15, but only in males; female littermates were unaffected (Fig. 9; Schlumpf et al., 1987b). The reader may remember that at PN 15, prenatally nicotine-exposed male pups differ from females by a reduction of DA turnover (Fig. 7), whereas NE turnover is affected in both sexes. These data appear to fit closely with the model proposed by Raskin and coworkers (1984). In adult offspring, the catecholamine system selectively affected in males is the noradrenergic one (Fig. 7). In view of the proposed relationship between lesions of NE systems and learning deficits (Raskin et al., 1984), it is then interesting to note that delayed effects of prenatal nicotine treatment on learning behavior have been found specifically in male offspring (Genedani et al., 1983; see below). There is yet another interesting aspect of the data on motor activity, i.e., the inversion of the nicotine-induced effect during the first two weeks of life (Fig. 9). A biphasic effect of prenatal nicotine treatment on the development of the electroshock seizure threshold, with an increase in the second and a decrease in the third postnatal week, has been reported by Hudson and coworkers (1973), without comment on pup sex. These effects could possibly be explained by temporal shifts in developmental processes (cf. next section), but they might also be related to abnormal transmitter turnover in specific systems.

Nicotine-induced changes in cerebral cell acquisition

Chronic prenatal nicotine exposure also affects DNA, RNA and protein metabolism in rat brain (Sershen et al., 1982; Slotkin et al., 1986, 1987b; see also Fig. 7). In an investigation based on daily nicotine injections, brain ornithine decarboxylase activity was increased during the last part of fetal life, indicating delayed cell maturation (Slotkin et al., 1986). Nucleotide and protein metabolism remained disturbed at least during prepubertal life, with region-specific differences. Moreover, ornithine decarboxylase values in this and a second study (Slotkin et al., 1987b) pointed to a disruption of the timing of control of macromolecule synthesis. Of special interest in the present context are data from the second study which used the osmotic minipump at a daily dose of 6 mg/kg. They can be compared with our transmitter data, though it should be noted that the study does not distinguish between sexes.

In lower brainstem and midbrain, which undergo a major phase of development and at the same time possess high numbers of nicotinic receptor sites during prenatal treatment with nicotine, DNA level, which provides an index of cell acquisition, was reduced at PN 7 but exhibited a rebound between PN 10 and PN 14. In contrast, cell acquisition was depressed in cerebral cortex and cerebellum at PN 14 (Slotkin et al., 1987b). In the rat, important developmental processes take place in these regions during postnatal life; also, they acquire a majority of their nicotinic binding sites after termination of the prenatal nicotine treatment. This suggests that changes in cortical cell acquisition may result in part from an indirect effect of nicotine. An effect of monoamines on neural cell differentiation has been repeatedly discussed (NE: König et al., 1983; 5-HT: Lauder et al., 1983) and could be taken into consideration in the present context in view of the marked reduction of forebrain NE turnover at PN 15, while the serotonin metabolite, 5-hydroxyindole acetic acid, is at control level in these

animals (Ribary, 1985). However, it remains uncertain whether an influence from a defined transmitter system would be general enough to become manifest in total regional DNA content, since in vitro studies indicate that catecholamines act selectively on certain types of neuron (König et al., 1986). Moreover, a considerable part of cell acquisition at this stage of development represents glial cells, for which a direct effect of catecholamines remains to be demonstrated.

The relative significance of general effects of nicotine on cell acquisition and of specific actions on certain transmitter systems, and the question of a possible relationship between these two sets of data, remain to be elucidated. Some of the effects of nicotine on brain growth may be linked with metabolic and endocrine effects of the drug (see following sections). Brain ornithine decarboxylase activity has proved to be a sensitive index of detrimental drug actions on brain development, but ornithine decarboxylase-dependent processes do not appear to represent the only pathogenetic mechanism. Thus, the sex-linked learning deficit produced by prenatal nicotine treatment (Genedani et al., 1983) is not mimicked by inhibition of ornithine decarboxylase during part of fetal development (Genedani et al., 1985).

Prenatal metabolic actions of nicotine

Nicotine may interfere with brain development in an indirect way through its action on a multitude of metabolic processes in maternal organism, placenta and fetus. Other components of tobacco smoke obviously contribute to the syndrome seen in humans. The consequences of maternal smoking for nutrition and oxygen supply of the fetus have recently been reviewed (Longo, 1982); only a few aspects will be outlined briefly in order to illustrate the potential significance of such indirect actions. Nicotine enhances the catabolic disposition present in late gestation; in rat, it increases maternal lipolysis and fetal body fat (Williams and Kanagasabai, 1984). Fasting in pregnancy is followed by greater than normal hypoglycemia and hyperketonemia (Felig and Lynch, 1970). Nicotine might exacerbate the ketosis. As shown by comparative studies on precocial (guinea pig) and non-precocial (rat) species, the significance of such a metabolic event would appear to depend upon the degree of maturation of individual brain regions, since the enzymes of ketone body metabolism are already active in immature nervous tissue, whereas characteristic enzymes of glucose metabolism develop later (Booth et al., 1980). Hence, one can speculate that the ketosis would be more critical for those neurons that had already switched to glucose metabolism. This example should illustrate that the significance of indirect metabolic effects of nicotine for brain development is also intimately linked with the developmental stage.

Nicotine affects placental function. It elicits a release of NE and epinephrine into the maternal blood (Quigley et al., 1979) and reduces placental blood flow, both in humans and in experimental animals (Lehtovirta and Forss, 1978; Philipp et al., 1984; Resnik et al., 1985). The drug did not seem to exert immediate effects on human fetal circulation when tested in late gestation (Jouppila et al., 1983). Some reports indicate that placental metabolism may also be disturbed. Nicotine reduces the uptake of alpha-aminoisobutyric acid by isolated placental tissue, which points to an interaction with amino acid transport (Rowell and Sastry, 1978; Fisher et al., 1984). However, the original idea of an interaction of the drug with the placental cholinergic system has not been supported by an analysis of this system (Rowell et al., 1986). Smoking also affects placental steroid metabolism, as shown by a lower conversion of dehydroepiandrosterone sulfate to estradiol (Mochizuki et al., 1984). Xenobiotic metabolism in human placenta is enhanced by smoking (Nebert et al., 1969; Manchester et al., 1984), but this effect results from the action of the polycyclic hydrocarbons of tobacco smoke.

Interaction of nicotine with developing neuroendocrine systems

The interaction of drugs with developing neuroendocrine systems is an important aspect of pre- and perinatal drug action (for review: Lichtensteiger and Schlumpf, 1984). Many neuroendocrine systems undergo a period of organization during fetal and – depending on the species – perinatal life. This period of organization has turned out to be quite sensitive to external influences. Since neuroendocrine regulation includes many brain functions, interactions with its organization may have widespread effects. Moreover, it seems possible that even drug actions of short duration may have lasting effects if they interfere with the organizational action of hormones during a critical period of development.

Although nicotine affects many hormone systems, lasting changes after prenatal treatment have so far only been documented for functions linked with the action of sex hormones. Also, it should be noted that corresponding human data are lacking. Prenatal nicotine exposure leads to two classes of alterations: on the one hand, certain normal manifestations of sexual dimorphism have been found to disappear, on the other hand, new abnormal sex differences appeared in the offspring. When time-pregnant rats were treated from GD 12 for one week with nicotine delivered by an osmotic minipump at the dose level discussed earlier (0.25 mg/kg × h or 6 mg/kg × day), their adult offspring showed a complete disappearance of the characteristic sexual dimorphism in the preference for saccharin-containing drinking water (Lichtensteiger and Schlumpf, 1985). Many mammals of both sexes prefer sweet solutions, but as a rule, females show a significantly higher preference (Valenstein et al., 1967; Wade, 1976). Adult, prenatally nicotine-exposed males exhibited the high degree of saccharin preference of females, whereas the performance of their female littermates corresponded to that of control females. The same treatment suppressed the rise in serum testosterone which typically occurs in male rat fetuses at GD 18. This initial testosterone peak is thought to be important for sexual brain differentiation (Weisz and Ward, 1980). Since prenatal stress also affects male fetal testosterone levels (Ward and Weisz, 1980), possible effects of the treatment schedule were checked, but testosterone levels corresponded to those of untreated controls after either sham operation at GD 12 or implantation of minipumps containing tartaric acid or saline. In a limited series of experiments, sex behavior of prenatally nicotine-exposed male offspring was also found to be markedly reduced (Ribary, 1985). Meanwhile, several important psychoactive drugs have been found to interfere with the pre- or perinatal organization of sexually dimorphic functions (mostly sex behavior) and/or with the development of the adrenal axis in rat, mouse and hamster. These are cannabinoids, phenobarbital, opiates, ethanol and diazepam (reviewed by Lichtensteiger and Schlumpf, 1984). All compounds active on the gonadal axis also caused a reduction of fetal male testosterone levels.

Prenatal nicotine exposure can also create new sex differences in the sense that abnormal behavior is seen only in one sex. Male offspring usually appear to be more affected. The sex-linked effect of prenatal nicotine exposure on motor activity of the rat during the first two weeks of life has already been described (Fig. 9). After prenatal administration of nicotine in the drinking water (6 mg/kg × day), Peters and Tang (1982) observed a reduction of rearing activity and of initial activity in the open field in adult male rat offspring. Females were unaffected. As mentioned above, a reduced acquisition of a two-way avoidance behavior was also seen exclusively in adult male offspring after prenatal nicotine treatment (2 × 0.25 mg/kg × day s.c. between GD 1 and GD 20), while learning behavior of the female littermates was normal (Genedani et al., 1983). These data can be compared with the sex differences in the effects of prenatal nicotine exposure on catecholamine metabolism (see above). In all cases, the offspring had been exposed to nico-

tine also during the early phase of organization of the male gonadal axis. It seems probable that the special sensitivity of the males is related to the interaction of the drug with this process, but the mechanism may be quite different from the one preventing the development of sexually dimorphic functions.

Summary and conclusions

Nicotine affects the materno-fetal unit through multiple actions. Specific direct actions of nicotine on the developing brain seem possible during a major part of prenatal life, since binding sites for [^{3}H]nicotine are already detectable in the central nervous system of the rat at late embryonic stages. As neural circuitry and the state of maturation of brain regions change continuously in the course of prenatal ontogeny, the drug may elicit different effects at different developmental stages. This aspect has received little attention so far. Acute effects of nicotine on central catecholamine neurons, which are typical targets for the drug in adulthood, have been demonstrated during the midfetal period. Prolonged prenatal exposure to the drug affects nicotinic binding sites, catecholamine systems and cell acquisition in various brain regions. When doses of nicotine are compared with drug levels in smokers and in human fetal blood at term, it is evident that neurochemical effects are obtained in experimental animals with moderate dose levels, in the absence of general toxic effects. Alterations are present also in postnatal life, after cessation of drug treatment. These delayed effects are not stable but change in relation to the developmental stage. Alterations in catecholamine metabolism, with differences between noradrenergic and dopaminergic systems, are present until adulthood, while the pre- and early postnatal increase in the number of nicotinic receptor sites is normalized in 2 week-old rat pups, with no further changes found at least until puberty. While some neurochemical consequences of prenatal nicotine exposure are thus known, the underlying pathogenetic mechanisms remain a matter of speculation. They are probably related to direct as well as indirect actions of the drug.

Actions of nicotine at central cholinergic receptor sites combine in a complex way with effects of the drug on circulation, metabolism and endocrine systems of mother and fetus. Data on placental function and lipid metabolism are briefly discussed. A potentially important pathogenetic mechanism is seen in interactions of nicotine with developing neuroendocrine systems, since even transient exposure to the drug may cause persistent changes in the developing brain by disturbing the organizing action of hormones. Like several other psychoactive drugs, nicotine interferes with the organization of the fetal male gonadal axis; in adult rat offspring, a typical sexual dimorphism in behavior (saccharin preference) is lost. Possible developmental effects on other hormone axes have not yet been tested. Prenatal nicotine exposure can also create new sex differences: in experimental animals, some types of abnormal behavior (motor behavior, learning) are encountered only in one sex, generally in males. These behavioral data are reflected by certain sex differences in nicotine-induced changes in catecholamine metabolism. The mechanisms underlying the latter group of defects may differ from the one preventing the development of sexually dimorphic brain functions.

Children of mothers who smoked during pregnancy display symptoms of minimal brain dysfunction or attention deficit disorder (ADD). Analogous behavioral abnormalities are found in prenatally nicotine-exposed animals. Certain alterations in behavior and central catecholamine metabolism of two-week-old and adult rat offspring correspond to what would be expected from other experimental data linking ADD to defects in dopaminergic and noradrenergic systems. Behavioral data suggest that with respect to brain development, nicotine is an important constituent of tobacco smoke, but one should not overlook possible contributions from components such as carbon monoxide. Other smoke constituents (polycyclic aromatic hydrocarbons, cadmium) can affect additional functions of the materno-placento-fetal unit.

Acknowledgements

The research of the authors was supported by Swiss National Science Foundation grants (nos. 3.519-0.83 and 3.238-0.85).

References

Aston-Jones, G., Ennis, M., Pieribone, V. A., Nickell, W. T. and Shipley, M. T. (1986) The brain nucleus locus coeruleus: Restricted afferent control of a broad efferent network. *Science*, 234: 734–737.

Baer, D. S., McClearn, G. E. and Wilson, J. R. (1980) Fertility, maternal care, and offspring behavior in mice prenatally treated with tobacco smoke. *Dev. Psychobiol.*, 13: 643–652.

Benowitz, N. L. and Jacob, P. III (1984) Nicotine and carbon monoxide intake from high- and low-yield cigarettes. *Clin. Pharm. Ther.*, 36: 265–270.

Bhagat, B. (1970) Influence of chronic administration of nicotine on the turnover and metabolism of noradrenaline in the rat brain. *Psychopharmacologia.*, 18: 325–332.

Booth, R. F. G., Patel, T. B. and Clark, J. B. (1980) The development of enzymes of energy metabolism in the brain of a precocial (guinea pig) and non-precocial (rat) species. *J. Neurochem.*, 34: 17–25.

Bruinink, A., Lichtensteiger, W. and Schlumpf, M. (1983) Pre- and postnatal ontogeny and characterization of dopaminergic D2, serotonergic S2 and spirodecanone binding sites in rat forebrain. *J. Neurochem.*, 40: 1227–1236.

Bruinink, A. and Lichtensteiger, W. (1984) Beta-adrenergic binding sites in fetal rat brain. *J. Neurochem.*, 43: 578–581.

Carr, L. A., Walters, D. E. and Meyer, D. C. (1985) Postnatal development in the rat following pre- or postnatal exposure to nicotine. *Res. Commun. Substances Abuse*, 6: 151–164.

Clarke, P. B. S., Schwartz, R. D., Paul, S. M., Pert, C. B. and Pert, A. (1985) Nicotinic binding in rat brain: autoradiographic comparison of [^{3}H]acetylcholine, [^{3}H]nicotine, and [^{125}I]α-bungarotoxin. *J. Neurosci.*, 5: 1307–1315.

Davie, R., Butler, N. and Goldstein, H. (1972) From Birth to Seven: The Second Report of the National Child Development Study (1958 Cohort). Longman in association with the National Children's Bureau. William Clowes & Sons, London.

Denson, R., Nanson, J. L. and McWatters, M. A. (1975) Hyperkinesis and maternal smoking. *Can. Psychiatr. Assoc. J.*, 20: 183–187.

Dunn, .G., McBurney, A. K., Ingram, S. and Hunter, C. M. (1977) Maternal cigarette smoking during pregnancy and the child's subsequent development: II: Neurological and intellectual maturation to the age of 6½ years. *Can. J. Pub Health*, 68: 43–50.

Felig, P. and Lynch, V. (1970) Starvation in human pregnancy: hypoglycemia, hypoinsulinemia, and hyperketonemia. *Science*, 170: 990–992.

Fishell, G. and van der Kooy, D. (1987) Pattern formation in the striatum: developmental changes in the distribution of striatonigral neurons. *J. Neurosci.*, 7: 1969–1978.

Fisher, S. E., Atkinson, M. and Van Thiel, D. H. (1984) Selective fetal malnutrition: the effect of nicotine, ethanol, and acetaldehyde upon in vitro uptake of alpha-aminoisobutyric acid by human term placental villous slices. *Dev. Pharmacol. Ther.*, 7: 229–238.

Floeter, M. K., and Jones, E. G. (1985) The morphology and phased outgrowth of callosal axons in the fetal rat. *Dev. Brain Res.* 22: 7–18.

Gavish, M., Avnimelech-Gigus, N., Feldon, J. and Myslobodsky, M. (1985) Prenatal chlordiazepoxide effects on metrazol seizures and benzodiazepine receptors density in adult albino rats. *Life Sci.*, 36: 1693–1698.

Genedani, S., Bernardi, M. and Bertolini, A. (1983) Sex-linked differences in avoidance learning in the offspring of rats treated with nicotine during pregnancy. *Psychopharmacology*, 80: 93–95.

Genedani, S., Bernardi, M. and Bertolini, A. (1985) Developmental and behavioral outcomes of perinatal inhibition of ornithine decarboxylase. *Neurobehav. Toxicol. Teratol.*, 7: 57–65.

Giorguieff, M.F., Le Floch, M.L., Westfall, T.C., Glowinski, I. and Besson, M.J. (1976) Nicotinic effect of acetylcholine on the release of newly synthesized [³H]dopamine in rat striatal slices and cat caudate nucleus. *Brain Res.*, 106: 117–131.

Hagino, N. and Lee, J. W. (1985) Effect of maternal nicotine on the development of sites for [³H]nicotine binding in the fetal brain. *Int. J. Dev. Neurosci.*, 3: 567–571.

Hara, Y., Shiosaka, S., Senba, E., Sakanaka, M., Inagaki, S., Takagi, H., Kawai, Y., Takatsuki, K., Matsuzaki, T. and Tohyama, M. (1982) Ontogeny of the neurotensin-containing neuron system of the rat: immunohistochemical analysis. I. Forebrain and diencephalon. *J. Comp. Neurol.*, 208: 177–195.

Hill, P., Haley, N.J. and Wynder, E.L. (1983) Cigarette smoking: carboxyhemoglobin, plasma nicotine, cotinine and thiocyanate vs self-reported smoking data and cardiovascular disease. *J. Chron. Dis.*, 36: 439–449.

Hudson, D.B., Meisami, E. and Timiras, P.S. (1973) Brain development in offspring of rats treated with nicotine during pregnancy. *Experientia*, 29: 286–288.

Johns, J.M., Louis, T.M., Becker, R.F. and Means, L.W. (1982) Behavioral effects of prenatal exposure to nicotine in guinea pigs. *Neurobehav. Toxicol. Teratol.*, 4: 365–369.

Jonsson, G. and Hallman, H. (1980) Effects of neonatal nicotine administration on the postnatal development of central noradrenaline neurons. *Acta Physiol. Scand. Suppl.*, 479: 25–26.

Jouppila, P., Kirkinen, P. and Eik-Nes, S. (1983) Acute effect of maternal smoking on the human fetal blood flow. *Br. J. Obstet. Gynecol.*, 90: 7–10.

Isaac, P.F. and Rand, M.J. (1972) Cigarette smoking and plasma levels of nicotine. *Nature*, 236: 308–310.

Kelly, J., Mathews, K.A. and O'Conor, M. (1984) Smoking in pregnancy: effects on mother and fetus. *Br. J. Obstet. Gynecol.*, 91: 111–117.

Kent, J.L., Pert, C.B. and Herkenham, M. (1982) Ontogeny of opiate receptors in rat forebrain: visualization by in vitro autoradiography. *Dev. Brain Res.*, 2: 487–504.

König, N., Serrano, J.-J., Szafarczyk, A. and Dememes, D. (1983) Role of catecholamines in nervous system development: effects of prenatal 6-hydroxydopa treatment on behavior and brain structures. In M. Schlumpf and W. Lichtensteiger (Eds.), *Drugs and Hormones in Brain Development Monogr. Neural Sci., Vol. 9*, S. Karger, Basel, pp. 11–19.

König, N., Drian, M.-J., Privat, A. and Pares-Herbute, N. (1986) Action of catecholamines on neuronal differentiation in vitro. *Inter. J. Dev. Neurosci., 4, Suppl.* 1: S40.

Landesman-Dwyer, S., and Emanuel, I. (1979) Smoking during pregnancy. *Teratology*, 19: 119–126.

Large, T.L., Lambert, M.P., Gremillion, M.A. and Klein, W.L. (1986) Parallel postnatal development of choline acetyltransferase activity and muscarinic acetylcholine receptors in the rat olfactory bulb. *J. Neurochem.*, 46: 671–680.

Lauder, J.M., Wallace, J.A., Wilkie, M.B., DiNome, A. and Krebs, H. (1983) Roles for serotonin in neurogenesis. In M. Schlumpf and W. Lichtensteiger (Eds.), *Drugs and Hormones in Brain Development. Monogr. Neural Sci., Vol. 9*, S. Karger, Basel, pp. 3–10.

Lauder, J.M., Han, V.K.M., Henderson, P., Verdoorn, T. and Towle, A.C. (1986) Prenatal ontogeny of the GABAergic system in the rat brain: an immunocytochemical study. *Neuroscience*, 19: 465–493.

Lehtovirta, P. and Forss, M. (1978) The acute effect of smoking on intervillous blood flow of the placenta. *Br. J. Obstet. Gynecol.*, 85: 729–731.

Lichtensteiger, W. and Schlumpf, M. (1984) Prenatal neuropharmacology: implications for neuroendocrine development. In F. Ellendorff, P.D. Gluckman and N. Parvizi (Eds.), *Fetal Neuroendocrinology. Research in Perinatal Medicine II*, Perinatology Press, Ithaca, pp. 59–70.

Lichtensteiger, W. and Schlumpf, M. (1985) Prenatal nicotine affects fetal testosterone and sexual dimorphism of saccharin preference. *Pharmacol. Biochem. Behav.*, 23: 439–444.

154

Lichtensteiger, W., Felix, D., Lienhart, R. and Hefti, F. (1976) A quantitative correlation between single unit activity and fluorescence intensity of dopamine neurones in zona compacta of substantia nigra, as demonstrated under the influence of nicotine and physostigmine. *Brain Research*, 117: 85–103.

Lichtensteiger, W. Hefti, F., Felix, D., Huwyler, T. Melamed, E. and Schlumpf, M. (1982) Stimulation of nigrostriatal dopamine neurons by nicotine. *Neuropharmacology*, 21: 963–968.

Lichtensteiger, W., Schlumpf, M. and Ribary, U. (1984) Effects of nicotine on the developing gonadal axis and on central catecholamine systems of the male rat fetus. In F. Caciagli, E. Giacobini and R. Paoletti (Eds.), *Developmental Neuroscience: Physiological, Pharmacological and Clinical Aspects*, Elsevier, Amsterdam, pp. 131–135.

Lichtensteiger, W., Schlumpf, M. and Ribary, U. (1987) Modifications pharmacologiques de l'ontogenese neuro-endocrine. Developpement de récepteurs, nicotine et catecholamines. *Ann. d'Endocrinol.*, 48: 393–399.

Lidov, H. G. W. and Molliver, M. E. (1982) An immunohistochemical study of serotonin neuron development in the rat: ascending pathways and terminal fields. *Brain Res. Bull.*, 8: 389–430.

Longo, L. D. (1982) Some health consequences of maternal smoking: issues without answers. *Birth Defects: Original Article Series, Vol. 18*, March of Dimes Birth Defects Foundation, pp. 13–31.

Luck, W., Nau, H., Hansen, R. and Steldinger, R. (1985) Extent of nicotine and cotinine transfer to the human fetus, placenta and amniotic fluid of smoking mothers. *Dev. Pharmacol. Ther.*, 8: 384–395.

Manchester, D. K., Parker, N. B. and Bowman, C. M. (1984) Maternal smoking increases xenobiotic metabolism in placenta but not umbilical vein endothelium. *Pediatric Res.*, 18: 1071–1075.

Marichich, E. S., Molina, V. A. and Orsingher, O. A. (1979) Persistent changes in central catecholaminergic system recovery of perinatally undernourished rats. *J. Nutr.*, 109: 1045–1050.

Marks, M. J., Burch, J. B. and Collins, A. C. (1983) Effects of chronic nicotine infusion on tolerance development and nicotinic receptors. *J. Pharmacol. Exp. Ther.*, 226: 817–825.

Martin, J. C. and Becker, R. F. (1971) The effects of maternal nicotine absorption or hypoxic episodes upon appetitive behavior of rat offspring. *Dev. Psychobiol.*, 4: 133–147.

McNabb, McK. E., Ebert, R. V. and McCusker, K. (1982) Plasma nicotine levels produced by chewing nicotine gum. *J. Am. Med. Assoc.*, 248: 865–868.

Mochizuki, M., Maruo, T., Masuko, K. and Ohtsu, T. (1984) Effects of smoking on fetoplacental-maternal system during pregnancy. *Am. J. Obstet. Gynecol.*, 149: 413–420.

Murrin, L. C., Ferrer, J. R., Zeug, W. and Haley, N. J. (1987) Nicotine administration to rats: Methodological considerations. *Life Sci.*, 40: 1699–1708.

Naeye, R. L. and Peters, E. C. (1984) Mental development of children whose mothers smoked during pregnancy. *Obstet. Gynecol.*, 64: 601–607.

Nebert, D. W., Winker, J. and Gelboin, H. V. (1969) Aryl hydrocarbon hydroxylase activity in human placenta from cigarette smoking and nonsmoking women. *Cancer Res.*, 29: 1763–1769.

Oke, A. F. and Adams, R. N. (1978) Selective attention dysfunctions in adult rats neonatally treated with 6-hydroxydopamine. *Pharmacol. Biochem. Behav.*, 9: 429–432.

Palacios, J. M., Pazos, A., Dietl, M. M., Schlumpf, M. and Lichtensteiger, W. (1987) The ontogeny of brain neurotensin receptors studied by autoradiography. *Neuroscience*, in press.

Peters, D. A. V. (1984) Prenatal nicotine exposure increases adrenergic receptor binding in the rat cerebral cortex. *Res. Commun. Chem. Pathol. Pharm.*, 46: 307–317.

Peters, D. A. V. and Tang, S. (1982) Sex-dependent biological changes following prenatal nicotine exposure in the rat. *Pharmacol. Biochem. Behav.*, 17: 1077–1082.

Peters, D. A. V., Taub, H. and Tang, S. (1979) Postnatal effects of maternal nicotine exposure. *Neurobehav. Toxicol.*, 1: 221–225.

Philipp, K., Pateisky, N. and Endler, M. (1984) Effects of smoking on uteroplacental blood flow. *Gynecol. Obstet. Invest.*, 17: 179–182.

Quigley, M. E., Sheehan, K. L., Wilkes, M. M. and Yen, S. S. C. (1979) Effects of maternal smoking on circulating catecholamine levels and fetal heart rates. *Am. J. Obstet. Gynecol.*, 133: 685–690.

Rantakallio, P. (1983) A follow-up study up to the age of 14 of children whose mothers smoked during pregnancy. *Acta Paediatr. Scand.*, 72: 747–753.

Raskin, L. A., Shaywitz, B. A., Shaywitz, S. E., Cohen, J. D. and Anderson, G. M. (1984) Early brain damage and attentional deficit disorder: an animal model. In C. R. Almly and S. Finger (Eds.), *Early Brain Damage, Vol. 1*, Academic Press, Orlando, pp. 111–125.

Resnik, R., Conover, W. B., Key, T. C. and VanVunakis, H. (1985) Uterine blood flow and catecholamine response to repetitive nicotine exposure in the pregnant ewe. *Am. J. Obstet. Gynecol.*, 151: 885–891.

Ribary, U. (1985) Nicotine in pregnancy: acute and persistent effects on central monoaminergic systems in rat fetus and offspring. Thesis No. 7939 Federal Institute of Technology, Zürich.

Ribary, U., Schlumpf, M. and Lichtensteiger, W. (1986) Analysis by HPLC-EC of metabolites of monoamines in fetal and postnatal rat brain. *Neuropharmacology*, 25: 981–986.

Rosenberg, E. C. and Chiu, T. H. (1981) Tolerance during chronic benzodiazepine treatment associated with decreased receptor binding. *Eur. J. Pharmacol.*, 70: 453–460.

Rosengarten, H. and Friedhoff, A.J. (1979) Enduring changes in dopamine receptor cells of pups from drug administration to pregnant and nursing rats. *Science*, 203: 1133–1135.

Rosenthal, R.N. and Slotkin, T.A. (1977) Development of nicotinic responses in the rat adrenal medulla and long-term effects of neonatal nicotine administration. *Br. J. Pharmacol.*, 60: 59–64.

Rowell, P.P. and Sastry, B.V.R. (1978) The influence of cholinergic blockade on the uptake of alpha-aminoisobutyric acid by isolated placental villi. *Toxicol. Appl. Pharmacol.*, 45: 79–93.

Rowell, P.P., Leventer, S.M. and Clark, M.J. (1986) The effect of cigarette smoking during pregnancy on the cholinergic system in isolated term human placental tissue. *Biol. Reprod.*, 34: 344–348.

Saxton, D.W. (1978) The behaviour of infants whose mothers smoke in pregnancy. *Early Human Dev.*, 2/4: 363–369.

Schlumpf, M. and Lichtensteiger, W. (1987) Regional ontogeny of drug binding sites in fetal rat and human brain as indication of neurotransmitter receptor formation. *IBRO Second World Congress of Neurosciences, Satellite Symposium on Developmental and Reactive Synaptogenesis*, Tihany, Abstracts, p. 15.

Schlumpf, M., Lichtensteiger, W., Shoemaker, W.J. and Bloom, F.E. (1980) Fetal monoamine systems: early stages and cortical projections. In J. Parvez and S. Parvez (Eds.), *Biogenic Amines in Development*, Elsevier, Amsterdam, pp. 567–590.

Schlumpf, M., Richards, J.G., Lichtensteiger, W. and Möhler, H. (1983) An autoradiographic study of the prenatal development of benzodiazepine binding sites in rat brain. *J. Neurosci.*, 3: 1478–1487.

Schlumpf, M., Palacios, J.M., Cortes, R., Pazos, A., Richards, J.G., Bruinink, A. and Lichtensteiger, W. (1984) Pre- and postnatal development of drug and neurotransmitter receptors: an autoradiographic study. In F. Caciagli, E. Giacobini and R. Paoletti (Eds.), *Developmental Neuroscience: Physiological, Pharmacological and Clinical Aspects*, Elsevier, Amsterdam, pp. 159–166.

Schlumpf, M., Palacios, J.M., Cortes, R., Pazos, A., Bruinink, A. and Lichtensteiger, W. (1985) Development of drug and neurotransmitter binding sites in fetal rat brain. *Society for Neuroscience Abstracts*, Vol. 11, Part 1: 602 (no. 177.17).

Schlumpf, M., Bruinink, A., Lichtensteiger, W., Cortes, R., Palacios, J.M. and Pazos, A. (1987a) Beta-adrenergic binding sites in fetal rat c.n.s. and pineal gland: their relation to other receptor sites. *Devl. Pharmacol. Ther.*, 10: 422–435.

Schlumpf, M., Gähwiler, M., Ribary, U. and Lichtensteiger, W. (1987b) A new device for monitoring early motor development: prenatal nicotine-induced changes. *Pharmacol. Biochem. Behav.*, in press.

Schwartz, R.D. and Kellar, K.J. (1983) Nicotinic cholinergic receptor binding sites in the brain: regulation in vivo. *Science*, 220: 214–216.

Sershen, H., Reith, M.E.A., Banay-Schwartz, M. and Lajtha, A. (1982) Effects of prenatal administration of nicotine on amino acid pools, protein metabolism, and nicotine binding in the brain. *Neurochem. Res.*, 7: 1515–1522.

Shaywitz, B.A., Yager, R.D. and Klopper, J.H. (1976) Selective brain dopamine depletion in developing rats: an experimental model for minimal brain dysfunction. *Science*, 191: 305–307.

Shoemaker, W.J. and Wurtman, R.J. (1971) Perinatal undernutrition: accumulation of catecholamines in rat brain. *Science*, 171: 1017–1019.

Slotkin, T.A., Greer, N., Faust, J., Cho, H. and Seidler, F.J. (1986) Effects of maternal nicotine injections on brain development in the rat: Ornithine decarboxylase activity, nucleic acids and proteins in discrete brain regions. *Brain Res. Bull.*, 17: 41–50.

Slotkin, T.A., Orband-Miller, L. and Queen, K.L. (1987a) Development of [^{3}H]nicotine binding sites in brain regions of rats exposed to nicotine prenatally via maternal injections or infusions. *J. Pharmacol. Exp. Ther.*, 242: 232–237.

Slotkin, T.A., Orband-Miller, L., Queen, K.L., Whitmore, W.L. and Seidler, F.J. (1987b) Effects of prenatal nicotine exposure on biochemical development of rat brain regions: maternal drug infusions via osmotic minipumps. *J. Pharmacol. Exp. Ther.*, 240: 602–611.

Specht, L.A., Pickel, V.M., Joh, T.H. and Reis, D.J. (1981) Light microscopic immunocytochemical localization of tyrosine hydroxylase in prenatal rat brain. I. Early ontogeny. *J. Comp. Neurol.*, 199: 233–253.

Svensson, T.H. and Engberg, G. (1980) Effect of nicotine on single cell activity in the noradrenergic nucleus locus coeruleus. *Acta Physiol. Scand. Suppl.*, 479: 31–34.

Taylor, P. (1985) Ganglionic stimulation and blocking agents. In A.G. Gilman, L.S. Goodman, T.W. Rall and F. Murad (Eds.) *The Pharmacological Basis of Therapeutics*, 7th edn., Macmillan Publishing Co., New York, pp. 215–221 and 1699.

Valenstein, E.S., Kakolewski, J.W. and Cox, V.C. (1967) Sex differences in taste preference for glucose and saccharin solutions. *Science*, 156: 942–943.

Wade, G.N. (1976) Sex hormones, regulatory behaviors, and body weight. In J.S. Rosenblatt, R.A. Hinde, E. Shaw and G.G. Beer (Eds.), *Adv. in the Study of Behavior, Vol. 6*, Academic Press, New York, pp. 201–279.

Wallace, J.A. and Lauder, J.M. (1983) Development of the serotonergic system of the rat embryo: an immunocytochemical study. *Brain Res. Bull.*, 10: 459–479.

Ward, I.L. and Weisz, J. (1980) Maternal stress alters plasma testosterone in fetal males. *Science*, 207: 328–329.

Weisz, J. and Ward, I.L. (1980) Plasma testosterone and progesterone titers of pregnant rats, their male and female fetuses, and neonatal offspring. *Endocrinology*, 106: 306–316.

Widmer, H.R., Schlumpf, M. and Lichtensteiger, W. (1986) The morphology and distribution of choline acetyltransferase (ChAT) containing neurons in early postnatal rat brain. In N. Elsner and W. Rathmayer (Eds.) *Beiträge zur 14. Göttinger Neurobiologentagung*, Georg Thieme Verlag, Stuttgart, 1986, p. 296.

Williams, C.M. and Kanagasabai, T. (1984) Maternal adipose tissue response to nicotine administration in the pregnant rat: effects on fetal body weight and cellularity. *Br. J. Nutr.*, 51: 7–13.

Discussion

J.M. Lauder: Since you have shown nicotinic receptors in the region of the developing serotonergic neurons of the raphe nuclei, I wonder if you have looked at effects of prenatal nicotine administration on serotonin and its metabolites?

W. Lichtensteiger: 5-HIAA (5-hydroxy-indoleacetic acid) was analysed simultaneously with the catecholamine metabolites. Acute administration of nicotine caused an increase of 5-HIAA in fetal rat forebrain of both sexes at gestational day (GD) 21. After chronic prenatal nicotine treatment, 5-HIAA was at control levels at GD 18 and postnatal (PN) 15 (adult levels were not studied; Ribary, 1985). Since we did not determine serotonin, we cannot be sure about possible changes in turnover of this amine. I believe the effects of nicotine on fetal catecholamine systems are of some behavioral importance, but I am also convinced that alterations could be found in additional transmitter systems. The catecholamine neurons may be taken as a model system.

T.A. Slotkin: As additional information I would like to remark that nicotine receptor supersensitivity does regress after birth (Slotkin et al., 1987). But I have a question as well. Is there relationship between the nicotine-induced changes in turnover of catecholamines and the effect on the prenatal testosterone level?

W. Lichtensteiger: Thank you for the information on nicotinic binding sites. However, I would like to mention that the adult condition has still not been examined.

With respect to your question there are actually two questions to be answered: (a) could damage to central catecholamine systems be responsible for the reduced testosterone level at GD 18, and (b) could interactions between steroid hormone and catecholamine systems be disturbed by the low testosterone level? At the present time, neither of the two questions can be definitely answered. We do not know what mechanism (brain, pituitary or other) causes the rise in fetal testosterone at GD 18 and whether the reduction of fetal plasma testosterone is due to a peripheral or central action of nicotine. Catecholamine fibers are present in the preoptic area at GD 16 (Lichtensteiger et al., 1982). Selective lesions of noradrenaline (NA) systems with intrafetal injections of DSP 4 (*N*-(2-chloroethyl)-*N*-ethylbromobenzylamine) (Lichtensteiger et al., 1982) so far have not provided a definite answer because testosterone levels at GD 18 were found to be affected by experimental manipulations at GD 16. A majority of catecholamine neurons are target cells for sex steroids, and some observations indicate that alpha- and beta-adrenergic mechanisms may play a role in sexual brain differentiation (see for references Lichtensteiger and Schlumpf, 1984). The postnatal sex differences in catecholamine metabolism of prenatally nicotine-exposed offspring also point to an influence of the hormonal environment. However, the underlying mechanisms remain obscure.

D.F. Swaab: In relation to the minipump data of Murrin et al. (1987), I should like to ask you how we have to choose for a neuroteratological dose in order to be clinically meaningful. Your dose was causing serum levels that were much higher than those in maternal or umbilical cord serum, and was chosen because it caused electrical changes in adulthood. On the other hand, human beings might be more sensitive than our experimental animals, as we have learned from the thalidomide tragedy (Schardein, 1985; cf. Swaab et al., Chapter 1 of this volume).

W. Lichtensteiger: I think the best information would be provided by a dose-response study. However, this is sometimes not possible in more elaborate types of analyses because of practical and legal limitations (need for restricting the number of animals). For teratological risk assessment (e.g. in drug screening), one may choose to first use a high dose which should increase the probability of developmental defects. Since we are primarily interested in a somewhat different aspect, i.e., the neurochemical background of behavioral disturbances caused by drug doses, we chose a dose within or close to the usual range. In this way, information is not only of theoretical interest, but is at the same time important in health and environmental politics. Lower doses need not necessarily produce smaller neurochemical changes; their effects could well be qualitatively different. Therefore, one should collect additional information, i.e. functional changes elicited by a given dose in a given animal. This we have tried to do when extrapolating from electrophysiological data.

I do not quite agree with your interpretation of our dose level. According to the correlative data by Murrin et al. (1987), the dose we (and others) have used should give a serum level corresponding to about 2 times the mean, or 1.5 times the upper level of adult smokers, or 4 times the cord blood levels (Luck et al., 1985). These levels lie within a realistic range. The s.c. implanted minipump released 0.25 mg/kg nicotine per h. Acute s.c. injection of 0.33 mg/kg nicotine to adult rats increased firing of substantia nigra zona compacta neurons by ca. 40% (Lichtensteiger et al., 1976). It is more difficult to account for the possibly higher sensitivity of developing systems.

References

Lichtensteiger, W., Felix, D., Lienhart, R. and Hefti, F. (1976) A quantitative correlation between single unit activity and fluorescence intensity of dopamine neurones in zona compacta of substantia nigra, as demonstrated under the influence of nicotine and physostigmine. *Brain Res.*, 117: 85-103.

Lichtensteiger, W., Schlumpf, M., Davis, M. D., Bruinink, A. and Otten, U. (1982) *Adv. in the Biosciences, Vol. 37*, M. Kohsaka et al. (Eds.), Pergamon Press, Oxford, pp. 313–325.

Lichtensteiger, W. and Schlumpf, M. (1984) Prenatal neuropharmacology: Implications for neuroendocrine development. In F. Ellendorf, P.D. Gluckman and N. Parvizi (Eds.), *Fetal Neuroendocrinology. Research in Perinatal Medicine II*, Perinatology Press, Ithaca, pp. 59–70.

Luck, W., Nau, H., Hansen, R. and Steldinger, R. (1985) Extent of nicotine and cotinine transfer to the human fetus, placenta and amniotic fluid of smoking mothers. *Dev. Pharmacol. Ther.*, 8: 384–395.

Murrin, L.C., Ferrer, J.R., Zeug, W. and Haley, N.J. (1987) Nicotine administration to rats: methodological considerations. *Life Sci.*, 40: 1699–1708.

Ribary, R. (1985) Nicotine in pregnancy: acute and persistent effects on central monoaminergic systems in rat fetus and offspring. Thesis No. 7939 Federal Institute of Technology, Zürich.

Schardein, J.L. (1985) *Chemically induced birth defects*, Marcel Dekker, New York and Basel.

Slotkin, T.A., Orband-Miller, L. and Queen, K.L. (1987) Development of [^{3}H]nicotine binding sites in brain regions of rats exposed to nicotine prenatally *via* maternal injections or infusions. *J. Pharmacol. Exp. Ther.*, 242: 232–237.

G.J. Boer, M.G.P. Feenstra, M. Mirmiran, D.F. Swaab and F. Van Haaren
Progress in Brain Research, Vol. 73
© 1988 Elsevier Science Publishers B.V. (Biomedical Division)

CHAPTER 11

Functional deprivation of noradrenaline neurotransmission: effects of clonidine on brain development

Majid Mirmiran, Matthijs G. P. Feenstra, Fred A. Dijcks*, Nico P. A. Bos and Frans Van Haaren

*Netherlands Institute for Brain Research, Meibergdreef 33, 1105 AZ Amsterdam ZO, The Netherlands, and *Department of CNS-Pharmacology, P.O. Box 20, Organon, Oss, The Netherlands*

Introduction

It has been shown that neurotransmitters have a trophic function in development and that a decrease or increase of these chemical messengers can induce disturbances in the brain (for review see Lauder, 1983; Mirmiran et al., 1985; Mirmiran, 1986b; Patel and Lewis, Chapter 25 of this volume). The goal of the present review is to provide the foundations for a working hypothesis on drug-induced functional neuroteratology. A class of centrally acting antihypertensive drugs, including clonidine, which are still being prescribed during pregnancy in humans is used as the model. Since centrally acting antihypertensives predominantly affect the noradrenaline (NA) system in the brain, the induced modifications of central NA neurotransmission will be emphasized.

Neurons show spontaneous activity that varies greatly as a function of the behavioral state of the organism. This has been demonstrated for noradrenergic neurons of the locus coeruleus (LC), serotonergic neurons of the dorsal raphe (DR), dopaminergic neurons of the substantia nigra (SN) and cholinergic neurons of the dorsolateral part of the pons and basal forebrain (Aston-Jones and Bloom, 1981a,b: Aston-Jones, 1985; Foote et al., 1983; Jacobs, 1985; Rasmussen et al.,

1986; Rasmussen and Jacobs, 1986; Sakai, 1984; also see McGinty and Drucker-Colin, 1982); the spontaneous activity of these neurons shows changes in the mean rates as well as in the patterns of discharges (e.g., phasic vs. tonic firing). NA neurons of the rat LC fire rapidly and tonically during quiet wakefulness, with bursts of firing in response to noxious or novel stimuli, slow down during quiet sleep and cease firing altogether at the transition to rapid-eye-movement (REM) sleep (Aston-Jones and Bloom, 1981a,b; Rasmussen et al., 1986). During REM sleep these neurons fire sporadically either in bursts or singly, with long and variable intervals. Such observations emphasize the existence of 'spontaneous fluctuations' in the activity of identified neurons across state and time.

A close correlation exists between single unit variations and NA metabolic changes in the LC (Hilaire et al., 1984). Using newly developed brain dialysis methods it has been shown that the basal release of NA (e.g., in cortical areas) involves depolarization and depends upon calcium availability; high-frequency medial forebrain bundle electrical stimulation increases, while interruption of impulse flow by tetrodotoxin abolishes the release of NA, similar to what is known for peripheral sympathetic neurons (L'Heureux et al., 1986). It should also be noted that the rate of the amine synthesis is dependent upon the level of LC activity. Following an action potential, the released neurotransmitter activates both pre- and post-synaptic receptors, the sensitivity of which together with the membrane potential of the neuron are key factors in the regulation of the on-going activity for a given neurotransmitter (for review see Starke, 1977; Langer, 1981; Andrade and Aghajanian, 1984a,b; Kalsner, 1985; Ennis and Aston-Jones, 1986; Simson and Weiss, 1987).

The sensitivity of neurotransmitter signal transduction has been shown to depend upon receptor density, which in turn may increase or decrease homeostatically in response to the available neurotransmitter (for review see Schwartz et al., 1978; Reisine, 1981; Sulser, 1984; Molinoff, 1984; Neve and Molinoff, 1986). It has been shown, in both developing and adult rats, that depletion of forebrain NA with 6-hydroxydopamine (6-OHDA) produces a compensatory increase in the number of postsynaptic beta-adrenergic receptors (e.g., Sporn et al., 1976; U'Prichard et al., 1980). Reserpine, an antihypertensive drug, depletes monoamines in the brain and also induces an NA-receptor supersensitivity (Baudry et al., 1976). On the other hand, chronic treatment with antidepressant agents which block the *reuptake* of monoamines leads to a decrease in the number of beta-receptors in adult (Banerjee et al., 1977; Vetulani and Sulser, 1975) as well as in developing rats (Del Rio et al., Chapter 12 of this volume). In addition, it was recently shown that chronic beta-receptor activation in the brain by isoprenaline also causes a reduction in the receptor density (Ordway et al., 1987).

Hypothesis

Neuronal spontaneous activity varies across time in a (behavioral) state-dependent manner, and so does the mean membrane potential and the amount of released neurotransmitter. If the level of neurotransmitter at the synaptic cleft is continuously high or low, so that fluctuations in membrane potential are largely eliminated, the overall receptor sensitivity will depart from its previous setting. In other words, a transmitter system would lose its capacity to maintain a steady-state level in the absence of the frequent variations in bioelectric activity.

State-dependent changes in neuronal activity have been demonstrated in monoaminergic neurons in developing rats and cats (e.g., Adrien and Lanfumay, 1984, 1986). However, since the set point (upon which the homeostatic response of a given neurotransmitter operates) is not yet fully established in the immature brain, interference with spontaneous variations in neurotransmitter release patterns would shift the homeostatic set-point for receptor sensitivity. More importantly, although effects of such functional disturbances on adults are generally transient in nature, changes induced during a critical period of development would be permanent.

Developmental observations on the noradrenaline system

The monoamines, NA, dopamine (DA) and serotonin (5-hydroxytryptamine; 5-HT), are among the first neurotransmitters present at early stages of brain development (Olson and Seiger, 1972; Seiger and Olson, 1973; Lauder and Bloom, 1974). The brain of a newborn rat is very immature, comparable to a 7-month-old human fetal brain (Dobbing and Sands, 1973, 1979). In the rat (the gestational period of which is about 21 days), NA neurons of the LC are born on days 10–13, while DA neurons of SN appear on days 11–15 of gestation. LC neuronal projections reach forebrain structures around days 15–16 of gestation in the rat (Schlumpf et al., 1980), whereas the time of appearance of monoamines in the human CNS is between 3 and 4 months in utero (Nobin and Björklund, 1973; Masudi and Gilmore, 1983).

High-affinity NA uptake first appears on day 18 of gestation in the rat (Coyle and Axelrod, 1971). NA fibers of newborn rats readily take up the neurotoxin 6-OHDA, resulting in a near-total destruction of NA axon terminals (e.g. Sachs and Jonsson, 1975; Brenner et al., 1987; Kostrzewa et al., Chapter 26 of this volume). Beta-adrenergic binding sites in fetal rat brain were first detectable on day 15 of gestation, and showed dissociation constants (K_d) values similar to those of adult rats by day 19 (Bruinink and Lichtensteiger, 1984). This finding suggests the possibility of β-receptor blockade in the fetal brain after use of antihypertensives such as propranolol. Alpha-receptor binding sites were detectable one day after birth in the rat brain (Morris et al., 1980). Nomura et al. (1984) have demonstrated that, although the number of clonidine (α_2-agonist) binding sites in the cerebral cortex at postnatal day 7 was still far below the adult level, the K_d values for the high- and low-affinity clonidine binding sites did not differ significantly from the adult values.

An interesting finding by Harden et al. (1977) was the differential development in the rat postsynaptic monoamine receptor responses in comparison with the presynaptic projections and the amine content of the cerebral cortex. The β-receptor-stimulated cyclic AMP accumulation in the cerebral cortex develops rapidly in early postnatal life, and reaches adult levels between day 7 and day 14. Cortical NA content develops more gradually, only reaching adult values at two months of age. It was concluded that cortical β-NA-receptor development is not closely correlated with the time-course of development either for NA content or for enzymes involved in NA synthesis (Coyle, 1974; Agrawal et al., 1966). Moreover, observations on the development of α_1- and α_2-NA-receptors failed to show any correlation between the increase in NA content and the increase in receptor binding, the latter being much more rapid (Morris et al., 1980). Receptor subtypes appear to develop independently even within a given brain area; for β_1- and β_2-NA-receptors different developmental patterns have been reported for both cerebral cortex and cerebellum (Minneman et al., 1979; Pittman et al., 1980).

The above-mentioned studies do not, generally speaking, provide any information about the functional state of neurons and receptors. It is important to know the extent to which NA is capable of being released, and how the development of this ability is related to the functional maturity of the receptors. Potassium-induced membrane depolarization is reported to cause a calcium-dependent release of cortical NA from day 18 of gestation (Nomura et al., 1982). The potassium-evoked NA release from brain slices of 2–3-day-old rats is equivalent to that in slices from adult animals (Nomura ct al., 1979), a finding which is corroborated by the fact that the concentration of the NA metabolite MHPG (3-methoxy-4-hydroxyphenylethylene glycol) does not significantly change after birth (Ribary et al., 1986).

Many electrophysiological, biochemical and behavioural studies have demonstrated the responsiveness of developing brain monoamines to pharmacological challenges. Drugs such as imipramine, which are able to inhibit NA uptake, have been shown to be already active in newborn rats (Nomura et al., 1978). Reserpine, which releases the amines from nerve terminal storage vesicles, is also able to do so in fetal brains (Tennyson et al., 1983; see also Patel and Lewis, Chapter 25 of this volume). Clonidine caused a 50% reduction in potassium-induced cortical NA release on days 7 and 70, but not on day 1, of postnatal life in the rat (Nomura et al., 1982). These workers concluded that presynaptic α_2-receptors which regulate NA release seem to become sensitive to α_2-agonists (such as clonidine) to reach functional maturity between postnatal days 1 and 7 in the rat cerebral cortex. Recently, the postnatal development of α-receptor-mediated auto-inhibition of rat LC neurons was demonstrated electrophysiologically to be established by postnatal day 9 (Kimura and Nakamura, 1987). Biochemical studies have demonstrated NA depletion in various brain regions by NA synthesis inhibition as early as day 4 postnatally (Kellogg and Lundborg, 1973) as well as the inhibition of such depletion by clonidine pretreatment (Kellogg and Wennerström, 1974), thus suggesting that the NA neurons are fully functional by that time. However, the behavioural outcome of clonidine treatment changes from hyperactivity on days 1–7 to hypoactivity on day 20 (Nomura, 1980) suggesting a further maturation of the neuronal networks in which NA participates. In summary, it can be concluded that not only is NA available in a functionally releasable pool at the nerve terminals of central noradrenergic neurons in the newborn rat but also it acts as a true adult neurotransmitter.

Although information about the functional reactivity of monoaminergic systems in the human brain to drugs such as antihypertensives is lacking, it seems likely that the effects found in rats during the 2nd and 3rd weeks of postnatal life will appear during the 2nd half of gestation in human fetal brain.

Behavioral states in development and the relationship with noradrenaline

As indicated above, the activity of LC neurons shows dramatic changes across different behavioral states. Local application of clonidine in the vicinity of LC neurons of adult rats drastically reduces REM and deep quiet sleep as well as causing a decreased frequency of spontaneous discharges in LC neurons (Abercrombie and Jacobs, 1987; De Sarro et al., 1987; Leppavuori and Putkonen, 1980). These effects are mediated by α_2-NA-receptors, which apparently are located on the NA cell bodies and mediate an inhibitory feedback response on NA release (Aghajanian and Van der Maelen, 1982). Clonidine also inhibits the evoked responses of pontine neurons to noxious stimuli; this effect is also α_2-mediated (O'Neill and Haigler, 1985; see also Simson and Weiss, 1987). Using in vivo voltammetry techniques in the rat LC, it was shown that clonidine reduces both the baseline and the stress-induced increase in catecholamine metabolic activity, in a dose-dependent manner, to less than 75% of control values (Quintin et al., 1986). NA release in the cerebral cortex measured by in vivo transcortical dialysis has demonstrated that clonidine does indeed reduce NA release in target brain areas (L'Heureux et al., 1986). Clonidine thus appears to induce a state of functional denervation of NA in target areas of the brain. These effects of clonidine, along with its action on behavioral states and on the associated characteristic pattern of spontaneous activity of central NA neurons, make this compound suitable for testing the hypothesis (see above) that changes of neurotransmitter activity have considerable developmental state-dependent significance.

Behavioral states become clearly differentiated in development during the second week of postnatal life in the rat (Jouvet-Monnier et al., 1969; Gramsbergen et al., 1970; Mirmiran and Corner, 1982). Although the exact time of differentiation of behavioral states in humans is still uncertain, it is generally accepted that the three major behavioral states, i.e. wakefulness, quiet and REM sleep, are distinguishable by 32–36 weeks in the human fetus (Dreyfus-Brisac, 1979; Nijhuis et al., 1982; Curzi-Dascalova et al., 1988). Moreover, the state dependency of monoaminergic neuronal activity in immature rats and cats has been shown to become fully established during the second postnatal week (e.g., Adrien and Lanfumay, 1984, 1986).

Chronic treatment with clonidine during the second and third weeks of life in rats is able to influence the behavioral states in the same fashion as in adults (Mirmiran et al., 1983a). Similar results were obtained with another antihypertensive drug, α-methyl-dopa, both in developing rats and in kittens (Saucier and Astic, 1973; Juvancz and Nowaczyk, 1975; Mirmiran et al., 1985). Simultaneous recordings of spontaneous activity from LC or other NA-containing neurons together with dialysis of the amount of neurotransmitter release (see above) are not yet feasible in very small animals. However, given (i) the similarity in developing and adult animals of clonidine effects on NA release in vitro and on behavioral states in vivo (Nomura et al., 1982; Mirmiran et al., 1983a), (ii) the early appearance of α_2-mediated auto-inhibition of LC neurons (Kimura and Nakamura, 1987), and (iii) the dramatic reduction of NA release found in the adult brain following clonidine administration (Quintin et al., 1986; L'Heureux et al., 1986), we must expect to find state-dependent abnormalities of NA input to forebrain target areas as a result of clonidine therapy in early life.

Neurochemical teratogenicity of clonidine

Studies on the role of neurotransmitters in general, and NA in particular, have often used surgical or chemical lesions (see e.g. Jonsson, 1980; Kostrzewa, Chapter 26 of this volume). A major drawback in interpreting the effect of NA lesions on brain development in adulthood is the fact that experimental animals still bear the lesion at the time of testing. It is thus difficult to causally relate the observed sequelae to the lack of central NA activity specifically during development. However, in the case of *functional* deprivation, induced by drugs such as clonidine, the acute effects of the treatment are terminated upon withdrawal of the drug, so that lasting developmental consequences can be examined. Since centrally acting antihypertensive drugs are also used during gestation in humans, the long-term consequences of these drugs also become interesting from a clinical perspective.

In a series of experiments (see below) male rat pups were injected subcutaneously with two daily doses of 100 $\mu g/kg$ of clonidine from postnatal day 8 to 21. This dose was chosen on the basis of the amount required to obtain physiological effects on behavior and blood pressure in rats equivalent to those found in humans (at much lower dosages: e.g., Autret, 1977; for a general discussion of interspecies differences in drug pharmacokinetics, see Boxenbum and Ronfeld, 1983). The period of 8–21 days after birth was selected on the basis of the above-mentioned developmental studies which document the time of appearance of functional activity in central NA

systems, and the period in which rapid brain growth is taking place in rats.

Biochemical measures

Measurements of the NA content of the brainstem (the area containing the NA cell bodies) and the cerebral cortex (one of the major projecting areas) of adult rats which have been treated neonatally with clonidine and saline, respectively, showed no significant differences (Mirmiran et al., 1983a), nor did measurements of DA or of adrenaline (unpublished results). In a second series of experiments, the turnover of NA and DA was estimated (on the basis of the amount of catecholamine depletion following inhibition of its synthesis by α-methyl-p-tyrosine) 10 days after termination of the treatment. The results suggested a decrease in NA but not DA turnover in the amygdala and hypothalamus, while neither of these amines showed any alterations in the cerebral cortex (Mirmiran et al., 1985). These results have been corroborated by an anatomically more detailed study (Feenstra et al., in preparation): NA depletion was retarded not only in the hypothalamus and amygdala but also in the brainstem and limbic basal forebrain (Table 1); no changes were observed in two neocortical areas or in the cerebellum, while in the hippocampus NA depletion was accelerated. An interesting finding was that the levels of free MHPG – another putative indication of NA turnover – were elevated in several brain regions, suggesting an increase in NA turnover. Further experiments are being carried out in order to reconcile these, in some respects apparently contradictory, results. In relation to the above-reviewed data on the functional maturation of central NA systems, it was found that after the last clonidine injection (i.e. on day 21 postnatally) free MHPG concentrations were indeed decreased in all brain regions, again suggesting a clonidine-induced decrease in NA neuronal activity during development.

TABLE 1

Relative depletion of noradrenaline following α-methyl-p-tyrosine in adult rats that have been exposed to clonidine treatment neonatally

	CXf	CXo	CB	Hpp	AM	LI	Hyp	BS
Control	59 ± 2	52 ± 3	53 ± 3	60 ± 2	58 ± 2	59 ± 4	56 ± 5	57 ± 2
Clonidine	58 ± 2	54 ± 3	49 ± 3	53 ± 3	65 ± 3	$73 \pm 5^*$	66 ± 6	$67 \pm 3^*$

Given are NA contents expressed as percentage ($\pm$ SEM; n = 6–8) of controls, measured in 3-month-old male rats 2 h after i.p. injection of 250 mg/kg α-methyl-p-tyrosine methylester HCl (αMPT). Two-way ANOVA testing showed significant interaction of clonidine and αMPT in the brainstem and in the limbic basal forebrain (asterisk). Abbreviations: AM, amygdala; BS, brainstem; CB, cerebellum; CXf, frontal cortex; CXo, occipital cortex; Hpp, hippocampus; Hyp, hypothalamus; LI, limbic basal forebrain. From Feenstra, Van Galen and Boer, unpublished results.

Micro-iontophoretic studies

There are several ways in which one can test the sensitivity of NA receptors, one of these being to measure the electrophysiological response at the cellular level of the micro-iontophoretically applied neurotransmitter. Adult rats neonatally injected with saline or clonidine were studied under intravenous urethane anesthesia. Neurons from different layers of the occipital cortex were recorded, using a single glass micropipette with a tip diameter of 0.5 μm. A 7-barrelled micropipette with a total average tip diameter of 12 μm was glued to the recording electrode, and used to eject different neurotransmitters via a 5-channel micro-iontophoresis unit. A data-processor and a micro-computer were used for acquisition and analysis of the data. Each neurotransmitter ejection at a fixed current level was cycled 3–5 times and the averaged response to the last three cycles was used for later analysis. The mean ejection time required to reach the half-maximal response (T_{50}) was used for making statistical comparisons between the two groups.

Our initial studies have shown variable responses to NA, although a clear-cut excitatory response to glutamate was observed in almost all of the neurons studied. It was decided, therefore, to test the effect of glutamate under baseline conditions as well as following constant application of NA (Figs. 1 and 2).

A type of effect, often seen as a result of NA application, was a reduction in responsiveness to glutamate administration (Fig. 1). This effect includes a reduced maximum firing rate as well as an increased latency in attaining that level, thus resulting in higher T_{50} values (Figs. 1 and 2). The magnitude of the reduction in glutamate response caused by NA was variable from one neuron to the next, the increase in T_{50} values varying from approx. 5% to more than 400%. In some neurons a decrease in background activity, with no enhancement of the response to glutamate, i.e., an increased 'signal-to-noise ratio', was also observed (Fig. 3). T_{50} values for glutamate response in control and experimental rats are presented in Table 2. These results indicate a non-significant 20% increase in NA response as a result of the early clonidine treatment. More experiments such as micro-iontophoretic studies in other brain regions are required before the conclusion that functional deprivation of NA neurotransmission during ontogeny has no significant effect on NA receptors can be accepted, especially for those brain regions where, in contrast to the cerebral cortex, biochemical changes have been found (see above).

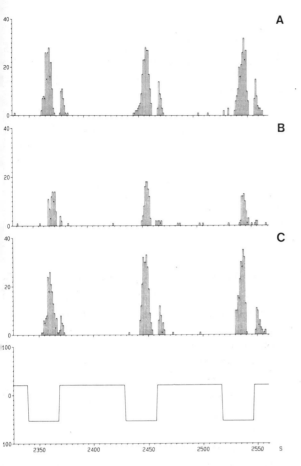

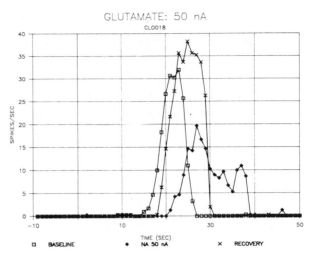

Fig. 2 Averaged response to glutamate (Glu) shift by nor-adrenaline (NA) and recovery to base-line value in a neuron extracellularly recorded at $610\,\mu m$ depth of the occipital cortex. Each response is an average of three cycles of either baseline ($\square$), NA ($\blacklozenge$) or recovery measurements ($\times$). The times taken to reach 50% of maximum response (i.e. T_{50}) derived from the averaged figures such as this were used for the final analysis presented in Table 2. In this neuron the latency of response to Glu is increased 10 s upon NA application. Other information is as in Fig. 1.

Fig. 1 Effect of noradrenaline (NA) on glutamate (Glu)-induced cortical neuronal activation. This neuron is recorded at $480\,\mu m$ occipital cortical depth in the rat. (A) baseline response to Glu pulses (50 nA; 0.25 M; pH 8), (B) response to Glu pulses under concomitant continuous NA application (50 nA; 25 mM; pH 4), (C) recovery to baseline values upon termination of NA application. Note depression of maximum firing rate as well as the longer latency of response to Glu in B. Ordinate, spike rate per second; abscissa, time in seconds. Bottom trace shows on the ordinate pulses of micro-iontophoretically applied Glu (in nA), ejected at 1-min intervals.

Clinical significance of experimental studies with antihypertensives

Potential neuroteratological hazards of antihypertensive therapy were first reported by Moar et al. (1978), who observed a smaller head circum-ference in children born to hypertensive mothers treated with α-methyl-dopa in comparison with non-treated hypertensive controls. The effect was found only in those children who had been exposed since mid-gestation, but no relationship to either the dose or the duration of α-methyl-dopa treatment could be established. Follow-up studies of these children at the age of 4 years showed a persistent smaller head circumference and a slight developmental delay in visual-motor performances (Ounsted et al., 1980).

Huisjes et al. (1986) compared children (with a mean age of 6.3 years) of hypertensive mothers treated with clonidine with children born to hypertensive mothers treated with diuretics and/or bed-resting. They did not find any differences in head circumference, neurological examinations, school performance, or in a number of behavioral characteristics except for a marginal hyperactivity and a higher incidence of sleep disturbances in the

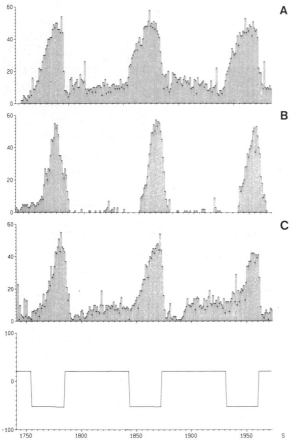

A

B

C

TABLE 2

T_{50} values of cortical neuron responses to micro-iontophoretically applied glutamate and relative T_{50} values for NA in adult rats neonatally treated with saline (10 rats) or clonidine (10 rats)

	T_{50} (Glu)	Relative T_{50} (NA)[a]
Saline	20 ± 1 (28)	0.88 ± 0.34 (16)
Clonidine	23 ± 2 (40)	1.07 ± 0.37 (17)

Data are means $\pm$ SEM (number of recorded neurons).
[a] Relative T_{50} (NA) = (T_{50} (Glu + NA) − T_{50} (Glu))/T_{50} (Glu).

Fig. 3 An example of increased 'signal-to-noise ratio' following noradrenalin (NA) application in cerebral cortical cells of rat. Peri-stimulus time histogram of the response to Glu of this neuron (recorded at 873 μm depth) is shown under baseline conditions (A), under constant NA application (B) and upon recovery (C). Note depression of background activity by NA resulting in an enhanced signal-to-noise ratio. Ordinate, spike rate per second; abscissa time in seconds. Bottom trace shows Glu pulses. Other information is as in Fig. 1.

treatment group. A single case report in Japan also showed sleep disturbances in a boy born to a hypertensive mother treated with α-methyl-dopa during gestation (Shimohira et al., 1986).

Our own studies with clonidine in male rats revealed hyperactivity and hyperanxiety in an open-field test, reduced attentional span in a Y-maze, reduced sexual performance, as well as sleep disturbances (Mirmiran et al., 1983a, 1985).

Comparable results were obtained with the antidepressant drug clomipramine, which also acts on monoaminergic systems (Mirmiran et al., 1981). However, as far as the learning ability of *animals* is concerned, our recent studies with α-methyl-dopa indicate that treating newborn rats during the first and second weeks of life with 300 mg/kg α-methyl-dopa (a dose well below the level required for total suppression of REM sleep) does not affect the adult rats' performances in either a Hebb-Williams or an 8-arm radial maze.

Another important characteristic of the developing brain is its 'plasticity', i.e., ability to undergo lasting changes as a function of environmental manipulations. It is well established that depriving the visual cortex of input from one eye leads to reorganization of cortical neurons in such a way that they respond preferentially to the non-deprived eye, together with a large deficit in binocular vision (Hubel and Wiesel, 1970). There exists a critical period in development in which such plasticity can occur. Recent studies in developing kittens have shown that chronic application of clonidine during this critical period blocks vision-induced abnormalities of the occipital cortex (Nelson et al., 1985). On the other hand, it is known that increasing environmental complexity during development by daily maze-training, or by exposure to an 'enriched environment', results in an increased number of synapses and an increased cortical thickness above the control level (Rosenzweig and Bennett, 1978). We were able to show that chronic clonidine application during early postnatal development in the rat reduces the ability of the cerebral cortex to respond to the 'beneficial' influences of enriched environmental rearing (Mirmiran and Uylings, 1983; Mirmiran et al., 1983b). If these results are generalizable in humans, we can expect that children born to hypertensive mothers (treated with clonidine and, probably, with other antihypertensives as well) will show changed responses to novel situations.

Although it is surely premature to draw any unequivocal conclusions from the available animal and human studies, the fact that hyperactivity and sleep disturbances have been found in both rat and man as a result of clonidine treatment in early life arouses strong suspicion that exposure of pregnant women to antihypertensives can induce subtle, but nevertheless partially disabling, physiological changes in their offspring.

Concluding remarks

A hypothesis was put forward in this review which proposes that behavioral state-dependent changes in monoaminergic neuronal firing levels and patterns play a key role during early ontogeny in regulating neuron membrane potential, neurotransmitter release and neurotransmitter receptor sensitivity patterns in adulthood. Clonidine, a centrally acting antihypertensive drug which reduces both NA neuronal activity and NA release, was used in order to test the biochemical and physiological sequelae of chronic functional deprivation of NA activity during postnatal development in the rat. An indication for reduced adult NA turnover following neonatal clonidine treatment was found. Furthermore, behavioral changes such as sleep disturbances are found in both rat and man as a result of early clonidine or α-methyl-dopa therapy. Such results suggest a functional 'teratogenic' potential for these and related compounds. Further studies are of course

required before one can make a firm statement about the biological consequences of blunting the state-dependent activities of brain NA neurons in early life (see also Brenner and Mirmiran, 1988).

An important consideration for future research is the use of spontaneously hypertensive rats as an improved animal 'model system' for investigating the hazards of antihypertensive use in human (Trippodo and Frohlick, 1981). A possible involvement of LC in the pathogenesis of hypertension is suggested by findings in which it was shown that both the spontaneous activity of LC neurons and their response to micro-iontophoretic application of epinephrine are reduced in hypertensive as compared with normotensive rats (Olpe et al., 1985; Berecek et al., 1987). Upon clonidine administration, spontaneously hypertensive rats show a much higher increase in growth hormone (GH) release than controls (Eriksson et al., 1986). An increase in the number of α_2-adrenoreceptors (up-regulation) in the hypothalamus of hypertensive rats has been suggested to be induced by NA dysfunction during development (Wijnen et al., 1980).

Furthermore, circadian variations in monoaminergic content in both LC and DR in normal rats have been demonstrated (Agren et al., 1986), and micro-iontophoretic responses to both 5-HT and NA are reported to show clear day–night changes (Brunel and de Montigny, 1987). In view of these facts, and since the differences between NA activity in the brains of hypertensive and normotensive rats have been found to be maximal at the end of the dark period (Wirz-Justice et al., 1983), circadian variations in these variables must be taken into consideration in future studies. It is worth mentioning in this regard that clonidine reduces the amplitude of circadian body temperature changes in adult rats (Lewis et al., 1986). In our own studies, rats were injected subcutaneously 2 or 3 times daily with clonidine, a treatment which induces high plasma peaks with long intervals of low drug levels. A more efficient treatment, and one which may be more comparable to the human clinical situation, would be continuous drug delivery (Conway and Jarrott, 1982; Lewis et al., 1986; Atkinson et al., 1986).

Although it is always difficult to extrapolate from animal studies to man (see Huisjes, Chapter 4 of this volume), it is important to point out the possible electrophysiological and biochemical mechanisms underlying the functional teratogenicity of antihypertensives (as well as other psychoactive drugs: see Swaab and Mirmiran, 1984; Mirmiran et al., 1985; Mirmiran and Swaab, 1987; Swaab et al., Chapter 1 of this volume). Clonidine-like antihypertensive drugs, in addition to their effects on monoaminergic systems, produce suppression of REM sleep and abnormalities in sleep-wake cycle (reviewed in Mirmiran, 1986a; Mirmiran and Swaab, 1987). It is not yet clear whether this also applies to fetal behavioral states in man. Monitoring fetal behavior in pregnant women, using the now routinely available ultrasound techniques, will be of great value in the assessment of drug effects on the fetus. This could even be used as a safety measure for monitoring the possible teratogenicity of such drugs since, from the reviewed animal studies, it is clear that doses well below the level required for substantial suppression of REM sleep will not be strongly teratogenic. Furthermore, receptor studies in humans (using placental tissues) might give additional insight into the possible functional teratogenicity of antihypertensive drugs in man (Perry et al., Chapter 13 of this volume). In conclusion, given the putative subtle abnormalities induced by antihypertensive drugs in the unborn child, these sequelae will need to be weighed against the effects of hypertension per se when discussing the medical treatment of hypertensive pregnant mothers.

Acknowledgements

The authors wish to thank Drs. G.J. Boer and M.A. Corner for their help in revising this manuscript.

References

Abercrombie, E.D. and Jacobs, B.L. (1987) Microinjected clonidine inhibits noradrenergic neurons of the locus coeruleus in freely moving cats. Neurosci. Lett., 76: 203–208.

Adrien, J. and Lanfumey, L. (1984) Neuronal activity of the developing raphe dorsalis: its relation with the states of vigilance. In A. Borbely and J.L. Valatx (Eds.), Sleep-Mechanisms, Experimental Brain Research Supplementary, Vol. 8, Springer Verlag, Berlin, pp. 67–78.

Adrien, J. and Lanfumey, L. (1986) Ontogenesis of unit activity in the raphe dorsalis of the behaving kitten: its relationship with the states of vigilance. Brain Res., 366: 10–21.

Aghajanian, G.K. and Van der Maelen, C.P. (1982) Alpha-2-adrenoreceptor-mediated hyperpolarization of locus coeruleus neurons: intracellular studies in vivo. Science, 215: 1394–1396.

Agrawal, H.C., Glisson, S.N. and Himwich, W.A. (1966) Changes in monoamines of rat brain during postnatal ontogeny. Biochim. Biophys. Acta, 130: 511–513.

Agren, H., Koulu, M., Saavedra, J.M., Potter, W.Z. and Linnoila, M. (1986) Circadian covariation of norepinephrine and serotonin in locus coeruleus and dorsal raphe nucleus in the rat. Brain Res., 397: 353–358.

Andrade, R. and Aghajanian, G.K. (1984a) Intrinsic regulation of locus coeruleus neurons: electrophysiological evidence indicating a predominant role for autoinhibition. Brain Res., 310: 401–406.

Andrade, R. and Aghajanian, G.K. (1984b) Locus coeruleus activity in vitro: intrinsic regulation by a calcium-dependent potassium conductance but not alpha-2 adrenoreceptors. J. Neurosci., 4: 161–170.

Aston-Jones, G. and Bloom, F.E. (1981a) Activity of norepinephrine-containing locus coeruleus neurons in behaving rats anticipates fluctuations in the sleep-wake cycle. J. Neurosci., 1: 876–886.

Aston-Jones, G. and Bloom, F.E. (1981b) Norepinephrine-containing locus coeruleus neurons in behaving rats exhibit pronounced responses to non-noxious environmental stimuli. J. Neurosci., 1: 887–900.

Aston-Jones (1985) Behavioral functions of locus coeruleus derived from cellular attributes. Physiol. Psychol., 13: 118–126.

Atkinson, J., Lambas-Senas, L., Parker, M., Boillat, N., Luthi, P., Sonnay, M., Seccia, M. and Renaud, B. (1986) Chronic clonidine treatment and its withdrawal: effects on blood pressure and catecholamine synthesizing enzymes in brain-stem nuclei. Eur. J. Pharmacol., 121: 97–106.

Autret, A. (1977) Effects of clonidine on sleep pattern in man. Eur. J. Clin. Pharmacol., 12: 319–322.

Banerjee, S.P., Kung, L.S., Riggi, S.J. and Chanda, S.K.

(1977) Development of beta-adrenergic receptor sub-sensitivity by antidepressants. *Nature*, 268: 455–456.

Baudry, M., Martres, M. P. and Schwartz, J. C. (1976) Modulation in the sensitivity of noradrenergic receptors in the CNS studied by the responsiveness of the cyclic AMP system. *Brain Res.*, 116: 111–124.

Berecek, K. H., Olpe, H. R., Mah, S. C. and Hofbauer, K. G. (1987) Alterations in responsiveness of noradrenergic neurons of the locus coeruleus in deoxycorticosterone acetate (DOCA)-salt hypertensive rats. *Brain Res.*, 401: 303–311.

Boxenbum, H. and Ronfeld, R. (1983) Interspecies pharmacokinetic scaling and the Dedrick plots. *Am. J. Physiol.*, 245: R768–R775.

Brenner, E. and Mirmiran, M. (1988) Functions of the noradrenergic innervation of the rat brain: coping with the unexpected. *Brain Dysfunction*, 1: in press.

Brenner, E., Mirmiran, M., Van Haaren, F., Theunisse, B. E., Feenstra, M. G. P., Lamur, A. A. and Van Eden, C. G. (1987) Central noradrenaline depletion during development and its effect on behaviour. *Physiol. Behav.*, 41: 163–170.

Bruinink, A. and Lichtensteiger, W. (1984) Beta-adrenergic binding sites in fetal rat brain. *J. Neurochem.*, 43: 578–581.

Brunel, S. and de Montigny, C. (1987) Diurnal rhythms in the responsiveness of hippocampal pyramidal neurons to serotonin, norepinephrine, GABA and acetylcholine. *Brain Res. Bull.*, 18: 205–212.

Conway, E. L. and Jarrott, B. (1982) Effects of clonidine infusion and withdrawal on blood pressure and behaviour in the rat. A preliminary study. *Clin. Exp. Hyper. Theory Practice*, 8: 1323–1334.

Coyle, J. T. (1974) Development of the central catecholaminergic neurons. In F. O. Schmitt and F. G. Worden (Eds.), *Neurosciences, Third Study Program*, MIT Press, MA, pp. 877–884.

Coyle, J. T. and Axelrod, J. (1971) Development of the uptake and storage of L-[^{3}H]norepinephrine in the rat brain. *J. Neurochem.*, 18: 2061–2075.

Curzi-Dascalova, L., Peirano, P. and More-Kahn, F. (1988) Development of sleep states in normal premature and full-term newborns. *Dev. Psychobiol.*, in press.

De Sarro, G. B., Ascioti, C., Froio, F., Libri, V. and Nistico, G. (1987) Evidence that locus coeruleus is the site where clonidine and drugs acting at alpha-1- and alpha-2-adrenoreceptors affect sleep and arousal mechanisms. *Br. J. Pharmacol.*, 90: 675–685.

Dobbing, J. and Sands, J. (1973) Quantitative growth and development of human brain. *Arch. Dis. Child.*, 48: 757–767.

Dobbing, J. and Sands, J. (1979) Comparative aspects of the brain growth spurt. *Early Human Dev.*, 3: 79–83.

Dreyfus-Brisac, C. (1979) Ontogenesis of brain electrical activity and sleep organization in neonates and infants. In F. Falkner and Tanner, J. M. (Eds.), *Human Growth,*

Neurobiology and Nutrition, Vol. 3, Plenum Press, New York, pp. 157–182.

Ennis, M. and Aston-Jones, G. (1986) Evidence for self- and neighbour-mediated postactivation inhibition of locus coeruleus neurons. *Brain Res.*, 374: 299–305.

Eriksson, E., Dellborg, M., Soderpalm, B., Carlsson, M. and Nilsson, C. (1986) Growth hormone responses to clonidine and GRF in spontaneously hypertensive rats: neuroendocrine evidence for an enhanced responsiveness of brain alpha-2-adrenoreceptors in genetical hypertension. *Life Sci.*, 39: 2103–2109.

Foote, S. L., Bloom, F. E. and Aston-Jones, G. (1983) The nucleus Locus Coeruleus: new evidence of anatomical and physiological specificity. *Physiol. Rev.*, 63: 844–914.

Gramsbergen, A., Schwartze, P. and Prechtl, H. F. R. (1970) The postnatal development of behavioral states in the rat. *Dev. Psychobiol.*, 3: 267–280.

Harden, T. K., Wolfe, B. B., Sporn, J. R., Perkins, J. P. and Molinoff, P. B. (1977) Ontogeny of beta-adrenergic receptors in rat cerebral cortex. *Brain Res.*, 125: 99–108.

Hilaire, G., Quintin, L. and Pujol, J. F. (1984) Metabolic activity closely parallels electrical activity in the rat locus coeruleus. *Soc. Neurosci. Abstr.*, 10: 679.

Hubel, D. H. and Weisel, T. N. (1970) The period of susceptibility to the physiological effects of unilateral eye closure in kittens. *J. Physiol.*, 206: 419–436.

Huisjes, H. J., Hadders-Algra, M. and Touwen, C. B. L. (1986) Is clonidine a behavioral teratogen in human? *Early Human Dev.*, 3: 79–83.

Jacobs, B. L. (1985) Overview of the activity of brain monoaminergic neurons across the sleep-wake cycle. In A. Wauquier, J. M. Gaillard, J. M. Monti and M. Radulovaki (Eds.), *Sleep: Neurotransmitters and Neuromodulators*, Raven Press, New York, pp. 1–14.

Jonsson, G. (1980) Chemical neurotoxins as denervation tools in neurobiology. *Annu. Rev. Neurosci.*, 3: 169–187.

Jouvet-Monnier, D., Astic, L., Lacote, D. (1969) Ontogenesis of the states of sleep in rat, cat and guinea pig during the first postnatal month. *Dev. Psychobiol.*, 2: 216–239.

Juvancz, P. and Nowaczyk, T. (1975) Effects of early postnatal alpha methyldopa treatment on behavior in the rat. *Psychopharmacology*, 42: 95–97.

Kalsner, S. (1985) Is there feedback regulation of neurotransmitter release by autoreceptors? *Biochem. Pharmacol.*, 34: 4085–4097.

Kellogg, C. and Lundborg, P. (1973) Inhibition of catecholamine synthesis during ontogenetic development. *Brain Res.*, 61: 321–329.

Kellogg, C. and Wennerström, G. (1974) An ontogenetic study on the effect of catecholamine receptor-stimulating agents on the turnover of noradrenaline and dopamine in the brain. *Brain Res.*, 79: 451–464.

Kimura, F. and Nakamura, S. (1987) Postnatal development of alpha-adrenoreceptor-mediated autoinhibition in the locus coeruleus. *Dev. Brain Res.*, 35: 21–26.

170

Langer, S.Z. (1981) Presynaptic regulation of the release of catecholamines. *Pharmacol. Rev.*, 32: 337–362.

Lauder, J.M. (1983) Hormonal and humoral influences on brain development. *Psychoneuroendocrinology*, 8: 121–155.

Lauder, J.M. and Bloom, F.E. (1974) Ontogeny of mono-amine neurons in the locus coeruleus, raphe nuclei and substantia nigra of the rat. *J. Comp. Neurol.*, 155: 469–481.

Leppavuori, A. and Putkonen, P.T.S. (1980) Alpha-adreno-ceptive influences on the control of the sleep-wake cycle in the cat. *Brain Res.*, 193: 95–115.

Lewis, S.J., Maccarrone, C. and Jarrott, B. (1986) Modifi-cation of the circadian body temperature rhythm of the spontaneously hypertensive rat during and following ces-sation of continuous clonidine infusion. *Brain Res.*, 385: 383–388.

L'Heureux, R.L., Dennis, T., Curet, O. and Scatton, B. (1986) Measurement of endogenous noradrenaline release in the rat cerebral cortex in vivo by transcortical dialysis: effects of drugs affecting noradrenaline transmission. *J. Neuro-chem.*, 46: 1794–1801.

Masudi, N.A. and Gilmore, D.P. (1983) Biogenic amine levels in the mid-term human fetus. *Dev. Brain Res.*, 7: 9–12.

McGinty, D.J. and Drucker-Colin, R.R. (1982) Sleep mecha-nisms: biology and control of REM-sleep. *Int. Rev. Neurobiol.*, 23: 391–436.

Minneman, K.P., Dibner, M.D., Wolfe, B.B. and Molinoff, P.B. (1979) Beta-1- and beta-2-adrenergic receptors in rat cerebral cortex are independently regulated. *Science*, 204: 866–868.

Mirmiran, M. (1986a) The importance of fetal/neonatal REM sleep. *Eur. J. Obstet. Gynecol. Reprod. Biol.*, 21: 283–291.

Mirmiran, M. (1986b) The role of the central monoaminergic system and rapid eye movement sleep in development. *Brain Dev.*, 8: 382–389.

Mirmiran, M. and Corner, M.A. (1982) Neuronal discharge patterns in the occipital cortex of developing rats during active and quiet sleep. *Dev. Brain Res.*, 3: 37–42.

Mirmiran, M. and Uylings, H.B.M. (1983) The environ-mental enrichment effect upon cortical growth is neu-tralized by concomitant pharmacological suppression of active sleep in female rats. *Brain Res.*, 261: 331–334.

Mirmiran, M. and Swaab, D.F. (1987) Influence of drugs on brain neurotransmitters and behavioral states during development. *Dev. Pharmacol. Ther.*, 10: 377–384.

Mirmiran, M., Van de Poll, N.E., Corner, M.A., Van Oyen, H. and Bour, H. (1981) Suppression of active sleep by chronic treatment with chlorimipramine during postnatal development: effects upon adult sleep and behavior in the rat. *Brain Res.*, 204: 129–146.

Mirmiran, M., Scholtens, J., Van de Poll, N.E., Uylings, H.B.M., Van der Gugten, J. and Boer, G.J. (1983a) Effects of experimental suppression of active (REM) sleep during early development upon adult brain and behavior in the rat. *Dev. Brain Res.*, 7: 277–286.

Mirmiran, M., Uylings, H.B.M. and Corner, M.A. (1983b) Pharmacological suppression of REM sleep prior to wean-ing counteracts the effectiveness of subsequent environ-mental enrichment on cortical growth in rats. *Dev. Brain Res.*, 7: 102–105.

Mirmiran, M., Brenner, E., Van der Gugten, J. and Swaab, D.F. (1985) Neurochemical and electrophysiological dis-turbances mediate developmental behavioral alterations produced by medicines. *Neurobehav. Toxicol. Teratol.*, 7: 677–683.

Moar, V.A., Jefferies, M.A., Mutch, L.M.M., Ounsted, M.K. and Redman, C.W.G. (1978) Neonatal head circum-ference and the treatment of maternal hypertension. *Br. J. Obstet. Gynecol.*, 85: 933–937.

Molinoff, P.B. (1984) Alpha- and beta-adrenergic receptor subtype properties, distribution and regulation. *Drugs*, 28: 1–15.

Morris, M.J., Dausse, J.P., Devynck, M.A. and Meyer, P. (1980) Ontogeny of alpha-1- and alpha-2-adrenoreceptors in rat brain. *Brain Res.*, 190: 268–271.

Nelson, S.B., Schwartz, M.A. and Daniels, J.D. (1985) Clonidine and cortical plasticity: possible evidence for noradrenergic involvement. *Dev. Brain Res.*, 23: 39–50.

Neve, K.A. and Molinoff, P.B. (1986) Effects of chronic administration of agonists and antagonists on the density of beta-adrenergic receptors. *Am. J. Cardiol.*, 57: 17F–22F.

Nijhuis, J.G., Prechtl, H.F.R., Martin, C.B. and Bots, R.S.G.M. (1982) Are there behavioral states present in the human fetus? *Early Human Dev.*, 6: 177–195.

Nobin, A. and Björklund, A. (1973) Topography of the monoamine neuron system in the human brain as revealed in the fetuses. *Acta. Physiol. Scand. Suppl.*, 388: 1–40.

Nomura, Y. (1980) The locomotor effect of clonidine and its interaction with alpha-flupenthixol or haloperidol in the developing rat. *Naunyn-Schmiedeberg's Arch. Pharmacol.*, 313: 33–37.

Nomura, Y., Tanaka, Y. and Segawa, T. (1978) Influences of sodium, ouabaine and tricyclic antidepressant drugs on L-[³H]norepinephrine uptake into synaptosomal fractions of developing rat brain. *Jpn. J. Pharmacol.*, 28: 501–504.

Nomura, Y., Yotsumoto, I. and Segawa, T. (1979) High potassium-induced, calcium-dependent monoamine re-lease from brain slices of the newborn rat. *Jpn. J. Pharma-col.*, 29: 847–854.

Nomura, Y., Yotsumoto, I. and Nishimoto, Y. (1982) Onto-geny of influence of clonidine on high potassium-induced release of noradrenaline and specific [³H]clonidine bind-ing in the rat brain cortex. *Dev. Neurosci.*, 5: 198–204.

Nomura, Y., Kawai, M., Mita, K. and Segawa, T. (1984) Developmental changes of cerebral cortical [³H]clonidine binding in rat: influences of guanine nucleotide and cations. *J. Neurochem.*, 42: 1240–1245.

Olpe, H.R., Berecek, K., Jones, R.S.G., Steinmann, M.W., Sonnenburg, C. and Hofbauer, K.G. (1985) Reduced activity of locus coeruleus neurons in SHR and DOCA-salt rats. *Neurosci. Lett.*, 6: 125–129.

Olson, L. and Seiger, A. (1972) Early prenatal ontogeny of central monoamine neurons in the rat: fluorescence histochemical observations. *Z. Anat. Entwicklungsgesch.*, 137: 301–316.

O'Neill, T. P. and Haigler, H. J. (1985) Effects of clonidine on neuronal firing evoked by a noxious stimulus. *Brain Res.*, 327: 97–103.

Ordway, G. A., Gambarana, C. and Frazer, A. (1987) Regionally selective reductions in the density of central beta-adrenoreceptors after chronic intracerebroventricular infusion of isoproterenol in rats. *Soc. Neurosci. Abstr.*, 13: 1342.

Ounsted, M. K., Moar, V. A., Good, F. J. and Redman, C. W. G. (1980) Hypertension during pregnancy with and without specific treatment; the development of the children at the age of four years. *Brit. J. Obstet. Gynecol.*, 87: 19–24.

Pittman, R. N., Minneman, K. P. and Molinoff, P. B. (1980) Ontogeny of beta-1 and beta-2 adrenergic receptors in rat cerebellum and cerebral cortex. *Brain Res.*, 188: 357–368.

Quintin, L., Gonon, F., Buda, M., Ghignone, M., Hilaire, G. and Pujol, J. F. (1986) Clonidine modulates locus coeruleus metabolic hyperactivity induced by stress in behaving rats. *Brain Res.*, 362: 366–369.

Rasmussen, K. and Jacobs, B. L. (1986) Single unit activity of locus coeruleus neurons in the freely moving cat. II. Conditioning and pharmacological studies. *Brain Res.*, 371: 335–344.

Rasmussen, K., Morilak, D. A. and Jacobs, B. L. (1986) Single unit activity of locus coeruleus neurons in the freely moving cat. I. During naturalistic behaviors and in response to simple and complex stimuli. *Brain Res.*, 371: 324–334.

Reisine, T. (1981) Adaptive changes in catecholamine receptors in the central nervous system. *Neuroscience*, 6: 1471–1502.

Ribary, U., Schlumpf, M. and Lichtensteiger, W. (1986) Analysis by HPLC-EC of metabolites of monoamines in fetal and postnatal rat brain. *Neuropharmacology*, 25: 981–986.

Rosenzweig, M. R. and Bennett, F. L. (1978) Experimental influences in brain anatomy and brain chemistry in rodents. In C. Gottlieb (Ed.), *Studies on the Development of Behavior and the Nervous System, Vol. 4*, Academic Press, New York, pp. 289–327.

Sachs, C. and Jonsson, G. (1975) Effects of 6-hydroxydopamine on central noradrenaline neurons during ontogeny. *Brain Res.*, 99: 277–291.

Sakai, K. (1984) Central mechanisms of paradoxical sleep. In A. Borbely and J. L. Valatx (Eds.), *Sleep Mechanisms, Experimental Brain Research Supplementary, Vol. 8*, Springer Verlag, Berlin, pp. 3–18.

Saucier, D. and Astic, L. (1973) Effets de l'alpha-methyl-dopa sur le sommeil du chat nouveau-né. *Psychopharmacology*, 52: 299–333.

Schlumpf, M., Shoemaker, W. J. and Bloom, F. E. (1980) Innervation of embryonic rat cerebral cortex by catecholamine-containing fibers. *J. Comp. Neurol.*, 192: 361–376.

Schwartz, J. C., Costentin, J., Martres, M. P., Protais, P. and Baudry, M. (1978) Modulation of receptor mechanisms in the CNS: hyper- and hyposensitivity of catecholamines. *Neuropharmacology*, 17: 665–685.

Seiger, A. and Olson, L. (1973) Late prenatal ontogeny of central monoamine neurons in the rat: fluorescence histochemical observations. *Z. Anat. Entwicklungsgesch.*, 140: 281–318.

Shimohira, M., Kohyama, J., Kawano, Y., Suzuki, H., Ogiso, M. and Iwakawa, Y. (1986) Effects of alpha-methyldopa administration during pregnancy on the development of the child's sleep. *Brain Dev.*, 8: 416–423.

Simson, P. E. and Weiss, J. M. (1987) Alpha-2 receptor blockade increases responsiveness of locus coeruleus neurons to excitatory stimulation. *J. Neurosci.*, 7: 1732–1740.

Sporn, J. R., Harden, R. K., Wolfe, B. B. and Molinoff, P. B. (1976) Beta-adrenergic receptor involvement in 6-hydroxydopamine-induced supersensitivity in rat cerebral cortex. *Science*, 194: 624–626.

Starke, K. (1977) Regulation of noradrenergic release by presynaptic receptor systems. *Rev. Physiol. Biochem. Pharmacol.*, 77: 1–24.

Sulser, F. (1984) Regulation and function of noradrenaline receptor systems in brain. *Neuropharmacology*, 23: 255–261.

Swaab, D. F. and Mirmiran, M. (1984) Possible mechanisms underlying the teratogenic effects of medicines on the developing brain. In J. Yanai (Ed.), *Neurobehavioral Teratology*, Elsevier, Amsterdam, pp. 55–71.

Tennyson, V. M., Gershon, P., Budininkas-Schoenenbeck, M. and Rothman, T. (1983) Effects of extended periods of reserpine and methyl-*p*-tyrosine treatment on the development of the putamen in the fetal rabbits. *Int. J. Dev. Neurosci.*, 1: 305–318.

Trippodo, N. C. and Frohlick, E. D. (1981) Similarities of genetic (spontaneous) hypertension in man and rat. *Circ. Res.*, 48: 309–319.

U'Prichard, D. C., Reisine, T. D., Mason, S. T., Fibiger, H. C. and Yamamura, H. T. (1980) Modulation of rat brain alpha- and beta-adrenergic receptor populations by lesion of the dorsal noradrenergic bundle. *Brain Res.*, 187: 143–148.

Vetulani, J. and Sulser, F. (1975) Action of various antidepressant treatment reduces activity of cyclic AMP-generating system in limbic forebrain. *Nature*, 257: 495–496.

Wijnen, J. H. L. M., Spierenburg, H. A., De Kloet, E. R., de Jong, W. and Versteeg, D. H. G. (1980) Decrease in noradrenergic activity in hypothalamic nuclei during the development of spontaneous hypertension. *Brain Res.*, 184: 153–162.

Wirz-Justice, A., Krauchi, K., Campbell, I.C. and Feer, H. (1983) Adrenoreceptor changes in spontaneous hypertensive rats: a circadian approach. *Brain Res.*, 262: 233–242.

Discussion

M.V. Johnston: Clonidine stimulates growth-hormone release (Eriksson et al., 1986). Have you studied effects of early clonidine treatment on later growth-hormone response, and clonidine effects on neurogenesis?

M. Mirmiran: You raised an important issue and I must say that, unfortunately, we were not able to measure growth-hormone release either during development or in adulthood in our rats. Moreover, I do not recall any study addressing this matter in animals pre- or postnatally treated with clonidine. In connection with the second part of your question, we have examined brain weight and regional brain tissue parameters of our neonatally clonidine-treated animals in adulthood (Mirmiran et al., 1983). The results showed a smaller brain, and a cerebral cortex lower in weight for protein but not for DNA content. However, Dr. Patel has some more data on actual neurogenesis in rats exposed to different drugs acting on the noradrenaline (NA) system during development.

A.J. Patel (comment): When various agonists and antagonists of the noradrenergic neurotransmitter system were tested, we observed dose-dependent reductions in DNA labelling by (–)-isoproterenol (β-agonist) and phenoxybenzamine (α-antagonist) but not by phenylephrine (α-agonist) or clonidine (α_2-agonist) in either the forebrain or the cerebellar slices in vitro (cf. Patel and Lewis, Chapter 25 of this volume).

M.V. Johnston: Which of the anti-hypertensive drugs clonidine, methyl-dopa or reserpine do you consider safest?

M. Mirmiran: I do not consider any of the above-mentioned antihypertensive drugs safe. In fact it is very difficult to rank the antihypertensive drugs on the basis of their safety, since this probably depends on what parameter you are measuring. Moreover, there are insufficient data with regard to children born from hypertensive mothers treated with one of the drugs. Another problem is the fact that mixed drugs were used in many instances. However, given the drastic changes induced in the monoaminergic system and the deleterious effects found in neurogenesis as a result of neonatal reserpine treatment (cf. Patel and Lewis, Chapter 25), this drug should perhaps be placed at the bottom of any list. Some clinicians believe that low doses of pindolol together with bed-resting, low-salt diet and diuretics might be the safest.

W. Lichtensteiger: The fact that NA turnover was differentially affected by clonidine in different brain regions suggests that these changes were the result of specific functional adaptive reactions to clonidine. Such adaptive reactions might be different during fetal and postnatal life. In view of drug use in humans, it would be interesting to compare consequences of pre- and postnatal drug application.

M. Mirmiran: Thank you for your very interesting comment. I should also add that since rats are altricial animals their prenatal lives are not comparable with humans, so, for the studies you have just mentioned, primates might be more appropriate to use.

References

Eriksson, E., Dellborg, M., Soderpalm, B., Carlsson, M. and Nilsson, C. (1986) Growth hormone responses to clonidine and GRF in spontaneously hypertensive rats: neuroendocrine evidence for an enhanced responsiveness of brain alpha-2-adrenoreceptors in general hypertension. *Life Sci.*, 39: 2103–2109.

Mirmiran, M., Scholtens, J., Van de Poll, N.E., Uylings, H.B.M., Van der Gugten, J. and Boer, G.J. (1983) Effects of experimental suppression of active (REM) sleep during early development upon adult brain and behavior in the rat. *Dev. Brain. Res.*, 7: 277–286.

G.J. Boer, M.G.P. Feenstra, M. Mirmiran, D.F. Swaab and F. Van Haaren
Progress in Brain Research, Vol. 73
© 1988 Elsevier Science Publishers B.V. (Biomedical Division)

CHAPTER 12

Long-lasting changes after perinatal exposure to antidepressants

Joaquín Del Río, Dolores Montero and María L. De Ceballos

Department of Neuropharmacology, Cajal Institute, CSIC, 28006-Madrid, Spain

A great interest has arisen in the last fifteen years in the possible effects of psychotropic drugs on the behavioural development of offspring. Instead of inducing gross physical alterations, the effects of drugs can be more subtle and neurochemical changes can be observed in progeny without apparent morphological alterations. The functional consequences of perinatal administration of drugs is the subject of functional neuroteratology or behavioural teratology. Even though the psychotropic drugs which are usually taken by a high percentage of pregnant women (e.g., Boethius, 1977) have a low teratogenic potential, some animal experiments cast a note of caution on the possible harmful effects of certain psychotropic drugs taken in critical periods of development.

The development of fetal brain results from a sequence of events – neurogenesis, migration and maturation – and the possible effects of drugs are dependent upon the stage of development at which they are administered. Thus, a drug may induce teratogenic effects if administered early in the development while behavioural alterations would occur if the exposure to the same drug was restricted to the final period of gestation. Indeed, the period of fetal susceptibility to drug-induced behavioural abnormalities is broader than that in which malformations of the nervous system may

occur. The term *pure behavioural teratogen* was defined by Vorhees et al. (1979) as the class of compound that produces behavioural alterations without interfering with growth development or modifying any physical parameter, even at high doses.

One of the aims of behavioural teratology is the detection of those drugs which can induce subtle deleterious effects on progeny. Regardless of the basic difficulties in correlating biochemistry and behaviour, it is assumed that, after intake of psychotropic drugs during gestation, any abnormal behaviour of the progeny would be induced by some disturbance in the dynamics of neurotransmitter function. Both classical and peptide neurotransmitters have been reported to play a role in cell proliferation and maturation in the central nervous system (Boer and Snijdewint, this volume) and psychotropic drugs may thus induce, by acting on neurotransmitter systems, slight changes in neuronal organization which would result in functional disturbances not easily detectable in the child but later in life. It seems at first glance an extremely complicated task to ascribe late functional disturbances in man to the use of a given drug during pregnancy; experiments in animals may help to reveal subtle but long-lasting neurochemical alterations which may be correlated in some cases with functional changes.

It is obviously difficult to extrapolate the findings obtained in animals to man, not only for the known differences among species in drug susceptibility or in drug pharmacokinetics but also because drugs may affect maternal behaviour, either directly or through changes induced in the behavioural pattern of the pups (Joffe, 1969; Leonard, 1981).

Antidepressant drugs seem a good case for neurobehavioural teratology studies. In 1971 it was estimated that around 20% of the numerous prescriptions of antidepressants were for females 15–44 years of age (Goldberg and DiMascio, 1978). Since then, new and more effective antidepressants have been developed so the use of these drugs has probably increased and it may be anticipated that a higher number of women use antidepressants during pregnancy. Although the mechanism of action of antidepressants is still obscure (Sugrue, 1983), most of these drugs show marked effects on central monoaminergic neurotransmitter systems, so it seems of interest to study these effects from the point of view of neurobehavioural and biochemical teratology. The effects of noradrenaline and serotonin on cell proliferation and differentiation in several tissues have been known for years (Lanier et al., 1976) and drugs acting on these neurotransmitters may produce permanent effects on the organization of neural circuitries.

Teratogenic and behavioural effects of perinatal antidepressants

The more classic tricyclic antidepressants are not teratogenic in humans (Goldberg and DiMascio, 1978). Likewise, no marked gross teratogenic effects have been generally described in rodents after prenatal administration of antidepressant drugs. The pioneering work of Harper et al. (1965) showed that the highest maternal and fetal toxicity of imipramine was found in rabbits, whereas no significant effect of high doses, up to 150 mg/kg, was found in mice. In rats, chronic administration of imipramine to female rats be-

fore mating reduced litter size and the number of pups weaned. This study clearly shows the marked differences in susceptibility to imipramine among species.

The effects of some tricyclic antidepressants given via different routes to rat dams either prenatally or at an early postnatal period are summarized in Table 1. The most dramatic decrease in litter size was found when imipramine was administered for a long period, before mating and during gestation. Litter size was not however affected when imipramine or amitriptyline were given in the last 2 weeks of pregnancy. On the other hand, pups from dams treated with antidepressants, either during gestation or in the nursing period, gained less weight than controls.

The behavioural alterations in the offspring after perinatal exposure to tricyclic antidepressants have also been analysed in different studies, many of them being summarized in Table 2. In general, the observed changes were not too marked and the most consistent finding was probably a reduction in exploratory activity and in open-field behaviour. In most of these studies no attempt was made to correlate the behavioural observations with alterations in central neurotransmitter systems. Moreover, only the so-called typical antidepressants (e.g., Maj, 1981) which inhibit noradrenaline and serotonin uptake were considered in these previous studies. In the absence of an unequivocally established mechanism of action for all classes of antidepressants (e.g., Sugrue, 1983) one cannot discard the possibility that the perinatal administration of a serotonergic and presynaptic α-adrenoceptor blocker such as mianserin (Van Riezen, 1972; Baumann and Maître, 1977) or of a very potent inhibitor of dopamine uptake such as nomifensine (Hunt et al., 1974) would differentially affect the behaviour of the offspring.

We have sought to determine some neurochemical alterations in rats after prenatal exposure to typical or atypical antidepressants. Where possible, a correlation with behavioural data has been pursued. The results obtained are

TABLE 1

Effect of perinatal administration to rats of antidepressants on litter size and body weight of the pups

Treatment	Dose (mg/kg), route	Time	Litter size	Body weight	References
IMI	5–15, p.o.	BM	↓	↓	Harper et al. (1965)
IMI	5–30, i.p.	BM + G	↓↓	=	Singer and Coyle (1973)
IMI	10, p.o.	BM	=	=	Broitman and Donoso (1978)
CMI	10, p.o.	BM	↓	=	Broitman and Donoso (1978)
IMI	15, p.o.	GD 8–20	=	↓	Jason et al. (1981)
AMI	4, i.p.	GD 8–21	=	=	Bigl et al. (1982)
IMI	10, p.o.	N	=	↓	Broitman and Donoso (1978)
CMI	10, p.o.	N	=	↓	Broitman and Donoso (1978)
CMI	3, p.o.	N	=	↑	Echandia and Broitman (1983)

Treatment: IMI, imipramine; CMI, chlorimipramine; AMI, amitriptyline. Time of administration: G, gestation; GD, gestational days; BM, before mating; N, administration to dams in the nursing period. ↑, increased; ↓, decreased; or =, identical to controls.

TABLE 2

Effects of perinatal administration to rats of antidepressants on the behaviour of offspring

Treatment	Dose (mg/kg), route	Time	Behavioural parameters	References
IMI	5–30, i.p.	BM + G	↓ Locomotor activity	Coyle and Singer (1975)
IMI	10, p.o.	BM	= eye opening, = open-field behaviour	Broitman and Donoso (1978)
CMI	10, p.o.	BM	↓ eye opening, = open-field behaviour	Broitman and Donoso (1978)
CMI	3, p.o.	BM + G	↑ digging, ↑ grooming, ↓ exploration, ↓ social behaviour	Echandia and Broitman (1983)
IMI	15, p.o.	GD 8–20	↑ eye-opening, ↓ righting reflex	Jason et al. (1981)
AMI	4, i.p.	GD 8–21	↓ open-field behaviour	Bigl et al. (1982)
IMI	5–10, s.c.	GD 8–20	↑ negative geotaxia, ↑ amphetamine-induced locomotor activity, ↓ startle reflex	Ali et al. (1986)
CMI	3, p.o.	G + N	abnormal digging and grooming, ↑ scratching, ↓ exploration	Echandia and Broitman (1983)
IMI	10, p.o.	N	↓ eye-opening, ↓ open-field behaviour	Broitman and Donoso (1978)
CMI	10, p.o.	N	↓ eye-opening, = open-field behaviour	Broitman and Donoso (1978)
CMI	3, p.o.	N	= eye-opening, = open-field behaviour, ↓ exploration, = social behaviour	Echandia and Broitman (1983)
CMI	30, i.p.	PND 8–21	↓ active sleep, ↓ open-field behaviour, ↓ sexual behaviour	Mirmiran et al. (1981)

PND, pups injected at the postnatal days indicated. For other abbreviations, see Table 1.

described in the following sections along with previous data on the neurochemical effects of perinatal antidepressants.

Neurochemical effects of perinatal antidepressants

Effects on brain noradrenergic systems

Noradrenergic systems develop early in the rat brain and both noradrenaline and β-adrenergic bindings sites are already detectable in the fetal brain at gestational day 15 (Bruinink and Lichtensteiger, 1984). Long-term changes in these systems may consequently be expected from early exposure to neuroactive drugs.

The levels of noradrenaline and some of its metabolites have been measured in different brain regions of rats whose mothers had been treated with imipramine for a long period, before mating and during the gestation and nursing period. No changes in noradrenaline or normetanephrine levels were recorded as compared to controls (Tonge, 1973), although it should be noted that the animals were 9 months old at the time of the experiments. No change in the hypothalamic content of noradrenaline was either observed at postnatal days 14 or 30 in the offspring of rat dams treated with imipramine during gestation (Jason et al., 1981), whereas an increase in the whole brain content of noradrenaline was found in 15-day-old rats prenatally exposed to amitriptyline (Leonard, 1981).

It is known that chronic administration of different antidepressants to adult rats reduces the density of β-adrenoceptors in the cerebral cortex (see review by Pandey and Davis, 1983). Since the beneficial effects of antidepressant therapy are only apparent after 1–3 weeks of daily administration, it is generally accepted that only those neurochemical changes found after chronic administration of the drugs may be related to their therapeutic efficacy. In this respect, the reduction in the activity of a noradrenaline-sensitive adenylate cyclase (Vetulani and Sulser, 1975) and

of the associated β-adrenergic receptors are probably the most consistent findings. However, the mechanism involved in this down-regulation of β-adrenoceptors awaits clarification (Sugrue, 1983). In adult animals, the reduced density of β-adrenergic binding sites does not persist for more than one week after cessation of treatment (Pandey and Davis, 1983). More persistent changes could be expected if the animals were exposed to antidepressants in the neurogenesis period.

In a previous study using prenatal exposure of rats to imipramine, Jason et al. (1981) found a decrease in the density of β-adrenoceptors at postnatal day 14, that was still observed 16 days later. In a more recent study, we (De Ceballos et al. 1985b) used not only the typical antidepressant chlorimipramine but also the atypical antidepressants mianserin, nomifensine (see above) and iprindole. This last antidepressant is a very weak inhibitor of the uptake of noradrenaline and serotonin (Maxwell, 1983). Another typical antidepressant, desipramine, was included initially in our study. However, daily subcutaneous injection of this drug induced a severe and persistent ulceration of the skin at the site of injection and the treatment was discontinued. The other four antidepressants were subcutaneously given daily to female rats from gestational day 6 to delivery. Neither drug treatment had any significant effect on the litter size or on the body weight of the pups. Moreover, preliminary experiments showed that there was no significant sex difference in the binding parameters of [^{3}H]dihydroalprenolol to rat cortical membranes; thus, the data from both sexes were pooled. The results obtained (Table 3) show that all of the antidepressants markedly reduced, following prenatal exposure, the density of cortical β-adrenoceptors in 25-day-old animals, whereas a single dose of any of the antidepressants given to animals of the same age did not modify the number of binding sites. The apparent affinity of [^{3}H]dihydroalprenolol binding was 1.2 nM in control animals, treated with distilled water, and was not significantly modified by any drug treatment.

TABLE 3

Effect of antidepressant treatment on the density of [^{3}H]-dihydroalprenolol-labelled β-adrenoceptors in rat cerebral cortex

	B_{max} (fmol/mg tissue)	
	Acute treatment	Prenatal exposure
Control	10.4 ± 1.3	12.1 ± 1.1
Chlorimipramine	9.1 ± 1.0	8.0 ± 1.0[a]
Iprindole	11.4 ± 1.7	8.5 ± 1.2[a]
Mianserin	9.3 ± 1.2	6.6 ± 1.3[a]
Nomifensine	13.0 ± 1.3	7.7 ± 0.4[a]

Membranes were prepared from animals of 25 days of age after either acute administration (10 mg/kg i.p., -1 h) or after prenatal exposure to the antidepressant (mothers injected with 10 mg/kg s.c., in gestational days 6–21).
[a] Significant difference vs. controls, $P < 0.05$ (Student's t test).
For further details see De Ceballos et al. (1985b).

The results of our work indicate that prenatal exposure of rats to different antidepressants induces a reduction in the number of β-adrenoceptors that is much more persistent than after chronic treatment of adult animals (Pandey and Davis, 1983). Furthermore, mianserin (Mishra et al., 1980) and nomifensine (De Ceballos et al., 1985b) do not induce a down-regulation of β-adrenoceptors after chronic administration to adult rats. The results confirm the vulnerability of the developing brain. It should be noted however that the present results indicate an effect more marked than in adult animals, but in the same direction. This is at variance with the results obtained with the dopaminergic blocker haloperidol. When this antipsychotic was given to pregnant rats, a reduction in [^{3}H]spiperone binding to dopaminergic receptors was found in the pups, whereas the opposite effect, i.e., increased dopamine receptor binding, was found when haloperidol was given to the nursing mothers (Rosengarten and Friedhoff, 1979). Obviously in the present case we are dealing with compounds with a less well defined mechanism of action (Maj, 1981; Sugrue, 1983). For instance, iprindole, a substance without conspicuous pharmacological effects on the noradrenergic systems, induced down-regulation of β-adrenoceptors, an effect not easily explainable in view of the pharmacological profile of this drug.

Effects on brain serotonergic systems

Traditionally, blockade of serotonin uptake by tricyclic antidepressants has been considered an important point in interpreting their efficacy in the treatment of depression (Schildkraut and Kety, 1967). The more classic antidepressants block to a different extent the re-uptake of 5-HT into nerve endings and it has been repeatedly suggested that the increase in the concentration of 5-HT in central synaptic clefts may underlie their antidepressant effectiveness. As previously mentioned, some more recently discovered antidepressants, e.g., iprindole or mianserin, do not block 5-HT re-uptake but interact in different ways with central serotonergic systems and yet are of value in treating depression (Maxwell, 1983).

The heterogeneity of central postsynaptic 5-HT receptors has been demonstrated and two types of binding sites termed 5-HT$_1$ (or S$_1$) and 5-HT$_2$ (or S$_2$) are recognized (Peroutka and Snyder, 1979), although a further heterogeneity has been suggested in more recent studies (e.g., Green 1987). The effects of chronic treatment with antidepressants on S$_1$ receptors are controversial (Anderson, 1983; Sugrue, 1983) but it has been generally reported that chronic administration of typical or atypical antidepressants down-regulates the number of S$_2$ recognition sites in the rat brain (Sugrue, 1983). The function of the S$_2$ receptors, labelled with [^{3}H]spiperone or [^{3}H]ketanserin, is not well known but it was suggested that they mediate the serotonin behavioural syndrome induced in rats by intense excitation of central 5-HT receptors (Peroutka et al., 1981).

From the point of view of functional neuroteratology, few studies have dealt in the past with the effects of antidepressants on the 5-HT systems of the offspring after perinatal exposure. No long-term change in 5-HT levels or 5-HT turnover was found in different regions of the brain of 9-month-old rats whose mothers had been treated with imipramine before conception and during the gestation and nursing periods (Tonge, 1974). When the early stages of postnatal development were studied in rats prenatally exposed to amitriptyline, 5-HT was significantly reduced in the brain of 1-day-old animals, whereas the levels of 5-HIAA, the major metabolite of 5-HT, were increased 8 days after birth (Bigl et al., 1982).

The ontogeny of S_2 binding sites for [^{3}H]-spiperone has been studied. These receptors are already detectable at embryonic day 15 (Bruinink et al., 1983), at the same stage of development as β-adrenergic binding sites. Since 5-HT systems appear to be involved in neurogenesis (Lauder and Krebs, 1984) and, on the other hand, S_2 receptors are down-regulated after chronic treatment of adult animals with antidepressants (see above), it was of interest to study the binding parameters of [^{3}H]spiperone to S_2 receptors of the frontal cortex of the rat after prenatal exposure to antidepressants. The schedule of treatment of rat dams and the antidepressants used were the same as in the above-mentioned study on β-adrenoceptors (De Ceballos et al., 1985b). The serotonergic syndrome (cf. Peroutka et al., 1981) induced by a combination of a MAO inhibitor and 5-HTP was also studied in the same animals.

The results obtained in S_2 binding assays are summarized in Table 4. Acute treatment with the antidepressants did not change the binding sites for [^{3}H]spiperone. On the contrary, prenatal exposure to the antidepressants chlorimipramine, iprindole or mianserin reduced by about 25% the number of binding sites in 25-day-old rats. The K_D in the binding experiments was 1.5 nM in control animals and was not modified by either acute or prenatal exposure to these drugs. These

TABLE 4

Effect of antidepressant treatment on the density of [^{3}H]-spiperone-labelled S_2 receptors in rat cerebral frontal cortex

	B_{max} (fmol/mg tissue)	
	Acute treatment	Prenatal exposure
Control	57.3 ± 4.4	55.3 ± 3.0
Chlorimipramine	54.8 ± 5.5	40.6 ± 2.5[a]
Iprindole	56.9 ± 5.5	42.0 ± 1.9[a]
Mianserin	53.2 ± 5.3	40.4 ± 4.2[a]
Nomifensine	59.4 ± 5.8	92.5 ± 6.6[a]

25-day-old rats after acute treatment (10 mg/kg i.p., −60 min) or following prenatal exposure to the antidepressants were used.

[a] Significant difference vs. controls, $P < 0.05$ (Student's t test).

For further details, see De Ceballos et al. (1985b).

data also demonstrate that the decreased binding was not due to any drug remaining in the brain 25 days after discontinuation of the treatment. By contrast, prenatal exposure to the atypical antidepressant nomifensine enhanced by approximately 60% the maximum number of binding sites and, at the same time, increased the K_D value to 3.8 nM. The long-lasting changes induced by prenatal exposure to antidepressants is an interesting finding that shows, as in the case of β-adrenoceptors, the greater vulnerability of the developing brain. It should be noted that the reduction in S_2 receptors after chronic treatment of adult rats with amitriptyline or mianserin reverts to control values in 10 days (Peroutka and Snyder, 1980; Blackshear and Sanders-Bush, 1982).

In order to study the duration of the down-regulation of S_2 receptors by prenatal exposure of rats to antidepressants, an additional experiment was carried out with chlorimipramine. The daily dose was 10 mg/kg p.o. and the antidepressant was given to rat dams in the last 15 days of gestation. Instead of [^{3}H]spiperone, [^{3}H]-ketanserin was used to more specifically label S_2

TABLE 5

Effect of prenatal exposure to chlorimipramine on [³H]ketanserin binding to S_2 receptors in rat frontal cortex

	PND 25		PND 90	
	B_{max}	K_D	B_{max}	K_D
Control	329 ± 24	0.65 ± 0.14	294 ± 35	0.48 ± 0.08
Chlorimipramine	234 ± 12[a]	0.47 ± 0.08	283 ± 48	0.63 ± 0.07

[³H]Ketanserin binding was measured in frontal cortex of 25- or 90-day-old rats, prenatally exposed to chlorimipramine (10 mg/kg, p.o.) for the last 15 days of gestation. Data are means $\pm$ S.E.M. of four to five Scatchards plots, each plot constructed with seven points in triplicate. The concentration range of [³H]ketanserin was 0.5–5 nM; specific binding was defined using cyproheptadine 30 μM.
[a] Significantly different vs. controls, $P < 0.01$ (Student's t test).

receptors (Leysen et al., 1982). Similar to the previous experiment, prenatal exposure to chlorimipramine significantly reduced the B_{max} without modifying the K_D in 25-day-old rats (Table 5).

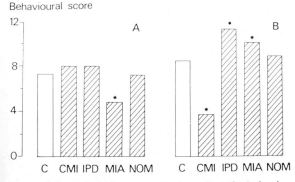

Behavioural score

Fig. 1. Effect of antidepressant treatment on the behavioural syndrome induced by combined administration of clorgyline (5 mg/kg i.p., – 60 min) and 5-HTP (25 mg/kg, i.p., 0 min) in 25-day-old rats. The behavioural syndrome included head-twitches, resting tremor, hind limb abduction, forepaw-treading and snake-tail. The different symptoms were scored from 0 to 3, 30 min after injection of 5-HTP for a 10 min period. A, acute antidepressant treatment (10 mg/kg i.p., – 30 min); B, prenatal exposure to antidepressants (drugs, 10 mg/kg s.c. given to the mothers during the last 15 days of gestation). The behavioural score is the mean value of eight to ten animals. Abbreviations: C, control; CMI, chlorimipramine; IPD, iprindole; MIA, mianserin; NOM, nomifensine. * $P < 0.02$ vs. controls (Mann-Whitney U-test).

However, the B_{max} in 90-day-old rats was not significantly different from controls. It remains to be established whether the previously used atypical antidepressants are able to induce longer-lasting changes on S_2 receptors.

Enduring changes in the serotonergic syndrome were also observed after prenatal exposure to antidepressants. However, the intensity of this behaviour was only antagonized by chlorimipramine, whereas iprindole and mianserin potentiated the syndrome (Fig. 1). On acute treatment, only mianserin, a potent 5-HT antagonist (Van Riezen, 1972), antagonized the abnormal behaviour. The varying effects of the antidepressants on the 5-HT syndrome are in keeping with previous reports (Mogilnicka and Klimek, 1979; Friedman et al. 1983) and probably reflect the different actions of the antidepressants used on serotonergic transmission (see above). Regardless of the mechanisms involved in the down-regulation of S_2 receptors, it is clear that the present results do not confirm the proposed mediation by S_2 receptors in the serotonergic syndrome.

Effects on brain dopaminergic systems

Dopamine has been traditionally disregarded as a crucial neurotransmitter in the mechanism of action of antidepressant drugs. In fact antidepressants barely have any effect on DA re-uptake (Friedman et al., 1977) and they do not displace ligand binding to DA receptors (Hall and Ögren, 1981). Nevertheless, chronic antidepressant treatment of adult rats may enhance the function of central dopaminergic systems, as demonstrated in electrophysiological and behavioural studies (Chiodo and Antelman, 1980; Spyraki and Fibiger, 1981; Martin-Iverson et al, 1983; Willner, 1983). There have been attempts to correlate these functional changes with increased dopamine receptor binding, but either no modification (Charney et al., 1981; Martin-Iverson et al., 1983) or decreased receptor density (Koide and Matsushita, 1981) have been reported after chronic antidepressant treatment.

Dopaminergic receptors in the rat brain are already detectable at embryonic day 17 (Bruinink et al., 1983) and as mentioned above, psychotropic drugs influencing dopaminergic mechanisms are able to induce profound behavioural and neurochemical alterations in the offspring when administered to pregnant rats. Even though the effects of antidepressants, except perhaps for

nomifensine (Hunt et al., 1974), on the dopaminergic systems are not pronounced, it appeared of interest to determine if the effects would be more marked after chronic prenatal exposure. Locomotor activity, a typical dopamine-mediated behaviour, was studied together with the eventual alterations in binding to dopaminergic receptors of striatal membranes (De Ceballos et al., 1985a).

In keeping with several previous studies (Table 2) spontaneous locomotor activity was significantly decreased by either acute treatment or prenatal exposure to chlorimipramine, iprindole or mianserin (Fig. 2). By contrast, nomifensine dramatically increased the spontaneous locomotion of 25-day-old rats after a single injection (Fig. 3A). When animals exposed in utero to nomifensine were studied, an increase in locomotor activity was still present (Fig. 3B). Since nomifensine is a potent blocker of DA uptake (Hunt et al., 1974), this property would be responsible for the increased locomotor activity. Similar results have been described following prenatal exposure to D-amphetamine (Bigl et al., 1982).

The effect of the different treatments on the

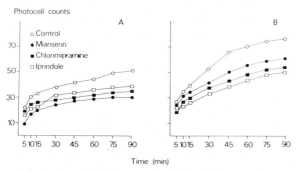

Fig. 2. Effect of antidepressant treatment on spontaneous locomotor activity of 25-day-old rats. A, acute antidepressant treatment (10 mg/kg i.p., – 60 min); B, prenatal exposure to antidepressant (10 mg/kg s.c.) during the last 15 days of gestation. Locomotion was measured for 90 min at different intervals, after a 5 min period of habituation to the photocell activity cages (Garzón et al. 1979). Data are means of eight to ten animals. S.E.M. (not shown) were always less than 15% of the mean.

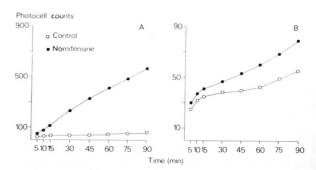

Fig. 3. Effect of nomifensine after either acute treatment (A, 10 mg/kg i.p., – 60 min) or prenatal exposure (B, 10 mg/kg s.c. given daily to the mothers during the last 15 days of gestation) on spontaneous locomotor activity of 25-day-old rats. Locomotion was measured for 90 min, after a 5 min period of habituation to the activity cages. Results are means of eight to ten animals. S.E.M. (not shown) were less than 15% of the mean.

hyperactivity induced by a moderate dose of the dopaminergic stimulant apomorphine (200 μg/kg) was subsequently studied. Following antidepressant treatment, only mianserin antagonized the locomotor activation induced by apomorphine (Fig. 4A), whereas prenatal exposure to all of the antidepressants, except mianserin, potentiated the apomorphine effect (Fig. 4B). These results appear to be indicative of supersensitive dopamine receptors induced by prenatal exposure to the antidepressants, the only exception being mianserin. This drug is endowed with multiple pharmacological actions including a marked sedative effect (Maj et al., 1983). It is yet possible to suppose that mianserin produces supersensitive dopamine receptors but there may be a masking effect, hypothetically mediated through simultaneous activation of central noradrenergic pathways (Baumann and Maître, 1977).

The behavioural supersensitivity to a dopaminergic stimulant should be correlated with an increased number of dopamine receptors. However, no antidepressant, either on acute treatment or prenatal exposure, modified the B_{max} or K_D of [^{3}H]spiperone binding to homogenates from rat corpus striatum (De Ceballos et al., 1985a). Different studies have suggested that functional changes in receptor sensitivity correlate better with alterations in agonist competition for [^{3}H]antagonist binding sites than with alterations in the parameters of binding of these [^{3}H]-antagonists (e.g.,Wessels et al., 1979). Competition curves for inhibition by dopamine of [^{3}H]-spiperone binding to striatal membranes were consequently constructed and the K_i calculated. While with acute treatment no antidepressant changed the K_i, prenatal exposure to any of the antidepressants significantly lowered this parameter (Table 6). This neurochemical change may explain the behavioural supersensitivity found in the present study. A more marked hyperactive response to amphetamine was also recently described in 21-day-old rats prenatally exposed to imipramine (Ali et al., 1986).

The results show once more the more persistent behavioural and neurochemical effects that

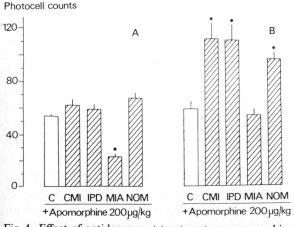

Photocell counts

Fig. 4. Effect of antidepressant treatment on apomorphine-induced hyperactivity. A, acute treatment, antidepressants were given 60 min before apomorphine (200 μg/kg s.c.); B, prenatal exposure, animals whose mothers were injected daily with the antidepressant (10 mg/kg s.c.) in the last 15 days of gestation. For further details, see De Ceballos et al. (1985a). C, controls; CMI, chlorimipramine; IPD, iprindole; MIA, mianserin; NOM, nomifensine. *Significant difference vs. controls (P < 0.05, Student's t test).

TABLE 6

Effect of antidepressant treatment on dopamine competition for [^{3}H]spiperone binding to rat striatal membranes

	K_i (μM)	
	Acute treatment	Prenatal exposure
Control	4.3 ± 0.6	4.5 ± 0.4
Chlorimipramine	5.4 ± 0.6	2.3 ± 0.5[a]
Iprindole	4.5 ± 0.6	1.7 ± 0.4[a]
Mianserin	5.9 ± 0.7	0.4 ± 0.0[a]
Nomifensine	4.2 ± 0.5	2.5 ± 0.6[a]

Animals of 25 days of age, after either acute treatment (10 mg/kg i.p., 60 min before sacrifice) or prenatal exposure to antidepressants (dams treated with 10 mg/kg s.c., from day 6 to delivery) were used in the experiments.
[a] Significant difference vs. controls, $P < 0.05$ (Student's t test).
For further details, see De Ceballos et al. (1985a).

can be obtained after prenatal exposure of rats to antidepressants. For instance, Spyraki and Fibiger (1981) found that the potentiation of the locomotor response to amphetamine in adult rats after chronic treatment with desipramine was only observed for 5 days after cessation of antidepressant treatment. By contrast, in the present study the potentiation of a dopaminergic agonist was observed at least 25 days after discontinuation of drug treatment. It must be stressed again that, at variance with antipsychotics (Rosengarten and Friedhoff, 1979), prenatal exposure to antidepressants produces effects which are much more marked than in adult animals, but qualitatively identical. With regard to the time course of the different behavioural and neurochemical changes found in our study, it is possible to suppose that none of the alterations are parallel but a given alteration may be produced by a previous, more crucial change. It is known, for instance, that lesions of central 5-HT axons prevent the down-regulation of β-adrenoceptors by desipramine (Brunello et al., 1982a) or lesions of central noradrenergic pathways block the potentiation of dopamine-mediated behaviour induced by repeated electroconvulsive shock (Green and Deakin, 1980). These examples are indicative of the importance of the interactions between mono-aminergic systems in the sequence of changes induced by antidepressants, an aspect not analysed in the present study.

Effects on [^{3}H]imipramine binding sites

High affinity [^{3}H]imipramine binding sites have been described in brain and platelets (Briley et al., 1980; Raisman et al., 1980). In general, antidepressants are potent displacers of [^{3}H]imipramine binding (Langer et al., 1980). These binding sites are associated with the serotonin uptake mechanism in serotonergic nerve endings (Langer et al., 1980; Brunello et al., 1982b). Perhaps one of the findings that raised more interest in this putative receptor is that its population is decreased in platelets from untreated depressed

patients (Briley et al., 1980; Langer et al., 1982) and in brains from depressed patients and suicide victims studied post-mortem (Paul et al., 1984).

Chronic antidepressant treatment has been found to decrease the density of [^{3}H]imipramine sites in brain, without changing their affinity (Raisman et al., 1980; Kinnier et al., 1980), but this effect was not confirmed in all subsequent studies (Plenge and Mellerup, 1982; Gentsch et al., 1984). Zimelidine, a potent serotonin uptake blocker, upon repeated administration increased, unlike typical antidepressants, the density of [^{3}H]imipramine binding sites (Fuxe et al., 1983) and, similarly, increased also the B_{max} for [^{3}H]imipramine binding in platelets from depressed patients (Wägner et al., 1987). These controversial results prompted us to examine [^{3}H]-imipramine binding after prenatal exposure, expecting more marked effects than in adult rats.

In this study, pregnant rats were treated with several typical and atypical antidepressants, including the selective serotonin re-uptake inhibitors, zimelidine and fluoxetine (Wong et al., 1975). Oral administration (via the drinking water) was preferred to s.c. administration of the drug to mimic the route used in Clinics. Target doses were 10 mg/kg per day, except for zimelidine and fluoxetine, which were used at a dose of 3 mg/kg because two pregnant rats treated with a higher dose of zimelidine (10 mg/kg) died on the day of delivery. Continuous oral administration of antidepressants to pregnant dams had no effect on the mothers' weight gain. Litter size or pup weight at 25 days of age was not affected either. Obviously, acute treatments were not considered in this part of the study due to the high affinity of most of these antipressants for the [^{3}H]imipramine binding sites (Raisman et al., 1979).

The effect of prenatal exposure to antidepressants on [^{3}H]imipramine binding in cortical membranes from 25-day-old rats is summarized in Table 7. Chlorimipramine and fluoxetine decreased the B_{max} without altering the K_D. The other drugs prenatally administered were without significant effect on the binding process. The sig-

TABLE 7

Effect of prenatal exposure to antidepressants on [³H]-imipramine binding in rat cortical membranes

	B_{max} (fmol/mg protein)	K_D (nM)
Control	491 ± 46	3.5 ± 0.4
Chlorimipramine	348 ± 19[a]	4.0 ± 0.5
Desipramine	466 ± 48	3.6 ± 0.9
Nomifensine	579 ± 48	4.6 ± 0.5
Zimelidine	534 ± 69	4.7 ± 0.5
Fluoxetine	326 ± 43[a]	4.3 ± 0.7

Animals of 25 days of age prenatally exposed to drugs. Mothers treated the last 15 days of gestation with 10 mg/kg p.o. of chlorimipramine, desipramine or nomifensine, or 3 mg/kg p.o. of zimelidine or fluoxetine. Results are means ± S.E.M. of six Scatchard plots, constructed with seven points in triplicate. The concentration range of [³H]-imipramine was 0.5–8 nM. Desipramine (10^{-6} M) was used as displacing drug.
[a] Significant difference vs. controls, $P < 0.01$ (Student's t test).

nificant difference in density of [³H]imipramine binding sites after prenatal chlorimipramine disappeared at 3 months of age (Controls: B_{max} 521 ± 46 fmol/mg protein, $n = 6$; prenatal exposure to chlorimipramine: B_{max} 490 ± 58 fmol/mg protein, $n = 5$). The effect is thus parallel to that obtained in the case of S_2 receptors. However, no generalization can be made regarding the duration of the effects of antidepressants on prenatal exposure since this 3-month study with chlorimipramine has not yet been extended to the other antidepressants.

The main finding of this study is consequently a decrease in the density of [³H]imipramine binding sites after prenatal exposure to chlorimipramine or fluoxetine. This effect is observed at least 25 days after discontinuation of the drug treatment. This finding suggests a possible involvement of the common serotonin uptake blocking activity. Chlorimipramine given to healthy subjects for one week also decreased

[³H]imipramine binding sites in human platelets and this decrease persisted 3 weeks after discontinuation of treatment (Poirier et al., 1985). On the contrary, zimelidine, another selective blocker of serotonin uptake, was without effect in the present study. In fact, much higher doses of this drug have been reported to increase the density of [³H]imipramine binding sites in rat cortical membranes (Fuxe et al., 1983).

The possible functional significance of [³H]-imipramine binding awaits further exploration. At variance with some of the other receptors studied, it appears that all types of antidepressant drugs do not act in a similar way on these recognition sites.

Summary and Concluding remarks

The mechanism(s) involved in the clinical effectiveness of antidepressant drugs is not well known but all of these drugs share some effects on different monoamine receptors of the rat brain upon chronic administration. Behavioural and neurochemical changes were studied in 25-day-old rats acutely treated or prenatally exposed to typical or atypical antidepressants. After prenatal exposure, chlorimipramine, iprindole and mianserin reduced the number of cortical β-adrenergic and 5-HT$_2$ receptors without modifying the K_D. Prenatal nomifensine also down regulated β-adrenoceptors but increased the density of 5-HT$_2$ receptors. Acute treatments were always ineffective. These four antidepressants did not modify binding of [³H]spiperone to striatal dopamine receptors but enhanced, upon prenatal exposure, the ability of dopamine to compete for these sites. The number of cortical binding sites for [³H]-imipramine was also decreased by prenatal exposure to chlorimipramine or fluoxetine but not to other antidepressants. With regard to behavioural changes, there was no correlation between the number of 5-HT$_2$ or dopamine receptors and the serotonin behavioural syndrome or the locomotor response to apomorphine, respectively. However, there was a good correlation between the locomotor response to apomorphine and the ability of dopamine to compete for binding of [³H]-spiperone to striatal membranes. In general, the neurochemical and behavioural changes after prenatal exposure of rats to antidepressants are more marked and longer-lasting than those induced by chronic treatment of adult rats. This approach may perhaps only contribute to unravel some aspects of the mechanism of action of antidepressants, but suggests also that a certain caution should be exercised in the intake of antidepressants by pregnant women.

Acknowledgements

This work was supported by grant from CAICYT, Spain. We thank Astra, Ciba-Geigy, Hoechst, Lilly, Organon and Wyeth for their gifts of drugs.

References

Ali, S. F., Buelke-Sam, J., Newport, G. D. and Slikker, W. Jr., (1986) Early neurobehavioural and neurochemical alterations in rats prenatally exposed to imipramine. *Neurotoxicology*, 7: 365–380.

Anderson, J. L. (1983) Serotonin receptor changes after chronic antidepressant treatments: Ligand binding, electrophysiological and behavioral studies. *Life Sci.*, 32: 1791–1801.

Baumann, P. A. and Maître, L. (1977) Blockade of presynaptic alpha receptors and amine uptake in the rat brain by the antidepressant mianserin. *Naunyn-Schmiedeb. Arch. Pharmacol.*, 300: 31–37.

Bigl, V., Dalitz, E., Kunert, E. Biesold, D. and Leonard, B. E. (1982) The effect of D-amphetamine and amitriptyline administered to pregnant rats on the locomotor activity and neurotransmitters of the offspring. *Psychopharmacology*, 77: 371–375.

Blackshear, M. A. and Sanders-Bush, E. (1982) Serotonin receptor sensitivity after acute and chronic treatment with mianserin. *J. Pharmacol. Exp. Ther.*, 221: 303–308.

Boethius, G. (1977) Recording of drugs prescription in the county of Jamtland, Sweden. (ii). Drug exposure of pregnant women in relation to course and outcome of pregnancy. *Eur. J. Clin. Pharmacol.*, 12: 37–42.

Briley, M. S., Langer, S. Z., Raisman, R., Sechter, D. and Zarifian E. (1980) Tritiated imipramine binding sites are decreased in platelets of untreated depressed patients. *Science*, 209: 303–305.

Broitman, S. T. and Donoso, A. O. (1978) Effects of chronic imipramine and clomipramine oral administration on maternal behaviour and litter development. *Psychopharmacology*, 56: 93–101.

Bruinink, A., Lichtensteiger, W. and Schlumpf, M. (1983) Pre- and postnatal ontogeny and characterization of dopaminergic D_2, serotonergic S_2, and spirodecanone binding sites in rat forebrain. *J. Neurochem.*, 40: 1227–1236.

Bruinink, A. and Lichtensteiger, W. (1984) β-Adrenergic binding sites in fetal rat brain. *J. Neurochem.*, 43: 578–581.

Brunello, N., Barbaccia, M. L., Chuang, D. M. and Costa, E. (1982a) Down-regulation of β-adrenergic receptors following repeated injections of desmethylimipramine: permissive role of serotonergic axons. *Neuropharmacology*, 21: 1145–1149.

Brunello, N., Chuang, D. M. and Costa, E. (1985b) Different synaptic localization of mianserin and imipramine binding sites. *Science*, 215: 1112–1115.

Charney, D. S., Menkes, D. B. and Heninger, G. R. (1981) Receptor sensitivity and the mechanism of action of antidepressants. *Arch. Gen. Psychiatr.*, 38: 1160–1165.

Chiodo, L. A. and Antelman, S. M. (1980) Repeated tricyclics induce a progressive dopamine autoreceptor subsensitivity independent of daily drug treatment. *Nature*, 287: 451–454.

Coyle, I. and Singer, G. (1975) The interactive effects of prenatal imipramine exposure and post-natal rearing conditions on behaviour and histology. *Psychopharmacologia*, 44: 253–259.

De Ceballos, M. L., Benedi, A., De Felipe, C. and Del Río, J. (1985a) Prenatal exposure of rats to antidepressants enhances agonist affinity of brain dopamine receptors and dopamine-mediated behaviour. *Eur. J. Pharmacol.*, 116: 257–262.

De Ceballos, M. L., Benedi, A., Urdín, C. and Del Río, J. (1985b) Prenatal exposure of rats to antidepressant drugs down-regulates beta-adrenoceptors and 5-HT$_2$ receptors in cerebral cortex. Lack of correlation between 5-HT$_2$ receptors and serotonin-mediated behaviour. *Neuropharmacology*, 24: 947–952.

Echandia, E. L. R. and Broitman, S. T. (1983) Effect of prenatal and postnatal exposure to therapeutic doses of chlorimipramine on emotionality in the rat. *Psychopharmacology*, 79: 236–241.

Friedman, E., Cooper, T. B. and Dallob, A. (1983) Effects of chronic antidepressant treatment on serotonin receptor activity in mice. *Eur. J. Pharmacol.*, 89: 69–76.

Friedman, E., Fung, F. and Gershon, S. (1977) Antidepressant drugs and dopamine uptake in different brain regions. *Eur. J. Pharmacol.*, 42: 47–51.

Fuxe, K., Ögren, S. O., Agnati, L. F., Benfenati, F., Fredholm, B., Andersson, K., Zini, I. and Eneroth, P. (1983) Chronic antidepressant treatment and central 5-HT synapses. *Neuropharmacology*, 22: 389–400.

Garzón, J., Fuentes, J. A. and Del Río, J. (1979) Antidepressants selectively antagonize the hyperactivity induced in rats by long-term isolation. *Eur. J. Pharmacol.*, 59: 293–296.

Gentsch, C., Lichtsteiner, M. and Feer, H. (1984) [^{3}H]-imipramine and [^{3}H]-cyano-imipramine binding in rat brain tissue: effect of long-term antidepressant administration. *J. Neural Transm.*, 59: 257–264.

Goldberg, H. L. and DiMascio, A. (1978) Psychotropic drugs in pregnancy. In M. A. Lipton, A. DiMascio and K. F. Killam (Eds.), *Psychopharmacology: A Generation of Progress*. Raven Press, New York, pp. 1047–1055.

Green, J. P. (1987) Nomenclature and classification of receptors and binding sites: the need for harmony. *Trends Pharmacol. Sci.*, 8: 90–94.

Green, A. R. and Deakin, J. F. W. (1980) Brain noradrenaline depletion prevents ECS-induced enhancement of serotonin- and dopamine-mediated behavior. *Nature*, 285: 232–234.

Hall, H. and Ögren, S. (1981) Effects of antidepressant drugs on different receptors in the brain. *Eur. J. Pharmacol.*, 70: 393–407.

Harper, K. H., Palmer, A. K. and Davies, R. E. (1965) Effect of imipramine upon the pregnancy of laboratory animals. *Arzneimittel-Forsch.*, 15: 1218–1221.

Hunt, P., Kannengiesser, M. H. and Raynaud, J. P. (1974) Nomifensine: a new potent inhibitor of dopamine uptake into synaptosomes from rat brain corpus striatum. *J. Pharm. Pharmacol.*, 26: 370–375.

Jason, K. M., Cooper, T. B. and Friedman, E. (1981) Prenatal exposure to imipramine alters early behavioral development and beta-adrenergic receptors in rats. *J. Pharmacol. Exp. Ther.*, 217: 461–466.

Joffe, J. M. (1969) *Prenatal Determinants of Behaviour*. Academic Press, New York.

Kinnier, W. J., Chuang, D. and Costa, E. (1980) Down regulation of dihydro-alprenolol and imipramine binding sites in brain of rats repeatedly treated with imipramine. *Eur. J. Pharmacol.*, 67: 289–294.

Koide, T. and Matsushita, H. (1981) An enhanced sensitivity of muscarinic cholinergic receptor associated with dopaminergic receptor subsensitivity after chronic antidepressant treatment. *Life Sci.*, 28: 1139–1145.

Langer, S. Z., Moret, C., Raisman, R., Dubocovich, M. L. and Briley, M. S. (1980) High affinity [^{3}H]imipramine binding in rat hypothalamus: association with uptake of serotonin but not of norepinephrine. *Science*, 210: 1133–1135.

Langer, S. Z., Zarifian, E., Briley, M., Raisman, R. and Sechter, D. (1982) High affinity [^{3}H]imipramine binding: A new biological marker in depression. *Pharmacopsychiatria*, 15: 4–10.

Lanier, L. P., Dunn, A. J. and Van Hartesveldt, C. (1976) Development of neurotransmitters and their function in brain. In S. Ehrempreis and I. J. Kopin (Eds.), *Reviews of Neuroscience, Vol. 2*, Raven Press, New York, pp. 195–256.

Lauder, J. M. and Krebs, H. (1984) Neurotransmitters and development as possible substrates for drugs of use and abuse. In J. Yanai (Ed). *Neurobehavioral Teratology*, Elsevier, Amsterdam, pp. 289–314.

Leonard, B. E. (1981) Effect of psychotropic drugs administered to pregnant rats on the behaviour of the offspring. *Neuropharmacology*, 20: 1237–1242.

Leysen, J. E., Neimegeers, C. J. E., Van Nueten, J. M. and Laduron, P. M. (1982) ^{3}H-Ketanserin (R41468), a selective ^{3}H-ligand for serotonin$_2$ receptor binding sites. *Mol. Pharmacol.*, 21: 301–314.

Maj, J. (1981) Antidepressant drugs: will new findings change the present theories of their action? *Trends Pharmacol. Sci.*, 2: 80–83.

Maj, J., Rogoz, Z., Skuza, G. and Sowinska, H. (1983) Reserpine-induced locomotor stimulation in mice chronically treated with typical and atypical antidepressants. *Eur. J. Pharmacol.*, 87: 469–474.

Martin-Iverson, M. T., Leclere, J. F. and Fibiger, H. C. (1983) Cholinergic-dopaminergic interactions and the mechanism of action of antidepressants. *Eur. J. Pharmacol.*, 94: 193–201.

Maxwell, R. A. (1983) Second generation antidepressants: the pharmacological and clinical significance of selected examples. *Drug Develop. Res.*, 3: 203–211.

Mirmiran, M., Van de Poll, N. E., Corner, M. A., Van Oyen, H. G. and Bour, H. L. (1981) Suppression of active sleep by chronic treatment with chlorimipramine during early postnatal development: effects upon adult sleep and behavior in the rat. *Brain Res.*, 204: 129–146.

Mishra, R., Janowsky, A. and Sulser, F. (1980) Action of mianserin and zimelidine on the norepinephrine receptor coupled adenylate cyclase system in brain: subsensitivity without reduction in β-adrenergic receptor binding. *Neuropharmacology*, 18: 983–987.

Mogilnicka, E. and Klimek, V. (1979) Mianserin, danitracen and amitriptyline withdrawal increases the behavioral responses of rats to 5-HTP. *J. Pharm. Pharmacol.*, 31: 704–705.

Pandey, G. N. and Davis, J. M. (1983) Treatment with antidepressants and down-regulation of β–adrenergic receptors. *Drug Develop. Res.*, 3: 393–406.

Paul, S. M., Rehavi, M., Skolnick, P. and Goodwin, F. K. (1984) High affinity binding of antidepressants to biogenic amine transport sites in human brain and platelets in depression. In R. M. Post and J. C. Ballenger (Eds), *Neurobiology of Mood Disorders, Vol. 1*, Williams and Wilkins, Baltimore, pp. 846–853.

Peroutka, S. J., Lebovitz, R. M. and Snyder, S. H. (1981) Two distinct central serotonin receptors with different physiological functions. *Science*, 212: 827–829.

Peroutka, S. J. and Snyder, S. H. (1979) Multiple serotonin receptors: Differential binding of ^{3}H-5-hydroxytryptamine, ^{3}H-lysergic acid diethylamide and ^{3}H-spiroperidol. *Mol. Pharmacol.*, 16: 687–699.

Peroutka, S. J. and Snyder, S. H. (1980) Regulation of serotonin (5-HT$_2$) receptors labeled with (^{3}H)spiroperidol by chronic treatment with the antidepressant amitriptyline. *J. Pharmacol. Exp. Ther.* 215: 582–587.

Plenge, P. and Mellerup, E.T. (1982) ³H-imipramine high-affinity binding sites in rat brain. Effects of imipramine and lithium. *Psychopharmacology*, 77: 94–97.

Poirier, M.F., Loo, H., Benkelfat, C., Sechter, D., Zarifian, E., Galzin, A.M., Schoemaker, H., Segonzac, A. and Langer, S.Z. (1985) ³H-Imipramine binding and ³H-5-HT uptake in human blood platelets: changes after one week chlorimipramine treatment. *Eur. J. Pharmacol.*, 106: 629–633.

Raisman, R., Briley, M. and Langer, S.Z. (1979) Specific tricyclic antidepressant binding sites in rat brain. *Nature*, 281: 148–150.

Raisman, R., Briley, M.S., Langer, S.Z. (1980) Specific tricyclic antidepressant binding sites in rat brain characterized by high-affinity ³H-imipramine binding. *Eur. J. Pharmacol.*, 61: 373–380.

Rosengarten, H. and Friedhoff, A.J. (1979) Enduring changes in dopamine receptor cells of pups from drug administration to pregnant and nursing rats. *Science*, 203: 1133–1135.

Schildkraut, J.J. and Kety, S.S. (1967) Biogenic amines and emotion. *Science*, 156: 21–30.

Singer, G. and Coyle, I.R. (1973) The effect of imipramine administered before and during pregnancy on litter size in the rat. *Psychopharmacologia*, 32: 337–342.

Spyraki, C. and Fibiger, H.C. (1981) Behavioural evidence for supersensitivity of postsynaptic dopamine receptors in the mesolimbic system after chronic administration of desipramine. *Eur. J. Pharmacol.*, 74: 195–206.

Sugrue, M.F. (1983) Do antidepressants possess a common mechanism of action? *Biochem. Pharmacol.*, 32: 1811–1817.

Tonge, S.R. (1973) Catecholamine concentrations in discrete areas of the rat brain after the pre- and neonatal administration of phencyclidine and imipramine. *J. Pharm. Pharmacol.*, 25: 164–165.

Tonge, S.R. (1974) Permanent alterations in 5-hydroxytryptamine metabolism in discrete areas of rat brain following exposure to drugs during the period of development. *Life Sci.*, 15: 245–249.

Van Riezen, H. (1972) Different central effects of the 5-HT antagonists mianserin and cyproheptadine. *Arch. Int. Pharmacodyn. Ther.*, 198: 256–269.

Vetulani, J. and Sulser, F. (1975) Action of various antidepressant treatments reduces reactivity of noradrenergic cyclic AMP-generating system in limbic forebrain. *Nature*, 257: 495–496.

Vorhees, C.V., Brunner, R.L. and Butcher, R.E. (1979) Psychotropic drugs as behavioral teratogens. *Science*, 205: 1220–1225.

Wägner, A., Aberg-Wistedt, A., Asberg, M., Bertilsson, L., Martensson, B. and Montero, D. (1987) Effects of antidepressant treatments on platelet ³H-imipramine binding in major depressive disorder. *Arch. Gen. Psychiat.*, 44: 870–877.

Wessels, M.R., Mullikin, D. and Lefkowitz, R.J. (1979) Selective alteration in high affinity agonist binding: a mechanism of β-adrenergic desensitization. *Mol. Pharmacol.*, 16: 10–15.

Willner, P. (1983) Dopamine and depression: A review of recent evidence. III. The effects of antidepressant treatments. *Brain Res. Rev.*, 6: 237–246.

Wong, D.T., Bymaster, F.P., Horng, J.S. and Molloy, B.B. (1975) A new selective inhibitor for uptake of serotonin into synaptosomes of rat brain: 3-(p-trifluoromethyl-phenoxy)-N-methyl-3-phenylpropylamine. *J. Pharmacol. Exp. Ther.*, 193: 804–810.

Discussion

M.V. Johnston: Since patients who are depressed typically do not improve for several weeks after therapy is begun (Gilman et al. 1980), have interactions between combined effects of hormonal change (e.g., increased corticosteroid levels) found in depression and antidepressants been looked for? Could the stress of severe depression itself been looked at as a teratogen? What is the best therapy for a severely depressed woman who is pregnant?

J. Del Rio: Antidepressant drugs have been reported to modify different hormone secretion patterns (e.g., prolactin, growth hormone, cortisol, thyroid-stimulating hormone) but no consistent hormonal changes have been found after chronic administration of the different classes of antidepressants. In regard to your other questions, I agree that certain forms of severe depression may represent a stressful condition for the mother and, as such, may be considered as a potential teratogen (Weinstock et al., Ch. 21, this volume). Depression should therefore be treated, and, if psychotherapy is not useful, then antidepressants should be given with a certain caution to the pregnant woman. There is not as yet any clear evidence for teratogenic effects of antidepressants, and nowadays we cannot but speculate on their possible adverse effects later in life. I think that the more classical tricyclic antidepressants should still be used in pregnant women.

J.W. Olney: As a psychiatrist I would like to suggest an additional perspective regarding the use of antidepressant drugs in pregnancy. First I would stress that if the depression is not serious (i.e., suicidal and life threatening), I would not use any treatment other than psychotherapy. If the depression is severe and life threatening, the treatment of choice may be electroconvulsive therapy. There is no evidence that electroconvulsive treatment of the mother is hazardous to the fetus but there is evidence that this mode of therapy is more effective than drugs in rapidly reversing depression and preventing suicide which in the case of a pregnant woman is also infanticide (Avery and Winokur, 1976). Moreover, rapid reversal of the depression may be beneficial for both the mother and baby.

J. Del Rio: As a pharmacologist, I would like to say that electroshock produces marked neurochemical changes in the brain of adult rats, as do chronic antidepressants (Sulser, 1979; Chiodo and Antelman, 1980; Kellar et al., 1981) I do not know whether maximal electroshock given to pregnant rats would induce also some neurochemical change in the brain of the pups, and this is interesting to investigate. On the other hand, although electroconvulsive therapy is not contraindicated in pregnancy, I think that there is always a certain risk in relation to previous medication.

G.J. Boer: Have you considered that in addition to the changes in receptor number (B_{max}), your treatments during development of the brain have changed post-receptor responses, i.e., have effected the second messenger system? This is anyhow the final message for the target cell on which behavior would be based.

J. Del Rio: Following chronic antidepressant treatment of adult rats, both beta-receptor number and noradrenaline-induced cAMP production are decreased (see review in Sulser, 1979). However, in some cases, e.g., mianserin, only the later response is changed (Mishra et al., 1980). In our study, prenatal exposure of rats to typical or atypical antidepressants, including mianserin, induced in all cases a long-lasting reduction in beta-adrenoreceptor density. In experiments with antidepressants in adult animals, a decreased number of beta-adrenoreceptors is always linked to a decreased sensitivity of the cyclase (Sulser, 1979) so we would expect that the second messenger response would also be affected in our study.

H.H. Swanson: In both your presentation and the one by Mirmiran et al. (Ch. 11, this volume), drugs which in humans counteract a clinical condition, i.e., hypertension or depression, were given to normal rats. You mentioned that depression effected certain neurotransmitters and that these deficits could be reversed by the drugs. Is it not possible, then, that the untreated disease could have more adverse effects on the fetus than the drugs used to treat the disease? Is the normal rat treated with pharmacological doses of drugs a good model for the clinical use of these drugs in human pregnancy?

J. Del Rio: The data from the study of Mann et al. (1986) that I have mentioned show an increased number of beta-adrenoreceptors and serotonergic type 2 receptors in the frontal cortices of suicide victims. These results are of interest because, if all of these suicide victims were indeed depressed subjects, this would provide a rationale for the therapeutic effect of antidepressants. I do not know of course whether this altered number of monoamine receptors would be involved in possible adverse effects on the progeny. With regard to your second question, it would probably be more appropriate to use chronically depressed animals, but I am afraid that no entirely valid animal model of human depression is presently available (cf. Willner, 1984).

J.M. Lauder: Have you looked at the effects of fluoxetine in a teratologic sense in your studies? I ask this because we have found that fluoxetine is a relatively potent teratogen for craniofacial development in cultured mouse embryos (Lauder et al., 1987).

J. Del Rio: In our hands, fluoxetine did not produce any overt teratogenic effect in rats prenatally exposed to the drug but we only used a relatively low dose of 3 mg/kg/day.

References

Avery, D. and Winokur, G. (1976) Mortality in depressed patients with electroconvulsive therapy and antidepressants. *Arch. Gen. Psychiatr.* 33: 1029–1037.

Chiodo, L. A. and Antelman, S. M. (1980) Electroconvulsive shock: Progressive dopamine autoreceptor subsensitivity independent of repeated treatment. *Science* 210: 799–801.

Gilman, A. G., Goodman, L. S. and Goodman, A. (1980) *The Pharmacological Basis of Therapeutics*, MacMillan Publishing Co., New York, p. 420.

Kellar, K. J., Cascio, C. S., Butler, J. A. and Kurtzke, R. N. (1981) Differential effects of electroconvulsive shock and antidepressant drugs on serotonin-2 receptors in rat brain. *Eur. J. Pharmacol.* 69: 515–518.

Lauder, J. M., Tamir, H. and Sadler, T. (1987) Sites of serotonin uptake and binding protein immunoreactivity in the cultured mouse embryo. Roles in morphogenesis? *Soc. Neurosci. Abstr.* 13: 254.

Mann, J. J., Stanley, M., McBride, A. and McEwen, B. S. (1986) Increased serotonin-2 and beta-adrenergic receptor binding in the frontal cortices of suicide victims. *Arch. Gen. Psychiatr.* 43: 954–959.

Mishra, R., Janowsky, A. and Sulser, F. (1980) Action of mianserin and zimelidine on the norepinephrine receptor coupled adenylate cyclase system in brain: subsensitivity without reduction in beta-adrenergic receptor binding. *Neuropharmacology* 19: 983–987.

Sulser, F. (1979) New perspectives on the mode of action of antidepressant drugs. *Trends Pharmacol. Sci.* 1: 92–94.

Willner, P. (1984) The validity of animal models of depression. *Psychopharmacology* 83: 1–16.

G.J. Boer, M.G.P. Feenstra, M. Mirmiran, D.F. Swaab and F. Van Haaren
Progress in Brain Research, Vol. 73
© 1988 Elsevier Science Publishers B.V. (Biomedical Division)

CHAPTER 13

Placental and blood element neurotransmitter receptor regulation in humans: potential models for studying neurochemical mechanisms underlying behavioral teratology

Bruce D. Perry

Department of Psychiatry, Division of Child and Adolescent Psychiatry and The Harris Center for Developmental Studies, The University of Chicago School of Medicine, 5841 S. Maryland Ave., Chicago, IL 60637, USA

Introduction

Pre- and perinatal exposure to drugs or chemicals can result in disruption of fetal growth often causing some developmental abnormality in the newborn. In recent years a number of investigators have determined that some of these developmental alterations do not manifest themselves as grossly obvious physical abnormalities but as subtle behavioral changes (Brent, 1974; Hutchings, 1978; Vorhees et al., 1979; Coyle et al., 1980). This 'behavioral' teratogenesis is clearly related to alterations of neural development (neuroteratology). The specific mechanisms underlying behavioral teratology in humans are unknown but research in animal models has demonstrated that low, non-neurotoxic doses of many psychoactive drugs can result in behavioral or functional teratogenesis. Many of the compounds demonstrated to be functional teratogens are known to have specific, selective high-affinity interactions at neurotransmitter receptors, or alter the intra-synaptic level of endogenous receptor agonist. Neurotransmitter/hormone receptor-mediated communication plays a key role in neuronal migration and differentiation (Sidman and Rakic, 1973; Deskin et al., 1981). Disruption of

'normal' receptor-mediated signals would be expected to alter development of the CNS and, potentially, alter the behavioral repertoire of the developing organism.

Examining the specific role played by neurotransmitter receptors in CNS development has been possible in animal models or cell culture preparations. Studying receptor-mediated mechanisms of neurochemical teratogenesis in humans has been difficult. The purpose of the present chapter is to describe studies of neurotransmitter receptor regulation in humans under conditions which may model those seen in neurochemical teratogenesis in an attempt to begin to study the critical role that the developmental milieu plays in determining the ultimate functional output (including behavior) of the developed human CNS.

Background

Alterations of the microenvironment (i.e., changing the timing, concentration or nature of the hormone or neurochemical afferentation of the developing neuron) can permanently alter the phenotypic neurochemistry of the cell (e.g., Lumsden and Davies, 1986; Helman et al., 1987). This has been demonstrated in cell culture systems in which exposure to, for example, nerve growth factor (NGF; Thoenen and Barde, 1980), gluco-corticoids (Helman et al., 1987), opiate antago-nist (Tempel et al., 1986) or other psychoactive drugs (Wolfe et al., 1981) results in the develop-ment of atypical cellular neurochemistry. Trans-plantation of cholinergic neurons to a 'permissive' environment, for example, results in phenotypic alteration of the neurons; they begin to manifest properties of adrenergic neurons (Coulombe and Bronner-Fraser, 1986). In primary cell culture reaggregates from neonatal murine telencephalon, the development of neurochemical properties of specific neuronal systems (e.g., dopamine-con-taining cells) are determined, in part, by the speci-fic 'microenvironment' provided by the brain region with which these cells are co-aggregated (Hemmendinger et al., 1981; Heller et al., 1983).

Similarly, using intact animal models, a num-ber of investigators have demonstrated specific alterations in certain CNS neurotransmitter sys-tems following administration of drug (or hor-mone) in the perinatal period. Prenatal opiate exposure has been demonstrated to change a variety of CNS neurochemical parameters (Peters, 1977), including ornithine decarboxylase levels (Slotkin et al., 1976), cortical adrenergic and opiate receptors (Tsang and Ng, 1980; Wang et al., 1986) and various parameters of the central norepinephrine system in rats (Slotkin et al., 1979; Sobrian, 1977; Zagon and McLaughlin, 1983). Prenatal exposure to diazepam alters the neurochemistry of central noradrenergic (Kellogg and Retell, 1986) and opiate systems (Watanabe et al., 1983) in the developed rat. Other drugs (among many) which result in specific neuro-chemical alterations in animals following peri-natal administration include phenobarbital (Gup-ta et al., 1980), reserpine ostensibly via gluco-corticoids (Jonakait et al., 1980), thyroid hor-mone (Patel et al., 1980), chlorpromazine (Ordy et al., 1966), amphetamine (Seliger, 1974), fen-fluramine (Vorhees et al., 1979), imipramine (Jason et al., 1981), naloxone (Zagon and McLaughlin, 1983), propoxyphene (Vorhees et al., 1979), phencyclidine (Tonge, 1973) and

other centrally acting drugs (Werboff and Kesner, 1963; Rosengarten and Friedhoff, 1979). In all of these models of neuroteratology, a likely mecha-nism by which the 'teratogen' acts is by changing intracellular functioning either directly via high-affinity interactions with specific receptor/effector systems or by altering neurotransmission and, in-directly, receptor/effectors. The critical timing of this intracellular change can determine the man-ner in which the cell differentiates and change the phenotypic properties of the developed neuron.

In parallel with the many studies examining the specific neurochemical alterations associated with exposing the developing CNS to centrally active drugs, the long-term functional concomi-tants have been examined as well. Many of the same pre- and perinatal drug exposures that result in neuroteratology result in 'behavioral' terato-genesis, among them methadone (Zagon and McLaughlin, 1978), phenothiazines (Werboff and Kesner, 1963), propoxyphene (Vorhees et al., 1979), morphine (Sobrian, 1977), chlorpromazine (Ordy et al., 1966), diazepam (Kellogg et al., 1980), imipramine (Jason et al., 1981) and pheno-barbital (Gupta et al., 1980). Implicit in these studies is that the prenatal drug exposure has resulted in neuroteratology in the CNS neuro-chemical systems mediating the altered behaviors.

In humans, studies of the behaviors of infants exposed in utero to drugs of abuse have suggested 'behavioral' teratogenesis. Infants prenatally ex-posed to opiates during pregnancy show behav-ioral abnormalities on the Brazelton Neonatal Assessment Scale (Chasnoff et al., 1980; Kron et al., 1975), disturbed sleep architecture (Dinges et al., 1980), and long-term perceptual and social-ization difficulties (Wilson et al., 1979) among other differences from 'control' populations (Ting et al., 1975; Kandall and Gartner, 1977; House-holder et al., 1982). Prenatal exposure to phen-cyclidine appears to influence neonatal 'irrita-bility' (Chasnoff et al., in press).

While these studies suggest that 'behavioral' teratogenesis occurs in humans, few studies have comprehensively examined subtle behavioral effects in children following prenatal exposure to centrally active compounds. Even fewer have addressed the neurochemistry which may underlie the 'behavioral' teratogenesis. Examining the mechanisms of behavioral teratology in humans has been difficult. In animal models one can control the prenatal environment, administer a drug, follow the behavior of the offspring, and do detailed neurochemical examinations of the CNS, clearly not possible in humans. Unfortunately, many mothers do take centrally active drugs (usually illicit) during pregnancy. In the early 1980s, we began studying the neurochemistry of receptor regulation in peripheral tissues (placenta and platelets) following perinatal drug exposure in substance-abusing mothers and their children. These studies, described in this chapter, assume that any observed neurochemical alterations seen in the placental or platelet neurotransmitter receptors which could be attributed to the chronic low-level psychotropic drug exposure might mirror similar changes in those same neurotransmitter receptor-effector systems in the CNS. The results of these studies are suggestive but overall demonstrated the complexities and frustrations inherent in neurochemical studies (particularly static or single-time studies) in human populations. A second set of experiments described in this chapter is an attempt to develop more physiological, dynamic assays of receptor regulation that can be employed in longitudinal clinical studies. The promise of studies of this sort is the potential to follow a high-risk population (e.g., offspring of drug-dependent mothers) over time in conjunction with standardized clinical rating tools and measures to assess 'behavioral' teratogenesis along with our neurochemical measures.

Placental neurotransmitter receptor studies

Screening studies

When these studies began in 1980, little work had been done previously with neurotransmitter receptors in placental tissues (see Schocken et al., 1980; Valette et al., 1980). In order to determine

which of the transmitter receptors would be characterized and followed, a series of screening studies in 'control' placentas was performed to determine the specific binding of a set of radio-ligands specific for neurotransmitter receptors of interest (Perry et al., 1984). These studies demonstrated small-to-moderate amounts of specific binding for tritiated quinuclidinylbenzilate (QNB), lysergic acid diethylamide (LSD), prazosin (PRAZ), spiroperidol and naloxone (NAL) (using modifications of the methods of Yamamura and Snyder, 1975; Peroutka and Snyder, 1979; Greengrass and Bremner, 1979; Pert and Snyder, 1973). Higher levels of specific binding were found for [^{3}H]rauwolscine (RAUW) and [^{125}I]cyanopindolol (ICYP) (Perry and U'Prichard, 1981; Engel et al., 1981). Characterization of the PRAZ, ICYP, NAL and RAUW binding sites in control placental tissue was performed to ensure that the binding of each ligand was specific for the receptor of interest. Competition studies indeed confirmed that placental RAUW, ICYP, PRAZ and NAL specific binding was alpha$_2$-, beta-, and alpha$_1$-adrenergic and mu-opiate specific, respectively.

Labor and receptor down-regulation

Single concentration assays in controls revealed that 30% higher concentrations of RAUW, NAL and ICYP binding were found in placentas from scheduled cesarean deliveries (no labor) when compared to either 'regular' vaginal deliveries (mean labor = 8 h) or cesarians performed following a difficult labor (mean labor = 16 h). Limited saturation studies in controls demonstrated significant differences (see Table 1) in the apparent number (B_{max}) of PRAZ, RAUW, ICYP and NAL placental binding sites seen in scheduled cesarean deliveries compared to 'emergency' cesareans (70% fewer PRAZ-, 40–50% fewer RAUW-, ICYP- and NAL-labeled sites). Placental tissue from vaginal deliveries demonstrated values intermediate to those of scheduled and 'emergency' cesareans. No statistically significant differences in the apparent affinity (K_d) of

TABLE 1

Adrenergic and opiate receptor binding sites in human placental membranes obtained from normal or cesarean delivery

	n	PRAZ		RAUW		ICYP		NAL	
		K_d	B_{max}	K_d	B_{max}	K_d	B_{max}	K_d	B_{max}
Cesarean, scheduled	5	0.57 ± 0.05	77 ± 16	2.1 ± 0.9	43 ± 12	0.06 ± 0.02	165 ± 34	1.2 ± 0.3	43 ± 5
Vaginal	8	0.45 ± 0.21	36 ± 13	2.8 ± 1.1	30 ± 10	0.10 ± 0.04	133 ± 25	1.0 ± 0.4	30 ± 6
Cesarean, emergency	4	0.49 ± 0.22	24 ± 9[a]	1.6 ± 0.4	21 ± 4[a]	0.08 ± 0.03	110 ± 12[a]	1.1 ± 0.2	27 ± 7[a]

Values represent means $\pm$ S.E.M. from 4–8 experiments each performed in triplicate. Five to seven concentrations of radioligand were incubated with placental membranes as described in Perry et al. (1984). For each ligand, concentration ranges were selected to bind to the 'high-affinity' component of binding.
K_d values for all ligands are in nM and all B_{max} values are in fmol/mg protein.
[a] $P < 0.05$ using Student's t-test.

the ligands for the placental binding sites were seen.

This observed down-regulation of placental opiate and adrenergic receptors in the 'control' population during labor was felt to be due to the massive outpouring of catecholamines and opioid peptides (e.g., beta-endorphin; Houck et al., 1980) seen during labor and delivery. The process of labor, particularly for primigravid women, may take 18–48 h, a period clearly long enough to induce down regulation in the adrenergic and mu-opiate receptor in other tissues (see Harden, 1983). In general, these results suggested that the longer and more difficult the labor and delivery, the more down-regulated the receptors (see Table 1). This raises a number of issues, including the role that the length of labor would play in the process of acquiring a suitable, reproducible 'control' set of radioligand binding parameters in placenta to be used in any group or case by case comparisons. A more interesting issue is the possibility of functional concomitants of the down-regulated (and likely desensitized) receptor/effector systems induced by the long labor. Are the findings in placenta mirrored in the CNS and, if so, do they play a role in the phenotypic expres-

sion of developing neuronal systems? The relationship between psychiatric disorder and 'difficulty of birth' has long been debated. Indeed, in studies of schizophrenics and other major neuropsychiatric disorders, longer labor (Jacobsen and Kenny, 1980) and pregnancy and birth complications (Taylor et al., 1985) are found more frequently than in control comparison groups. Is difficult birth (and the 'neurochemical' milieu associated with it) a significant 'expressor' of a 'genetically predisposed' set of maladaptive or restricted behaviors such as psychiatric disorder? Do short-term exposures to these levels of agonist have permanent effects, are there critical, more vulnerable periods for certain neurochemical systems around birth? What effects would long-term prenatal exposure to 'higher than control' levels of catecholamine (and other subtle neuroendocrinopathies) seen in affective disorders (Roy et al., 1985) have on the development and phenotypic expression of receptors? The demonstration of significant, labor-related placental receptor down-regulation, which may be mirrored in the CNS, suggests a neurochemical mechanism worthy of further study in relation to these questions.

Placental receptor 'regulation' following prenatal drug exposure

Following the initial characterization studies described above, placental tissue was collected from a wide variety of substance-abusing women (Perry et al., 1984). In order to attempt to control for the labor-related receptor regulation, all substance-abuse placentas were from vaginal deliveries (mean labor of 10 h). Control and substance-abuse mothers were comparable with regard to socioeconomic, age, race, pregravid health and prenatal health care characteristics. The experimental population was subdivided into five major groups, depending upon the specific drug of abuse: (a) opiate, primarily methadone-maintenance mothers (some of whom used heroin i.v. during the first trimester), (b) ethanol, moderate to heavy ethanol abusers (2–6 1 ounce drinks per day), (c) amphetamine, 10–100 mg/day during the majority of the pregnancy, and (d) phencyclidine, unquantified abuse during the entire pregnancy, and (e) polysubstance abuse, generally a combination of ethanol, marijuana and opiates. All substance-abuse mothers were cigarette smokers, while 30% of the controls smoked.

RAUW, ICYP, PRAZ and NAL saturation isotherms were generated in 'substance-abuse' placentas (see Fig. 1). No significant population differences in the affinity (K_d) of any of the ligands for binding sites were seen (Table 2). In general the B_{max} values obtained in the substance-abuse groups were different from controls; however, within-group differences were also large (e.g., RAUW binding, opiate subject 1 = 80 fmol/mg protein, opiate subject 2 = 22 fmol/mg protein). These results were much more variable than those obtained in 'control' tissues. In the opiate group ICYP binding sites (beta-adrenergic) appeared to be decreased from 133 to 56 fmol/mg protein and NAL binding sites (mu-opiate) increased from 30 to 66 fmol/mg protein. The ethanol population appeared to have few differences from control except a possible decrease in PRAZ (alpha$_1$-adrenergic) binding sites from 36 to 15 fmol/mg protein. The polysubstance abuse group had a decrease in RAUW binding sites (alpha$_2$-adrenergic). Within-group variability was great (see the S.E.M. values in Table 2), with some subjects having near-normal values for each receptor but with others demonstrating very large differences

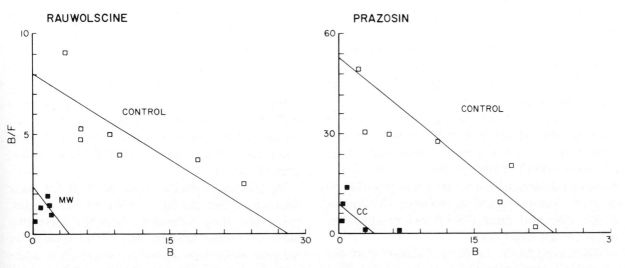

Fig. 1 Scatchard transformations of rauwolscine and prazosin saturation isotherms in placental tissue from 'ethanol-abusing' and 'control' women (from Perry et al., 1984). MW and CC represent placental tissue from two ethanol-abusing patients (closed squares). Control tissue (open squares). Values represent one experiment performed in triplicate. B/F: bound/free radioligand.

TABLE 2

Adrenergic and opiate receptor binding sites in human placental membranes from vaginal deliveries of substance-abusing mothers

	n	PRAZ		RAUW		ICYP		NAL	
		K_d	B_{max}	K_d	B_{max}	K_d	B_{max}	K_d	B_{max}
Control	8	0.45 ± 0.21	36 ± 13	2.8 ± 1.1	30 ± 10	0.10 ± 0.04	133 ± 25	1.0 ± 0.4	30 ± 6
Opiate	6	0.51 ± 0.13	23 ± 12	1.7 ± 0.4	33 ± 26	0.12 ± 0.10	56 ± 21	1.7 ± 0.5	66 ± 36
Ethanol	4	1.00 ± 0.11	15 ± 13	2.1 ± 0.7	21 ± 20	0.09 ± 0.03	111 ± 24	1.8 ± 0.3	35 ± 12
Polysubstance	4	0.55 ± 0.11	32 ± 10	1.7 ± 0.4	16 ± 10	0.07 ± 0.05	143 ± 65	1.4 ± 0.5	40 ± 23
Amphetamine	2	–	–	2.2 ± 0.1	133 ± 51	0.14 ± 0.04	122 ± 23	0.9	91
Phencyclidine	1	–	–	1.1	62	no binding detected		1.6	51

Values represent means $\pm$ S.E.M. for the number of experiments signified, each performed in triplicate. See further legend Table I.

K_d values are in nM and B_{max} values are in fmol/mg protein. B_{max} values of substance-abuse populations were so variable that statistical comparison to control values was deferred.

from control in binding (see ICYP binding for the phencyclidine subject and Fig. 1).

The demonstration of 'altered' adrenergic and mu-opiate receptors in the substance-abusing population is difficult to comment on definitively because of the lack of consistent within-group findings. This lack of consistent differences from control implies that a number of superimposing variables, including the use of psychotropic drugs, influence the expression of the receptors examined. In this regard, the current number of subjects was too small to accurately assess the influence of such factors as (a) the exact dosage and schedule of illicit drug use, (b) the specific timing of the drug use during pregnancy (some mothers abused more heavily during the first trimester) or (c) maternal 'emotional' state (Ferreira, 1965). These preliminary results do, however, demonstrate that prenatal exposure to centrally active drugs does influence the way in which placental (and CNS?) neurotransmitter receptors are expressed.

The comparison of these findings with the existing animal literature on brain receptor changes following prenatal drug use reveals some interesting findings which raise further questions

regarding the mechanisms responsible for the expression of placental receptors. In our studies on the effects of perinatal methadone on alpha$_2$-adrenergic and opioid receptors in rats two general conclusions were that the effects of methadone on brain receptor expression were dependent upon the brain region examined and the timing of the exposure to methadone (see Wang et al., 1986). In contrast to the increased values obtained in human placental tissues (Table 2), fewer opiate binding sites were seen in both hypothalamus and cortex of rats prenatally exposed to methadone. Fewer cortical alpha$_2$ binding sites were also seen following prenatal methadone in rat (Wang et al., 1986) but in the opiate-abuse human group no difference from control was observed in placental RAUW binding sites (Table 2).

A number of factors may account for these differences, not the least of which are species, tissue and drug differences between these two models. Understanding the determinants of receptor expression, however, would allow a less speculative interpretive comparison of these data. Currently the developmental determinants of neurotransmitter receptor expression in neural tissues are not well understood. Studies have suggested that at certain stages of development, the expression of a set of neurotransmitter receptors is determined, in part, by the presence of the neurotransmitter active at that receptor/effector system. Higher amounts of transmitter lead to higher concentrations of the receptor expressed in the membrane (e.g., Slotkin et al., 1979). After a certain, as yet uncharacterized, point in development the amount of receptor expressed can be decreased by higher levels of transmitter (see Wolfe et al., 1981; Tempel et al., 1986). One assumes that at the earliest point of synaptogenesis, the cell expresses receptors which have been able to 'communicate' with the cell, and will not express receptors for which there has been no 'signal'. Following maturation of the synapse, the more familiar homeostatic mechanisms which determine membrane receptor expression (i.e., agonist-induced down-regulation) come into play and excesses of agonist or antagonist regulate receptor/effector mechanisms as in the adult. The nature of CNS development (caudal to rostral) then, dictates that the same treatment (i.e., drug exposure) will result in different effects in different regions when given at the same point in development, and further, more important, that the effects of any drug exposure are exquisitely sensitive to the stage of CNS development. One might predict then, for example, that third-trimester exposure to a sympathomimetic (causing increased noradrenergic agonism) might increase the number of adrenergic receptors expressed in cortical tissues where synaptogenesis would be at a relatively less developed stage, and on the other hand decrease the number of medullary-pontine adrenergic receptors where local synaptogenesis and receptor-effector functioning would be at a more mature stage.

The studies in placental tissues provided some preliminary evidence to suggest that, under certain well-controlled conditions, peripheral receptor studies might provide a useful neurochemical 'marker' by which possible neurochemical dysfunction related to 'behavioral teratogenesis' could be examined. In order to follow the development of behavior (and the possibility of teratogenesis) in these high-risk offspring, longitudinal studies are needed and, if receptor-effector functioning was to be the neurochemical marker employed, other tissues than placenta would have to be used. The next section therefore describes platelet alpha$_2$-adrenergic receptor assays designed to allow longitudinal studies of receptor-effector functioning in clinical populations which, when coupled with behavioral assessments using standardized clinical rating tools, will provide a more powerful paradigm for examining neurochemical and 'behavioral' teratogenesis in human populations.

Platelet alpha$_2$-adrenergic receptor regulation

As with alpha$_2$-receptors in other tissues, there are multiple membrane components of the platelet alpha$_2$-adrenergic receptor-effector system: (a) the receptor/recognition site (R) with the agonist (and antagonist) binding sites, and (b) the Ni component, a protein heterotrimer which links the R and the catalytic moiety of adenylate cyclase (AC). In radioligand binding studies, the free R is labeled with low affinity by agonists. This binding site is also called the alpha$_2$-(L) affinity state. The R-Ni complex is labeled with higher affinity by agonists, thus it is called the alpha$_2$-(H) affinity state. The antagonist RAUW labels these sites with inverse affinities (see Perry and U'Prichard, 1984): the high-affinity component of RAUW binding is the free R (or alpha$_2$-(L) affinity state), while the low affinity component of RAUW binding is the R-Ni complex (or alpha$_2$-(H) affinity state). In the placental studies (see above), apparent agonist-induced 'down-regulation' had been observed for the alpha$_2$-receptors. The following studies describe a more detailed examination of the alpha$_2$-adrenergic receptor-effector changes under conditions of chronic agonist exposure in a clinical population.

Chronic agonist exposure: PTSD

Post-traumatic stress disorder (PTSD) is a psychiatric disorder characterized by (among

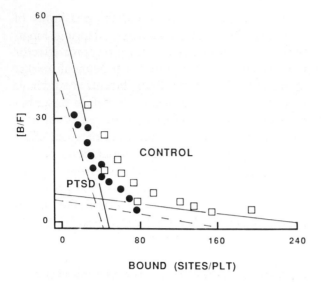

BOUND (SITES/PLT)

Fig. 2 Representative Scatchard transformation of [³H]-rauwolscine (RAUW) specific binding in platelet membranes in post-traumatic stress disorder (PTSD). Platelet membranes were prepared from a control (open squares) and a PTSD (closed circles) subject and the RAUW saturation study was performed between 0.12 and 40.0 nM as described previously (Perry and U'Prichard, 1984). Data were analysed using LIGAND (Munson and Rodbard, 1980; McPherson, 1985); the two components of binding are indicated by the lines (control: continuous line, PTSD: broken line). PLT: platelet, B/F: bound/free radioligand.

other things) symptoms of increased sympathetic arousal and lability (Am. Psych. Assoc., 1980; Horowitz et al., 1980). Kosten et al. (1987) have demonstrated that these subjects have chronically elevated urinary catecholamines, probably secondary to elevated circulating catecholamines. The platelet alpha$_2$-adrenergic receptor-effector systems in this population have been exposed chronically to these elevated levels of catecholamine, offering an opportunity to examine the effects of chronic 'higher than control' agonist exposure on the alpha$_2$-adrenergic receptor (see Perry et al., 1987).

Saturation studies using [³H]RAUW (Fig. 2, Table 3) demonstrate fewer platelet alpha$_2$-adrenergic receptors in this population (from 230 to 136 sites/platelet). Furthermore, LIGAND analysis of the RAUW saturation isotherm reveals two sites of interaction (see curvilinear Scatchard in Fig. 2.) for both control and PTSD subjects. No population differences are seen in the affinity (K_d) of RAUW for either site. The observed decrease in total number of RAUW sites is due to fewer of the site 2 (alpha$_2$-(H)) in the PTSD subjects (Table 2). Similar findings are seen by examining (−)-epinephrine competition studies (Table 4). Epinephrine appears to be a less potent inhibitor of RAUW specific binding in the

TABLE 3

Platelet alpha$_2$-adrenergic receptor affinity states determined by rauwolscine saturation studies in post-traumatic stress disorder (PTSD)

	n	Site 1		Site 2		Total sites	Ratio of sites[b]
		K_d	B_{max}	K_d	B_{max}		
Control	24	0.40 ± 0.16	24 ± 11	27 ± 9	205 ± 94	230 ± 93	13 ± 6
PTSD	21	0.44 ± 0.19	47 ± 27[a]	25 ± 9	112 ± 41[a]	136 ± 52[a]	23 ± 8[a]

Platelet membranes were incubated with 12 concentrations of RAUW (0.12–40.0 nM) in duplicate for 45 min at 25 °C. Parallel incubations with 100 μM (−)-norepinephrine defined specific binding. K_d values are in nM and B_{max} values are in sites/platelet. Values are means $\pm$ S.D.
[a] $P < 0.02$ using Student's t-test.
[b] Ratio = B_{max} Site 1/B_{max} Site 2 $\times$ 100.

TABLE 4

Platelet alpha$_2$-adrenergic receptor affinity states determined by epinephrine displacement studies in post-traumatic stress disorder (PTSD)

	n	Site 1		Site 2		Ratio[b]
		K_i	% sites	K_i	% sites	
Control	8	142 ± 32	67 ± 4	4.2 ± 2.4	33 ± 4	207 ± 18
PTSD	8	132 ± 23	81 ± 6[a]	3.1 ± 3.3	20 ± 2[a]	413 ± 33[a]

Membranes were incubated with 4.0 nM RAUW and 12 concentrations of unlabeled (−)-epinephrine. K_i values are in nM and K_i and % sites values were computer-derived using LIGAND. Specific binding was defined by 100 μM (−)-norepinephrine.
[a] $P < 0.02$ using Student's t-test.
[b] Ratio = (% sites Site 1/% sites Site 2) × 100.

PTSD membranes: the competition curve is somewhat steeper and shifted to the right. LIGAND analysis of the (−)-epinephrine competition curves revealed two sites of interaction. No population differences in the affinity of (−)-epinephrine for the two sites were seen. More of the total alpha$_2$-adrenergic receptors were in the (−)-epinephrine low-affinity state (alpha$_2$-(L)) and fewer in the high-affinity state (alpha$_2$-(H)) in the PTSD membranes, accounting for the observed apparent decreased potency. Again the observed difference in the relative prevalence of the alpha$_2$ affinity states was reflected by the ratio (as above) in PTSD being twice the control value (see Table 4).

The attempts to look more closely at membrane receptor changes in human platelets following chronic exposure to agonist demonstrated a number of interesting findings similar to those reported for the adrenergic receptor in, for example, placental tissues (Perry et al., 1983): in both, an apparent 'down-regulation' of alpha$_2$-adrenergic receptors was found and could be related to chronic exposure to (agonistic) 'drug'. Chronic exposure to an agonist as in the PTSD subjects also appeared to change the equilibria between the affinity states (R and R-Ni), which is reflected as an increase of the ratio of alpha$_2$-(L) to alpha$_2$-(H) (Table 3). The equilibria between

the multiple affinity states of the alpha$_2$-receptor are complex but in general the ratio of affinity states derived from membrane binding studies is thought to reflect the efficiency of the receptor-effector coupling and therefore is a more physiologically significant measure of receptor-effector functioning (Kent et al., 1980; Supiano et al., 1987). In this case, the equilibria change so that the decrease in total receptor shows up as a selective loss of the R-Ni complex or alpha$_2$-(H) affinity state.

Other clinical states in humans with increased circulating catecholamine have demonstrated similar (but less characterized) results in platelet alpha$_2$-receptors, i.e., congestive heart failure (Weiss et al., 1983), aging (Supiano et al., 1987), hypertension (Hollister et al., 1986) and 'in vivo' administration of catecholamine (Hollister et al., 1981). With regard to neurochemical teratogenesis, a down-regulated, less efficiently coupled system might result in altered neurochemical afferentation and thus phenotypic expression. Indeed, in a brain cell preparation, by changing the timing and 'intensity' of beta-receptor stimulation by exogenous isoproterenol the final developed expression of the beta-adrenergic receptor population is altered (Wolfe et al., 1981).

The next studies demonstrate how agonist exposure, both acute and chronic, can alter the intracellular mechanisms involved in the expression of alpha$_2$-receptors in the membrane.

Acute agonist exposures: 'in vitro' dysregulation studies

The number of receptors present in the membrane and 'available' for agonist is dependent upon a variety of complex intracellular processes (see Fig. 3). Standard radioligand binding assays

will 'freeze' a moment and will reflect a summation of a set of dynamic events. The following studies attempted to examine some of the dynamic processes involved in receptor regulation by using an 'in vitro' incubation of intact platelets with agonist.

Intact, isolated platelets from controls were incubated with (−)-epinephrine for 1, 2.5 and 5 h. Binding studies were performed to assess the

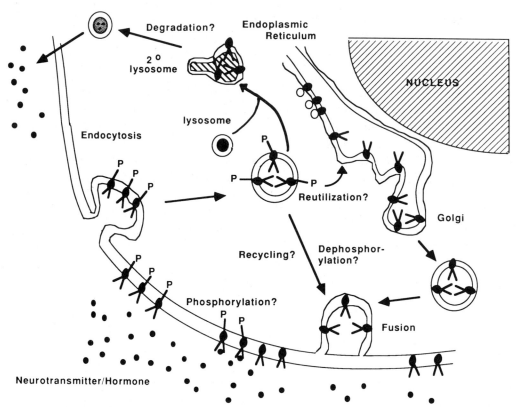

Fig. 3 Schematic representation of the regulation of membrane neurotransmitter/hormone receptors. This cartoon illustrates some of the major steps in the 'life cycle' of many membrane-bound receptors (including beta and probably alpha$_2$-adrenergic). The receptor recognition site is synthesized from mRNA in the endoplasmic reticulum, and post-translational changes (e.g., adding carbohydrate moieties) take place in the Golgi. The 'new' receptors are transported to the cell membrane surface, where they are added to the available pool of receptors. Agonist binds to the receptor, triggering a complex set of interactions with other membrane proteins and second messengers (see text). The receptor may be phosphorylated, which appears to trigger (or at least increase the probability of) internalization. The internalized receptor may be 'recycled', 'reutilized' or degraded. The complex equilibria between the various steps described above determine the amount of receptor in the membrane available to agonist and the fraction of available receptor that is phosphorylated (less active or 'desensitized'?). In addition, the set of second messengers (e.g., cAMP, Ca^{2+}, diacylglycerol) produced by any agonistic stimuli have the potential to ultimately effect other intracellular mediators which have intranuclear effects which help determine the phenotypic expression of the cell. Platelets have no nucleus, but they do have the other intracellular 'machinery' involved in the internalization process.

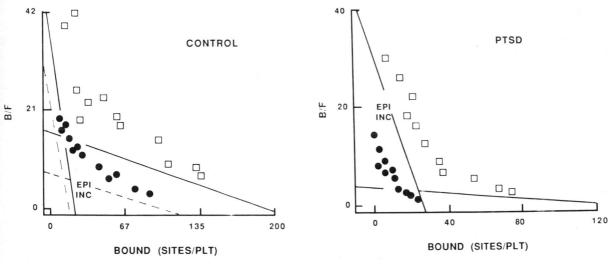

Fig. 4 Representative Scatchard transformations of [³H]rauwolscine specific binding to platelet membranes before and after epinephrine incubation in post-traumatic stress disorder (PTSD). Platelet membranes were prepared from intact platelets following a 5 h incubation with (closed circles, broken lines) or without (open squares, solid lines) 1.0 μM (–)-epinephrine (EPI INC). Saturation studies were then performed as described in the legend to Fig. 2.

changes in receptor binding parameters. Saturation studies demonstrated loss of RAUW specific binding sites (Figs. 4 and 5) in the membranes prepared from both control and PTSD subjects. Again, biphasic saturation isotherms were obtained, and no changes in the affinity of RAUW for the two sites of interaction were observed in either the PTSD or the control membranes following incubation (data not shown). The progressive loss of RAUW binding sites observed in both controls and PTSD during epinephrine incubation was due primarily to the loss of RAUW site 2, or the alpha₂-(H) affinity state: no change was seen in the RAUW site 1 or alpha₂-(L) state. The ratio of affinity states (see above) changed dramatically with incubation (Fig. 5). Competition studies also demonstrated a significant change in the relative prevalence of alpha₂-affinity states with agonist incubation (Table 5), with an increase in epinephrine low-affinity state (alpha₂-(L)) and a decrease in the high affinity state (alpha₂-(H)).

Acute incubation in controls results in a decrease in receptor number, shift in equilibria

between R and R-Ni (reflected as an increase in the ratio) and an apparent 'selective' loss of R-Ni, so that the control binding parameters following

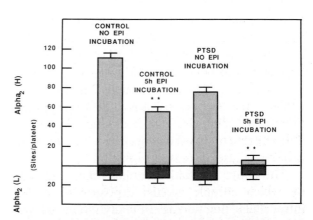

Fig. 5 Loss of alpha₂-(H) sites from platelet membranes following incubation in epinephrine in post-traumatic stress disorder (PTSD). This histogram illustrates the LIGAND-derived B_{max} values (expressed as sites/platelet) obtained following a 5 h incubation of intact, isolated platelets in (–)-epinephrine (EPI; cf. Fig. 4). Values are means from saturation studies in five experiments, each performed in triplicate using tissues from six controls and six PTSD subjects.

TABLE 5

Displacement of rauwolscine specific binding in platelet membranes by epinephrine: changes following 5 h incubation of intact platelets with agonist

	n	Site 1		Site 2		Ratio
		K_i	% sites	K_i	% sites	
Incubation, no agonist	5	154 ± 34	67.0 ± 0.5	3.4 ± 1.1	33.0 ± 0.5	204 ± 25
Incubation, agonist	5	123 ± 33	80.9 ± 2.1	3.1 ± 1.1	19.0 ± 2.1	425 ± 32

Intact platelets were incubated, and epinephrine competition studies were performed as described in Perry et al. (1987). K_i values are in nM $\pm$ S.D. Ratio is (% sites Site 1/% sites Site 2) $\times$ 100.

acute agonist exposure look very much like the PTSD subjects at baseline. These findings are similar to those seen following acute agonist exposure in other receptor-linked adenylate cyclase systems (e.g., Chioffi and El Fakahany, 1986).

These studies also suggested, among other things, that the rate of loss of RAUW binding in the PTSD membranes was increased relative to controls. In order to directly study this, the specific binding of a single concentration of RAUW (3.0–4.0 nM) in platelet membranes prepared from the intact platelets incubated for various times was examined (Table 6). In controls, the rate and extent of loss in RAUW specific binding was quite reproducible, with a 40–50% loss at 5 h, with a $t_{1/2}$ of approximately 2 h. In PTSD subjects, the extent of loss is greater, with approximately a 60–80% decrease from original values at 5 h. The rate of loss showing up as a 2-component process is also increased (Table 6).

The above incubation studies reflect one way by which chronic agonist exposure may alter intracellular functioning. In many intact cell systems (Harden, 1983) and 'in vivo' (Perry et al., 1983), enhanced levels of agonist result in downregulation of adrenergic membrane receptors. Critical in regulating the number of receptors in the membrane is the complex process of receptor 'internalization' (see Fig. 3 and Harden, 1983). The rate of internalization is dependent upon a

variety of factors, among them agonist concentration, duration of exposure, rate of degradation, rate of phosphorylation, and other as yet unidentified processes. The present studies demonstrate that chronic exposure to agonist 'induces', in an unknown fashion, the processes that increase internalization. The PTSD subjects had a more rapid and extensive apparent internalization following agonist incubation which was accompanied by a very large increase in the 'ratio' (more rapidly 'uncoupled' from cyclase; more free R in a membrane preparation and, 'in vivo', probably

TABLE 6

Rate constants of the loss of rauwolscine specific binding from platelet membranes following incubation of intact platelets with agonist: post-traumatic stress disorder (PTSD) vs. control

	n	Component 1	Component 2
Control	8	0.30 ± 0.01	0.13 ± 0.03
PTSD	5	0.72 ± 0.02[a]	0.21 ± 0.01[a]

Rate constants (h^{-1}) were computer-derived using KINETIC (McPherson, 1985). The loss of binding from membranes best fit a 2-component model. Values are means $\pm$ S.E.M. from the number of experiments signified above, each performed in triplicate.
[a] $P < 0.05$ using Student's t-test.

less capable of interacting with Ni). Chronic exposure to high levels of agonist in PTSD results in a 'fatigued' receptor-effector system less capable of tolerating a transient stressor. The platelet alpha$_2$-adrenergic receptor-effector system in the PTSD subjects was 'overtaxed' and easily 'fatigued'. Does this chronic exposure to agonist alter in a more permanent fashion the ability of the cell to express receptor? Permanent intraneuronal changes which change the expression of receptors in the membrane do take place with 'agonism' in mature neuronal systems and provide the molecular basis for 'memory' and learning (Kandel and Schwartz, 1982). Are similar processes taking place in PTSD which may result in the 'fatigued' alpha$_2$-adrenergic system in the CNS? A recent study suggests that this is likely (see Krystal et al., in press). Similar neurochemical mechanisms may be involved in neuroteratology. The functional concomitants of a fatigued system in the developed CNS are unknown but may be related to some of the symptoms seen in PTSD (see Krystal et al., in press), while in the developing CNS they may be related to functional teratogenesis.

Implications, speculations and questions

In the developing human CNS, both in utero and postnatally, the neurochemical 'milieu' plays a role in determining ultimate functional capacity. Brain development in humans continues beyond birth. The role of the 'macro-environment' (including such 'intangibles' as parenting style) in inducing an internal neurochemical milieu in the developing infant, and the subsequent development of the CNS (and behavioral patterns), has been under-explored. The pioneering work of Spitz (1945) with institutionalized, 'under-parented' children and the work of Harlow and Harlow (1962) with maternally deprived primates have demonstrated clearly one end of the spectrum with regard to the behavioral effects of the affectively or somatically deprived postnatal en-

vironment. What are the neuroendocrine or neurochemical concomitants of maternal deprivation (or other postnatal, early developmental experiences) and what role do they play in determining the ultimate phenotypic characteristics of the CNS and, thereby, behavior? The primary and persistent nature of behavioral patterns developed in infancy and childhood is clear. As the environment (macro- and micro-) shapes the ultimate phenotypic expression of neural systems in the developed CNS so it shapes the behavioral patterns which result from this phenotype. The ability to identify certain prenatal and perinatal factors (including drug exposure) that result in neurochemical 'teratology' and, as a result, less adaptive or compromised behaviors suggests that there may be ways to optimize neurochemical 'development' and behavior. Certainly those factors which can be identified that result in an adversely altered neurochemical development should be avoided when possible in pregnant mothers (e.g., use of centrally active agents when not absolutely necessary). In the future, 'preventative' psychiatry may be directed at minimizing factors which may contribute to the expression of any genetically inherited diathesis for a psychiatric disorder.

Summary and future directions

The studies outlined in this chapter attempted to examine possible mechanisms of neurochemical and 'behavioral' teratology in human populations. A goal of this research would be to develop a suitable model in which to examine more closely mechanisms of receptor-mediated alterations in CNS development induced by centrally active substances (exogenous and endogenous) which, when well-characterized, might allow case-by-case longitudinal investigations in high-risk populations (e.g., substance-abuse or psychiatrically ill). The present studies, while preliminary, suggest that placental and blood element receptor regulation in humans is similar to that in other more completely characterized tissues (including neural tissues; see U'Prichard et al., 1983, 1984).

Specific points of interest in these studies include: (a) evidence for the down-regulation of placental adrenergic and opiate receptors by endogenous agonist during labor; (b) regulation (or disruption) of placental neurotransmitter receptors by prenatal exposure to centrally active compounds (drugs of abuse); (c) down-regulation of platelet $alpha_2$-adrenergic receptors in PTSD, presumably a result of chronic endogenous agonist exposure; and, most interestingly, (d) the alteration of intracellular mechanisms related to receptor regulation apparently induced by this chronic 'higher than control' exposure to agonist.

The complexity of the developmental processes involved in determining the ultimate functional capabilities of the CNS dictates that future research directions must include a variety of approaches. The application of peripheral models such as those presented in this chapter must be coupled with appropriate studies in animal and cell culture models. The critical questions regarding the neurochemical processes underlying neuroteratology will need to come from a better understanding of the determinants of normal neural (and behavioral) development. There are probably many molecular mechanisms in a developing neural system which, if 'disturbed' (via receptor-mediated or other processes), will result in a different (though not necessarily dysfunctional) phenotypic expression and, potentially, behavioral repertoire. Preliminary evidence in peripheral models such as placental tissue and platelets shows that neurotransmitter receptor expression (and function?) is influenced by low-level exposure to centrally active substances. This may be a mechanism by which neuroteratology occurs. Interpretation of the results from human studies must be cautious but the complexity of the problems need not preclude careful investigation. Further studies are needed to clarify and extend those presented in this review. In combination with well-controlled extensive longitudinal behavioral measures, these peripheral receptor 'markers' may ultimately provide a method by which both brain development and the molecular processes of receptor regulation may be studied in human populations.

Acknowledgements

The author would like to acknowledge his co-workers and collaborators in the various projects described in this chapter. Drs. Sidney Schnoll, David U'Prichard and Daniel Pesavento participated in the placental receptor studies carried out at Northwestern University in Chicago, IL. Drs. Earl Giller, Jr. and Steven Southwick participated in the platelet dysregulation studies carried out at Yale University in New Haven, CT. Excellent technical assistance was provided by Paul Kussie, Alex Ackles, Janet Giunti and Helen Spencer. These studies were supported in part by an ADAMHA fellowship award MH-08834 to B.P.D., by Veterans Administration funds and by the Harris Center for Developmental Studies at The University of Chicago.

References

American Psychiatric Association (1980) *Diagnostic and Statistical Manual of Mental Disorders* (3rd edn.) (DSM-III), APA Press, Washington, DC, pp. 236–238.

Brent, R.L. (1974) Environmental effects on the embryos and fetuses of experimental animals. *Pediatrics*, 53: 821.

Chasnoff, I.J., Hatcher, R., Burns, W.J. (1980) Early growth patterns of methadone-addicted infants. *Am. J. Dis. Child.*, 134: 1049–1051.

Chasnoff, I.J., Burns, W.J. and Hatcher, R. Phencylidine: effects on the fetus and neonate. *Dev. Pharmacol. Ther.*, in press.

Cioffi, C.L. and El Fakahany, E.E. (1986) Short term desensitization of muscarinic cholinergic receptors in mouse neuroblastoma cells: selective loss of agonist low affinity and pirenzepine high-affinity binding sites. *J. Pharmacol. Exp. Ther.*, 238: 916–923.

Coulombe, J.N. and Bronner-Fraser, M. (1986) Cholinergic neurones acquire adrenergic neurotransmitters when transplanted into an embryo. *Nature*, 324: 569–571.

Coyle, I., Wayner, M. and Singer, M. (1980) Behavioral teratogenesis: a critical evaluation. In T.V.N. Persaud (Ed.), *Advances in the Study of Birth Defects: Vol. 4, Neural and Behavioral Teratogenesis*, Academic Press, New York, pp. 110–129.

Deskin, R., Seidler, F. J., Whitmore, W. L. and Slotkin, T. A. (1981) Development of alpha-noradrenergic and dopaminergic receptor systems depends on maturation of their presynaptic nerve terminals in the rat brain. *J. Neurochem.*, 36: 1683–1690.

Dinges, D. R., Davis, M. M. and Glass, P. (1980) Fetal exposure to narcotics: neonatal sleep as a measure of nervous system disturbance. *Science*, 209: 619–621.

Engel, G., Hoyer, D., Berthold, R. and Wayne, H. (1981) [^{125}Iodo]cyanopindolol, a new ligand to beta-adrenoceptors: identification and quantitation of subclasses of beta-adrenoceptors in guinea pig. *Naunyn-Schmied. Arch Pharmacol.*, 317: 227–285.

Ferreira, A. J. (1965) Emotional factors in prenatal environment: a review. *J. Nerv. Ment. Dis.*, 141: 108–118.

Greengrass, P. and Bremner, R. (1979) Binding characteristics of [^{3}H]prazosin to rat brain alpha$_1$-adrenergic receptors. *Eur. J. Pharmacol.*, 55: 323–326.

Gupta, C., Sonawane, B. R., Yaffe, S. J. and Shapiro, B. H. (1980) Phenobarbital exposure in utero: alterations in female reproductive function in rats. *Science*, 208: 508–510.

Harden, T. K. (1983) Agonist-induced desensitization of the beta-adrenergic receptor-linked adenylate cyclase. *Pharmacol. Rev.*, 35: 5–32.

Harlow, H. F. and Harlow, M. K. (1962) Social deprivation in monkeys. *Sci. Am.*, 207: 136–146.

Heller, A., Hoffmann, P. C., Kotake, C. and Shalaby, I. (1983) Regulation of the morphologic and biochemical differentiation of embryonic dopamine neurons in vitro. *Psychopharm. Bull.*, 19: 311–316.

Helman, L. J., Thiele, C. J., Linehan, W. M., Nelkin, B. D., Baylin, B. and Israel, M. A. (1987) Molecular markers of neuroendocrine development and evidence of environmental regulation. *Proc. Natl. Acad. Sci. USA*, 84: 2336–2339.

Hemmendinger, L. M., Garber, B. B., Hoffman, P. C. and Heller, A. (1981) Target neuron-specific process formation by embryonic mesencephalic dopamine neurons in vitro. *Proc. Natl. Acad. Sci. USA*, 78: 1264–1268.

Hollister, A. S., Fitzgerald, G. A. and Robertson, D. (1981) Reduction in platelet alpha$_2$-receptor agonist affinity by endogenous and exogenous catecholamines in man. *Clin. Res.*, 29: 819A.

Hollister, A. S., Onrot, J., Lonce, S., Nadeau, J. L. J. and Robertson, D. (1986) Plasma catecholamine modulation of adrenoreceptor agonist affinity and sensitivity in normotensive and hypertensive human platelets. *J. Clin. Invest.*, 77: 1416–1421.

Horowitz, M. J., Wilner, N., Kaltredder, N. and Alvarez, W. (1980) Signs and symptoms of post-traumatic stress disorder. *Arch. Gen. Psychiatry*, 37: 85–92.

Houck, J. C., Kimball, C., Chang, C., Pedigo, N. W. and Yamamura, H. (1980) Placental beta-endorphin-like peptides. *Science*, 207: 78–80.

Householder, J., Hatcher, R., Burns, W. and Chasnoff, I. (1982) Infants born to narcotic-addicted mothers. *Psychol. Bull.*, 453–468.

Hutchings, D. E. (1978) Behavioral teratology: embryopathic and behavioral effects of drugs during pregnancy. In G. Gottlieb (Ed.), *Studies on the Development of Behavior and the Nervous System*, Academic Press, New York, pp. 7–30.

Jacobsen, B. and Kinney, D. K. (1980) Perinatal complications in adopted and non-adopted schizophrenics and their controls: preliminary results. *Acta Psychiatr. Scand.*, (Suppl. 285) 62: 337–346.

Jason, K. M., Cooper, T. B. and Friedman, E. (1981) Prenatal exposure to imipramine alters early behavioral development and beta-adrenergic receptors in rats. *J. Pharmacol. Exp. Ther.*, 217: 461–466.

Jonakait, G. M., Bohn, M. C. and Black, I. B. (1980) Maternal glucocorticoid hormones influence neurotransmitter phenotypic expression in embryos. *Science*, 210: 551–553.

Kandall, S. R. and Gartner, L. M. (1977) The narcotic-dependent mother: fetal and neonatal consequences. *Early Hum. Dev.*, 1: 159–169.

Kandel, E. R. and Schwartz, J. H. (1982) Molecular biology of an elementary form of learning: modulation of transmitter release by cyclic AMP. *Science*, 218: 433–443.

Kellogg, C. K. and Retell, T. M. (1986) Release of [^{3}H]norepinephrine: alteration by early developmental exposure to diazepam. *Brain Res.*, 366: 137–144.

Kellogg, C., Tervo, D., Ison, J., Parisi, T. and Miller, R. (1980) Prenatal exposure to diazepam alters behavioral development in rats. *Science*, 207: 205–207.

Kent, R. S., DeLean, A. and Lefkowitz, R. J. (1980) A quantitative analysis of beta-adrenergic receptor interactions: resolution of high and low affinity states of the receptor by computer modeling of ligand binding data. *Mol. Pharmacol.*, 17: 14–21.

Kosten, T. R., Mason, J. W., Giller, E. L., Ostroff, R. B. and Harkness, L. (1987) Sustained urinary norepinephrine and epinephrine elevation in post-traumatic stress disorder. *Psychoneuroendocrinology*, 12: 13–20.

Kron, R. E., Finnegan, L. P., Kaplan, S. L., Litt, M. and Phoenix, M. D. (1975) The assessment of behavioral change in infants undergoing narcotic withdrawal. Comparative data from clinical and objective methods. *Addict. Dis.*, 2: 257–263.

Krystal, J. H., Kosten, T., Perry, B. D., Southwick, S. M., Mason, J. and Giller, E. L. Neurobiological aspects of post-traumatic stress disorder: review of clinical and preclinical studies. *Behav. Ther.*, in press.

Lumsden, A. G. S. and Davies, A. M. (1986) Chemotropic effect of specific target epithelium in the developing mammalian nervous system. *Nature*, 323: 538–539.

McPherson, G. A. (1985) *KINETIC, EBDA, LIGAND, LOWRY: a collection of radioligand analysis programs, manual.* Elsevier-Biosoft, Elsevier, Amsterdam.

Munson, P.J. and Rodbard, D. (1980) LIGAND: a versatile computerized approach for the characterization of ligand binding systems. *Anal. Biochem.*, 107: 220–239.

Ordy, J.M., Samorajski, T., Collins, R.L. and Rolsten, C. (1966) Prenatal chlorpromazine effects on liver, survival, and behavior of mice offspring. *J. Pharmacol. Exp. Ther.*, 151: 110–116.

Patel, A.J., Smith, R.M., Kingsbury, A.E., Hunt, A. and Balazs, R. (1980) Effects of thyroid states on brain development: muscarinic acetylcholine and GABA receptors. *Brain Res.*, 198: 389–402.

Peroutka, S.J. and Snyder, S.H. (1979) Multiple serotonin receptors: differential binding of [^{3}H]5-hydroxytryptamine, [^{3}H]lysergic acid diethylamide and [^{3}H]spiroperidol. *Mol. Pharmacol.*, 16: 687–699.

Perry, B.D. and U'Prichard, D.C. (1981) [^{3}H]Rauwolscine (alpha-yohimbine): a specific antagonist radioligand for brain alpha$_2$-adrenergic receptors. *Eur. J. Pharmacol.*, 76: 461–464.

Perry, B.D. and U'Prichard, D.C. (1984) Alpha-adrenergic receptors in neural tissues: methods and applications of radioligand binding assays. In P.J. Marangos, I. Campbell and R.M. Cohen (Eds.), *Brain Receptor Methodologies Part A: General Methods and Concepts, Amines and Acetylcholine*, Academic Press, New York, pp. 256–284.

Perry, B.D., Stolk, J.M., Vantini, G., Guchhait, R.B. and U'Prichard, D.C. (1983) Strain differences in rat brain epinephrine synthesis and alpha-adrenergic receptor number: apparent 'in vivo' regulation of brain alpha-adrenergic receptors by epinephrine. *Science*, 221: 1297–1299.

Perry, B.D., Pesavento, D.J., Kussie, P.H., U'Prichard, D.C. and Schnoll, S.H. (1984) Prenatal exposure to drugs of abuse in humans: effects on placental neurotransmitter receptors. *Neurobehav. Toxicol. Teratol.*, 6: 295–301.

Perry, B.D., Southwick, S.M. and Giller, E.L., Jr. (1987) Altered platelet alpha-adrenergic receptor affinity states in post-traumatic stress disorder. *Am. J. Psychiatry*, 144: 1511–1512.

Pert, C.B. and Snyder, S.H. (1973) Properties of opiate-receptor binding in rat brain. *Proc. Natl. Acad. Sci. USA*, 70: 2243–2247.

Peters, M.A. (1977) The effect of maternally administered methadone on brain development in the offspring. *J. Pharmacol. Exp. Ther.*, 203: 340–346.

Rosengarten, H. and Friedhoff, A.J. (1979) Enduring changes in dopamine receptor cells of pups from drug administration to pregnant and nursing rats. *Science*, 203: 1133–1135.

Roy, A., Pickar, D., Linnoila, M. and Potter, W.Z. (1985) Plasma norepinephrine level in affective disorders. *Arch. Gen. Psych.* 42: 1181–1186.

Schocken, D.D., Caron, M.G. and Lefkowitz, R.J. (1980) The human placenta, a rich source of beta-adrenergic receptors: characterization of the receptors in particulate and solubilized preparations. *J. Clin. Endocrinol. Metab.*, 50: 1082–1088.

Seliger, D.L. (1974) Prenatal maternal d-amphetamine effects on emotionality and audiogenic seizure susceptibility of rat offspring. *Dev. Psychobiol.*, 8: 261–268.

Sidman, R.L. and Rakic, P. (1973) Neuronal migration, with special reference to developing human brain: a review. *Brain Res.*, 62: 1–35.

Slotkin, T.A., Lau, C. and Bartolome, M. (1976) Effects of neonatal or maternal methadone administration on ornithine decarboxylase activity in brain and heart of developing rats. *J. Pharmacol. Exp. Ther.*, 199: 141–148.

Slotkin, T.A., Whitmore, W.L., Salvaggio, M. and Seidler, F.J. (1979) Perinatal methadone addiction affects the brain synaptic development of biogenic amine systems in the rat. *Life Sci.*, 24: 1223–1230.

Sobrian, S.K. (1977) Prenatal morphine administration alters behavioral development in the rat. *Pharmacol. Biochem. Behav.*, 7: 285–288.

Spitz, R. (1945) Hospitalism: an inquiry into the genesis of psychiatric conditions in early childhood. *Psychoanal. Study Child*, 1: 53–74.

Supiano, M.A., Linares, O.A., Halter, J.B., Reno, K.M. and Rosen, S.G. (1987) Functional uncoupling of the platelet alpha$_2$-adrenergic receptor adenylate cyclase complex in the elderly. *J. Clin. Endocrinol. Metab.*, 64: 1161–1164.

Taylor, D.J., Howie, P.W., Davidson, J., Davidson, D. and Drillen, C.M. (1985) Do pregnancy complications contribute to neurodevelopmental disability? *Lancet*, i: 713–716.

Tempel, A., Crain, S.M., Peterson, E.R., Simon, E.J. and Zukin, R.S. (1986) Antagonist induced opiate receptor upregulation in cultures of fetal mouse spinal cord explants. *Dev. Brain Res.*, 25: 287–291.

Thoenen, H. and Barde, Y.A. (1980) Nerve growth factor. *Physiol. Rev.*, 60: 1284–1335.

Ting, R., Keller, A., Berman, P. and Finnegan, L. (1975) Follow-up studies of infants born to methadone-dependent mothers. *Pediatric Res.*, 8: 346–355.

Tonge, S.R. (1973) Some persistent effects of the pre- and neonatal administration of psychotropic drugs on noradrenaline metabolism in discrete areas of rat brain. *Br. J. Pharmacol.*, 48: 364–365.

Tsang, D. and Ng, S.C. (1980) Effect of antenatal exposure to opiates on the development of opiate receptors in rat brain. *Brain Res.*, 21: 199–206.

U'Prichard, D.C., Mitrius, J.C., Kahn, D.J. and Perry, B.D. (1983) The alpha$_2$-adrenergic receptor: multiple affinity states and regulation of a receptor inversely coupled to adenylate cyclase. In T. Segawa, H.L. Mayamura, K. Kuriyama (Eds.), *The Molecular Pharmacology of Neurotransmitter Receptor Systems: Advances in Biochemical Psychopharmacology, Vol. 36*, Raven Press, New York, pp. 53–75.

U'Prichard, D. C., Perry, B. D., Wang, C. H., Mitrius, J. C. and Kahn, D. J. (1984) Molecular aspects of regulation of alpha$_2$-adrenergic receptors. In E. Usdin, M. Goldstein, P. Georgotas (Eds.), *Frontiers in Neuropsychiatric Research*. MacMillan Press, London, pp. 65–82.

Valette, A., Reme, J. M., Pontonnier, G. and Cros, J. (1980) Specific binding for opiate-like drugs in the placenta. *Biochem. Pharmacol.*, 29: 2657–2661.

Vorhees, C. V., Brunner, R. L. and Butcher, R. E. (1979) Psychotropic drugs as behavioral teratogens. *Science*, 205: 1220–1225.

Wang, C., Pasulka, P., Perry, B. D., Pizzi, W. J. and Schnoll, S. H. (1986) Effect of perinatal exposure to methadone on brain opioid and alpha$_2$-adrenergic receptors. *Neurobehav. Toxicol. Teratol.*, 8: 399–402.

Watanabe, Y., Shibuya, T., Salafsky, B. and Hill, H. F. (1983) Prenatal and postnatal exposure to diazepam: effects on opioid receptor binding in rat brain cortex. *Eur. J. Pharmacol.*, 96: 141–144.

Weiss, R. T., Tobes, M., Wertz, C. E. and Smith, C. B. (1983) Platelet alpha$_2$-adrenoceptors in chronic congestive heart failure. *Am. J. Cardiol.*, 52: 101–105.

Werboff, J. and Kesner, R. (1963) Learning deficits of offspring after administration of tranquilizing drugs to the mothers. *Nature*, 197: 106–107.

Wilson, G. S., McCreary, R., Klan, J. and Baxter, J. C. (1979) The development of preschool children of heroin-addicted mothers: a controlled study. *Pediatrics*, 63: 135–141.

Wolfe, B. B., Augustyn, D. H., Majocha, R. E., Dibner, M. D., Molinoff, P. B., Baldessarini, R. J. and Walton, K. G. (1981) Effects of isoproterenol on the development of beta adrenergic receptors in brain cell aggregates. *Brain Res.*, 207: 174–177.

Yamamura, H. I. and Snyder, S. H. (1975) Muscarinic cholinergic receptor binding in the longitudinal muscle of the guinea pig ileum with [^{3}H]quinuclidinyl benzilate. *Mol. Pharmacol.*, 10: 861–867.

Zagon, I. S. and McLaughlin, P. J. (1978) Perinatal methadone exposure and its influence on the behavioral ontogeny of rats. *Pharmacol. Biochem. Behav.*, 9: 665–672.

Zagon, I. S. and McLaughlin, P. J. (1983) Increased brain size and cellular content in infant rats treated with an opiate antagonist. *Science*, 221: 1179–1180.

Discussion

A. J. Patel: One observes big changes in platelet receptor numbers obtained from the same person at different times. Would you suggest, from your experience, how to normalize these variations?

B. D. Perry: We also have found approximately 20% variability in the 'number' of sites per platelet in individuals. The values which do *not* vary much, unless we observe a state change, are the affinity constants of the ligand for the multiple states of the alpha$_2$-receptor, and, more reliably, the ratio of the two affinity constants. We also find that with extended saturation studies, all measures, including B_{max}, vary much less in an individual.

D. F. Swaab: Did the receptors on the placenta change with gestational age? How did you estimate gestational age in the drug abusers, since they usually seem to deliver preterm?

B. D. Ferry: We did not do enough studies in placental tissues out of the 36–42 week period to assess change with gestational age. I suspect from our preliminary results that we would have seen variable changes, with some systems increasing and others decreasing with gestational age. Gestational age was estimated by ultrasonographic measures such as femur length and head size.

G.J. Boer, M.G.P. Feenstra, M. Mirmiran, D.F. Swaab and F. Van Haaren
Progress in Brain Research, Vol. 73
© 1988 Elsevier Science Publishers B.V. (Biomedical Division)

CHAPTER 14

Benzodiazepines: influence on the developing brain

Carol K. Kellogg

Department of Psychology, University of Rochester, Rochester, NY 14627, USA

Introduction

The concept that drugs elicit their effects through combination with specific receptors was proposed at the turn of this century by Langley (1906). In recent years, neural receptors mediating the pharmacological effects of many neuroactive drugs have been identified. Of particular pertinence to this discussion, specific neural binding sites for the anxiolytic benzodiazepine (BDZ) compounds have been identified (Squires and Braestrup, 1977; Mohler and Okada, 1977), and the interaction of these drugs with their binding sites correlates well with their anxiolytic, anticonvulsant, sedative and muscle-relaxant properties (Braestrup and Squires, 1978). If occupancy of specific neural receptors mediates the actions of neuroactive drugs in adult organisms, then the presence of specific receptors in the developing brain could render the developing brain vulnerable to the presence of exogenous compounds.

Precisely how a drug will influence developing nervous systems cannot be predicted, however, based simply on the presence of recognition sites for the drug. Receptor function depends not only on the presence of a specific, high-affinity recognition site but also on the existence of effector mechanisms that translate the interaction of a drug with its binding site into a response in the receptive cell. Studies on the development of transmitter receptors in the brain indicate that, whereas some early appearing sites are linked to active effector mechanisms, other early appearing receptors are unable to mediate appropriate effector responses (see Miller et al., 1987, for review). Additionally, effector mechanisms present during development may differ from those present in the adult.

The full expression of drug interaction with neural receptors during development will also depend upon the neural interactions that receptive cells make with other neurons and upon the maturational state of specific neural circuitry. Because neuroactive drugs can influence chemical neurotransmission, the developmental profile of specific neurotransmitters may be an important determinant of the effect of early developmental drug exposure. The processes underlying chemical transmission in specific neural populations are known to appear early in fetal rat brain (Coyle, 1977), and these early developing systems respond in a predictable manner to many psychoactive drugs (Coyle and Henry, 1973). A role for these early differentiating chemically defined neurons in regulation of cell proliferation (Patel et al., 1983) or as differentiation signals (Lauder and Krebs, 1978) has been proposed. The complexities of neural development, therefore, make it difficult to predict the consequences of drug exposure during development.

Evidence accumulated from developmental studies using specific neurotoxins to destroy selective neurotransmitter systems, however, has provided important guidelines for designing tests to evaluate the effects of developmental exposure to neuroactive drugs that have specific sites of interaction with the central nervous system (CNS). These studies have indicated that the effects of any drug can be expected to be very selective and dependent upon the timing of exposure. Functional tests that take into account the known pharmacological effects of the drug as well as the known anatomical distribution of the neural sites of interaction are likely to be more sensitive in detecting the effects of developmental drug exposure than behavioral tests which may reflect parallel underlying neural systems (see Miller et al., 1987, for review).

Developmental exposure to BDZs has been associated with neural, physiological and behavioral alterations in both clinical and experimental studies (Weber, 1985). In this review, mechanisms and interactions that may be responsible for these alterations will be presented. We will consider alterations at the level of the receptor itself, biochemical effects that may be mediated by drug-receptor interaction and neural systems that may be influenced. The scope of the discussion will be limited to the presentation of results of research on the effects of in utero exposure to BDZs in rats. An extensive literature also exists on the effect of postnatal exposure to BDZs. The neural mechanisms underlying the functional effects of postnatal exposure in all likelihood will differ from those involved in mediating the effects of prenatal exposure because of the different developmental stage of the organism. The reader is referred to other reviews for a presentation of postnatal exposure (Tucker, 1985).

In utero drug exposure: important considerations

In any study considering the consequences of prenatal drug exposure on the offspring there are difficulties in determining whether any alterations apparent in the offspring are related to a direct action of the drug on the fetus or result from a secondary response in the fetus following a direct action in the dam. In order to develop hypotheses concerning neural alterations resulting from drug-receptor interactions in the fetus, certain information must be obtained that will support a direct action in the fetus.

At the very least, it is necessary to demonstrate the presence of drug in the brains of the offspring following administration of the drug to the dam. We have shown that diazepam (DZ) is present in the brain of the offspring at birth (following administration of DZ at 2.5 mg/kg over gestational days 13–20) and persists for up to 10 days postnatal age (Simmons et al., 1983). Furthermore, Scatchard analysis of ligand binding to BDZ binding sites in the brain of dam and offspring 1 h following an s.c. injection of DZ (2.5 mg/kg) to the dam (on day 20 of gestation) demonstrated a similar effect on binding in the two groups (Pleger and Kellogg, unpublished observation). Under control conditions the K_d of the binding site for the ligand ([^{3}H]flunitrazepam) was 1.5 nM in the dam and 1.47 nM in the fetal brain. However, following DZ, the K_d in both dam and fetal tissue increased; to 4.67 nM in the dam and to 2.14 nM in the fetal tissue. This increase resulted from the presence of unlabelled drug which competed with the radiolabelled ligand for the recognition site. The presence of the drug did not alter density: B_{max} was 1.28 and 1.33 pmol/mg protein in control and injected dams, respectively and 0.44 and 0.40 pmol/mg protein in the fetal tissue. The assumption, therefore, that DZ is at least present in fetal brain and can interact with appropriate binding sites seems justified.

To fully understand the implications that binding of drug to specific sites in fetal brain may have, it will be necessary to demonstrate a response in the fetal brain to the presence of the drug. Studies are currently in progress in our laboratory to evaluate an effector response in fetal tissue following the interaction of DZ with specific binding sites. The results of these studies will assist in understanding the initial mechanisms that may be responsible for long-term consequences.

For interpretation of results obtained in studies of prenatal drug exposure, it is also important to determine the plasma levels of drug achieved in the pregnant dam. This is essential for cross-study as well as cross-species extrapolation. Using ^{14}C-labelled DZ (at a dose of 2.5 mg/kg given s.c. to the dam), the level of radioactivity in the plasma of the dam plateaued at a level of 115 pmol/μl from 1 to 6 h following injection (Simmons, Miller and Kellogg, unpublished observation). Total plasma radioactivity reflects activity in both parent compound and metabolites. If one assumes that 90% of the activity at 1 h is DZ and its active metabolite N-desmethyldiazepam, the plasma level reached is approximately 0.26 μg/ml, which is comparable to levels reported in clinical studies following DZ administration during pregnancy and labor (Yeh et al., 1974; Cree et al., 1973). While the dosages given in experimental studies may seem high when compared to clinical doses, one must keep in mind that the clearance rate of the compound differs between species. Approximately 55% of the total injected drug was eliminated in the feces and urine of the dam over 8 days of exposure to DZ at 2.5 mg/kg/day (Simmons et al., 1983).

Therefore, with respect to prenatal administration of DZ to the pregnant rat, we have demonstrated that the plasma level of drug reached in the dam at the mid-range dose used in most of our studies is not high relative to clinical reports, that DZ is present in the brain of the offspring, and that the drug is capable of interacting with specific neural receptors in fetal brain. For DZ, the hypothesis that neuroreceptors to specific drugs may provide points of access through which drugs may influence the course of neural development seems valid.

The benzodiazepine-GABA receptor complex

Before considering the effects of prenatal BDZ exposure, some background on BDZ binding sites needs to be presented. A major portion of the benzodiazepine recognition sites (BZR) in the CNS appear to be part of a polymolecular complex which contains, in addition to BZR the recognition site for the inhibitory neurotransmitter γ-aminobutyric acid (GABA) and the chloride ionophore protein which has recognition sites for various compounds (Schoch et al., 1985; Ticku, 1983; Tallman and Gallager, 1985). In particular, BDZ binding sites appear to be associated with a low-affinity GABA site. Interaction of BDZs at specific binding sites facilitates the action of GABA on the chloride ionophore. Conversely, the presence of GABA at its binding site facilitates the binding of BDZs.

The BZR mediating the classic pharmacological actions of the BDZs (and considered to be linked to the GABA receptor) are generally referred to as central-type BZR. The pharmacological profile of these sites is unique to BDZ binding in the CNS, thereby accounting for the name. Through the use of selective drugs, such as the triazolopyridazine CL 218-872, regional heterogeneity of BDZ binding kinetics has been demonstrated (Klepner et al., 1979), but the functional significance of this regional difference in binding kinetics is not understood.

Benzodiazepines also bind to sites in peripheral organs, and this binding has a different pharmacological profile from central-type BZR; hence, these sites are termed peripheral-type BZR. The peripheral-type BZR are also present in the CNS, and while these sites are present in glial elements in the brain (Shoemaker et al., 1982; Owen et al., 1983), peripheral-type BZR have also been localized to neuronal elements (Anholt et al., 1984). Recent evidence has linked the peripheral binding subtype to the mitochondrial outer membrane in the adrenal gland (Anholt et al., 1986), and subcellular distribution studies in the brain have indicated a high density of peripheral-type receptors in mitochondrial fractions (Marangos et al., 1982; Doble et al., 1987).

Hence, in considering the effect of developmental exposure to BDZs, the possibility of interaction with several different binding sites must be considered. Recent evidence has demonstrated the presence of endogenous substances in the brain that bind to BZR, some of which appear to act as classic BDZ agonists (Sangameswaran and DeBlass, 1985; Sangameswaran et al., 1986) and others which act as inverse agonists (Ferrero et al., 1984; Alho et al., 1985), i.e., they are anxiogenic. There is no information available on the development of these ligands, but the possibility of competition from exogeneous substances must be considered in evaluating the consequences of prenatal exposure to BDZs.

Developmentally, BZR have been identified by the beginning of the third week of gestation in the rat (Braestrup and Nielsen, 1978). Autoradiographic analysis indicates that BZR appear earliest in the brain stem and hypothalamus in the rat, but by birth BDZ binding is present in all areas of the CNS (Schlumpf et al., 1983). In human fetal tissue, BDZ binding is present by 12 weeks conceptual age (Aaltonen et al., 1983; Brooksbank et al., 1982).

Postnatally, development of BZR is rapid and adult densities are reached between the second and fourth week in the rat (Braestrup and Nielsen, 1978; Candy and Martin, 1979). The affinity of the BZR for the typical ligands is adult-like from the earliest appearance of the binding sites. However, displacement with CL 218-872 indicates that binding subtype development is regionally specific (Chisholm et al., 1981; Lippa et al., 1981). Because BZR appear early in fetal development, the possibility that exposure to BDZ compounds could alter binding characteristics of specific BZR, thereby accounting for some of the functional alterations, has been approached by several investigators.

In utero exposure to benzodiazepines: characteristics of later binding to BZR

In utero exposure to neuroactive drugs such as neuroleptic and antidepressant compounds has been associated with altered binding characteristics of relevant receptor sites (Rosengarten and Friedhoff, 1979; Jason et al., 1981). However, even in naive adult animals, altered BDZ

binding does not necessarily follow chronic BDZ exposure (Creese and Sibley, 1980; Gallager et al., 1985). While the results have not been entirely consistent, in utero exposure to BDZs such as diazepam likewise does not induce dramatic changes in ligand binding affinity (K_d) or in maximal receptor density (B_{max}) in exposed offspring. The membrane binding characteristics for the ligand [^{3}H]flunitrazepam for tissue from Long Evans rats exposed over days 13–20 of gestation to diazepam (2.5 or 10 mg/kg, subcutaneous injection) or vehicle are presented in Table 1. The data are presented only for binding to membrane preparations from newborn and 3-month-old adult animals. Binding was also carried out on membrane preparations from animals 7, 14, 21, 28, 35 and 56 days of age. An overall analysis of the data indicated that prenatal exposure to DZ did not exert a significant effect on the characteristics of [^{3}H]flunitrazepam binding. However, observation of the data presented in Table 1 does indicate that prenatal DZ exposure induced a 25% increase in the K_d (demonstrating, therefore, a decrease in affinity of BZR for the ligand) and a 20% decrease in B_{max} in adult offspring. Taken together, these two characteristics suggest that prenatal DZ exposure might induce a subsensitivity in BZR that becomes apparent in the adult organism.

Braestrup et al. (1979) reported no effect of prenatal DZ exposure on [^{3}H]diazepam binding to membrane preparations from 12- and 17-day-old rats exposed to DZ (40 mg/kg p.o.) from 10 days before birth to 7 days after birth. Likewise, Massotti et al. (1980) found no effect on the K_d or B_{max} for [^{3}H]diazepam binding in rat offspring over the first two weeks of life following exposure throughout pregnancy to DZ at 100 mg/kg (p.o., b.i.d.). These reports are consistent with our observations of no effect of the exposure during early development. One study, however, has reported an increase in the maximal density of [^{3}H]diazepam binding in exposed rats at 1–21 days postnatal age following in utero exposure (either over the first half or the latter half

TABLE 1

Characteristics of benzodiazepine binding in the forebrain

	Control		Prenatal DZ	
	Birth	Adult	Birth	Adult
Equilibrium dissociation constant, K_d (nM)	1.41 ± 0.09	1.39 ± 0.06	1.95 ± 0.31	1.73 ± 0.28
Maximal number of binding sites, B_{max} (pmol/mg protein)	0.72 ± 0.08	1.45 ± 0.21	0.94 ± 0.23	1.16 ± 0.03
Maximal stimulation by GABA, % increase over binding with no GABA	66 ± 9	70 ± 10	60 ± 2	102 ± 19

The K_d and B_{max} were obtained from Scatchard analysis of binding over 7 concentrations of [^{3}H]flunitrazepam. Specific binding was determined by displacement with clonazepam (10 μM). Control values include data from both uninjected and vehicle-injected groups and the prenatal DZ group includes data from animals exposed to either 2.5 or 10 mg/kg/day on gestational days 13–20. Animals from 2–3 litters were analysed for each experimental condition. Data are presented as means ± S.E.M. Binding analyses were also carried out at weekly intervals up to 56 days of age. From Kellogg et al., 1983a.

of gestation) to diazepam (20 mg/kg) administered subcutaneously to the dam (Shibuya et al., 1986). No differences were seen between DZ-exposed and control animals at 90 days of age. Certainly, the dose used in the latter study is higher than that administered subcutaneously in the study reported in Table 1. We have shown that following in utero exposure to DZ at 2.5 mg/kg (via subcutaneous administration), the drug persists in the brains of the offspring until day 10 postnatal age (Simmons et al., 1983). Hence, it is possible that following exposure to 20 mg/kg, a higher level of drug persists, perhaps for a longer time, and its presence, perhaps in competition or in cooperation with endogenous ligands, may stimulate development of binding sites during the period of normally occurring increases in the density of BZR. Whether a subcutaneous injection of 20 mg/kg to the dam results in higher and more persisting fetal levels of BDZs than oral exposure at 40 to 100 mg/kg is unknown. A major weak point in most studies evaluating the effect of prenatal exposure to drugs is the lack of information on drug levels reached in the offspring. This absence of information makes between-study as well as cross-species extrapolation exceedingly difficult.

A decrease in both the K_d and the B_{max} for [^{3}H]diazepam binding has been reported in the thalamus of one-year-old rat offspring exposed in utero to DZ at 5.0–7.5 mg/kg (via subcutaneous injection) over days 15–20 of gestation (Livezey et al., 1985). It is difficult to interpret the effect that these changes would have on BZR function. The decrease in K_d reflects an increase in the affinity of the binding site for the ligand, and this change in affinity could counteract any impact that might result from the decrease in receptor density. In view of studies showing a delay in the appearance of functional and neural changes until adulthood in offspring exposed in utero to DZ (see below), altered binding characteristics in year-old offspring could have functional implications. However, the inconsistencies in BDZ binding characteristics reported following prenatal exposure to DZ suggest that aspects of BZR other than binding need to be evaluated.

Another aspect of BDZ binding to be considered is whether developmental exposure to DZ and related drugs alters the heterogeneity of binding kinetics. As can be seen in Table 2, exposure to DZ (2.5 mg/kg) over gestational days 13–20 did not alter the displacing ability of the triazolo-pyridazine CL 218-872 in 70-day-old offspring

TABLE 2

Displacement of [^{3}H]flunitrazepam (1 nM) binding in the brain by CL 218-872: effect of prenatal exposure to DZ

Prenatal treatment (days 13–20)	IC$_{50}$ (nM)	Hill coefficient
No drug	483 ± 58.1	0.65 ± 0.03
Vehicle	600 ± 9.7	0.68 ± 0.06
DZ (2.5 mg/kg)	590 ± 58.0	0.68 ± 0.02

Data (means ± S.E.M.) presented are from the hippocampus of 70-day-old rats. Analysis was also carried out in the cortex and cerebellum and at postnatal days 0, 7, 14, 21, 35 and 90. No effect of the prenatal exposure was noted at any age or in any region. From Chisholm, 1982.

(Chisholm, 1982). The displacing ability was also examined in offspring at birth and up to 35 days (data not included), and no effect of prenatal DZ exposure was noted at any age.

One might also question whether DZ exposure altered binding at the GABA recognition site. Both work from our laboratory (Kellogg et al., 1983a) and the study by Massotti et al. (1980) suggest that binding to the high-affinity GABA site is unaltered by prenatal DZ exposure. However, since it is a low-affinity GABA binding site that appears linked to specific BZR, binding to the GABA site must be reevaluated for an effect of early DZ exposure.

Aspects of BDZ-GABA receptor interaction other than binding characteristics of the recognition sites may be more critically related to DZ-induced alterations in the offspring. Continuous exposure of adult rats to DZ induces a subsensitivity phenomenon at the level of the BDZ-GABA complex (Gallager et al., 1985). Precisely when a functional linkage between BZR and the GABA recognition site occurs developmentally is not known. However, it is conceivable that early occupancy of the BZR could alter the functional relationship between the two recognition sites. Considering this relationship, Massotti et al. (1980) reported a reduction in the ability of the GABA agonist muscimol to stimulate ^{3}H-DZ

binding to neural membranes from rat offspring (at 1, 7 and 14 days) following in utero exposure to DZ at 100 mg/kg (per os, b.i.d.). As can be seen in Table 1, exposure during late gestation to DZ at 2.5 or 10 mg/kg (by subcutaneous injection) leads to a somewhat greater increase in the maximal stimulation of [^{3}H]flunitrazepam binding by GABA (100 μM) in 90-day-old adult offspring.

These observations, however, still do not address the question of whether the prenatal exposure altered effector responses initiated by receptor occupancy. Clearly, such information is necessary. It is possible, e.g., that an altered receptor/effector response at the level of the complex is responsible for the altered behavioral responses observed in prenatally exposed offspring administered DZ as adults (Kellogg et al., 1983a). Studies measuring chloride flux, an effector response of the BDZ-GABA receptor complex, are now in progress in the laboratory.

To summarize, studies on the effect of in utero exposure to BDZs on BDZ binding indicate that permanent effects on the brain will probably not be most obviously expressed as changes in the density of binding sites or in the affinity of the binding sites for standard ligands. However, permanent alterations in the functional link between the BDZ-GABA sites is a possible lasting consequence.

In utero DZ exposure: effects on cellular metabolism

The previous section considered the possibility that the lasting effects induced in the CNS by early developmental exposure to BDZs might be related to permanent alterations in the BDZ-GABA receptor complex. However, the possibility must be addressed that binding of the drug in utero, via activation of effector responses, elicits specific biochemical changes in receptive cells. These changes may become permanent or may be altered as the organism matures. The possibility of a mitochondrial location for peripheral-type BZR implicates those sites in modulation of

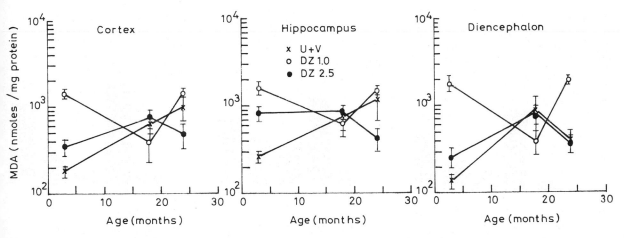

Fig. 1 Changes in levels (means ± S.E.M.) of malondialdehyde (MDA)-like material from young adult to old age in three brain regions of Long Evans rats. MDA levels were also measured in the telencephalic basal ganglia, cerebellum and midbrain. The control group (U + V) consists of both animals uninjected prenatally and those whose dams were injected with the vehicle used to suspend DZ. Prenatal injections of diazepam (DZ; 1.0 or 2.5 mg/kg/day) or vehicle were made subcutaneously into the nape of the neck of pregnant dams over gestational days 14–20 (with day 0 representing the day a vaginal smear tested sperm-positive). From Miranda and Kellogg, 1987.

mitochondrial function and intracellular metabolism. Peripheral-type sites may work in conjunction with central-type sites.

Recent work in our laboratory has demonstrated that in utero exposure to DZ altered cellular metabolism in the exposed offspring (Miranda and Kellogg, 1987). Levels of malondialdehyde (MDA) were selected as the index of cellular metabolism. Malondialdehyde is an end-product of a series of nonenzymatic autocatalytic lipid peroxidation reactions and reflects a composite of intracellular activity. As demonstrated in Fig. 1, brain MDA levels in nonexposed rats increased with normal aging. There were regionally specific differences noted, however, in the aging-related patterns. While MDA levels increased throughout aging in forebrain regions and in the cerebellum, the levels in the midbrain and diencephalon decreased from 18 to 24 months, following an initial increase from 3 to 18 months.

Prenatal exposure to DZ altered both MDA levels at 3 months and aging-related changes in levels in a dose-specific manner (Fig. 1). Early DZ exposure led to an elevation of MDA levels at 3 months, with the lower exposure dose (1 mg/kg)

producing a greater effect than the higher dose (2.5 mg/kg). The levels at 18 months did not differ from control values in either exposure group. Hence, in the lower exposure group, MDA levels decreased from 3 to 18 months, and in the higher exposure group they increased. The changes in MDA levels from 18 to 24 months were also dose-specific. In the group exposed to the lower dose, the MDA levels increased in all brain regions, an aging pattern resembling the changes seen in control forebrain regions and cerebellum. However, in animals exposed to the higher dose, the MDA levels decreased in all regions, yielding a pattern seen in control diencephalon and midbrain.

These initial results implicate BZR in the regulation of cellular metabolic processes and suggest that regulation of metabolic activity by BZR is a dynamic process relative to age. The different aging patterns in the two prenatal exposure groups, which resemble regionally specific changes in metabolism with aging in control animals, suggest that regional differences in BDZ binding subtypes, endogenous ligands and receptor interactions exist. The ability of in utero expo-

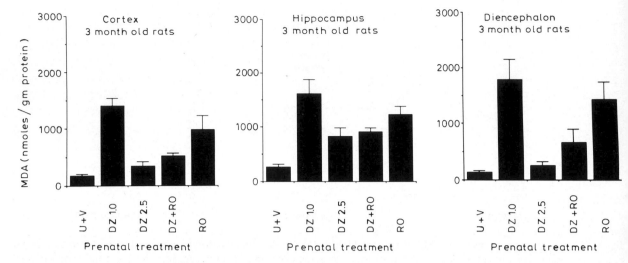

Fig. 2 Changes in brain levels (means ± S.E.M.) of MDA-like material at 3 months of age as a function of in utero drug exposure to diazepam (DZ) (over days 14–20 of gestation). Levels were also measured in the telencephalic basal ganglia, cerebellum and midbrain. U + V = combined uninjected plus vehicle-injected control animals; DZ 1.0 = DZ exposure at 1.0 mg/kg/day; DZ 2.5 = DZ exposure at 2.5 mg/kg/day; DZ + Ro = DZ exposure at 2.5 mg/kg/day in combination with Ro 15-1788 at 10 mg/kg/day; Ro = exposure to Ro 15-1788 only (at 10 mg/kg/day). From Miranda and Kellogg, 1987.

sure to DZ to influence metabolism into aging suggests that BZR are quite plastic during the exposure period and can be 'tuned' for interaction with specific ligands depending upon exposure level.

The rather generalized effect across brain regions on cellular metabolism following in utero exposure to DZ might suggest a nonspecificity of effect. However, if the BDZ-GABA complex is involved in initiating the effect, then the widespread changes are not surprising. GABA has been implicated as the neurotransmitter in 25–45% of all nerve endings (Belin et al., 1980) and, while the distribution of BZR in the brain is not uniform in density, BDZs bind to membranes in all brain regions. Within regions, selected cells will be influenced as determined by the location of BZR in any particular region.

To determine whether the lasting influence on cellular metabolism induced by in utero exposure to DZ was related to the interaction of DZ with selective BZR, the effect of co-exposure to DZ and BDZ antagonists was evaluated (Fig. 2). Coadministration of the central-type BDZ antagonist Ro 15-1788 (Hunkler et al., 1981) with DZ (2.5 mg/kg/day to the dam) did not prevent the influence of DZ on MDA levels measured in 3-month-old offspring, and in utero exposure to Ro 15-1788 alone led to far greater increases in MDA levels in the young adults than did exposure to DZ (Miranda and Kellogg, 1987).

While previous reports suggest that the drug Ro 15-1788 may have agonist or even inverse agonist (i.e., anxiogenic) as well as antagonist effects on the brain (File and Pellow, 1986), these different effects have generally been observed at different doses of the compound. In other studies from our laboratory (see below), prenatal exposure to Ro 15-1788 at the same dose utilized in the metabolism studies completely prevented the particular effect of DZ under evaluation, and by itself was without effect. Hence, a far more realistic explanation for the effect of prenatal exposure to Ro 15-1788 on later cellular metabolism would seem to be that during the exposure period the drug antagonized the effect of a particular endogenous ligand which interacts in a specific manner with BDZ binding sites. Ro 15-

1788 does appear to be specific to central-type binding sites, since the drug does not displace binding to sites in peripheral organs. Hence, the effect of Ro 15-1788 on metabolism may be initiated at a central-type binding site (where it probably acts as an antagonist to DZ), but a central site that is linked to another site, such as a peripheral-type site. Endogenous ligands may serve as the link between the two sites.

In summary, these investigations into the effects of prenatal drug exposure on cellular metabolism represent an approach not often taken. These studies have demonstrated that in utero drug exposure can have effects that are related to and altered by the aging process. The suggestion was made previously that prenatal DZ exposure may accelerate aging-related processes (Marczynski and Livezey, 1986). The data presented above indicate that such a generalized statement may be in error; exposure dose is critical and the interpretations one might make from the data would be dependent upon age of the animal at examination. In terms of accelerated mortality rates, none was observed regardless of exposure level or compound.

In utero exposure to DZ: effects on neuronal systems

Consideration will now be given to the concept that lasting effects on the brain from developmental exposure to drugs may be expressed as changes in the function of neuronal systems in which the various components may develop simultaneously. The decision of what systems to study is best directed by knowledge of the action of the particular drug under question. Hence, for anxiolytic drugs one would want to analyse those neural pathways involved in stress and anxiety. Since the neural pathways underlying behavioral expressions of stress and anxiety are not clearly understood, the suggestion might appear absurd. However, as Selye (1976) proposed, stressors induce two classes of responses: one, called the stress response, that is common to all stressors, and the second consisting of responses appropriate to individual stressors. One of the common stress responses is the release of ACTH from the pituitary via influence from the hypothalamus. ACTH then stimulates release of corticosteroids from the adrenal glands. Therefore, the hypothalamic-pituitary-adrenal axis provides a system that is likely to be influenced by developmental exposure to BDZs. Certainly, in rats, the plasma corticosterone response to stress, as well as behavioral responses, is altered by BZDs (Lahti and Barsuhn, 1975; LeFur et al., 1979).

Several neuropeptides that are produced in the hypothalamus influence ACTH release (Reisine et al., 1986). Additionally, norepinephrine (NE)-containing fibers which project to the hypothalamus from cell bodies in the brain stem exert a major influence over stress-influenced plasma corticosterone levels (Fuxe et al., 1973; Hedge et al., 1976). Precisely how that influence is mediated is not known, but the mechanisms could conceivably involve hypothalamic neuropeptides. Various stressors induce an increase in the turnover rate of hypothalamic NE (Corrodi et al., 1968), and BZDs prevent that stress-induced increase (Corrodi et al., 1971; Taylor and Laverty, 1969). Whether the blunting of the stress-induced increase in plasma corticosterone caused by BZDs is related to their effect on the NE projection to the hypothalamus is not known. The two effects may be independent, but development of the two stress-related responses could occur in parallel. Whether the two responses are linked or independent, prenatal exposure to anxiolytic compounds could affect both responses. Indeed, results from a series of experiments conducted in this laboratory have demonstrated this to be true.

Prior to analysing the effects of prenatal DZ exposure on stress responses, the effect on the hypothalamic NE projection was examined. Analysis of the effect of late gestational exposure to DZ on NE levels in the brain indicated that hypothalamic NE levels were significantly reduced in a dose-related manner (between 1 and 10 mg/kg) in adult prenatally exposed offspring

(Simmons et al., 1984a). No effect was observed on catecholamine levels in the cortex or hippocampus. Furthermore, the effect of the prenatal exposure on NE levels in the hypothalamus was not apparent until after 4 weeks postnatal age (Fig. 3A).

Measurement of the functional state of the NE neurons, by following the decrease in NE levels after inhibition of the limiting enzyme of synthesis, tyrosine hydroxylase, demonstrated that prenatal exposure to DZ induced a decrease in the kinetics of NE turnover in the hypothalamus of adult offspring (Table 3). Moreover, the effects of prenatal exposure to DZ (2.5 mg/kg) on NE levels and turnover could be prevented by coexposure in utero to the BDZ antagonist Ro 15-1788. The antagonist elicited no effect when administered alone.

These initial studies demonstrated that the noradrenergic innervation to the hypothalamus was selectively affected by the in utero exposure to DZ. The NE projections to this region arise predominantly (70%) from the A_1 cell group in the caudal ventrolateral medulla. A smaller group of fibers (20%) arise from cells within the nucleus of the solitary tract (A_2 cell group) and a few fibers arise from the locus coeruleus (Swanson et al., 1986). Hence, the noradrenergic projections to the hypothalamus represent a very different group of cells from the noradrenergic projection to the cortex and hippocampus, which arises from cells in the locus coeruleus. The selectivity of the prenatal exposure to DZ may reside in the uniqueness of the noradrenergic innervation to the hypothalamus.

The altered NE turnover rate measured in the adult prenatally exposed offspring could be reflecting many changes in the NE projections to the hypothalamus, such as altered activity within the cells of origin or alterations in molecular mechanisms regulating turnover at the level of the terminals. To differentiate among the possibilities, the depolarized release of [³H]NE measured in vitro was evaluated (Kellogg and Retell, 1986). Depolarization was induced by incubation of the

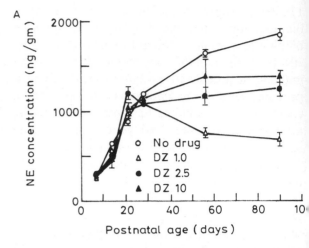

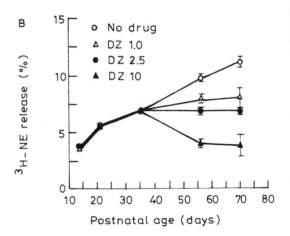

Fig. 3 (A) Changes in norepinephrine (NE) concentration (means ± S.E.M.) in the hypothalamus of Long Evans rats as a function of postnatal age and prenatal exposure to DZ at 1.0, 2.5 or 10.0 mg/kg/day (over gestational days 13–20). From Simmons et al., 1984a. (B) Changes in depolarized release of ³H-NE (induced by incubation in 25 mM potassium) in isolated hypothalamus of Long Evans rats as a function of postnatal age and prenatal exposure to DZ at 1.0, 2.5 or 10.0 mg/kg/day (over gestational days 13–20). Data are expressed as means ± S.E.M.. From Kellogg and Retell, 1986.

tissues in 25 mM potassium. This study demonstrated that prenatal exposure to DZ induced a dose-related decrease in depolarized release of [³H]NE from the isolated hypothalamus of adult offspring (Table 4). No effect of the exposure was observed on NE release from the hippocampus or cerebellum. The effect on release from the hypo-

TABLE 3

NE levels and turnover in the hypothalamus of adult rats: effect of prenatal exposure to DZ and/or Ro 15-1788

Prenatal exposure days 13–20	n	NE levels (ng/g)	Turnover rate (ng/g/h)	Turnover rate constant (h^{-1})
Uninjected	15	1719 ± 138	292	0.17 ± 0.01
Ro 15-1788 10.0 mg/kg	15	1695 ± 152	278	0.16 ± 0.02
Ro 15-1788 10 mg/kg + diazepam 2.5 mg/kg	15	1662 ± 133	288	0.17 ± 0.01
Diazepam 2.5 mg/kg	15	1298 ± 112[a]	117	0.09 ± 0.01[a]

n = number of animals. Data are presented as means ± S.E.M. From Simmons et al., 1984a.
[a] Significantly different from control value, $P < 0.05$.

thalamus was prevented by concurrent in utero exposure to the central-type BDZ antagonist Ro 15-1788.

The development of stimulated release from the hypothalamus was investigated and is presented in Fig. 3B. As observed for the development of NE levels, no effect of the prenatal exposure on stimulated release of [^{3}H]NE was apparent until after a prolonged period of apparently normal development.

That the influence of prenatal exposure on function of the NE projections to the hypothalamus could be detected even in an isolated tissue preparation suggests that the effect of the prenatal exposure was directed at the level of the hypothalamus. To determine whether BZR may have a unique relationship with NE terminals in this region compared to other regions, the ability of DZ to alter the stimulated release of [^{3}H]NE from unexposed adult tissue was examined (Harary and Kellogg, 1987). In vitro incubation with diazepam (10^{-5} M) did elicit a significant decrease in stimulated release of [^{3}H]NE from the hypothalamus while having no effect in the cerebellum (Table 5). Furthermore, the effect of DZ in the hypothalamus was antagonized by coincubation with the central-type BDZ antagonist Ro 15-1788 and by the GABA antagonist

TABLE 4

Depolarized release of [^{3}H]NE from adult Long Evans rat hypothalamus: effect of prenatal exposure to diazepam and/or Ro 15-1788

Prenatal exposure days 13–20	n	Depolarized release (%) (mean ± S.E.M.)
Uninjected	5	11.5 ± 0.4
Diazepam 1.0 mg/kg	6	8.3 ± 1.0[a]
Diazepam 2.5 mg/kg	6	7.5 ± 0.2[a]
Diazepam 10.0 mg/kg	6	3.0 ± 0.8[a]
Diazepam 2.5 mg/kg + Ro 15-1788 10 mg/kg	4	11.7 ± 0.3

n = number of animals.
From Kellogg and Retell, 1986.
[a] Significant difference from uninjected animals, $P < 0.01$.

TABLE 5

Depolarized release (means ± S.E.M.) of [^{3}H]NE from adult Long Evans rat brain: effect of in vitro incubation with diazepam

Drug	Hypothalamus		Cerebellum	
	n	Release (%)	n	Release (%)
No drug	17	15.2 ± 0.48	12	24.7 ± 1.09
Diazepam, 10^{-5} M	4	10.22 ± 0.39[a]	4	21.6 ± 1.14
Diazepam, 10^{-4} M	3	10.25 ± 1.05[a]	3	23.0 ± 1.58
Diazepam, 10^{-5} M + Ro 15-1788, 10^{-5} M	6	14.08 ± 0.9		–
Diazepam, 10^{-5} M + biccuculine, 10^{-5} M	4	15.95 ± 1.11		–

n = number of animals.
From Harary and Kellogg, 1987.
[a] Significant difference from no drug, $P < 0.01$.

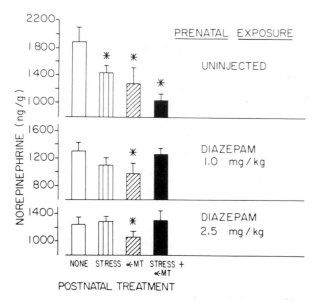

Fig. 4 Norepinephrine concentration in the hypothalamus of 90-day-old Long Evans rats as a function of prenatal drug exposure (over gestational days 13–20) and postnatal restraint stress and/or inhibition of catecholamine synthesis. Restraint stress (alone or in combination with synthesis inhibition) was imposed for 2 h. Catecholamine synthesis was inhibited by administration of α-methyl-*p*-tyrosine methyl ester hydrochloride (αMT, 250 mg/kg) 2 h prior to analysis of NE. NE levels presented as a function of adult manipulation in uninjected control animals or animals exposed in utero to DZ at 1.0 or 2.5 mg/kg.day. * indicates a significant difference (*P* < 0.05) from the basal NE level for the respective prenatal exposure group.

bicuculine. Since DZ added in vitro to normal adult hypothalamus had the same effect on depolarized release of [³H]NE as did in utero exposure, central-type BZR which are in a position to influence the function of NE terminals in the hypothalamus must be present and effective during the in utero exposure period. The critical period for DZ exposure to influence these NE projections can be as short as exposure over days 17–20 of gestation (Simmons et al., 1984a). Certainly, BZR are present in the hypothalamus at this time (Schlumpf et al., 1983), NE terminals are apparent in that region (Specht et al., 1981), and GABA terminals have been identified (Lauder et al., 1986). Hence, all of the necessary

components for a response to be initiated at appropriate BZR appear to be available.

Are the appropriate BZR located presynaptically on the NE terminals to this region? Data obtained following both in vitro and in vivo exposure to neurotoxins specific for catecholamine neurons indicated that the magnitude of decrease in BDZ binding correlated highly with the magnitude of reduction in hypothalamic NE (Harary and Kellogg, 1987). In the cerebellum and cortex, neurotoxin exposure elicited a far greater reduction in NE levels than in BDZ binding. While not conclusive evidence, these data do imply that a high proportion of BZR in the hypothalamus may be presynaptically located on NE terminals. That relationship between BZR and NE fibers may be unique to this noradrenergic projection system.

Since the NE projection to the hypothalamus is influenced by prenatal exposure to DZ, will some of the organism's stress responses be altered? In approaching this question, we evaluated the influence of prenatal DZ exposure on stress-induced changes in the hypothalamic NE projection and in plasma corticosterone levels (Simmons et al., 1984b). Whereas 2 hours of restraint stress induced a significant decrease in NE levels in the hypothalamus of control animals, no decrease was observed in adult prenatally exposed rats (Fig. 4). Since levels of neurotransmitters reflect the steady state between synthesis and utilization of transmitter, the decrease in control animals suggest that synthesis of NE could not keep pace with utilization. Likewise, the lack of effect of stress on NE levels in prenatally exposed animals suggests that stress did not increase NE utilization in these animals.

To evaluate that suggestion, the effect of restraint stress on NE levels measured in the presence of synthesis inhibition was analysed. While synthesis inhibition alone significantly reduced NE levels in all groups, the magnitude of decrease, as previously observed, was less in the exposed animals. A major difference in response to stress was observed, however, between control and exposed rats. Stress further reduced the NE

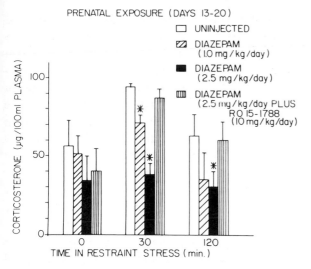

PRENATAL EXPOSURE (DAYS 13-20)

☐ UNINJECTED

▨ DIAZEPAM
(1.0 mg / kg / day)

■ DIAZEPAM
(2.5 mg / kg / day)

▥ DIAZEPAM
(2.5 mg / kg / day PLUS
RO 15-1788
(10 mg / kg / day)

Fig. 5 Plasma corticosterone levels in 90-day-old Long Evans rats under basal conditions and following 30 or 120 min of restraint stress. * indicates a significant difference from the uninjected value at each individual time period. Data are presented as means ± S.E.M.. From Simmons et al., 1984b.

levels in control rats beyond that reduction induced by synthesis inhibition alone, indicating that stress enhanced NE utilization in these animals. However, in the prenatally exposed rats, NE levels following 2 hours of restraint stress (in the presence of a synthesis inhibitor) were not significantly different from basal levels (Fig. 4). In other words, stress did not increase NE utilization but actually seemed to decrease it below basal rates, since in the basal state synthesis inhibition induced a significant decrease in NE levels. Coexposure in utero to the central-type antagonist prevented these effects of prenatal DZ exposure (Simmons et al., 1984b).

In addition to this altered CNS response to stress, prenatal DZ exposure also attenuated the stress-induced increase in plasma corticosterone levels (Fig. 5). While basal corticosterone levels were high, they did not differ among the exposure groups. Stress induced a 68% increase in corticosterone levels in the control group (measured after 30 min of stress). However, this increase was only 39% and 12% in animals exposed in utero to DZ

at 1.0 or 2.5 mg/kg, respectively. Concurrent exposure to the antagonist and DZ (2.5 mg/kg) in utero again prevented the effect of DZ. As hypothesized, therefore, two separate stress responses known to be influenced by administration of anxiolytic drugs to naive adult rats were also influenced by in utero exposure.

The observation that the NE projection to the hypothalamus developed normally up to at least 5 weeks of age, but showed alterations by 8 weeks, suggests that function within this system is modified by the events of puberty. Prenatal exposure to DZ may have influenced the manner in which those events could influence the NE projection. Interestingly, steroids have been shown to exert an effect on the BZ-GABA-chloride ionophore complex (Majewska et al., 1986). As an organism goes through puberty, the presence of sex steroids may influence specific BZR or interact with selective endogenous ligands to bring about an alteration in this specific neural pathway. If function in this particular pathway is altered by puberty, then because this pathway is involved in the stress response, the organism's response to stressful situations may likewise be altered by puberty. Prenatal exposure to DZ may alter the early developmental organization of these responses, so that the adult organism can no longer make appropriate responses to a stressor.

That different BDZ binding sites (or effector responses) must be mediating the effects of prenatal DZ exposure presented so far should be apparent. In utero exposure to the central antagonist Ro 15-1788 influenced the hypothalamic and adrenal measurements quite differently from the way it influenced cellular metabolism. The antagonist prevented the effect of prenatal exposure to DZ on measures of NE function in the hypothalamus and was ineffective when given alone. On the other hand, Ro 15-1788 was not effective in preventing DZ-induced effects on MDA levels and, given alone, Ro 15-1788 elicited an increase in MDA levels measured in young adult rats. Taken together, these results demonstrate that BDZs can interact with different populations of binding subtypes or initiate different effector responses. The effect of DZ on the hypothalamic NE projection and on the plasma corticosterone response appears to be mediated via the classic central-type receptor, linked to a GABA recognition site. On the other hand, the effect of the antagonist on metabolism suggests that the BDZs also bind to a central site that may be linked to another site, perhaps a peripheral-type site located on mitochondria. Perhaps by blocking the action of an endogenous ligand at the central-type site the ligand is displaced to another site.

Few other laboratories have analysed neural systems for an effect of prenatal BDZ exposure. Fujii et al. (1983) did examine the effects of exposure to DZ (0.2 or 2.0 mg/kg injected subcutaneously) over gestational days 15–21 on function of the hypothalamic-pituitary-thyroid axis on the offspring. Adult female exposed rats (10–12 weeks of age) elicited an enhanced thyrotropin response when administered thyrotropin stimulating hormone. Basal serum thyroxine levels were unchanged in the exposed offspring, whereas at 3 and 6 weeks of age the basal levels were decreased in both male and female prenatally exposed offspring. The observations made in that report support the suggestion that early developmental exposure to BDZs may interfere with the development of neural systems, even into adulthood. Alterations in functioning of the hypothalamic-pituitary-thyroid axis may reflect similar mechanisms responsible for the alterations in the hypothalamic-pituitary-adrenal axis.

In utero exposure to DZ: functional deficits

Several functional deficits have been reported following early developmental exposure to DZ. However, the relationship of these deficits to the neural consequences of prenatal exposure must be addressed.

Measurement of locomotor activity in the offspring is a common test in most studies evaluating the effect of in utero exposure to exogenous chemicals. Since drugs can influence locomotor activity by acting on several different neurotransmitter systems and neural pathways, it is very difficult to interpret effects or lack of effects on activity following prenatal drug exposures. However, development of spontaneous locomotor activity in rodents (tested in isolation) follows a pattern characterized by a sudden increase in activity around postnatal days 14–15 followed by an abrupt decline in activity on days 17–18 (Campbell et al., 1969). This brief phase of locomotor hyperactivity may reflect different rates of maturation of specific excitatory and inhibitory neural systems, and prenatal exposure to DZ, because of the link between BZR and specific GABA receptors, could alter this developmental phase.

As demonstrated in Fig. 6, the developmental phase of locomotor hyperactivity was attenuated in a dose-related manner by prenatal exposure to DZ (Kellogg et al., 1980). There was no effect of the exposure on locomotor activity measured after the phase of hyperactivity. Shore et al. (1983) also observed a decrease in activity at postnatal day 15 only, following prenatal exposure to DZ at 1 or 5 mg/kg (via gavage). Related to these observations, Frieder et al. (1984) observed that postnatal exposure to DZ (10 mg/kg) from day 3 to 18 induced hyperactivity in offspring at days 20 and 35. DZ exposure in that study occurred during the phase of normal developmental locomotor hyperactivity. Considered together, these results suggest that the neural systems underlying developmental locomotor hyperactivity may involve the BDZ-GABA receptor complex. Prenatal exposure to DZ, perhaps by 'tuning' specific BZR to respond differently to selective endogenous ligands or by altering the functional link between the BDZ site, the GABA site and the chloride ionophore, may alter relevant neural systems.

Long-lasting functional deficits induced by early developmental drug exposure are more readily observed when tests requiring complex neural processing are employed. Tests have been developed in this laboratory to evaluate sensory processing. These tests involve measuring sensory

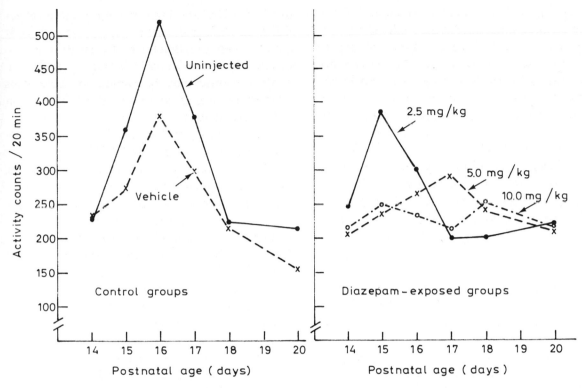

Fig. 6 Spontaneous locomoter activity measured in isolated Long Evans rats over postnatal days 14–20 as a function of prenatal DZ exposure (over gestational days 13–20). Each animal was tested for a 20-min period on each testing day. Rats prenatally uninjected or exposed to the vehicle (left). Animals prenatally exposed to DZ at 2.5, 5.0 or 10.0 mg/kg/day (right). From Kellogg et al., 1980.

and sensory-motor function within the auditory system by evaluating the acoustic startle reflex and its modification by brief acoustic stimuli. The neural pathway underlying the acoustic startle reflex itself is reasonably well specified (Davis et al., 1982), and several auditory nuclei involved in the reflex and in its modification are densely populated with BZR (Kuhar and Young, 1979; Richards et al., 1982).

The initial study (Kellogg et al., 1980) demonstrated that prenatal DZ exposure interfered with the development of noise potentiation of the acoustic startle process (Fig. 7). This response could be detected in control groups by 12 days of age, but was not evident in exposed groups even at 20 days of age. Additionally, the amplitude of the acoustic startle response itself was depressed

by prenatal DZ exposure. The disruption in this function was shown to be unrelated to a primary sensory deficit. Since potentiation of the acoustic startle response by background noise is presumed to result from activation of an arousal system, the neural systems underlying the development of noise potentiation may be similar to those underlying developmental locomotor hyperactivity.

Recent studies have demonstrated that potentiation of the acoustic startle response by background noise is normal in adult (70–90 days of age) prenatally exposed animals (Sullivan and Kellogg, 1985; Fig. 8A). It may be that different underlying neural systems are involved in this function in the mature organism than during development, just as with locomotor activity. The amplitude of the basal acoustic startle response, however, was still significantly altered in the prenatally exposed animals. Animals exposed to the intermediate dose (2.5 mg/kg) appeared hypersensitive to the startle stimulus, whereas animals exposed to the higher dose (10 mg/kg) were hyposensitive, relative to controls. This nonlinear dose-response effect is not unique to this function: recall that such a relationship was also evident at the biochemical level. The levels of MDA in exposed animals followed divergent directions (with respect to dose) with aging. And as was observed with the biochemical response, concurrent prenatal exposure to the central antago-

nist Ro 15-1788 and DZ did not prevent the effect of DZ on the basal startle response (Fig. 8B). It appears, therefore, that the particular BDZ receptor/effector system via which DZ influences the startle response may be similar to those sites involved in mediation of the effect of DZ on cellular metabolism.

Work from other laboratories has also provided evidence that prenatal DZ exposure may interfere with arousal processes. For example, 1-year-old cats exposed in utero to DZ demonstrated interference with post-reinforcement synchronization of the EEG (Livezey et al., 1986). Additionally, adult rats exposed to DZ (5.0–7.5 mg/kg) during late gestation demonstrated impaired sleep EEG patterns, suggestive of impaired synchronization (Livezey et al., 1985). Synchronized EEG patterns may be dependent upon neural circuits involving GABA-containing interneurons. Interference with these patterns by early DZ exposure is consistent with action of the drug at selective BZR.

Prenatal exposure to DZ also impairs performance on more complex sensory-motor tasks and on tasks related to learning. Work from our laboratory has demonstrated alterations in the development and mature function of auditory temporal resolution, as measured by evaluating the ability of gaps in background noise to inhibit the acoustic startle response (Kellogg et al., 1983b). Studies of auditory temporal resolution in humans show that individual differences in this function are related to speech perception in adults (Trinder, 1979) and to language and learning disabilities in children (McCrosky and Kidder, 1980). Auditory temporal resolution was measured in rats at weekly intervals up to 70 days of age. Statistical analysis revealed significant effects of prenatal DZ exposure on gap detection at 28 days, the age that the function emerged in control animals, and again at 70 days. Furthermore, the analysis indicated that the interference at 28 days differed from that at 70 days.

In other reports, in utero exposure to DZ over a prolonged period of gestation (Gai and Grimm,

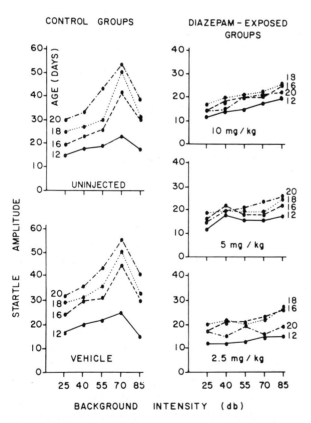

Fig. 7 Development of facilitation of the acoustic startle response by background noise as a function of prenatal exposure to DZ (2.5, 5 or 10 mg/kg) or vehicle over gestational days 13–20. Testing was conducted on postnatal days 12, 16, 18 and 20. The startle stimulus was a 110-dB, 10-kHz, 20-ms tone. From Kellogg et al., 1980.

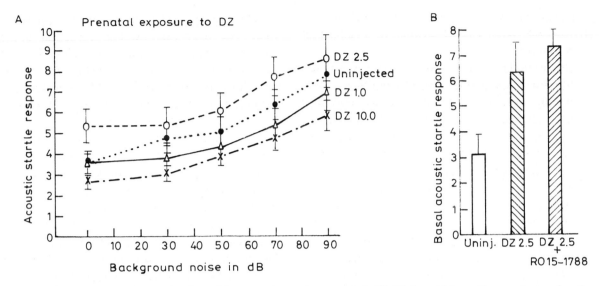

Fig. 8 (A) Facilitation, by background noise, of the acoustic startle response in 70–90-day-old Long Evans rats as a function of prenatal exposure to DZ (1.0, 2.5 or 10 mg/kg) over gestational days 13–20. The startle stimulus was a 120-dB, 10-kHz tone burst of 25 ms duration. (B) Basal acoustic startle response (no added background noise) in 70–90-day-old rats as a function of prenatal exposure to DZ (2.5 mg/kg/day) or DZ plus Ro 15-1788 (10 mg/kg).

TABLE 6

Effect of adult exposure to DZ and Ro 15-1788 on the noise-potentiated acoustic startle response: influence of prenatal DZ exposure

Prenatal exposure	No drug	DZ (2.5 mg/kg)	Ro 15-1788 (10 mg/kg)
A. Basal response (volts)			
Uninjected (n = 5)	4.05 ± 0.65	3.54 ± 0.48	4.35 ± 0.49
DZ 2.5 mg/kg (days 13–20) (n = 6)	5.57 ± 0.60	4.24 ± 0.71	5.70 ± 0.5
B. Slope of potentiated response[a]			
Uninjected (n = 5)	1.01 ± 0.08	0.53 ± 0.04	0.84 ± 0.15
DZ 2.5 mg/kg (days 13–20) (n = 6)	1.18 ± 0.07	0.71 ± 0.17	0.50 ± 0.09

Data are presented as means ± S.E.M. Drugs were administered sequentially every 60 min. Testing began 30 min after each drug.
[a] Background noise levels and intensity of the startle stimulus were the same as indicated in Fig. 8A.

1982) or only over days 14–20 (at 10 mg/kg; Frieder et al., 1984) induced deficits in adult offspring in a complex simultaneous-choice discrimination maze. No effect was observed if the prenatal exposure was limited to days 8–14 of gestation, and there was no effect from any exposure period on simple motor learning or in simple maze performance. The precise neural impairments leading to the deficit in the complex task are not understood, but could involve impairment at the level of processing of sensory information.

Analysis of auditory reflex functions has also shown that rats prenatally exposed to DZ have altered response as adults when challenged with drugs that interact with BZR. As can be seen in Table 6, while DZ reduces the acoustic startle response potentiated by noise (as indicated by the slope of the potentiated response) in both control and prenatally exposed adult rats, the antagonist was capable of reversing the effect of DZ only in control animals. This inability of Ro 15-1788 to reverse the effect of DZ in prenatally exposed rats does not appear to be related to a difference in the affinity of the antagonist for BZR, as indicated by displacement of [³H]flunitrazepam binding by Ro 15-1788 (Kellogg and Birnbaum, unpublished observation).

Other studies from our laboratory have shown a different effect of DZ administration to adult prenatally exposed rats on auditory temporal acuity (Kellogg et al., 1983b). These altered responses to drugs acting at BZR do not appear to relate to altered binding characteristics. Differences in receptor/effector systems and/or endogenous ligand interaction seem to be more likely candidates.

In summary, functional changes induced by prenatal exposure to DZ appear to be most apparent when the organism is challenged, either with complex behavioral tasks or pharmacologically. And, as was evident at the neural level, the impact of the prenatal exposure on functioning of the organism is dependent upon the age of the organism at testing.

Conclusion

It is now quite clear that early developmental exposure to DZ will induce long-lasting effects on the CNS and on function in animal models. The charge to investigators is now to elucidate the mechanisms whereby DZ interacts with the brain during development and whereby the early action on the brain becomes translated into functional alterations as the organism matures. The significance for the human condition of the effects induced in animal models by DZ exposure in utero will rest in the understanding of mechanisms via which exogenous substances may influence the developing brain.

From both neurochemical and behavioral observations following prenatal DZ exposure, the most sensitive period for inducing the long-term effects appears to be the last week of gestation in the rodent. The fact that the last four days of gestation is the critical period for the effect on the hypothalamic NE projection suggests that synaptogenesis and/or the formation of specific neural circuits may be most vulnerable to these neuroactive compounds.

The time period in human fetal development over which DZ could exert effects similar to those seen in rodents could conceivably extend from the second trimester into postnatal life. The observation, however, that postnatal DZ exposure of the rat elicits effects different from prenatal exposure (Frieder et al., 1984) suggests that in humans the second trimester may be the most vulnerable period for induction of effects similar to those seen following prenatal exposure in rats. Based upon selected biochemical indices, the rat brain at birth has been compared to a human brain around 20 weeks of gestation (Dobbing, 1974). Maturational events during late gestation in humans may be comparable to those events taking place during the first postnatal week in rats. Studies on human fetal brain development indicate that the sequencing of many specific neural events is similar to that in the rodent. That is, catecholamine-containing neurons begin chemical differentiation at 7–10 weeks conceptual age (Olson et al., 1973; Nobin and Bjorklund, 1973). And as noted above, BZR are present by 12 weeks of gestation. Hence, as in rats, two chemically defined systems that appear to interact begin to develop early and sequentially in human fetal development. Thus, as in rodents, the appropriate substrates for specific drug-CNS interactions are present developmentally in humans; therefore, long-lasting effects of such exposures would be predicted.

Many different types of functional deficit have been reported in rats following prenatal DZ exposure: alterations in stress responses, EEG synchronization, potentiated startle responses and complex maze tasks. All of these functions may reflect interference from the prenatal exposure with specific underlying neural circuitry, particularly that involved in arousal-attention and/or stress-related functions. Because of the association of a substantial proportion of BZR with GABA receptors, and because of the widespread distribution of GABA-containing synapses, the framework exists for an extensive impact of BDZs on neural function. Lauder et al. (1986) have shown that the outgrowth of GABA fibers during development, first apparent in the brain stem on gestational day 13, correlates well with the pattern of development of BZR (as reported by Schlumpf et al., 1983). The possible presence of BZR on subcellular membranes may augment responses initiated by binding of DZ to sites on the neuronal membrane.

Of particular note is the fact that the effects induced on the organism following prenatal exposure to DZ have a dynamic quality. It is not the case that once an alteration appears, that same alteration will always be observed. Impairment in locomotor activity is only evident during the stage of developmental locomotor hyperactivity. Decrements in NE level and turnover in the hypothalamus do not appear until young adulthood. The interference with auditory reflex functions that is observed during development of these functions differs from those impairments seen in the adult offspring. And the effects of the prenatal exposure on cellular metabolism change as the organism moves from young adulthood into aging. These observations suggest that BZR are associated with neural events that define transitional stages in the life span of the organism: e.g., from neonatal stages to juvenile periods, from the juvenile state into adolescence, from adolescence into young adulthood, and from mature adulthood into old age. It is critically important, therefore, for studies evaluating the effect of substances that may interact with BZR or the polymolecular complex to cover a wide range of ages in the lifespan of the organism, because the influence of the prenatal exposure appears to be most apparent at transition stages.

Clearly, a great deal more work is needed to understand not only the mechanisms whereby drugs such as DZ exert their lasting influences on the brain but also the role of the BDZ-GABA complex in normal development and function. Studies to date, though, have served to confirm the hypothesis that early drug exposure can indeed elicit a lasting imprint on neural function.

Acknowledgements

The considerable contribution from the following present or former students is gratefully acknowledged: Jane A. Chisholm, Norma Harary, Rajesh Miranda, Todd M. Retell, Steven M. Shamah, Roy D. Simmons and Donna M. Tervo. The generous support and assistance from my colleagues, Dr. Richard K. Miller, Dr. James R. Ison, Dr. G. Pleger and Dr. R. Guillet, have contributed significantly to the work reported.

Research reported in this paper was supported by Grant MH-31850 from the U.S. Public Health Service and by an award from Hoffmann-LaRoche, Inc., Nutley, NJ. Diazepam and Ro 15-1788 were generously supplied by Dr. William Scott and Dr. Peter Sorter, Hoffmann-LaRoche, Nutley, NJ. I wish to thank Ursula Hagen and Maryann Gilbert for their assistance in preparation of this manuscript.

References

Aaltonen, L., Erkkola, R. and Kanto, J. (1983) Benzodiazepine receptors in the human fetus. *Biol. Neonate*, 44: 54–57.

Alho, H., Costa, E., Ferrero, P., Fujimoto, M. and Cosenza-Murphy, D. (1985) Diazepam binding inhibitor: a neuropeptide located in selected populations of rat brain. *Science*, 229: 179–182.

Anholt, R. R. H., Murphy, K. M. M., Mack, G. E. and Snyder, S. H. (1984) Peripheral-type benzodiazepine receptors in the central nervous system: localization to olfactory nerves. *J. Neurosci.*, 4: 593–603.

Anholt, R. R. H., Petersen, P. L., De Souza, E. B. and Snyder, S. H. (1986) The peripheral benzodiazepine receptor: localization to the mitochondria outer membrane. *J. Biol. Chem.*, 261: 576–583.

Belin, M. F., Gamrani, H., Agnera, M., Calas, A. and Pujol, J. F. (1980) Selective uptake of [^{3}H]gammaaminobutyrate by rat supra- and subependymal nerve fibers: histologic and high resolution radioautographic studies. *Neuroscience*, 5: 241–254.

Braestrup, C. and Nielsen, M. (1978) Ontogenetic development of benzodiazepine receptors in the brain. *Brain Res.*, 147: 170–173.

Braestrup, C. and Squires, R. (1978) Pharmacological characterization of benzodiazepine receptors in the brain. *Eur. J. Pharmacol.*, 48: 263–270.

226

Braestrup, C., Nielsen, M. and Squires, R.F. (1979) No changes in rat benzodiazepine receptors after withdrawal from continuous treatment with lorazepam and diazepam. *Life Sci.*, 24: 347–350.

Brooksbank, B.W.L., Atkinson, D.J. and Balazs, R. (1982) Biochemical development of the human brain. III. Benzodiazepine receptors, free gamma-aminobutyrate (GABA) and other amino acids. *J. Neurosci. Res.*, 8: 581–594.

Campbell, B.A., Lytle, L.D. and Fibiger, H.C. (1969) Ontogeny of adrenergic arousal and cholinergic inhibitory mechanisms in the rat. *Science*, 166: 635–637.

Candy, J.M. and Martin, I.L. (1979) The postnatal development of the benzodiazepine receptor in the cerebral cortex and cerebellum of the rat. *J. Neurochem.*, 32: 655–658.

Chisholm, J.A. (1982) Benzodiazepine-displacing potency of a triazolopyridazine: brain regional ontogeny and susceptibility to alteration during development. Doctoral Dissertation, University of Rochester.

Chisholm, J., Kellogg, C. and Lippa, A. (1983) Development of benzodiazepine binding subtypes in three regions of rat brain. *Brain Res.*, 267: 388–391.

Corrodi, H., Fuxe, K. and Hokfelt, T. (1968) The effect of immobilization stress on the activity of central monoamine neurons. *Life Sci.*, 7: 107–112.

Corrodi, H., Fuxe, K., Lidbrink, P. and Olsen, L. (1971) Minor tranquilizers, stress and central catecholamine neurons. *Brain Res.*, 29: 1–16.

Coyle, J.T. (1977) Biochemical aspects of neurotransmission in the developing brain. *Int. Rev. Neurobiol.*, 20: 65–103.

Coyle, J.T. and Henry, D. (1973) Catecholamines in fetal and newborn rat brain. *J. Neurochem.*, 18: 2061–2075.

Cree, J.E., Meyer, J. and Hailey, D.M. (1973) Diazepam in labour: its metabolism and effect on the clinical condition and thermogenesis of the newborn. *Br. Med. J.*, 4: 251–255.

Creese, I. and Sibley, D.R. (1980) Receptor adaptations to centrally acting drugs. *Annu. Rev. Pharmacol. Toxicol.*, 21: 357–391.

Davis, M., Gendelman, D.L., Tischler, M.D. and Gendelman, P.M. (1982) A primary acoustic startle circuit: lesion and stimulation studies. *J. Neurosci.*, 2: 791–805.

Dobbing, J. (1974) Prenatal nutrition and neurologic development. In J. Crovido, L. Hambraeus and B. Vahlquist (Eds.), *Early Malnutrition and Mental Development*, Almquist and Wiksel, Stockholm, pp. 96–110.

Doble, A., Malgouris, C., Daniel, M., Daniel, N., Imbault, F., Basbaum, A., Uzan, A., Gueremy, C. and LeFur, G. (1987) Labeling of peripheral-type benzodiazepine binding sites in human brain with [^{3}H]PK 11195: anatomical and subcellular distribution. *Brain Res. Bull.*, 18: 49–61.

Ferrero, P., Guidotti, A., Conti-Tronconi, B. and Costa, E. (1984) A brain octadecaneuropeptide generated by tryptic digestion of DBI (diazepam binding inhibitor) functions as a proconflict ligand of benzodiazepine recognition sites. *Neuropharmacol.*, 23: 1359–1362.

File, S.E. and Pellow, S. (1986) Intrinsic actions of the benzodiazepine receptor antagonist Ro 15–1788. *Psychopharmacology*, 88: 1–11.

Frieder, B., Epstein, S. and Grimm, V.E. (1984) The effects of exposure to diazepam during various stages of gestation or during lactation on the development and behavior of rat pups. *Psychopharmacology*, 83: 51–55.

Fujii, T., Yamamoto, N. and Fuchino, K. (1983) Functional alterations in the hypothalamic-pituitary-thyroid axis in rats exposed prenatally to diazepam. *Toxicol. Lett.*, 16: 131–137.

Fuxe, K., Hokfelt, T., Jonsson, G. and Lofstrom, A. (1973) Brain and the pituitary-adrenal interaction: studies on central monoamine neurons. In A. Brodish and E.S. Redeetel (Eds.), *Brain-Pituitary-Adrenal Interrelationships*, S. Karger, Basel, pp. 239–269.

Gai, N. and Grimm, V.E. (1982) The effect of prenatal exposure to diazepam on aspects of postnatal development and behavior in rats. *Psychopharmacology*, 78: 225–229.

Gallager, D.W., Malcolm, A.B., Anderson, S.A. and Gonsalves, S.F. (1985) Continuous release of diazepam: electrophysiological, biochemical and behavioral consequences. *Brain Res.*, 342: 26–36.

Harary, N. and Kellogg, C.K. (1987) The relationship of benzodiazepine binding sites to the norepinephrine projection to the hypothalamus in the adult rat. Submitted.

Hedge, G.A., Van Ree, J.M. and Versteeg, D.H.G. (1976) Correlation between hypothalamic catecholamine synthesis and ether stress-induced ACTH secretion. *Neuroendocrinology*, 21: 236–246.

Hunkler, W., Mohler, H., Pieri, L., Bonnetti, E., Cumin, R., Schaffner, R. and Haefely, W. (1981) Selective antagonists of benzodiazepines. *Nature* (Lond.), 290: 514–516.

Jason, K.M., Cooper, T.B. and Friedman, Z. (1981) Prenatal exposure to imipramine alters early behavioral development and Beta adrenergic receptors in rats. *J. Pharmacol. Exp. Ther.*, 217: 461–466.

Kellogg, C.K. and Retell, T.M. (1986) Release of [^{3}H]norepinephrine: alteration by early developmental exposure to diazepam. *Brain Res.*, 366: 137–144.

Kellogg, C., Tervo, D., Ison, J., Parisi, T. and Miller, R.K. (1980) Prenatal exposure to diazepam alters behavioral development in rats. *Science*, 207: 205–207.

Kellogg, C.K., Chisholm, J., Simmons, R.D., Ison, J.R. and Miller, R.K. (1983a) Neural and behavioral consequences of prenatal exposure to diazepam. *Monogr. Neural Sci.*, 9: 119–129.

Kellogg, C., Ison, J.R. and Miller, R.K. (1983b) Prenatal diazepam exposure: effects on auditory temporal resolution in rats. *Psychopharmacology*, 79: 332–337.

Klepner, C.A., Lippa, A.S., Benson, D.I., Sano, M.C. and Beer, B. (1979) Resolution of two biochemically and pharmacologically distinct benzodiazepine receptors. *Pharmacol. Biochem. Behav.*, 11: 457–462.

Kuhar, M.J. and Young, W.S. (1979) Radiohistochemical localizations of benzodiazepine receptors in rat brain. *J. Pharmacol. Exp. Ther.*, 212: 337–346.

Lathi, R.A. and Barsuhn, C. (1975) The effect of various doses of minor tranquilizers on plasma corticosteroids in stressed rats. *Res. Commun. Chem. Pathol. Pharmacol.*, 11: 595–603.

Langley, J.N. (1906) On nerve-endings and on special excitable substances in cells. *Proc. R. Soc. Lond. Series B*, 78: 170–194.

Lauder, J.M. and Krebs, H. (1978) Serotonin as a differentiation signal in early neurogenesis. *Dev. Neurosci.*, 1: 13–30.

Lauder, J.M., Han, V.K.M., Henderson, P., Verdoorn, T. and Towle, A.C. (1986) Prenatal ontogeny of the GABAergic system in the rat brain: an immunocytochemical study. *Neuroscience*, 19: 465–493.

Le Fur, G., Guillout, F., Mitrani, N., Mizoule, J. and Uzan, A. (1979) Relationships between plasma corticosteroids and benzodiazepines in stress. *J. Pharmacol. Exp. Ther.*, 211: 305–308.

Lippa, A.S., Beer, B., Sano, M.C., Vogel, R.A. and Meyerson, L.R. (1981) Differential ontogeny of type 1 and type 2 benzodiazepine receptors. *Life Sci.*, 28: 2343–2347.

Livezey, G.T., Radulovacki, M., Isaac, L. and Marczynski, T.J. (1985) Prenatal exposure to diazepam results in enduring reactions in brain receptors and deep slow wave sleep. *Brain Res.*, 334: 361–365.

Livezey, G.T., Marczynski, T.J. and Isaac, L. (1986) Enduring effects of prenatal diazepam on the behavior, EEG, and brain receptors of the adult cat progeny. *Neurotoxicology*, 7: 319–333.

Majewska, M.D., Harrison, N.L., Schwartz, R.D., Barker, J.L. and Paul, S.M. (1986) Steroid hormone metabolites are barbiturate-like modulators of the GABA receptor. *Science*, 232: 1004–1007.

Marangos, P.J., Patel, J., Boulenger, J. and Clark-Rosenberg, R. (1982) Characterization of peripheral-type benzodiazepine binding sites in brain using [^{3}H]Ro 5-4864. *Mol. Pharmacol.*, 22: 26–32.

Marczynski, T.J. and Livezey, G.T. (1986) Prenatal diazepam: enduring receptor and behavioral deficits. In *Transactions of the American Society for Neurochemistry*, No. 17, Abstr. No. 323, p. 254.

Massotti, M., Alleva, F.R., Balazs, T. and Guidotti, A. (1980) GABA and benzodiazepine receptors in the offspring of dams receiving diazepam: ontogenetic studies. *Neuropharamacology*, 19: 951–956.

McCroskey, R.L. and Kidder, H.C. (1980) Auditory fusion among learning disabled, reading disabled, and normal children. *J. Learn. Disabil.*, 13: 18–25.

Miller, R.K., Kellogg, C.K. and Saltzman, R.A. (1987) Reproductive and perinatal toxicology. In W.O. Berndt and W. Haley (Eds.), *Fundamentals of Toxicology*, Hemisphere Pub. Corp., Washington, DC, pp. 195–309.

Miranda, R.C. and Kellogg, C.K. (1987) Early developmental exposure to diazepam alters brain intracellular metabolic activity in young adult and aged rats. Submitted.

Mohler, H. and Okada, T. (1977) Benzodiazepine receptor: demonstration in the central nervous system. *Science*, 198: 849–851.

Nobin, A. and Bjorklund, A. (1973) Topography of the monoamine neuron systems in the human brain as revealed in fetuses. *Acta Physiol. Scand. Suppl.*, 388: 1–38.

Olson, L., Boreus, L.O. and Seiger, A. (1973) Histochemical demonstration and mapping of 5-hydroxytryptamine and catecholamine-containing neuron systems in human fetal brain. *Z. Anat. Entwicklungsgesch.*, 139: 259–282.

Owen, F., Poulter, M., Waddington, J.L., Mashal, R.D. and Crow, T.J. (1983) [^{3}H]Ro 5-4864 benzodiazepine binding in kainate lesioned striatum and in temporal cortex of brains from patients with senile dementia of the Alzheimer type. *Brain Res.*, 278: 373–375.

Patel, A.J., Barochovsky, O., Borges, S. and Lewis, P.D. (1983) Effects of neurotropic drugs on brain cell replication in vivo and in vitro. *Monogr. Neural Sci.*, 9: 99–110.

Reisine, T., Affolter, H.-I., Rougon, G. and Barbet, J. (1986) New insights into the molecular mechanisms of stress. *Trends Neurosci.*, 9: 574–579.

Richards, J.G., Mohler, H. and Haefely, W. (1982) Benzodiazepine binding sites: receptors or acceptors. *Trends Pharmacol. Sci.*, 3: 233–235.

Rosengarten, H. and Friedhoff, A.J. (1979) Enduring changes in dopamine receptor cells of pups from drug administration to pregnant and nursing rats. *Science*, 203: 1133–1135.

Sangameswaran, L. and DeBlass, A. (1985) Demonstration of benzodiazepine-like molecules in the mammalian brain with monoclonal antibodies to benzodiazepines. *Proc. Natl. Acad. Sci. USA*, 82: 5560–5564.

Sangameswaran, L., Fales, H.M., Friedrich, P. and DeBlass, A.L. (1986) Purification of benzodiazepine from bovine brain and detection of benzodiazepine-like immunoreactivity in human brain. *Proc. Natl. Acad. Sci. USA*, 83: 9236–9240.

Schlumpf, M., Richards, J.G., Lichtensteiger, W. and Mohler, H. (1983) An autoradiographical study of the prenatal development of benzodiazepine binding sites in rat brain. *J. Neurosci.*, 3: 1478–1487.

Schoch, P., Richards, J.G., Haring, P., Takacs, B., Stahli, C., Staehelin, T., Haefely, W. and Mohler, H. (1985) Co-localization of GABA$_A$ receptors and benzodiazepine receptors in the brain shown by monoclonal antibodies. *Nature*, 314: 168–171.

Selye, H. (1976) *Stress in Health and Disease*, Butterworth, Boston.

Shibuya, T., Watanabe, Y., Hill, H.F. and Salafsky, B. (1986) Developmental alterations in maturing rats caused by chronic prenatal and postnatal diazepam treatments. *Japan J. Pharmacol.*, 40: 21–29.

Shoemaker, H., Morelli, M., Deshmukh, P. and Yamamura, H.I. (1982) [^{3}H]Ro 5-4864 benzodiazepine binding in the kainate-lesioned rat striatum and Huntington's diseased basal ganglia. *Brain Res.*, 248: 396–401.

Shore, C.O., Vorhees, C.V., Bornschein, R.L. and Stemmer, K. (1983) Behavioral consequences of prenatal diazepam exposure in rats. *Neurobehav. Toxicol. Teratol.*, 5: 565–570.

Simmons, R.D., Miller, R.K. and Kellogg, C.K. (1983) Prenatal diazepam: distribution and metabolism in perinatal rats. *Teratology*, 28: 181–188.

Simmons, R.D., Kellogg, C.K. and Miller, R.K. (1984a) Prenatal diazepam exposure in rats: long-lasting, receptor-mediated effects on hypothalamic norepinephrine-containing neurons. *Brain Res.*, 293: 73–83.

Simmons, R.D., Miller, R.K. and Kellogg, C.K. (1984b) Prenatal exposure to diazepam alters central and peripheral responses to stress in adult rat offspring. *Brain Res.*, 307: 39–46.

Specht, L.A., Pickel, V.M., Joh, T.H. and Reis, D.J. (1981) Light microscopic immunocytochemical localization of tyrosine hydroxylase in prenatal rat brain. II. Late ontogeny. *J. Comp. Neurol.*, 199: 255–276.

Squires, R. and Braestrup, C. (1977) Benzodiazepine receptors in brain. *Nature*, 266: 732–734.

Sullivan, A.T. and Kellogg, C.K. (1985) Dose-related effects of diazepam on noise-induced potentiation of the acoustic startle reflex: disclosure of several underlying mechanisms. *Abstr. Neurosci.*, 11: 1289, No. 377.4

Swanson, L.W., Sawchenko, P.E. and Lind, R.W. (1986) Regulation of multiple peptides in CRF parvocellular neurosecretory neurons: implications for the stress response. *Prog. Brain Res.*, 68: 169–190.

Tallman, J.F. and Gallager, D.W. (1985) The GABAergic system: a locus of benzodiazepine actions. *Annu. Rev. Neurosci.*, 8: 21–44.

Taylor, K.M. and Laverty, R. (1969) The effect of chlordiazepoxide, diazepam and nitrazepam on catecholamine metabolism in regions of the rat brain. *Eur. J. Pharmacol.*, 8: 296–301.

Ticku, M.K. (1983) Benzodiazepine-GABA receptor-ionophore complex. *Neuropharmacology*, 22: 1459–1470.

Trinder, E. (1979) Auditory fusion: a critical test with implications in differential diagnosis. *Br. J. Audiol.*, 13: 143–147.

Tucker, S.C. (1985) Benzodiazepines and the developing rat: a critical review. *Neurosci. Behav. Rev.*, 9: 101–111.

Weber, L.W.D. (1985) Benzodiazepines in pregnancy – academical debate or teratogenic risk? *Biol. Res. Pregnancy*, 6: 151–167.

Yeh, S.Y., Paul, R.H., Cordero, L. and Hon, E.H. (1974) A study of diazepam during labor. *Obstet. Gynecol.*, 43: 363–373.

Discussion

B.S. McEwen: What stressors have you used to show effects of prenatal benzodiazepines and how profound are their effects on the time course of the stress response?

C.K. Kellogg: The data presented were obtained using restraint stress. For hormonal assays, plasma was analysed at 30, 60, 90 and 120 minutes of stress. In control animals, a peak response of 68% increase in plasma corticosterone was measured at 30 min and values had returned to baseline by 120 min. In animals prenatally exposed to diazepam (DZ) at 1 mg/kg, there was only a 39% increase in corticosterone, again measured at 30 min. Exposure to DZ at 2.5 mg/kg essentially blocked the response.

D.F. Swaab: If you really want to claim an effect on aging, you should try to keep your animals a little longer. The moment of 50% survival rate is a well-accepted point (Mos and Hollander, 1987). This will be rather around 30 than around 24 months of age.

C.K. Kellogg: Twenty-four to twenty-six months is certainly longer than any other prenatal exposure study that I am aware of has been carried out. If changes in metabolism that can be observed from 3 months to 18 months to 24 months are not related to aging, then what are they related to? The rat is getting older! Dramatic changes seen between 18 and 24 months in the exposed rats suggest that the animals have gone through a transition stage.

B. Weiss: Your data are a powerful argument for conducting functional assessments late in the lifespan to determine the consequences of prenatal chemical exposure. Often, for safety assessment, 2-year toxicity studies are conducted, at the end of which the animals are sliced up for pathology. I don't see why late functional assessment could not be pursued in such a context without expanding the safety protocols unduly.

C.K. Kellogg: Newer methods, such as ^{31}P-nuclear magnetic spectroscopy, allow one to obtain metabolic information over the lifespan of the animal. These methods should be considered more often in these kinds of studies.

Reference

Mos. J. and Hollander, C.F. (1987) Analysis of survival data on aging rats cohorts: pitfalls and some practical considerations. *Mech. Ageing Dev.*, 38: 89–105.

G.J. Boer, M.G.P. Feenstra, M. Mirmiran, D.F. Swaab and F. Van Haaren
Progress in Brain Research, Vol. 73
© 1988 Elsevier Science Publishers B.V. (Biomedical Division)

CHAPTER 15

Anticonvulsants and brain development

Charles V. Vorhees, Daniel R. Minck and Helen K. Berry

Institute for Developmental Research, Children's Hospital Research Foundation, and University of Cincinnati, Cincinnati, OH 45229, USA

Introduction

It has been recognized for a number of years that epileptic women receiving anticonvulsant medication bear children with major malformations at rates 2–3 times that in the general population (Hill et al., 1974: Kalter and Warkany, 1983; Kelly, 1984). Whether this increase is related to the anticonvulsant drugs or to indirect effects arising from epilepsy itself is not resolved (Monson et al., 1973: Shapiro et al., 1976). Nakane (1979) has provided evidence that epileptics who were untreated did not have a higher than normal risk of birth defects among their children, while those who were treated did. Furthermore, the risk of malformation in the treated group was related to both the number and type of anticonvulsant drug(s) taken. Animal research confirms this, directly implicating the drugs rather than the presence of a seizure disorder in causing malformations (Finnell, 1981; Finnell et al., 1987).

A shift in the perspective on fetal anticonvulsant effects occurred in 1975 when Hanson and his colleagues described a cluster of symptoms associated with two specific drugs and termed the conditions the fetal hydantoin syndrome (Hanson and Smith, 1975) and the fetal trimethadione syndrome (Zackai et al., 1975). Children with both conditions were described as having characteristic features involving growth, facial morphology and CNS/functional integrity.

Similar to the fetal alcohol syndrome in certain respects, children exposed prenatally to anticonvulsants were found to be significantly smaller at birth and to grow poorly postnatally, to have multiple minor dysmorphic facial features, and to exhibit CNS effects ranging from developmental delay to mental retardation.

The embryopathy associated with trimethadione has been confirmed by other investigators (Feldman et al., 1977). This, combined with the advent of alternative drugs for the treatment of absence seizure, has largely eliminated the clinical use of trimethadione. Phenytoin, by contrast, continues to be the most widely prescribed anticonvulsant drug (Kelly et al., 1984), although its link to embryopathy is still undetermined (cf. Kelly et al., 1984, and Hanson, 1986). Several investigators have suggested that phenytoin's effects are equivocal if it is taken alone, but significantly deleterious when combined with phenobarbital (Majewski et al., 1981: Majewski and Steger, 1984; Hill and Tennyson, 1986).

Unlike the situation with the fetal alcohol syndrome, the incidence of fetal anticonvulsant syndrome (FACS) cases is not established. Hanson et al. (1976) found that approximately 11% of infants exposed in utero to phenytoin exhibited the full syndrome, while 31% revealed partial expressions. Estimates of epilepsy in the general population range from 0.33 to 0.52% (Kalter and Warkany, 1983; Kelly, 1984). In the United States there are 3.6 million births per year. There-

230

fore, using the conservative estimate of the prevalence of epilepsy, there are approximately 11 880 births per year to epileptic women in the USA. Prospective studies reveal that 95% of epileptic women in the USA are on anticonvulsant medications and, therefore, 11 286 births per year are exposed in utero to anticonvulsants. If we extrapolate from Hanson et al.'s (1976) data and presume that the incidence of all FACSs is the same as for the fetal hydantoin syndrome, then there may be as many as 1 241 new FACS cases occurring per year, with almost another 3 500 partial syndromes per year just in the USA. Investigations confirming such estimates are needed.

The symptoms of all the FACSs are similar, including those of the recently described fetal valproate syndrome (DiLiberti et al., 1984; Jager-Roman et al., 1986). A composite list of symptoms from several sources for the FACSs is shown in Table 1. The consistency with which

delay in the attainment of neurobehavioral milestones and mental development has been reported with these syndromes is striking. We became interested in these syndromes and began to develop a model to examine the effect of these drugs on brain development. There were several reasons for this interest. First, we have been interested for some time in the dose-effect relationship between structural malformations and more subtle functional CNS injury (Vorhees and Butcher, 1982; Vorhees, 1986); second, we were interested in the characteristics of agents which cause CNS injury at sub-malforming doses; and third, we have been interested in models of early brain injury and what they can teach us about CNS development, recovery and mechanisms of neurotoxic insults. The focus of this review will be upon trimethadione, phenobarbital, valproic acid and phenytoin (Vorhees, 1983, 1987a,b). Emphasis will be placed on phenytoin because more

TABLE 1

Fetal anticonvulsant syndromes (FACS)

Symptom[a]	Phenytoin	Trimethadione	Phenobarbital	Primidone	Valproate
Mental subnormality	+	+	+	+	+
Growth retardation	+	+	+	+	
Short nose	+		+		+
Low nasal bridge	+		+		+
Hypertelorism	+		+		
Ptosis	+		+		
Epicanthus	+	+		+	+
Cleft palate/lip	+	+		+	
Abnormal ear position		+	+	+	+
V-shaped eyebrows		+		+	
Hypoplastic digits	+		+		
Long upper lip					+
Shallow philtrum					+
Thin upper vermilion					+
Downturned mouth					+
Other defects	±	±	±	±	±

[a] Reported symptom found in clinical case reports cited in the Introduction. Listing of a symptom is not intended to imply that all reported cases possess all symptoms, but rather that multiple cases have shown the characteristic in question. Mental subnormality is used here as a generic term and includes a range of reported effects from mental retardation defined using standardized IQ test instruments, to descriptive terms such as 'mental' or 'developmental' delay.

research is available on this drug and because it remains the most widely used anticonvulsant in the world.

Perspective

As mentioned, the clinical description of several fetal anticonvulsant syndromes altered the direction of research on these drugs away from their possible role in causing major malformations and towards their possible functional effects. Laboratory research on functional effects has been dominated by investigations on phenobarbital. This research has come primarily from the laboratories of Middaugh et al. (1975a,b, 1981a,b, 1983), Yanai (1984) and Martin et al. (1979, 1985). Middaugh (1986) has recently reviewed this literature and concluded that the offspring of dams given doses comparable to human anticonvulsant doses show persistent reductions in habituation and increased reactivity to environmental novelty. He notes that reductions in neuron numbers in the hippocampus and cerebellum are induced by prenatal phenobarbital exposure, but that attempts to find a neurochemical basis for these effects remains to be found. This situation exists despite the fact that a number of laboratories have reported neurochemical changes. Unfortunately, agreement among different investigators regarding the nature of these changes has been conspicuously lacking.

As for the other anticonvulsants, only one credible early report on phenytoin exists (Vernadakis and Woodbury, 1969). No functional animal studies on trimethadione or valproic acid existed.

Our goal was to develop a rodent model of the fetal anticonvulsant syndromes which would enable us to examine the long-term CNS effects resulting from prenatal exposure. In order to attain this goal we reasoned that the model should meet several criteria. First, to evaluate the behavioral teratogenic effects of these drugs, doses should be used which, under our experimental conditions, would be at or below those producing teratogenensis as measured by conventional near-term fetal autopsy methods. Second, the model should provide a marker for comparisons to other species, viz., humans. For this purpose, three alternative approaches seemed plausible: (a) administration of doses comparable to those used to treat epilepsy in humans; (b) administration of doses equally effective pharmacologically to doses used in humans, i.e., doses that inhibit seizure activity, and (c) administration of doses which would produce comparable human therapeutic tissue drug concentrations. Of these approaches, (a) is not reliable because of well-known pharmacokinetic scaling problems between different species. This problem makes equal doses unequal in efficacy (Boxenbaum and Ronfeld, 1983), e.g., rats metabolize many drugs more rapidly than do humans. Approach (b) is plausible, but the problem is that rodent tests of a drug's anticonvulsant potential using induced seizures do not necessarily provide valid estimates of human therapeutic dose levels. Rather, these procedures are designed for screening new agents to determine whether they possess anticonvulsant activity (Swinyard and Woodhead, 1982; Loscher et al., 1984). Therefore, we chose option (c). Finally, our third consideration was to develop a model that produced minimal or no maternal toxicity in order to avoid the interpretational problems which complicate causal inference for investigations of teratogenicity (Khera, 1984).

Phenytoin is insoluble in aqueous vehicles, and its gastrointestinal absorption is known to be variable (Woodbury, 1982). Sodium phenytoin is usually used in humans to enhance absorption, but since the administered dose was irrelevant to the criteria established above, we opted to suspend phenytoin in propylene glycol. The same vehicle was then maintained for trimethadione, phenobarbital and, later, valproic acid. In order to meet the initial criterion that the dose of these drugs for behavioral teratological analysis not be embryopathic, a conventional teratology study was first conducted. These data will not be reviewed in detail here (see Vorhees, 1983). In brief, a dose of 500 mg/kg of phenytoin administered by gavage on gestation (G) days 7–18 was severely maternally toxic and produced 100% embryonic resorption. A dose of 250 mg/kg of phenytoin was not significantly teratogenic, but was maternally toxic, embryotoxic (increased resorptions) and ponderally teratogenic (reduced fetal weight). Finally, a dose of 200 mg/kg of phenytoin was not teratogenic or embryotoxic. Maternal weight was reduced, but this reduction was not severe (21% reduction on day G20). Finally, fetal weight was reduced by only 15% on day G20. It was concluded that the 200 mg/kg dose was not teratogenic by standard criteria (resorptions, skeletal or visceral malformations), but was a threshold dose based on fetal weight reduction. This dose was chosen, therefore, as our initial test dosage for postnatal evaluation, with lower doses of 50 and 5 mg/kg also included. Similar procedures were followed for trimethadione, phenobarbital and valproic acid. The final dose chosen for trimethadione by this approach was 250 mg/kg, with lower doses selected of 50 and 5 mg/kg. For phenobarbital the highest dose chosen was 80 mg/kg, with lower doses of 50 and 5 mg/kg also included. For valproic acid the threshold teratogenic dose chosen was 200 mg/kg and a lower dose of 150 mg/kg was also included. The results will be presented first for phenytoin, followed by those for trimethadione, phenobarbital and valproic acid.

There were no published behavioral teratology studies on phenytoin when we began our first experiment in 1980, although, while our study was in progress, Elmazar and Sullivan (1981) published a set of two experiments on this topic. They administered phenytoin as the sodium salt, and the dose used was 100 mg/kg administered by gavage on days G6–18. They found delayed dynamic righting development, decreased rotorod performance, impaired narrow-path walking, and shortened jump latencies from elevated platforms. They also noted modest reductions in postnatal body weight and, among culled offspring, slight delays in bone ossification.

In the experiments reviewed below the following experimental questions were evaluated. (1) What neurobehavioral, mortality and ponderal effects are produced by our highest dose of phenytoin? (2) Are there critical periods for these effects? (3) Are there linear or non-linear dose-effect relationships. (4) What is the relationship between dose and maternal and fetal plasma drug concentrations? (5) What are the pathological and biochemical bases of the observed functional effects, and how long do the behavioral effects persist?

In most experiments rats were gavaged with phenytoin on days 7–18 of gestation. This exposure period was selected as one which would span all of organogenesis and include a significant portion of the fetal period in order to encompass more of neurogenesis (Rodier, 1980). In a later experiment exposure days were G7–10, G11–14 or G15–18. Following this we returned to the G7–18 exposure period, but different groups received 100, 150 or 200 mg/kg of phenytoin on each day of treatment. The most recent experiment examined the long-term effects of phenytoin as well as several more specific hypotheses. A similar but less extensive set of investigations was conducted on the other three anticonvulsants.

Prenatal effects of phenytoin

Table 2 summarizes the effects observed in the offspring derived from the first behavioral experiment in the 200 mg/kg group. Note that for pivoting locomotion, dramatic increases were observed on this measure on test days PN9 and 11, but not on day 7. As will be seen later, this finding was replicated in subsequent experiments.

For swimming ontogeny, significant delays on all three measures of rated swimming development were found. The scales of swimming performance were swimming direction, angle (orientation in the water, primarily of the head) and paddling (limb usage). Particularly noteworthy was the marked delay seen in the development of swimming direction. This effect was character-

TABLE 2

Summary of significant behavioral effects of offspring from exposure to 200 mg/kg phenytoin on days G7–18 in rat

Tests	Effect obtained
Surface righting	No effect
Pivoting locomotion	Increased
Negative geotaxis	No effect
Olfactory orientation	No effect
Swimming ontogeny	Delayed
Auditory startle emergence	Delayed
Preweaning figure-8 activity	No effect
Home-cage T-maze learning	No effect
Postweaning figure-8 activity	Increased
Postweaning figure-8 rearing	Decreased
M-maze brightness discrimination	No effect
Straight channel swimming time	No effect
Biel maze errors	Increased
Biel maze times	Increased
Spontaneous alternation	No effect
Passive avoidance acquisition	No effect
Passive avoidance retention	Impaired
Cage side observation	Abnormal circling behavior (only some animals affected)

ized by a persistent circling pattern in phenytoin offspring at ages when controls had progressed to the adult phase of straight-line swimming. The significance of this observation was only understood later. For auditory startle, a delay in the ontogeny of this reflex was observed in the phenytoin offspring. No change in the adult auditory startle reflex was obtained in subsequent experiments. Inhibition of adult tactile startle response was noted, however. The figure-8 meter provides a test of spontaneous locomotor activity in an environment shaped as the name implies. The phenytoin offspring exhibited increased locomotor activity and, concomitantly, reduced rearing frequency.

Prior to water maze testing, a straight channel test of performance was conducted to assess performance factors. No difference in straight chan-

nel performance of phenytoin offspring was observed. Subsequently, testing in a complex multiple-T maze was divided into two phases. One phase was in path A and one in path B of the maze. Phenytoin offspring committed more errors and spent longer in the maze on path A than controls. When tested on path B, controls exhibited the typical increase in errors on the first two trials, followed by a pattern of rapid elimination of errors. By contrast, the phenytoin offspring exhibited a much larger increase in errors on the first two path B trials, and a very slow elimination of errors on subsequent trials. The net effect was that the phenytoin offspring committed in total about three times more errors than controls. Time spent in the maze showed a similar pattern, i.e., increased maze times in the phenytoin-exposed group.

No effect of phenytoin was seen on initial step-through latency on the passive avoidance task, or on trials to criterion scores. This was observed despite the phenytoin group's notable hyperactivity. However, a reduction in latency scores was seen in the phenytoin group when retested two weeks later for retention of the learned response.

Finally, in postweaning rats, a percentage of animals was noted to exhibit circling behavior. After completion of the experiment, groups were decoded, and out of the 10 treatment groups, only the phenytoin 200 mg/kg group contained animals that exhibited the unusual circling behavior. No effect of phenytoin on any functional test was observed at the lower doses of 50 or 5 mg/kg.

The next experiment was designed to detect a critical-period effect in the production of the functional effects observed in the previous experiment. In order to maximize comparability between the two experiments, the tests, test ages, test procedures and examiners were held constant. The dose was 200 mg/kg.

Pivoting locomotion effects in phenytoin offspring were again observed, but they were confined to those exposed on days G11–14 or G15–18, and were not apparent in those exposed on days G7–10. Swimming ontogeny was again delayed in the phenytoin groups, and all exposure intervals produced a delay on one or more of the three measures used on this test. However, the G11–14 exposure group was the most affected of the three exposure groups. Figure-8 activity was also affected by phenytoin exposure and, as before, the effect was increased postweaning activity with no effect on the same measure prior to weaning. Furthermore, the effect did not occur in all exposure groups, but was limited to the phenytoin group exposed on days G11-14. In Biel water maze performance, the same pattern as before emerged. There were no differences in straight channel swimming times, but increased errors and times in the maze. The effects obtained were only significant in the phenytoin G11-14 group. The effect of phenytoin on passive avoidance performance was again the same as previously noted. There was no effect of pheny-

toin on initial step-through latencies and no difference on trials to criterion, but a reduction in latency scores was observed when retention for the response was assessed two weeks after reaching the acquisition criterion. This effect was confined to only one phenytoin group, i.e., those exposed on days G11–14.

Not only did the results of this experiment confirm the same abnormalities as seen previously, it was also the case that the same tests which showed no phenytoin-related differences in the previous experiment also showed no phenytoin-induced changes in this experiment. The tests showing no effects in either experiment are listed in Tables 2 and 3 along with those that did show effects.

The results of the next experiment are summarized in Table 4. This experiment had three purposes: (1) to determine whether linear dose-dependent behavioral effects occurred; (2) to relate performance to maternal and fetal plasma drug concentrations during treatment; and (3) to attempt to replicate the air-righting delay caused

TABLE 3

Summary of significant behavioral effects on offspring from exposures to 200 mg/kg phenytoin on days G7–10, 11–14 or 15–18

Test	Effect obtained	Affected groups(s)
Surface righting	No effect	
Pivoting locomotion	Increased	11–14, 15–18 groups
Negative geotaxis	No effect	
Olfactory orientation	No effect	
Swimming ontogeny	Delayed	All groups (11–14 most affected)
Preweaning figure-8 activity	No effect	
Home-cage T-maze learning	No effect	
Postweaning figure-8 activity	Increased	11–14 group
Postweaning figure-8 rearing	No effect	
M-maze brightness discrimination	No effect	
Straight channel swimming times	No effect	
Biel maze errors	Increased	11–14 group
Biel maze times	Increased	11–14 group
Spontaneous alternation	No effect	
Passive avoidance acquisition	No effect	
Passive avoidance retention	Impaired	11–14 group

TABLE 4

Summary of significant behavioral effects on offspring from exposure to 100, 150 or 200 mg/kg phenytoin on days G7–18

Test	Effect obtained	Affected group(s)
Pivoting locomotion	Increased	Dose-dependent
Early photocell activity	Increased	Dose-dependent
Air righting	Delayed	Dose-dependent
Figure-8 locomotor activity	Increased	200 mg/kg group
Figure-8 rearing frequency	No effect	
Open-field locomotor activity	Increased	200 mg/kg group
Hole-board horizontal activity	Increased	200 mg/kg group
Hole-board vertical activity	No effect	
Straight channel swimming times	No effect	
Biel maze errors	Increased	Dose-dependent
Cincinnati maze errors	Increased	Dose-dependent
Acoustic startle response	No effect	
Tactile startle response	Reduced	200 mg/kg group
Rated circling behavior	Present	Partially dose-dependent

by prenatal phenytoin that was first described by Elmazar and Sullivan (1981). In this experiment the doses were 100, 150 or 200 mg/kg administered on days G7–18. Early locomotion was measured by two independent methods. Both methods revealed dose-related increases in locomotion and confirmed the pivoting effects observed previously.

The results of air-righting development revealed that, using two different scoring criteria, the phenytoin offspring exhibited a delay in the maturation rate of this response. Further, this effect was linearly dose-dependent, so that the high dose showed the largest delay, and the middle and low doses step-wise smaller delays. Postweaning activity was assessed using figure-8, open-field and hole-board tests. The tests showed complete convergence at the highest dose, all revealing a phenytoin-related hyperactivity and no drug × test-order interaction. Biel water maze testing revealed no effects of phenytoin on pre-maze straight channel swimming times. This experiment replicated the effects of previous experiments, however, showing increased errors and time spent in the maze. In addition, a second and more complex water maze test was conducted at the same time on a subset of littermates. The same pattern of increased errors and times in phenytoin offspring was observed. Adult acoustic startle testing revealed no effects associated with phenytoin exposure. Results in the same test apparatus with a tactile stimulus, however, showed a small phenytoin-associated reduction in startle amplitude. This effect was most consistent in the high dose group.

The circling behavior observed previously was systematically evaluated in this experiment. When the groups were decoded at the end of the study, a dose-effect trend was observed in the number of affected individuals and in the number of litters containing at least one affected individual. The pattern was not linear, however, in that the two lower dose groups showed similar incidences of affected individuals, while the high dose group showed a sharp increase in the percentage affected. The 200 mg/kg group had 18% of the offspring exhibiting circling, while the lower dose groups each had 4–5% affected. Among all the rats showing circling about 59% turned left and 41% turned right. As for sex differences, 55% of all those circling were females and 45% were males.

Mean serum concentrations 4 hours after the last drug dose on day G18 were 24.0 ± 2.2 (n = 10) in the high dose group, 20.1 ± 1.6 (n = 4) in the middle dose group, and 9.8 ± 0.8 (n = 4) μg/ml in the low dose group. Human therapeutic serum concentrations are generally regarded as 10–20 μg/ml, with toxicity developing at 30 μg/ml or above. Twenty-four-hour maternal

TABLE 5

Brain weight, body weight and brain protein of 80-day-old female rats born from phenytoin-exposed pregnant rat mothers

	Treatment group		Phenytoin group	
	Control	Phenytoin	Non-circlers	Circlers
n^a	11	17	9	8
Brain weight (mg)	1874.2 (30.7)	1854.9 (23.8)	1869.1 (38.4)	1838.9 (27.8)
Body weight (g)	231.7 (6.1)	242.3 (4.5)	244.2 (6.5)	240.1 (6.6)
Brain protein (mg/g)	90.6 (1.2)	90.0 (1.5)	89.4 (2.0)	90.5 (2.2)

Data are means (SE).
[a] Number of female progeny assayed. Multiple litters are represented within each group.

TABLE 6

Brain amino acid neurotransmitters of 80-day-old female rats born from phenytoin-exposed mothers

	Treatment group		Phenytoin group	
	Control	Phenytoin	Non-circlers	Circlers
n^a	11	17	9	8
GABA (I)[b]	25.6 (0.6)	27.2 (0.6)	27.3 (1.0)	27.1 (0.8)
Glycine (I)	12.0 (0.3)	12.5 (0.2)	12.7 (0.3)	12.2 (0.4)
Taurine (I)	56.4 (1.0)	57.1 (1.5)	57.0 (1.9)	56.6 (1.0)
Glutamic acid (E)	117.7 (1.4)	122.9 (2.1)	123.0 (3.2)	122.7 (2.8)
Aspartic acid (E)	38.8 (1.0)	39.2 (0.9)	39.7 (1.2)	38.6 (1.5)

Values are expressed as mmol/mg protein and given as means (SE).
[a] Number of female progeny assayed. Multiple litters are represented within each group.
[b] I = Inhibitory or E = excitatory neurotransmitter.

and fetal serum phenytoin levels revealed that fetal concentrations were a consistent fraction (approximately 50%) of maternal serum values. Such values are above the levels expected, based upon published data on the free fraction of this drug in serum in rats.

A subset of female offspring from the high dose group was killed by decapitation; the brains were removed on dry ice, weighed, and later analysed for protein and amino acids. In a preliminary smaller sample we previously reported several changes in the phenytoin offsprings' brain amino

TABLE 7

Brain amino acid neurotransmitter precursors of 80-day-old female rats born from phenytoin-exposed mothers

	Treatment group		Phenytoin group	
	Control	Phenytoin	Non-circlers	Circlers
n^a	11	17	9	9
Serine (Gly)[b]	8.7 (0.2)	9.0 (0.2)	9.2 (0.3)	8.8 (0.4)
Glutamine (Glu)	48.4 (1.9)	52.0 (2.0)	48.8 (2.9)	55.5 (2.4)
Alanine (β-Ala)	6.8 (0.3)	7.0 (0.2)	7.4 (0.3)	6.6 (0.3)
Tyrosine (CA)	0.6 (0.1)	0.5 (0.1)	0.5 (0.1)	0.6 (0.1)
Phenylalanine (CA)	0.4 (0.05)	0.5 (0.04)	0.4 (0.05)	0.6 (0.02)[c]
Histidine (Hist)	0.7 (0.03)	0.8 (0.04)	0.6 (0.06)	0.9 (0.09)[d]

Values are expressed as mmol/mg protein and given as means (SE).
[a] Number of female progeny assayed. Multiple litters are represented within each group.
[b] Indicates neurotransmitter for which each listed amino acid is the precursor. Gly = glycine, Glu = glutamic acid, β-Ala = β-alanine, CA = catecholamines, Hist = histamine.
[c] $P < 0.01$.
[d] $P < 0.05$.

TABLE 8

Brain amino acids of 80-day-old female rats born from phenytoin-exposed mothers

	Treatment group		Phenytoin group	
	Control	Phenytoin	Non-circlers	Circlers
n^a	11	17	9	8
Threonine	6.2 (0.3)	6.2 (0.3)	6.3 (0.2)	6.1 (0.4)
Valine	1.1 (0.07)	1.1 (0.04)	0.8 (0.1)	1.2 (0.1)[b]
Leucine	0.8 (0.05)	0.7 (0.06)	0.8 (0.06)	0.6 (0.09)[b]
Isoleucine	0.4 (0.05)	0.4 (0.04)	0.4 (0.06)	0.5 (0.06)
Methionine	0.3 (0.01)	0.3 (0.02)	0.3 (0.03)	0.3 (0.02)
Cystathionine	0.6 (0.03)	0.6 (0.04)	0.6 (0.06)	0.6 (0.06)
Ornithine	0.4 (0.03)	0.4 (0.03)	0.3 (0.03)	0.4 (0.04)
Lysine	3.4 (0.1)	3.1 (0.2)	3.3 (0.3)	3.0 (0.2)
Arginine	1.2 (0.2)	1.6 (0.1)	1.4 (0.2)	1.8 (0.2)
Phosphoethanolamine	12.2 (0.3)	12.5 (0.4)	13.2 (0.6)	11.8 (0.6)

Values are expressed as mmol/mg protein and given as means (SE).
[a] Number of female progeny assayed. Multiple litters are represented within each group.
[b] $P < 0.05$.

acid profile, including a reduction in total brain protein and changes in several amino acids' concentrations, e.g., an increase in GABA levels (Vorhees, 1985). In the larger series reported here for the first time, and more importantly drawn from more litters, these preliminary observations were not confirmed. No differences in brain weight, total brain protein or in body weight of females were seen at 80 days of age (Table 5). Brain amino acid neurotransmitters in these same animals are shown in Table 6. As can be seen, no group differences occurred. Amino acids which are precursors for neurotransmitters are shown in Table 7. Again, no group differences were found. Other amino acids measured in brain are shown in Table 8. No group differences were found. In the right halves of Tables 5–8 the phenytoin group is subdivided into those exhibiting circling behavior and those not. In Table 7 it can be seen that phenytoin offspring exhibiting circling showed an increase in brain phenylalanine and histidine as compared to non-circlers. In Table 8

it can be seen that circlers exhibited an increase in brain valine and a decrease in leucine. If these effects are specific to the circling behavior and not to phenytoin, then non-circlers should be similar to controls for these amino acid concentrations. This expectation holds for the changes in phenylalanine, histidine and leucine, but not for valine. In the case of valine, it is the non-circlers that differ most from controls, suggesting that the valine difference is not related to the phenytoin treatment.

Long-term effects of prenatal phenytoin

The results of our most recent experiment are summarized in Table 9. The results confirm the previous findings of phenytoin-induced increased early locomotion and adolescent figure-8 and open-field activity, combined with decreased rearing frequency. In addition, the open-field results showed that the phenytoin offspring exhibited significantly less habituation to the test environ-

TABLE 9

Summary of significant behavioral effects in adulthood of offspring from exposure to 200 mg/kg phenytoin on days G7–18 in rat

Test	Effects obtained
Early photocell activity	Increased
Figure-8 locomotor activity	Increased
Figure-8 rearing frequency	Decreased
Open-field locomotor activity	Increased
Open-field activity habituation	Decreased
Straight channel swimming times	Slowed
Cincinnati maze errors	Increased
Cincinnati maze times	Increased
Acoustic startle response	No effect
Tactile startle response	Reduced
Prepulse startle inhibition	No effect
Gap-induced startle inhibition	No effect
Morris hidden platform maze learning	Decreased
Cincinnati maze errors (16 mo. retention)	Increased
Straight channel swimming times (16 mo.)	No effect
Cincinnati maze errors (16 mo. acquisition)	Increased
Rated circling behavior	Present[a]

[a] Effect seen only when animal was assessed in a confined environment.

tested in a slightly modified version of the Morris hidden platform maze test of spatial memory. Phenytoin offspring required significantly longer to find the platform than controls across successive trials. Phenytoin offspring also spent less time in the target quadrant on test trials when the platform was removed. Lastly, the phenytoin offspring had longer latencies on the shift trials when the platform was moved to the opposite quadrant.

At 16 months of age, those rats that had been tested in the Cincinnati maze at 2 months were re-tested for retention using a re-acquisition paradigm. Since these rats had last received path B trials in the maze, their retention was assessed by giving them additional path B trials. Phenytoin offspring committed more errors than controls on these trials. They were then given additional trials in path A. Again, the phenytoin offspring committed more errors. The remaining littermates that had not received water maze testing at 2 months were tested for the first time at 16 months using the original test procedure. These maze-naive phenytoin offspring did not differ in straight channel swimming times, but they committed more errors and took more time in path A and path B

ment than controls. The results in the Cincinnati water maze test confirmed previous findings, in that the phenytoin offspring were found to commit more errors and spend more time in the maze than controls. In a departure from previous maze data, however, the phenytoin offspring in this experiment swam the pre-maze straight channel slower than controls.

Tests of startle revealed that, as before, the phenytoin offspring showed no effect on acoustic startle, but showed reduced tactile startle. Two startle modification test paradigms, one using an acoustic prepulse and another using a gap in a constant background signal, showed that phenytoin did not alter performance under either of these more complex startle procedures.

At approximately 14 months of age rats were

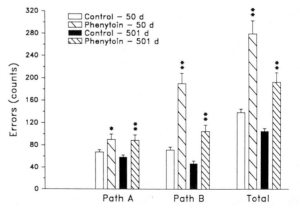

Fig. 1. Mean ($\pm$ SE) number of errors committed in the Cincinnati water maze by offspring of dams treated prenatally with phenytoin (200 mg/kg on days G7–18) or vehicle (controls). Half of the males and females in each litter were tested beginning at 50 days of age and the other half at 501 days. *P < 0.05, **P < 0.01.

than controls. Total errors in rats tested at 2 and 16 months on path A and B are shown in Fig. 1. As can be seen, the maze performance deficit in the phenytoin rats persists even at the later age. Furthermore, the data provide no support for the concept that a prenatal-induced impairment might worsen with advancing age.

Finally, the circling behavior described previously was seen again in this experiment. One additional characteristic noted about this behavior was that rats exhibiting the effect only revealed it when placed in confined spaces. When rats were allowed to ambulate in an open environment the behavior was generally absent and, when swimming in an open pool, the behavior was markedly suppressed. In small environments or swimming in narrow channels, however, the circling behavior unfolded.

In all of these experiments, prenatal phenytoin did not significantly reduce offspring growth or weight, but did increase postnatal mortality. The latter effect was confined to the high dose group and to the preweaning period. Preweaning mortality rates were highest in our early studies (25–33%) and were sharply lower (0–12%) when we switched to a pathogen-free rat from the same supplier (Charles River Sprague-Dawley CD). We are currently investigating this shift in toxicity but the exact reason for the shift is not yet understood.

Effects of phenytoin on inner ear development

In reflecting upon the unusual circling behavior seen in these rats, we were struck by its resemblance to behavioral defects described in certain inbred mutant strains of mice. In particular, we believed that the circling phenytoin rats shared several behavioral features with mouse mutants, such as the pallid trait, first described by Lyon (1951, 1953) and studied extensively since by Erway and associates (Erway et al., 1966, 1971, 1986; Lim and Erway, 1974). The homozygotically affected pallid mouse (pa/pa) exhibits several characteristic behavioral abnormalities. These include head tilting, turning in circles and ataxic gait. Some show gross disruptions in swimming, including swimming under water in head-over-heel loops, or swimming on their sides. Such animals exhibit large delays or complete inability to perform dynamic righting. The phenytoin-circlers did not exhibit ataxia, but a few did show slight head tilt. All phenytoin circlers did acquire the dynamic righting reflex, but as a group they were delayed compared to controls. Phenytoin circlers did not exhibit underwater swimming, but they did swim in circles and the most severely affected showed episodic disorientations in the water. Such disorientations sometimes led them to roll over one or more times in rapid succession before regaining proper orientation.

Erway et al. (1966) have shown that the behaviors seen in the pallid mouse are associated with a congenital absence of otoliths in the inner ear. They have also shown that tilted-head mutant mice show similar behavioral defects and also have abnormal otolith development (Lim et al., 1977). These same authors reported that the area covered by the otoconial crystals of the otoliths had to be reduced by more than 80% before abnormal behavior was observed. At reductions exceeding 80% of visible otoconia, the severity of the behavioral defect and the degree of otoconial deficiency were correlated. The authors went on to demonstrate that in the pallid mutant the congenital otoconial deficiency could be prevented by supplementing the diet with manganese (Erway et al., 1966; Lim and Erway, 1971; Shrader et al., 1973). When the otoconial deficiency was prevented by administering manganese, the behavioral defects were also prevented.

As a result of the behavioral similarities between these inbred mutant mice and our phenytoin circlers, we hypothesized that phenytoin was interfering with formation of otoconia in the utriculus and sacculus of the otic capsule. We recognized that this hypothesis was at variance with the published data on the teratogenicity of phenytoin, inasmuch as there were no reports of inner ear defects associated with this drug in experimental animals. We reasoned, however, that despite the extent to which the teratogenicity of phenytoin had been investigated, two circumstances made it unlikely that an otolith defect would have been detected by previous investigations. First, most of the teratological studies have focused upon gross malformations resulting from phenytoin exposure and on mechanisms of these defects, e.g., phenytoin's antagonism of folate metabolism and utilization. The teratological literature contains no studies of more subtle effects of phenytoin, and the methods of examination used to detect malformations were too gross to detect a change in a structure as small and inaccessible as fetal otoconia. Second, until the study by Elmazar and Sullivan (1981), no report in the literature on phenytoin had allowed the offspring to be delivered and develop postnatally. Therefore, no experiments had been conducted that could have revealed the behavioral symptoms which might lead one to suspect injury to vestibular system structures.

Based on our hypothesis, we examined the offspring from the last experiment in this series at approximately 18 months of age for otolith morphology. The results have been presented in preliminary form elsewhere (Minck et al., 1987), and revealed a positive relationship between circling behavior in the phenytoin offspring and deficiency of otoconia. Phenytoin offspring not exhibiting circling also did not exhibit an otoconial deficiency. Controls had completely normal otoconial development. We are currently in the process of determining the extent to which the otoconial deficiency correlates with the broad range of behavioral defects observed in these animals. Otoconial deficiency may account for the circling behavior. It is less clear whether this defect can account for all of the behavioral abnormalities, because even phenytoin non-circlers show significant reductions in complex water maze learning (Vorhees, 1987c) and impairments in memory as measured in the Morris maze. Significantly, Douglas et al. (1979) found that mice with congenital otoconial deficiency show many similarities to animals with hippocampal lesions, and the hippocampus contributes to spatial learning and memory. Douglas et al. (1979) hypothesized that hippocampal function may rely upon vestibular system inputs arising, in part, from the static balance organs of the inner ear. In the absence of such input, animals might exhibit memory impairments very similar to animals with direct hippocampal lesions. We have new data which might be viewed as converging with this idea, because we have found that phenytoin offspring exhibit reduced plasma synaptic membrane order using the fluorescent probe 1,6-diphenyl-1,3,5-hexatriene in the hippocampus, but not in other brain regions (Vorhees, Rauch and Hitzemann, unpublished observations).

In order to test the hypothesis that otolith defects could account for the behavioral abnormalities, we have just completed the first part of a two-part study. In part one, we administered phenytoin to rats on days G7–18 as before to one group, and phenytoin and manganous sulfate to another group. Fetuses were removed on day G20 and prepared for examination of otoconia. In the second part of this study, we are allowing litters similarly treated to be delivered for postnatal evaluation. The offspring will be assessed functionally as before and than their otoliths examined for confirmation of otoconial reduction in the phenytoin-only group or protection from reduction in the phenytoin-manganese group. We will test the hypothesis that phenytoin and manganese will result in either (a) completely normalized behavior, or (b) partially normalized behavior. The latter finding would support the view that phenytoin has multiple effects, some of which are not mediated through changes in inner ear structures.

Developmental effects of other anticonvulsants

Trimethadione was found to produce several functional effects similar to those seen in the phenytoin offspring. For example, trimethadione offspring exposed to 250 mg/kg exhibited delayed swimming ontogeny, hyperactivity in the figure-8 meter and more Biel water maze errors. Unlike the phenytoin offspring, however, the trimethadione progeny showed reduced spontaneous alternation, but no effects on startle, pivoting or passive avoidance tests, and no abnormal circling behavior. Also, the magnitude of the effects from trimethadione were consistently smaller than those seen among the phenytoin offspring. No effects of trimethadione at 50 or 5 mg/kg were seen.

Phenobarbital at 80 mg/kg produced delayed development of one aspect of swimming ontogeny and a suggestive trend towards reduced spontaneous alternation, but no other functional effects. No effects were seen at doses of 50 or 5 mg/kg of phenobarbital.

Finally, valproic acid produced reduced locomotion on open-field central and hole-board horizontal measures of activity. Valproic acid offspring also exhibited slower straight channel swimming, increased swimming maze errors (females only), reduced spontaneous alternation frequency and reduced startle amplitude across stimulus modalities. These effects were generally dose-dependent at the 200 and 150 mg/kg doses.

Synthesis and concluding remarks

Functional experiments with trimethadione, phenobarbital and valproic acid have not progressed as far as those with phenytoin, making it difficult to compare their effects. While there are some common trends in the findings, it is too early to determine whether these are more than superficial. For example, both phenytoin and trimethadione induced figure-8 hyperactivity, but the pattern and magnitude of the effects appear to be different. Moreover, the phenytoin effect on locomotion may be a by-product of disorientation resulting from otoconial deficiency and may not be a primary product of central nervous system injury. A second comparison is that both trimethadione and valproic acid produced reduced spontaneous alternation frequency. Whether this reflects a similar deficiency in inhibitory control centers remains to be tested using other measures of this function. Finally, we have recently found that prenatal valproic acid reduces anisotropy in brain synaptic plasma membrane preparations similar to that we have recently seen from prenatal phenytoin exposure (Vorhees, Rauch and Hitzemann, unpublished observations). Whether this marker of membrane fluidity indicates a commonality of mechanism is currently unknown. The only common thread that can be ascertained from this early stage of our work which spans all of the anticonvulsants we have investigated thus far is that all four of these drugs appear to be CNS functional teratogens at doses that do not produce conventional evidence of teratogenicity. Given these agents' related therapeutic profiles, but diverse chemical structures, there may be a lesson to be derived from such an observation. It is clear that future investigations on these drugs should be aimed at their mechanisms of action on embryonic tissues, with functional studies providing a new source of guidance in this endeavor.

Acknowledgements

The authors wish to express their appreciation to Dr. L. C. Erway for his collaboration in the examinations of inner ear structures, to M. S. Moran and C. A. Blanton in the conduct of the experiments, and to Dr. E. Mollnow for critical comments on the manuscript. Supported by grants DAR/BNS79–24710 from the National Science Foundation and AA06032 and HD19090 from the National Institutes of Health.

References

Boxenbaum, H. and Ronfeld, R. (1983) Interspecies pharmacokinetic scaling and the Dedrick plots. *Am. J. Physiol.*, 245: R768–R775.

DiLiberti, J.H., Farndon, P.A., Dennis, N.R. and Curry, C.J.R. (1984) The fetal valproate syndrome. *Am. J. Med. Genet.*, 19: 473–781.

Douglas, R.J., Clark, G.M., Erway, L.C., Hubbard, D.G. and Wright, C.G. (1979) Effects of genetic vestibular defects on behavior related to spatial orientation and emotionality. *J. Comp. Physiol. Psychol.*, 93: 467–480.

Elmazar, M.M.A. and Sullivan, F.M. (1981) Effect of prenatal phenytoin administration on postnatal development of the rat: a behavioral teratology study. *Teratology* 24: 115–124.

Erway, L.C., Hurley, L.S. and Fraser, A. (1966) Neurological defect: manganese in phenocopy and prevention of a genetic abnormality of inner ear. *Science*, 152: 1766–1768.

Erway, L.C., Fraser, A.S. and Hurley, L.S. (1971) Prevention of congenital otolith defect in pallid mutant mice by manganese supplementation. *Genetics*, 67: 97–108.

Erway, L.C., Purichia, N.A., Netzler, E.R., D'Amore, M.A., Esses, D. and Levine, M. (1986) Genes, manganese, and zinc in formation of otoconia: labeling, recovery, and maternal effects. *Scan. Electron Microscopy*, IV: 1681–1694.

Feldman, G.L., Weaver, D.D. and Lovrien, E.W. (1977) The fetal trimethadione syndrome. *Am. J. Dis. Child.*, 131: 1389–1392.

Finnell, R.H. (1981) Phenytoin-induced teratogenesis: a mouse model. *Science*, 211: 483–484.

Finnell, R.H., Shields, H.E., Taylor, S.M. and Chernoff, N.F. (1987) Strain differences in phenobarbital-induced teratogenesis in mice. *Teratology*, 35: 177–185.

Hanson, J.W. (1986) Teratogen update: fetal hydantoin effects. *Teratology*, 33: 349–353.

Hanson, J.W. and Smith, D.W. (1975) The fetal hydantoin syndrome. *J. Pediatr.*, 87: 285–290.

Hanson, J.W., Myrianthopoulos, N.C., Sedgwick-Harvey, M.S. and Smith, D.W. (1976) Risks to the offspring of women treated with hydantoin anticonvulsants, with emphasis on the fetal hydantoin syndrome. *J. Pediatr.*, 89: 662–668.

Hill, R.M. and Tennyson, L.M. (1986) Maternal drug therapy: effect on fetal and neonatal growth and neurobehavior. *Neurotoxicology*, 7: 121–140.

Hill, R.M., Verniaud, W.M., Horning, M.G., McCulley, L.B. and Morgan, N.M. (1974) Infants exposed in utero to antiepileptic drugs: a prospective study. *Am. J. Dis. Child.*, 127: 645–653.

Jager-Roman, E., Deichl, A., Jakob, S., Hartmann, A.-M., Koch, S., Rating, D., Steldinger, R., Nau, H. and Helge, H. (1986) Fetal growth, major malformations, and minor anomalies in infants born to women receiving valproic acid. *J. Pediatr.*, 108: 997–1004.

Kalter, H. and Warkany, J. (1983) Congenital malformations: etiological factors and their role in prevention. *N. Engl. J. Med.*, 308: 424–431 and 491–497.

Kelly, T.E. (1984) Teratogenicity of anticonvulsant drugs. I: Review of the literature. *Am. J. Med. Genet.*, 19: 413–434.

Kelly, T.E., Edwards, P., Rein, M., Miller, J.Q. and Dreifuss, F.E. (1984) Teratogenicity of anticonvulsant drugs. II: A prospective study. *Am. J. Med. Genet.*, 19: 435–443.

Khera, K.S. (1984) Maternal toxicity – possible factor in fetal malformations in mice. *Teratology*, 29: 411–416.

Lim, D.J. and Erway, L.C. (1974) Influence of manganese on genetically defective otolith: a behavioral and morphological study. *Ann. Otolaryngol.*, 83: 565–581.

Lim, D.J., Erway, L.C. and Clark, D.L. (1977) Titled-head mice with genetic otoconial anomaly. Behavioural and morphological correlates. In J.D. Hood (Ed.), *Vestibular Mechanisms in Health and Disease*, Academic Press, London, pp. 195–206.

Loscher, W., Nau, H., Marescaux, C. and Vergnes, M. (1984) Comparative evaluation of anticonvulsant and toxic potencies of valproic acid and 2-en-valproic acid in different animal models of epilepsy. *Eur. J. Pharmacol.*, 99: 211–218.

Lyon, M.F. (1951) Hereditary absence of otoliths in the house mouse. *J. Physiol.*, 114: 410–418.

Lyon, M.F. (1953) Absence of otoliths in the mouse: an effect of the pallid mutant. *J. Genet.*, 51: 638–650.

Majewski, F. and Steger, M. (1984) Fetal head growth retardation associated with maternal phenobarbital/primidone and/or phenytoin therapy. *Eur. J. Pediatr.*, 141: 188–189.

Majewski, F., Steger, M., Richter, B., Gill, J. and Rabe, F. (1981) The teratogenicity of hydantoins and barbiturates in humans, with considerations of the etiology of malformations and cerebral disturbances in the children of epileptic parents. *Biol. Res. Preg.*, 2: 37–45.

Martin, J.C., Martin, D.C., Lemire, R. and Mackler, B. (1979) Effects of maternal absorption of phenobarbital upon rat offspring development and function. *Neurobehav. Toxicol.*, 1: 49–55.

Martin, J.C., Martin, D.C., Mackler, B., Grace, R., Shores, P. and Chao, S. (1985) Maternal barbiturate administration and offspring response to shock. *Psychopharmacology*, 85: 214–220.

Middaugh, L.D. (1986) Prenatal phenobarbital: effects on pregnancy and offspring. In E.P. Riley and C.V. Vorhees (Eds.), *Handbook of Behavioral Teratology*, Plenum, New York, pp. 243–266.

Middaugh, L.D., Santos, C.A. and Zemp, J.W. (1975a) Effects of phenobarbital given to pregnant mice on behavior of mature offspring. *Dev. Psychobiol.*, 8: 305–313.

Middaugh, L.D., Santos, C.A. and Zemp, J.W. (1975b) Phenobarbital during pregnancy alters operant behavior of offspring in C57 BL/6J mice. *Pharmacol. Biochem. Behav.*, 3: 1137–1139.

Middaugh, L.D., Simpson, L.W., Thomas, T.N. and Zemp, J.W. (1981a) Prenatal maternal phenobarbital increases reactivity and retards habituation of mature offspring to environmental stimuli. *Psychopharmacology*, 74: 349–352.

Middaugh, L.D., Thomas, T.N., Simpson, L.W. and Zemp, J.W. (1981b) Effects of prenatal maternal injections of phenobarbital on brain neurotransmitters and behavior of young C57 mice. *Neurobehav. Toxicol. Teratol.*, 3: 271–275.

Middaugh, L.D., Zemp, J.W. and Simpson, L.W. (1983) Reaction of mature mice to phenobarbital after *in utero* exposure. *Teratology*, 27: 63A.

Minck, D.R., Erway, L.C. and Vorhees, C.V. (1987) Effects of prenatal phenytoin exposure: relationship between inner ear development and behavior. *Teratology*, 35: 9B.

Monson, R.R., Rosenberg, L., Hartz, S.C., Shapiro, S., Heinonen, O.P. and Slone, D. (1973) Diphenylhydantoin and selected congenital malformations. *N. Engl. J. Med.*, 289: 1049–1052.

Nakane, Y. (1979) Congenital malformation among infants of epileptic mothers treated during pregnancy – the report of a collaborative study group in Japan. *Folia Psychiatr. Neurol. Jpn.*, 33: 363–369.

Rodier, P.M. (1980) Chronology of neuron development: animal studies and their clinical implications. *Dev. Med. Child Neurol.*, 22: 525–545.

Shapiro, S., Slone, D., Hartz, S.C., Rosenberg, L., Siskind, V., Monson, R.R., Mitchell, A.A., Heinonen, O.P., Idanpaan-Heikkila, J., Haro, S. and Saxen, L. (1976) Anticonvulsants and parental epilepsy in the development of birth defects. *Lancet*, i: 272–275.

Shrader, R.E., Erway, L.C. and Hurley, L.S. (1973) Muco-polysaccharide synthesis in the developing inner ear of manganese-deficient and pallid mutant mice. *Teratology*, 8: 257–266.

Swinyard, E.A. and Woodhead, J.H. (1982) General principles: experimental detection, quantification, and evaluation of anticonvulsants. In D.M. Woodbury, J.K. Penry and C.E. Pippenger (Eds.), *Antiepileptic Drugs*, 2nd edn., Raven, New York, pp. 111–126.

Vernadakis, A. and Woodbury, D.M. (1968) The developing animal as a model. *Epilepsia*, 10: 163–178.

Vorhees, C.V. (1983) Fetal anticonvulsant syndrome in rats: dose- and period-response relationships of prenatal diphenylhydantoin, trimethadione, and phenobarbital exposure on the structural and functional development of the offspring. *J. Pharmacol. Exp. Ther.* 227: 274–287.

Vorhees, C.V. (1985) Fetal anticonvulsant syndrome in rats: effects on postnatal behavior and brain amino acid content. *Neurobehav. Toxicol. Teratol.*, 7: 471–482.

Vorhees, C.V. (1986) Principles of behavioral teratology. In E.P. Riley and C.V. Vorhees (Eds.), *Handbook of Behavioral Teratology*, Plenum, New York, pp. 23–48.

Vorhees, C.V. (1987a) Teratogenicity and developmental toxicity of valproic acid in rats. *Teratology*, 35: 195–202.

Vorhees, C.V. (1987b) Behavioral teratogenicity of valproic acid: selective effects on behavior after prenatal exposure to rats. *Psychopharmacology*, 92: 173–179.

Vorhees, C.V. (1987c) Fetal hydantoin syndrome in rats: dose-effect relationships of prenatal phenytoin on postnatal development and behavior. *Teratology*, 35: 287–303.

Vorhees, C.V. (1987d) Maze learning in rats: a comparison of performance in two water mazes in progeny prenatally exposed to different doses of phenytoin. *Neurotoxicol. Teratol.*, 9: 235–241.

Vorhees, C.V. and Butcher (1982) Behavioral teratogenicity.

In K. Snell (Ed.), *Developmental Toxicology*, Praeger, New York, pp. 247–298.

Woodbury, D.M. (1982) Phenytoin: absorption, distribution, and excretion. In D.M. Woodbury, J.K. Penry and C.E. Pippenger (Eds.), *Antiepileptic Drugs*, 2nd edn., Raven, New York, pp. 191–207.

Yanai, J. (1984) An animal model for the effect of barbiturate on the development of the central nervous system. In J. Yanai (Ed.), *Neurobehavioral Teratology*, Elsevier, Amsterdam, pp. 111–132.

Zackai, E.H., Mellman, W.J., Neiderer, B. and Hanson, J.W. (1975) The fetal trimethadione syndrome. *J. Pediatr.* 87: 280–284.

Discussion

M.V. Johnston: Would free phenytoin levels in your animal model be useful to relate to the levels found in human?

C.V. Vorhees: Yes, although there is debate in the human literature as to whether the phenytoin free fraction is in fact any better than total plasma concentration for predicting either therapeutic efficacy or toxicity in epileptics.

M.V. Johnston: Is the cerebellum disrupted by prenatal phenytoin administration?

C.V. Vorhees: I cannot yet answer this because we have not yet examined the cerebellum histologically. However, we find no gross changes in the cerebellum in terms of wet weight, protein content, in plasma membrane order (using the fluorescent probe diphenylhexatriene), or in terms of behaviors that would be expected to be affected by cerebellar damage.

J.M. Lauder: Have you considered the possibility that the circling behavior could be related to an effect on the dopaminergic system?

C.V. Vorhees: Yes, we were in fact planning to pursue this possibility; however, when we thought about it we felt it was appropriate to pursue and eliminate the more peripheral mechanisms, effect on otic capsule, first, then move towards more central mechanisms. Of course, what we found was that there was an effect of phenytoin on otoconical development; we have therefore decided to pursue that finding and have postponed investigations of possible extrapyramidal sites of injury until a later time.

J.M. Lauder: At what times did you administer phenytoin in animals where you saw the otoconial crystal defects? I ask because we have found that the developing otocyst has an uptake site for serotonin just in the vestibular portion (Chapter 24 of this volume), which might possibly be affected by your treatment.

C.V. Vorhees: We found the otoconia deficiencies in offspring exposed to phenytoin on days 7–18 of gestation. Your finding of serotonin uptake sites in the otocyst is quite interesting.

244

We also believe manganese may be involved, since manganese deficiency in mice is also known to result in a deficiency of otoconial development (Erway et al., 1971).

H. J. Romijn: Did you also study the effect of valproic acid on polarization of synaptic membranes in analogy to phenytoin?

C. V. Vorhees: Yes, but we do not yet have the results, but the samples are in our freezer and will be analysed in the near future.

Reference

Erway, L.C., Fraser, A.S. and Hurley, L.S. (1971) Prevention of congenital otolith defect in pallid mutant mice by manganese supplementation. *Genetics* 67: 97–108.

G.J. Boer, M.G.P. Feenstra, M. Mirmiran, D.F. Swaab and F. Van Haaren
Progress in Brain Research, Vol. 73
© 1988 Elsevier Science Publishers B.V. (Biomedical Division)

CHAPTER 16

Neuropeptides and functional neuroteratology

Gerard J. Boer, Frank G. M. Snijdewint and Dick F. Swaab

Netherlands Institute for Brain Research, Meibergdreef 33, 1105 AZ Amsterdam ZO, The Netherlands

Introduction

Nowadays it is clear that neurotransmission in the nervous system is brought about by a variety of endogene substances, including nucleotides, acetylcholine, amino acids, catecholamines, serotonin, histamine and neuropeptides. The number of neuropeptides outnumbers by far the other more 'classical' neurotransmitters. Although amino acid and aminergic neurons provide anatomically a prominent and extensive innervation of the central nervous system, the large neuropeptide variety as well as the great number of centrally regulated functions in which they are potently incorporated also make neuropeptides a very important class of neuro-messengers. This might also be illustrated by a recent paper by Zadina et al. (1986), who bibliographed the journal *Peptides* from 1980 to 1985; 40 pages were needed to describe the functions of over 40 neuropeptides. Neuropeptides have been recognized as brain messengers only in recent decades but many of them were previously known to have hormonal effects or to be present in the non-mammalian CNS (cf. Swaab, 1980). Consequently many peptides have dual characteristics, i.e., endocrine and as neurotransmitter or neuromodulator, depending on the site of synthesis and release within the organism.

Both neurotransmitters and hormones have been shown to influence ontogenic processes in the brain and to affect the sequence of neuronal proliferation, migration, maturation, differentia-

tion and the organization of functional circuitries. Since different types of neuron are generated in different brain regions and stages of development (Altman, 1969; Rodier, 1977), the well-defined timing of events in neuronal network formation becomes disturbed and will give rise to an altered organization of the brain at the cellular level. It was therefore regarded as likely (Swaab, 1980) that the potently neuroactive neuropeptides, in their role as hormone or neurotransmitter, might also influence neural development (cf. Boer and Swaab, 1983, 1985).

The present review provides evidence that many neuropeptides actually influence brain development and that abnormalities in the levels of neuropeptide may lead to permanent dysfunction of the nervous system, i.e. to functional neuroteratology. In the present paper particular emphasis will be given to the possible role of vasopressin in normal and abnormal development.

The early presence of neuropeptides

Some neuropeptides can be demonstrated immunochemically early in rat development (Swaab and Terborg, 1981). In fact, peptidergic neurons often show gene expression almost immediately after their birth dates (cf. Whitnall et al., 1985). Data available for catecholamines and serotonin demonstrating the presence of these neurotransmitter compounds prior to the first peak of neurogenesis in which the aminergic and serotonergic neurons are born (cf. Lauder, Chapter 24

TABLE 1

The developmental appearance of several vasopressin systems in the rat brain, exemplifying their separate generation and maturation

Cell bodies	Birth date	Immunodetection cell bodies	Target area	Immunodetection fibers in target areas
SON/PVN (magnocellular)	dpc 13	dpc 16	Neural lobe	dpc 16
PVN (parvocellular)	< dpc 18	Unknown	Median eminence	dpc 19
SCN	dpc 15	dpc 21	OVLT	dpc 21
			PVS	dpn 7
			DMH	> dpn 14
BNST	< dpc 18	Unknown	LS	dpn 10
			LH	dpn 10
LC	dpc 12	Unknown	Unknown	–
Amygdala	< dpc 18	Unknown	Hippocampus	dpc 20
Unknown	–	–	Olfactory bulb	dpc 17
			Amygdala	dpc 18
			Arcuate nucleus	dpc 21

Cell bodies found to be VP-synthesizing following blockade of axonal transport in adults were not investigated during development. They are indicated as unknown for earliest immunocytochemical detection.
Abbreviations: dpc, days postcoitally; dpn, days postnatally; SON, supraoptic nucleus; PVN, paraventricular nucleus; SCN, suprachiasmatic nucleus; BNST, bed nucleus of the stria terminalis; LC, locus coeruleus; OVLT, organum vasculosum laminae terminalis; PVS, periventricular area of the thalamus; DMH, dorsomedial area of the hypothalamus; LS, lateral septum; LH, lateral habenula.
Data based on Buys et al. (1980), De Vries et al. (1981, 1985), Caffé et al. (1987) and review by Boer (1987).

of this volume) are lacking for the neuropeptides. However, neuropeptides can certainly be demonstrated shortly after this peak. Neuropeptide Y is assayable on gestational day 13 in rat (Foster and Schultzberg, 1984) and somatostatin and substance P on day 14 (McGregor et al., 1982). Vasopressin (VP) and oxytocin (OT) are assayable from fetal day 14 and 17 onwards, respectively (cf. review Boer, 1987). Peptides of the proopiomelanocortin family are present on gestational day 15 (Bayon et al., 1979), somatostatin on gestational day 16 (Inagaki et al., 1982), both thyroid stimulating hormone releasing hormone (TRH) and corticotrophin releasing factor (CRF) on day 18 (Conklin et al., 1973; Bugnon et al., 1982) and luteinizing hormone releasing hormone (LHRH) on day 20 (Daikoku et al., 1978). Vasointestinal polypeptide (VIP) and bombesin appeared later, i.e., on the day of rat birth (McGregor et al., 1982). However, since neuro-

peptide levels in the brain are generally in the picomole range, further improvement of the sensitivity and detection limit of the immunoassays might reveal even earlier synthesis of these compounds.

Not much is known yet about the ontogenic appearance of neuropeptidergic pathways. The VP neurons are certainly the most well-described in this respect and revealed a rapid maturation process which differed for the various VP cells studied (see review, Boer, 1987). The axons of the magnocellular VP neurons of the hypothalamus, for instance, reveal immunodetection of VP in their neurohemal organ – the neural lobe of the pituitary – on the same fetal day 16 on which the cell bodies were found to stain. The fibers of the parvocellular VP cells of the paraventricular nucleus (PVN), which project neurohemally to the median eminence, appear 1 day later, whereas it takes one or more days (up to 1 week) before synapses of axonal endings of the extra- and exohypothalamic VP pathways are stainable. The latter exemplifies the fact that several VP-cell-containing nuclei in the brain have their own time-table of development (Table 1).

Notwithstanding the incomplete information about the early immunohistochemical presence of neuropeptide pathways, indications of the early development of the receptor site have become increasingly prominent, due to the rapid developments in the receptor assays for neuropeptides. Brain opiate receptors, as possible target sites for endorphins, were described as being already present on rat fetal day 14 (Clendeninn et al., 1976). More recent studies show somatostatin receptors to be detectable on fetal day 15 (Gonzalez et al., 1987), CRF receptors on day 17 (Insel et al., 1987), binding sites of VP and OT on fetal day 20 and postnatal day 1, respectively (Petracca et al., 1986; Snijdewint et al., 1987), cholecystokinin (CCK) receptors not later than rat birth (Hays et al., 1981) and brain LHRH receptors on postnatal day 6 (Reubi et al., 1986). One may even speculate that, due to technical improvements, in the near future ontogenic studies of several other neuropeptide binding sites in the brain will reveal an even earlier appearance. Anyhow, one can say that the early presence of neuropeptide receptors makes them accessible for agonistic and antagonistic action during the early phase of maturation (cf. Csaba, 1986).

For several neuropeptides a possible temporary activation has been described during normal brain ontogeny on either the pre- or the postsynaptic site. For instance, the levels of VP, α-melanocyte stimulating hormone (α-MSH), β-endorphin and somatostatin are (regionally) at certain periods of development higher than later on or in adulthood (Bayon et al., 1979; Boer et al., 1980b; Buijs et al., 1980; Inagaki et al., 1982; Bugnon et al., 1982; Alessi and Quinlan, 1985). For enkephalin it has even been shown that immunoreactivity is present only in the germinative cells of the cerebellum and not in adult cells (Zagon et al., 1985). Sometimes binding sites also

appeared to be expressed only transiently. This is seen for VP binding in the cingulate cortex (Petracca et al., 1985) and lateral reticular nucleus of the rat (Fig. 1), for OT binding in the dorsal hippocampus and parietal and cingulate cortex (Snijdewint et al., unpublished observations), and for somatostatin receptors in the cerebellum (Gonzalez et al., 1987). The latter observation is intriguing, since additionally no peptidergic synapses are involved, and one might think of a temporarily neurotrophic action of neuropeptides in a non-neurotransmitter fashion. Such a mechanism is also supposed for the aminergic neurotransmitters (cf. Lauder, Chapter 24 of this volume).

Approaches to reveal a peptidergic role in brain development

Research with steroid and thyroid hormones has shown that manipulation of the endocrine environment of the developing rat can have effects on body growth as well as organizational effects on the nervous system (De Kloet et al., Chapter 8, and Vaccari, Chapter 6 of this volume). The same holds for catecholamine neurotransmitters (cf. Patel and Lewis, Chapter 25, and Kostrzewa, Chapter 26). The approach to unravel a similar role for neuropeptides in brain development has followed the same line of investigation, including its neuroteratological aspects. On the one hand, cell generation and maturation are measured in relation to early alterations in the availability of neuropeptides, on the other hand organizational effects on the neuropeptidergic system and its target sites are studied.

The approach of looking for general growth effects is also justified by the trophic actions of certain neuropeptides. VP, for instance, has a mitogenic action on several cell systems, and may interfere with a variety of metabolic pathways (see review, Boer and Swaab, 1985) and with the release of other hormonal systems (cf. Hedge and Huffman, 1987) that might in turn affect brain growth. A recent report showed that VP may also

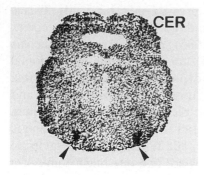

Fig. 1. Autoradiography of [³H]vasopressin binding in the lateral reticular nucleus (arrow heads) of the medulla oblongata of a day 20 fetal rat, a binding which disappeared after postnatal day 15. Autoradiogram of transversal brain section. CER, cerebellum (cf. Snijdewint et al., 1987).

promote neuritic growth of cultured embryonic neurons (Brinton and Gruener, 1987). α-MSH and ACTH (adrenocorticotrophic hormone) also have potent trophic effects on nervous cells. α-MSH-related compounds are particularly potent in inducing central (Swaab et al., 1977) and peripheral nerve cell maturation (Frischer et al., 1985), as well as in regenerating of peripheral (Strand and Kung, 1980; Bijlsma et al., 1983a,b) and central nervous system lesions (Veldhuis et al., 1985). VIP probably has a role in mediating a neuron-glia-neuron interaction which influences the trophic regulation of neuronal survival (Brenneman et al., 1987). Endogene opiates such as Met-enkephalin also seem to be involved in nerve cell proliferation but rather by an inhibitory mechanism (Zagon and McLaughlin, 1987; see also below).

Organizational effects are determined by testing the aberrations on the anatomical, biochemical and behavioral level. Receptor imprinting processes appeared to be an important aspect of such effects (Csaba, 1986; Miller and Friedhoff, Chapter 31) and the usual strategy is to test the mature animal for perturbations in the physiological systems, including behavior, in which the neuropeptide is known to play a role (Handelmann, Chapter 32). It goes without saying that if a particular peptidergic system is affected by early

manipulation, such changes might have consequences for interrelated systems (cf. Bakke et al., 1978; Lichtensteiger and Schlumpf, 1985).

The levels of neuropeptides may be increased by treatment of the pregnant female, fetus or neonate with the native peptide and decreased by the use of antisera. Congeners of certain peptides (e.g. VP and OT, α-MSH and ACTH) and other compounds with agonist or antagonist activity are also useful in developmental studies. As will be shown below, the effect of imbalance of neuropeptide levels has its vulnerable period for long-lasting effects. In addition, the timing of the exposure to neuropeptide changes also appears to be critical for the type of anomaly induced (see below). Changes in the offspring induced by maternal treatment with neuropeptides can rather be interpreted as indirect effects, since neuropeptides do not efficiently pass the placental barrier (e.g. Oosterbaan et al., 1985a).

Long-lasting effects upon early neuropeptide changes

This section will only summarize long-lasting effects of neuropeptides, since several reviews are available providing a profound insight into this rapidly broadening field with clinical implications (cf. Boer and Swaab, 1983, 1985; Zagon and McLaughlin, 1983; Handelmann, 1985). Moreover, it will focus on the functional *neuro*-teratological aspects, i.e. on brain impairments that have a long-term character (Table 2).

Endogene opiates. Studies on the developmental effects of opiates provided the first examples of peptide neuroteratology because of the occurrence of narcotic use by pregnant women. Most investigations, however, concern the manipulation of the early perinatal opiate environment in the rat by the use of opiate agonists (methadone, morphine, heroin) or antagonists (naltrexone, naloxone) rather than direct alterations in endogene opiates such as Met-enkephalin and β-endorphin.

In general, the studies on *prenatal*, i.e. mater-

TABLE 2

Brain functional teratology of neuropeptides in rats

	Treatment	Effects	References
β-Endorphin ↑	Pups	Hyperanalgesia	Sandman et al. (1979) Zadina and Kastin (1986)
		Decreased β-endorphin content	Moldow et al. (1981)
		Reduced opiate receptors	Zadina and Kastin (1986)
		Socio-sexual behavior influenced	Meyerson (1985)
		Reduced body weight	Zadina et al. (1985)
	Mother	Opiate receptors increased	Zadina et al. (1985)
Met-enkephalin ↑	Pups	Facilitation maze performance	Kastin et al. (1980)
		Decreased neurogenesis	Zagon and McLaughlin (1987)
		Hyperanalgesia	Handelmann (Chapter 32)
α-MSH ↑	Pups	Improved learning, memory and attention tasks	Nyakas (1975) Nyakas et al. (1981) Champney et al. (1976) Beckwith et al. (1977a,b)
		Accelerated motor behavior	V.d. Helm-Hylkema (1973)
		Advances eye opening	V.d. Helm-Hylkema and De Wied (1973)
		Reduced feedback of MSH on accelerated motor behavior	Lichtensteiger and Schlumpf (1985)
		Improved T-maze learning	Acker et al. (1985)
α-MSH ↓	Antibody into fetus	Disturbed brain cell maturation	Swaab et al. (1977)
VP ↑	Mother	Impaired memory in brightness discrimination test	Tinius et al. (1987)
		Impaired memory retrieval in passive avoidance test (males)	
VP ↓	Genetic deficiency (Brattleboro rat)	Disturbed brain growth	Boer et al. (1982) Greer et al. (1982)
		Earlier eye opening	Boer et al. (1980a)
		Changed catecholamine innervation	Versteeg et al. (1978)
		'Memory' deficits	cf. Van Wimersma Greidanus (1982)
		Impaired temperament-related tests	cf. Gash et al. (1987)
		Hyperresponsiveness	Warren and Gash (1983)
		Hyperanalgesia	Bodnar et al. (1980)
		etc. etc.	
	Antibody in pups	Hyperanalgesia	Moratella et al. (1986)
		Impaired memory in retrieval in passive avoidance test	Moratella et al. (1987)
		Impaired acquisition in active avoidance test	
VT ↑	Pups	Disturbed brain growth	Goldstein and Rodica (1986)
		Increased REM sleep	

TABLE 2 (continued)

Brain functional teratology of neuropeptides in rats

	Treatment	Effects	References
CRF ↑	Pups	Earlier eye opening Reduced body weight	Zadina and Kastin (1986)
		Increased rearing Body temperature regulation affected	Zadina et al. (1985)
		Increased exploration open field Better recovery following stress	Insel et al. (1987)
CCK ↑	Mother	Eye opening delayed Impaired active avoidance test Impaired memory retrieval in passive avoidance test Decreased rearing in open field Altered monoamine levels	Telegdy et al. (1986)
Substance P ↑	Pups	Increased brain substance P receptors Reduced pain threshold	Handelmann et al. (1987) Handelmann et al. (1984)
TRH ↑	Pups	Increased weight hypothalamus Impaired T-maze learning	Stratton et al. (1976)

Abbreviations: α-MSH, α-melanocyte stimulating hormone; VP, vasopressin; VT, vasotocin; CRF, corticotrophin releasing factor; CCK, cholecystokinin; TRH, thyroid hormone releasing hormone.

nal, treatment with opiates such as morphine or methadone showed retardation of somatic and neurobiological development (cf. Zagon and McLaughlin, 1983) and altered the [³H]Met-enkephalin and [³H]naloxone binding in the nervous system of the offspring (Tsang and Ng, 1980; Kirby, 1983). On the other hand, there is a report showing that morphine delayed normal cell death in the ciliary ganglion of the chick embryo (Meriney et al., 1985). Maternal naloxone, an opiate antagonist, appeared to evoke opposite effects, i.e., it accelerated post-weaning growth and postnatal behavioral development of the offspring in many tests (Vorhees, 1981). However, it induced long-term impairments of learning behavior. Prenatal treatment of rat mothers with β-endorphin also decreased somatic growth and temporarily reduced [³H]naloxone binding in the brain (Zadina et al., 1985). In the latter study one might wonder whether β-endorphin has a direct effect on the developing fetus, since no aber-

rations were found in a tail flick test measuring analgesic responsiveness known to be affected by maternal treatment with morphine (Steele and Johannesson, 1975; cf. also Zagon and McLaughlin, 1983).

Postnatal exposure to the endogenously present opiates β-endorphin or Met-enkephalin has been performed in a limited number of studies. Neonatal β-endorphin administration was shown to (a) cause long-term elevation in the threshold for thermal pain (Sandman et al., 1979; Zadina and Kastin, 1986), (b) lower concentrations of β-endorphin in the brain (Moldow et al., 1981), (c) alter the responsiveness to β-endorphin in socio-sexual behavior tests (Meyerson, 1985) and (d) reduce the number of brain [³H]naloxone (mu) and [³H]DADLE (delta) opiate receptors (Zadina et al., 1985; Zadina and Kastin, 1986), whereas no changes were observed in the somatic development (Meyerson, 1985; Zadina and Kastin, 1986). Neonatal Met-enkephalin treat-

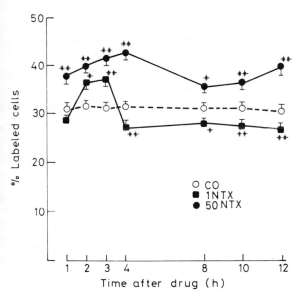

Fig. 2. Influence of a single injection of naltrexone on cell proliferation in the cerebellar external granular layer of a 6-day-old rat. Naltrexone (NTX) blocking the opiate receptor either shortly (1 mg/kg) or for 24 h (50 mg/kg) had temporally related effects on the incorporation of [³H]thymidine into the DNA of the cells. The high dose stimulated incorporation by preventing the inhibitory role of endogenic opiates, whereas the low dose does so only transiently followed by a period of decreased incorporation. The latter may be induced by short-term receptor down-regulation (from Zagon and McLaughlin, 1987).

ment (a) decreased neurogenesis in the cerebellum (Zagon and McLaughlin, 1987), (b) facilitated later performance in maze tasks (Kastin et al., 1980) and (c) elevated pain threshold as well (Handelmann, Chapter 32). Studies using opiate agonists or antagonists revealed a lot of additional information. Zagon and McLaughlin (1987) demonstrated that opioid receptor blockade in the developing brain increased cell division, indicating that the endogenous opiate system takes part in the orchestration of neurogenesis (Fig. 2). At the same time, maturation of neurons increased, as seen by increased dendritic growth and spine formation (Hauser et al., 1987). The opiate mu receptors are probably not involved in the inhibitory action on neurogenesis of endogenic opiates

(Zagon and McLaughlin, 1986), since the specific mu antagonist β-funaltrexamine failed to stimulate brain growth as did naltrexone. However, upon neonatal application it blocks later analgesia like naltrexone, indicating that lasting changes in mu receptors are probably involved. Methadone and morphine treatment of rat pups similarly affected the pain threshold in adulthood (Zagon and McLaughlin, 1982; Handelmann and Dow-Edwards, 1985) but Handelmann and Quirion (1983) were not able to relate this directly to mu or delta opiate receptor changes in brain regions involved in this behavior.

It is clear that opiate agonists and antagonists affect rat development in a variety of behavioral measures (cf. Zagon and McLaughlin, 1983, 1985), and that the involved manipulation of the endogenic opiate environment has severe and lasting functional teratological effects both pre- and postnatally. This is clearly reflected, e.g. following perinatal administration of methadone, when severe deficits in the neurochemistry of the biogenic amine systems are observed (Slotkin et al., 1979, 1982 and Chapter 17). It seems that dividing cells of germinal zones of the nervous system may be controlled by endogenous opiates (Zagon and McLaughlin, 1987), while organizational effects on the function of the opiate system also occur.

ACTH and its fragments. Several trophic actions of ACTH, α-MSH (*N*-acetyl-ACTH-(1–13)-amide) and other fragments such as ACTH-(4–10), ACTH-(4–9), etc., have been reported (see above). None of these compounds has ever been shown to affect postnatal somatic growth, but α-MSH antibodies inhibit prenatal body and brain growth (Swaab et al., 1976, 1977). When these antibodies were injected subcutaneously into rat fetuses, the size of the brain but not the number of cells (total DNA content) was affected, suggesting a maturation role for endogenic α-MSH activity. No other anatomical, neurochemical or functional change in adulthood due to prenatal (or maternal) treatment with ACTH-derived compounds has been reported. In a study by Peruzović and Milković (1986), however, following maternal treatment with metopirone, which causes fetal adrenal hyperplasia by inhibition of corticosterone synthesis and increases ACTH, a facilitation of two-way avoidance behavior was found in adulthood. Brain growth data were not reported in this study.

The latter result is in line with early postnatal exposure studies. Generally, treatment with ACTH, α-MSH or derivatives seems to improve performance in learning, memory and attention tasks. Early enhanced levels of ACTH result in improved acquisition of passive avoidance behavior, an effect opposite to that found after corticosterone treatment (Nyakas, 1975). Consequently, it was supposed that ACTH possessed an extra-adrenal influence on the development of this behavior. Similarly, early administration of α-MSH facilitated a lever-press learning task, and improved two-way active avoidance and brightness discrimination performance (Beckwith et al., 1977a), while females but not males exhibited greater body contact in adulthood (Beckwith et al., 1977b). Studies with early postnatal exposure to α-MSH, ACTH, ACTH-(1–24) and ACTH-(1–10) showed an acceleration of motor behavior of rat (Van der Helm-Hylkema, 1973; Saint-Côme et al., 1982), whereas treatment with ACTH-(4–10) (Nyakas et al., 1981; Acker et al., 1985), and ACTH-(4–9) (Champney et al., 1981) and its analogue Org 2766 (Acker et al., 1985) showed later improvement of passive avoidance behavior, T-maze learning and attention tasks.

Suppression of the α-MSH serum peak in 5–6-day-old rat pups impaired the development of the α-MSH feedback on the tubero-hypophyseal dopamine neurons (Lichtensteiger and Schlumpf, 1985). These dopamine neurons remained unresponsive in adulthood, possibly due to affected α-MSH receptor number in this circuitry.

So far, it may be concluded that ACTH-related peptides facilitate fetal brain growth by a mechanism unrelated to nerve cell proliferation but comparable with its trophic action on nerve fiber regeneration (cf. Bijlsma et al., 1983a,b; Edwards et al., 1986; Gispen et al., 1987) or its facilitation action on motor development (see above). The latter is brought about by a more rapid maturation of the neuromuscular junction (Frischer et al., 1985) and one may speculate that a more rapid maturation of synapse formation in the brain by neonatal ACTH compounds may underlie the organizational changes revealed by permanently changed behavior of adult rats.

Vasopressin and congeners. Although VP has frequently been described as a mitogen (see above), it failed to act this way when given to the

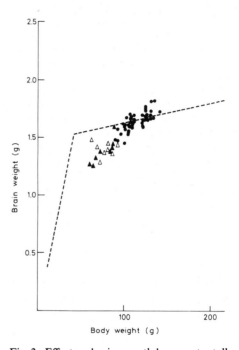

Fig. 3. Effect on brain growth by a postnatally applied vasopressin antagonist. The 3-week treatment with twice daily 2.5 μg dP[Tyr(Me)^2]VP, a central antagonist of vasopressin (VP) had affected body and brain weight of Wistar pups killed on day 32. Brains of treated pups are too small for their body size since the data points were below the (dashed) reference line of the allometric brain/body relationship. Thus, brain development was particularly affected. Co-treatment of VP in the same dose was not able to counteract the growth impairments, which possibly indicates a non-competitive effect of the antagonist (from Snijdewint and Boer, 1988a). ●, controls; △, treated with dP[Tyr(Me)^2]VP; ▲ treated with VP + dP[Tyr(Me)^2]VP.

rat in its perinatal period. On the contrary – at high dosages (daily μg quantities) – it may disrupt somatic growth (Oosterbaan et al., 1985b; Snijdewint and Boer, 1986) possibly by its vaso-constrictive action. Nevertheless, the genetic absence of VP in the Brattleboro rat (Boer et al., 1982) or postnatal treatment with a centrally act-ing VP antagonist in Wistar rat (Snijdewint and Boer, 1988a; Fig. 3) results in disturbed brain growth. Decreased availability of VP may there-fore be disruptive for nervous system ontogeny. The neuropeptides structurally related to VP, such as OT and [Lys^8]VP (LVP), did not result in severe alterations of postnatal brain growth (Boer and Kruisbrink, 1984; Snijdewint and Boer, 1986), but the precursor peptide vasotocin (VT) in 0.1 ng amounts daily given the first week neo-natally induced a remarkable decrease in brain weight and total brain lipid and galactolipids at the end of the treatment on day 8 as well as a reduction in active sleep (Goldstein and Rodica, 1986). Similar effects were found in kittens but not following application of VP, OT or LVP (Goldstein, 1984). Pharmacological evidence is given that these effects by VT on brain maturation are mediated by GABA mechanisms (Table 3),

TABLE 3

Vasotocin (VT) effects on early brain development of rat: mediation by a GABA mechanism

	REM sleep (% total)	Brain weight (g)	Total lipids (% weight)
–	67	0.78	8.0
VT	92*	0.60*	5.9*
VT + picrotoxin	64	0.75	8.2
VT + valproic acid	100*	0.61*	4.1*
Valproic acid	86*	0.81	6.1*

Daily i.p. treatment of neonatal rat between days 2 and 8 with 100 pg VT and/or 50 ng picrotoxin (GABA antagonist) or 1 ng valproic acid (GABA agonist). Assays were performed immediately after the treatment period. Asterisk indicates statistical significant difference from control treatment. Data summarized from Goldstein and Rodica (1986).

but their permanent character has not been in-vestigated so far.

Abnormalities in adult behavior of VP-defi-cient Brattleboro rats and other strains in which the mutation was transferred by cross-breeding (cf. reviews Van Wimersma-Greidanus, 1982; Gash et al., 1987) point to a possible role for VP in the organization of the central nervous system, the more so since many of these abnormalities could not be restored by VP supplementation (cf. review Gash et al., 1987). However, some be-havioral deficits in, for example passive avoidance behavior (De Wied et al., 1975; cf. Baily and Weiss, 1979; Carey and Miller, 1982) are not consistently found among several investigators (see further Gash et al., 1987). The age at which the later tests were performed might be of influence (Van Haaren et al., 1986), but it might also well be that the problematic breeding of these animals and the special care they need because of their severe polyurea have resulted in Brattleboro rat stocks with different behavioral patterns. Environment, handling and previous behavioral tests interfering with functional and chemical development of the brain may also play a role but are too often ignored (cf. Uphouse et al., 1983). Herman et al. (1986) have indeed reported avoid-ance responses to be significantly different between VP-deficient Brattleboro rat groups obtained from various animal suppliers (including even the results seen for the Long-Evans con-trols).

Recently administration of VP to pregnant rat has been shown to improve performance in a brightness discrimination test of their offspring (Ermisch et al., 1986; Tinius et al., 1987), but to impair memory retrieval of a 25-day-retention passive avoidance response at 2 months of age (Tinius et al., 1987). Early postnatal treatment with VP had no influence on a 1-day-retention passive avoidance test nor on open-field behavior at 2 months of age (Boer et al., unpublished observation). Interestingly, a single injection with antiserum to VP in 2-day-old rat pups also impaired this passive avoidance response at

TABLE 4

Controversies in the change of passive avoidance behavior of adult rats in which the vasopressin levels have been manipulated neonatally

Rat strain	VP treatment		Behavioral testing		Reference
	Dosage	Period	Age	Outcome	
Sprague-Dawley	1 μg/24 h by osmotic minipump s.c.	Gestational day 13–19	2 months	Latency of test trial shortened (25-day retention)	Tinius et al. (1987)
Wistar	5 μg twice daily injections s.c.	Postnatal day 1–9	2 months	No effect (1-day retention)	Boer et al. (unpublished data)
Wistar	100 μl purified immunoglobulin of VP antiserum s.c.	Postnatal day 2	3–4 months	Latency of test trial shortened (1-day retention)	Moratella et al. (1987)

3–4 months (as well as the acquisition in a 2-way active avoidance test; Moratella et al., 1987). The outcomes of the passive avoidance test in these investigations have so far been difficult to match, since the same defect, i.e., shortened latency for entering in the post-shock trial, was found following opposite changes of neonatal VP levels (Table 4). An effect of the age of testing, the test protocol and the difference in dosage might be involved. However, one could also imagine that during the subsequent stages in the long maturation process of the various VP neuronal subsystems (Table 1), different manipulations of the VP levels may have altered the organization of the neuronal system involved differently but with the same behavioral outcome. Moratella et al. (1986, 1987) additionally described their neonatally VP antiserum-treated rats to be hyperanalgesic and hypertensive, and pointed out that the latter lasting change in blood pressure might have modified the pathways for pain control and memory processes. Whether VP receptor changes are involved in such changes still has to be established (see below).

Other neuropeptides. Developmental and neuroteratological studies on other endogene neu-

ropeptides are very limited. Zadina et al. (1985) reported on the effects of maternally or postnatally administered CRF in rat. CRF-treated pups showed the most dramatic changes, including decreased body weight, accelerated eye opening and, in adulthood, increased open-field rearing behavior and altered temperature control.

Another single study reported brain developmental changes upon perinatal CCK exposure (Telegdy et al., 1986). Both the sulfated and the non-sulfated forms were applied maternally and postnatally. Body growth and active and passive avoidance behavior appeared to be affected only after the prenatal maternal treatment of the non-sulfated CCK and more clearly so in males. Additionally, regional monoamine transmitter levels were changed, yet in a sex-independent way.

Postnatal substance P treatment has been shown to affect later pain threshold, and increased substance P binding capacity in various, but not all, brain areas (Handelmann et al., 1984, 1987). Prenatal treatment with Tyr-MIF-1, an endogene neuropeptide with opiate-modulatory effects, increased postnatal body weight gain (Zadina et al., 1985). Finally, thyrotropin-releasing hormone (TRH) appears to facilitate brain growth, in particular of the hypothalamus, when given in the first neonatal week, but impaired later T-maze learning (Stratton et al., 1976).

In conclusion, neuropeptides join the growing group of neuroactive compounds that play a role in brain development (Table 2). Or, in other words, imbalances of these peptides during the strict time-table of events in brain ontogeny might lead to permanent anomalies in the anatomical and neurochemical organization, which will indubitably underlie the behavioral changes seen in adulthood. These observations support the hypothesis proposed by Swaab (1980) that any compound which acts on the adult nervous system would have long-term effects on brain growth and maturation when given at some vulnerable point in early life.

Vasopressin's influences explored in the Brattleboro rat

VP has a great variety of functions both peripherally and centrally. Nowadays it is even known that VP is not only synthesized in the brain, but also – though at low levels – in peripheral organs such as adrenal, testis, ovary and thymus. The time course of maturation of all these VP sources is not well-known (cf. Boer, 1987) but various VP neuron groups are known to develop at different times (Table 1). The same is possibly true for the receptors in target sites located either centrally or peripherally. So, following increased or decreased availability of VP during development one might have to investigate functional teratogenicity of different regulatory systems. The hereditary VP-deficient Brattleboro rat has been chosen as a model to unravel the role of VP in brain development, the rationale being that the functional changes in these animals will be due to the absence of VP from the onset of life (cf. Boer, 1985).

As mentioned above, the Brattleboro rat exhibits impaired body and brain growth, and the particular etiology of stunted brain growth seems to support VP's role in brain cell generation.

Based on regional DNA and [3H]thymidine incorporation studies, the main effects on postnatal brain cell mitosis exist in the cerebellum (Boer et al., 1982; Boer and Patel, 1983). Attempts to correct these deficits by long-term neonatal VP supplementation have failed so far (Wright and Kutscher, 1977; Boer et al., 1984a). No effects on the growth of the Brattleboro offspring were seen upon long-lasting VP treatment of pregnant Brattleboro mothers (Boer, 1985; Snijdewint et al., 1985). The latter studies were initiated as brain and cerebellar growth deficits were already evident at birth (Boer et al., 1984b). However, partial recovery was observed when LVP, instead of VP, was used as a therapy. Seven-fold-enhanced blood levels of VP in pregnant Wistar rats failed to induce passage to the fetal compartment (Oosterbaan et al., 1985a). Moreover, such high maternal VP levels reduced fetal growth. The results with LVP are therefore not easy to explain. Placental transfer might be different or the action of LVP might have its own specificity (this was also found for the ancestor peptide of both, i.e., VT; Goldstein, 1984).

Evidence that VP is a missing factor in brain cell proliferation of Brattleboro rat is therefore still incomplete. Nutritional and several other humoral and trophic factors (thyroid hormones, corticosterone, growth hormone, insulin-like growth factor) were largely ruled out as playing a role in the stunting of Brattleboro growth, but it is not possible to eliminate other still-unrecognized factors which might be related to the VP deficiency (cf. Boer, 1985, 1987). The continuously 2-fold-enhanced OT levels in these rats could be such a detrimental factor, since these levels are not sensitive to neonatal VP treatment (Boer et al., 1988) whereas maternal OT has already been shown to have some transient inhibitory effects on early body growth of Wistar rats (Boer and Kruisbrink, 1984).

In view of the mitogenic actions of VP in non-neuronal cells in vitro and in vivo (cf. review Boer, 1985), there are a few peculiar findings related to [3H]thymidine incorporation into the brain DNA of young Brattleboro rats which could be VP-dependent but have not yet been investigated as such. The tissue availability and breakdown of [³H]thymidine is enhanced (Boer and Patel, 1984; Snijdewint and Boer, 1988b) and the fate of DNA labelled on day 11 postnatally suggested enhanced cell death in the cerebellum, olfactory bulb and medulla oblongata (Fig. 4).

Another interesting aspect in the Brattleboro rat brain concerns the setting of VP receptors. These are undoubtedly present and appear as early and in the same brain regions as seen in controls (Petracca et al., 1986; Ravid et al., 1987; Snijdewint et al., 1987, and in preparation). In

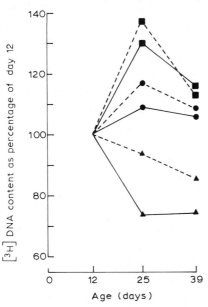

Fig. 4. Changes of brain cell turnover in young rats of the Brattleboro strain. On day 11 postnatally a subcutaneous injection of [³H]thymidine was given to label the dividing brain cells. On days 12, 25 and 39, the [³H]DNA content of several brain regions was determined and plotted here as percentage of day 12 data in order to compare VP-deficient homozygote (----) Brattleboro rats with their control heterozygote (——) strain mates. Relative [³H]DNA levels of day-25 VP-deficient rats were always higher due to increased tissue availability of [³H]thymidine on day 12; the steeper slopes between day 25 and 39 indicate more cell loss, or enhanced cell turnover for the VP-deficient Brattleboro rat (Snijdewint and Boer, 1988b). ●, cerebellum; ▲, medulla oblongata; ■, olfactory.

adults, however, the number of [³H]VP binding sites is increased and receptor affinity is lowered (Shewey and Dorsa, 1986). This up-regulation of receptor number is also seen in liver and adenohypophysis, but not in kidney (Koch and Lutz-Bucher, 1985; Shewey and Dorsa, 1986). Opposite changes, i.e. lasting down-regulation of [³H]VP binding sites of kidney, have been reported upon neonatal exposure of normal rat to VP (Handelmann and Sayson, 1984). VP receptors therefore seem to be subject to receptor imprinting (Csaba, 1986) which could explain the organizational effects of perinatal VP on several types of behavior (see before).

So far the VP-deficient Brattleboro rat has only been partially useful for exploring the role of VP in development. Additional perinatal VP treatment studies in both the Brattleboro rat (supplementation for VP defect) and normal rat (enhanced VP action) as well as antagonist and antibody treatment studies (decreased VP action) have therefore to be performed to further establish growth-related and organizational mechanisms. With respect to supplementation of VP in the Brattleboro rat, the question can be raised whether exogenously applied peptide can really replace the physiological function of VP cells. It might be better to supplement VP cells by using fetal graft techniques (Boer et al., 1985). Another approach might be to selectively kill the VP neurons in developing normal rat. Monoclonal antibodies to VP were recently shown to penetrate VP neurons (Burlet et al., 1987). A covalently coupled cytotoxin might this way be targeted to eliminate (particular) VP cells and the early and later consequences for brain and behavioral parameters could be investigated.

Clinical significance of rat perinatal neuropeptide studies

The question might be raised to what extent neuropeptides might also affect nervous system development in human. The data reviewed above on long-lasting effects of early neuropeptide exposure were usually obtained by the administration of relatively high dosages to the rat mother or to the pups. Many of these studies were moreover not primarily meant to investigate functional neuroteratological effects, but rather were initiated to substantiate the role of a neuropeptide in a particular physiological process of the organism. On the other hand, there are many situations in which human serum neuropeptide levels become considerably increased under physiological, pathological and environmental conditions. For instance, at birth, maternal and newborn plasma levels of VP, OT, ACTH and β-endorphin become very high (Csontos et al., 1979; Facchinetti et al., 1982; Oosterbaan, 1985), and smoking and stress are also potent releasers of neuropeptides (cf. Seyler et al., 1986; Weinstock et al., Chapter 21). It goes without saying that opiate addiction during pregnancy also leads to dramatic activity changes in the endogenic opioid systems (Zagon and McLaughlin, 1983). Finally, trials on the therapeutic use of neuropeptides have started and have shown that they can enhance endogenic peptides considerably above physiological levels. To mention only a few examples of the clinical use of neuropeptides during human development: OT is in use to initiate birth in late human pregnancy (Cerutti et al., 1979) and to promote lactation (Ruis et al., 1982), β-endorphin is used as an analgesic at the time of delivery (Oyama et al., 1980), VP and its analogues are administered to mentally retarded children (Andersen et al., 1979) and children with learning disorders (Eisenberg et al., 1984) or brain trauma (Wit et al., 1986), angiotensin is used in the early diagnosis of hypertensive disorders in pregnancy (Oney and Kaulhausen, 1982), and growth-hormone releasing hormone (GHRH) to treat GH-deficient children (Smith et al., 1986). Detrimental effects of enhanced neuropeptide levels might also be expected, because of the often greater sensitivity of human beings than of rat to teratological effects (Swaab et al., Chapter 1), a generally lower clearance rate of peptides in human (Lauson, 1974), an immature blood-brain barrier in young children

(Saunders, 1977), and the transfer of neuropeptides from mother to offspring via milk intake (pig; Weström et al., 1987a) followed by intestinal transmission into the circulation, a pathway which is still present during development (rat; Weström et al., 1987b).

Although neuropeptide receptors have not been recognized in rat fetal stages before the first peak of neurogenesis (see before), Friedler (1974) reported that deleterious effects might even be transferred by the sperm or occur at the stage of the egg-cell. Morphine treatment of male or female rats prior to mating resulted in hyperanalgesia in their offspring, and the rate of weight gain was found to be reduced, even in a second generation (cf. Sonderegger et al., 1979). Thus, functional neuroteratological effects of neuropeptide exposure may have transgenerational aspects (see review, Campbell and Perkins, Chapter 33 of this volume), which should make us even more aware of the possibilities and stimulate us to carry out thorough basic and clinical studies on functional neuroteratology also for the class of behaviorally active neuropeptides.

Summary

Neuropeptides form a relatively recently recognized putative class of centrally active neurotransmitters which formerly were only known as mammalian or non-mammalian hormones. These compounds are very potent in inducing behavioral changes in mature mammals and in their variety they outnumber the other (classical) neurotransmitters. Neuropeptides are synthesized early in brain development and binding sites appear in the same period. Imbalances in hormonal as well as aminergic neurotransmitter levels in ontogeny have shown to be deleterious for brain development, both anatomically, neurochemically and functionally. Because neuropeptides have hormonal as well as neurotransmitter characteristics and because many of them are present early in ontogeny, it was reasonable to suppose that such compounds play a role in brain ontogeny as well.

Moreover, several neuropeptides have been found to have trophic actions in a variety of cell proliferation or regeneration studies. The present review summarizes the growing evidence that changes in the neuropeptidergic environment of the perinatal rat can indeed result in long-lasting or life-long alterations in the nervous system, and consequently in behavioral changes. This supports the hypothesis (Swaab, 1980) that any chemical which can act functionally on the adult brain will affect brain organization when given at certain vulnerable stages of development.

Perinatal exposure to neuropeptides, even when these are given to the mother and therefore probably do not reach the fetus in large amounts, may affect neural cell proliferation and maturation on the one hand, and may have organizational effects on the developing neuropeptidergic system on the other hand. Neuropeptides may possibly alter the homeostatic set-point for their receptor synthesis, which is seen as an ontogenetic imprinting mechanism that has also been shown for peptide hormonal (Csaba, 1986) and catecholamine receptor systems (Miller and Friedhoff, Chapter 31). Such effects would also explain why often particularly those behavioral aspects are affected by the perinatally applied neuropeptide in which the compound has a regulatory or modulatory role in adulthood (cf. Handelmann, Chapter 32).

Neuropeptides and their agonist and antagonist analogues are therefore potential neuroteratogens which upon perinatal use can alter the brain in a subtle but long-lasting way. This aspect should also alert clinicians who intend to use these compounds therapeutically in pregnant mothers and young children.

Acknowledgements

The authors wish to thank Dr. M. G. P. Feenstra for evaluating the manuscript and Ms. Tini Eikelboom for editorial help.

References

Acker, G. R., Berran, J. and Strand, F. L. (1985) ACTH neuromodulation of the developing motor system and neonatal learning in rat. *Peptides*, 6, Suppl. 2: 41–49.

Alessi, N. E. and Quinlan, P. (1985) Postnatal development of ACTH and α-MSH in the medulla oblongata of rat: α-MSH is the predominant peptide. *Peptides*, 6, Suppl. 2: 137–141.

Altman, J. (1969) DNA metabolism and cell proliferation. In *Handbook of Neurochemistry, Vol. 2*, New York, Plenum Press, pp. 137–182.

Anderson, L. T., David, R., Bonnet, K. and Dancis, J. (1979) Passive avoidance learning in Lesch-Nyan disease: effect of 1-desamino-8-arginine-vasopressin. *Life Sci.*, 24: 905–910.

Baily, W. H. and Weiss, J. M. (1979) Evaluation of a 'memory deficit' in vasopressin-deficient rats. *Brain Res.*, 162: 174–178.

Bakke, J. L., Lawrence, N. L., Robinson, S. A., Bennett, J. and Bowers, C. (1978) Late endocrine effects of L-dopa, 5-HTP, and 6-OH-dopa administered to neonatal rats. *Neuroendocrinology*, 25: 291–302.

Bayon, A., Shoemaker, W. J., Bloom, F. E., Maus, A. and Guillemin, R. (1979) Perinatal development of the endorphin- and enkephalin-containing systems in the rat brain. *Brain Res.*, 179: 93–101.

Beckwith, B. E., Sandman, C. A., Hothersall, D. and Kastin, A. J. (1977a) Influence of neonatal injections of α-MSH on learning, memory and attention in rats. *Physiol. Behav.*, 18: 63071.

Beckwith, B. E., O'Quin, R. K., Petro, M. S., Kastin, A. J. and Sandman, C. A. (1977b) The effects of neonatal injections of α-MSH on the open-field behavior of juvenile and adult rats. *Physiol. Psychol.*, 5: 295–299.

Bodnar, R. J., Zimmerman, E. A., Nilaver, G., Mansour, A., Thomas, L. W., Kelly, D. D. and Glusman, M. (1980) Dissociation of cold-water swim and morphine analgesia in Brattleboro rats with diabetes insipidus. *Life Sci.*, 26: 1581–1590.

Boer, G. J. (1987) Development of vasopressin systems and their functions. In D. M. Gash and G. J. Boer (Eds.), *Vasopressin, Principles and Properties*, Plenum Press, New York, pp. 117–175.

Boer, G. J. and Kruisbrink, J. (1984) Effects of continuous administration of oxytocin by an Accurel device on parturition in the rat and on development and diuresis in the offspring. *J. Endocrinol.*, 101: 121–129.

Boer, G. J. and Patel, A. J. (1983) Disorders of cell acquisition in the brain of rats deficient in vasopressin (Brattleboro mutant). *Neurochem. Int.*, 5: 463–469.

Boer, G. J. and Swaab, D. F. (1983) Long-term effects on brain and behavior of early treatments with neuropeptides.

In G. Zbinden, V. Cuomo, G. Racagni and B. Weiss (Eds.), *Application of Behavioral Pharmacology in Toxicology*, New York, Raven Press, pp. 251–263.

Boer, G.J. and Swaab, D.F. (1985) Neuropeptide effects on brain development to be expected from behavioral teratology. *Peptides*, 6, Suppl. 2: 21–28.

Boer, G.J., Buijs, R.M., Swaab, D.F. and De Vries, G.J. (1980a) Vasopressin and the developing rat brain. *Peptides*, 1: 203–209.

Boer, G.J., Swaab, D.F., Uylings, H.B.M., Boer, K., Buijs, R.M. and Velis, D.N. (1980b) Neuropeptides in rat brain development. *Prog. Brain Res.*, 53: 207–227.

Boer, G.J., Van Rheenen-Verberg, C.M.F. and Uylings, H.B.M. (1982) Impaired brain development of the diabetes insipidus Brattleboro rat. *Dev. Brain Res.*, 3: 557–575.

Boer, G.J., Kragten, R., Kruisbrink, J. and Swaab, D.F. (1984a) Vasopressin fails to restore postnatally the stunted brain development in the Brattleboro, but affects water metabolism permanently. *Neurobehav. Toxicol. Teratol.*, 6: 103–109.

Boer, G.J., Dozy, M.H. and Uylings, H.B.M. (1984b) Cerebellar DNA and tissue water changes in the brain of diabetes insipidus Brattleboro rats are already present at birth. *Int. J. Dev. Neurosci.*, 2: 301–304.

Boer, G.J., Gash, D.M., Dick, L. and Schluter, N. (1985) Vasopressin neuron survival in neonatal Brattleboro rat; critical factors in graft development and innervation of the host brain. *Neuroscience*, 15: 1087–1109.

Boer, G.J., Van Heerikhuize, J.J. and Van der Woude, T.P. (1988) Elevated serum oxytocin of the vasopressin-deficient Brattleboro rat is present throughout life and is not sensitive to treatment with vasopressin. *Acta Endocrinol.*, 118.

Brenneman, D.E., Neale, E.A., Foster, G.A., D'Autremont, S.W. and Westbrook, G.L. (1987) Nonneuronal cells mediate neurotrophic action of vasoactive intestinal peptide. *J. Cell Biol.*, 104: 1603–1610.

Brito, G.N.O., Thomas, G.J., Gingold, S.I. and Gash, D.M. (1980) Behavioral characteristics of vasopressin-deficient rats (Brattleboro strain). *Brain Res. Bull.*, 6: 71–75, 1980.

Brinton, R.E. and Gruener, R. (1987) Vasopressin promotes neurite growth in cultured embryonic neurons. *Synapse*, 1: 329–334.

Bugnon, C., Fellmann, D., Gouget, A. and Cardot, J. (1982) Ontogeny of the corticoliberin neuroglandular system in rat brain. *Nature*, 298: 159–161.

Burlet, A.J., Leon-Henri, B.P., Robert, F.R., Arahmani, A., Fernette, B.M.L. and Burlet, C.R. (1987) Monoclonal anti-vasopressin (VP) antibodies penetrate into VP neurons, in vivo. *Exp. Brain Res.*, 65: 629–638.

Buijs, R.M., Velis, D.N. and Swaab, D.F. (1980) Ontogeny of vasopressin and oxytocin in the fetal rat. *Peptides*, 1: 315–324.

Bijlsma, W.A., Jennekens, F.G.I., Schotman, P. and Gispen, W.H. (1983a) Stimulation by ACTH[4–10] of nerve fibre regeneration following sciatic nerve crush. *Muscle Nerve*, 6: 104–112.

Bijlsma, W.A., Schotman, P., Jennekens, F.G.I. and Gispen, W.H. (1983b) The enhanced recovery of sensorimotor function in rats is related to the melanotropic moiety of ACTH/MSH neuropeptides. *Eur. J. Pharmacol.*, 92: 231–236.

Caffé, A.R., Van Leeuwen, F.W. and Luiten, F.G.M. (1987) Vasopressin cells in the medial amygdala of the rat project to the lateral septum and the ventral hippocampus. *J. Comp. Neurol.*, 261: 237–252.

Carey, R.J. and Miller, M. (1982) Absence of learning and memory deficits in the vasopressin-deficient rat (Brattleboro strain). *Behav. Brain Res.*, 6: 1–13.

Cerutti, R., Stoppa, G., Drago, D., Terrin, P., Spada, A., Gambato, M. and Di Giannantonio, E. (1979) Oxytocin and feto-neonatal stress. In L. Zichella and P. Pancheri (Eds.), *Psychoneuroendocrinology in Reproduction*, Elsevier/North-Holland Biomed. Press, Amsterdam, pp. 529–532.

Champney, T.F., Sahley, T.L. and Sandmann, C.A. (1976) Effects of neonatal cerebral ventricular injection of ACTH 4–9 and subsequent adult injection in learning in male and female albino rats. *Pharmacol. Biochem. Behav.*, 5: 3–9.

Clendeninn, N.J., Petraitis, M. and Simon, E.J. (1976) Ontological development of opiate receptors in rodent brain. *Brain Res.*, 118: 157–160.

Conklin, P.M., Schindler, W.J. and Hull, S.F. (1973) Hypothalamic thyrotropin releasing factor. Activity and pituitary responsiveness during development of the rat. *Neuroendocrinology*, 11: 197–211.

Csaba, G. (1986) Receptor ontogeny and hormonal imprinting. *Experientia*, 42: 750–759.

Csontos, K., Rust, M., Höllt, V., Mahr, W., Kromer, W. and Teschemacher, H.J. (1979) Elevated plasma α-endorphin levels in pregnant women and their neonates. *Life Sci.*, 25: 835–844.

Daikoku, S., Kanano, H., Matsumura, H. and Saito, S. (1978) In vivo and in vitro studies on the appearance of LHRH neurons in the hypothalamus of perinatal rats. *Cell Tiss. Res.*, 194: 433–445.

De Vries, G.J., Buijs, R.M. and Swaab, D.F. (1981) Ontogeny of the vasopressinergic neurons of the suprachiasmatic nucleus and their extrahypothalamic projections in the rat brain. Presence of a sex difference in the lateral septum. *Brain Res.*, 218: 67–78.

De Vries, G.J., Buijs, R.M., Van Leeuwen, F.W., Caffé, A.R. and Swaab, D.F. (1985) The vasopressinergic innervation of the brain in normal and castrated rats. *J. Comp. Neurol.*, 233: 236–254.

De Wied, D., Bohus, B. and Van Wimersma-Greidanus, Tj.B. (1975) Memory deficit in rats with hereditary diabetes insipidus. *Brain Res.*, 85: 152–156.

Eisenberg, J., Chazan-Gologorsky, S., Hattab, J. and Belmaker, R.H. (1984) A controlled trial of vasopressin treatment of childhood learning disorder. *Biol. Psychiatry*, 19: 1137–1141.

Edwards, P.M., Kuiters, R.R.F., Boer, G.J. and Gispen, W.H. (1986) Recovery from peripheral nerve transection is accelerated by local application of α-MSH by means of microporous Accurel^R polypropylene tubes. *J. Neurol. Sci.*, 74: 171–176.

Ermisch, A., Kock, M. and Barth, T. (1986) Learning performance of rats after pre- and postnatal application of arginine-vasopressin. *Monogr. Neural Sci.*, 12: 142–147.

Facchinetti, F., Bagnoli, F., Bracci, R. and Genazzani, A.R. (1982) Plasma opioids in the first hours of life. *Pediatr. Res.*, 16: 95–98.

Foster, G.A. and Schultzberg, M. (1984) Immunohistochemical analysis of the ontogeny of neuropeptide Y immunoreactive neurons in the fetal rat brain. *Int. J. Dev. Neurosci.*, 2: 387–407.

Friedler, G. (1974) Long-term effects of opiates. In J. Dancis and J.C. Hwang (Eds.), *Perinatal Pharmacology: Problems and Priorities*, Raven Press, New York.

Frischer, R.E., El-Kawa, N.M. and Strand, F.L. (1985) ACTH peptides as organizers of neuronal patterns in development: maturation of the rat neuromuscular junction as seen by scanning electron microscopy. *Peptides*, 6, Suppl. 2: 13–19.

Gash, D.M., Hermans, J.P. and Thomas, G.J. (1987) Vasopressin and animal behavior. In D.M. Gash and G.J. Boer (Eds.), *Vasopressin, Principles and Properties*, Plenum Press, New York, pp. 517–548.

Gispen, W.H., De Koning, P., Kuiters, R.R.F., Van der Zee, C.E.E.M. and Verhaagen, J. (1987) On the neurotrophic action of melanocortins. *Prog. Brain Res.*, 72: 319–331.

Goldstein, R. (1984) The involvement of arginine vasotocin in the maturation of the kitten brain. *Peptides*, 5: 25–28.

Goldstein, R. and Rodica, B. (1986) Pharmacological evidence that effects of vasotocin on brain maturation are mediated by GABA mechanisms. *Int. J. Dev. Neurosci.*, 4: 305–309.

Gonzalez, B.J., Leroux, P., Laquerriere, A., Bodenant, C. and Vaudry, H. (1987) Transient expression of somatostatin receptors in the rat cerebellum. Proc. Symp. 'Neuropeptides, from gene to behavior', Paris, p. 108.

Greer, E.R., Diamond, M.C. and Tang, J.M.W. (1982) Effect of age and enrichment on certain brain dimensions in Brattleboro rats deficient in vasopressin. *Exp. Neurol.*, 75: 11–22.

Handelmann, G.E. (1985) Neuropeptide effects on brain development. *J. Physiol. Paris*, 80: 268–274.

Handelmann, G.E. and Dow-Edwards, D. (1985) Modulation of brain development by morphine: effects on central motor systems and behavior. *Peptides*, 6, Suppl. 2: 29–34.

Handelmann, G.E. and Quirion, R. (1983) Neonatal expo-

sure to morphine increases mu opiate binding in the adult forebrain. *Eur. J. Pharmacol.*, 94: 357–358.

Handelmann, G.E. and Sayson, S.C. (1984) Neonatal exposure to vasopressin decreases vasopressin binding sites in the adult kidney. *Peptides*, 5: 1217–1219.

Handelmann, G.E., Selsky, J.H. and Helke, C.J. (1984) Substance P administration to neonatal rats increases adult sensitivity to substance P. *Physiol. Behav.*, 33: 297–300.

Handelmann, G.E., Shults, W.W. and O'Donohue, T.L. (1987) A developmental influence of substance P on its receptor. *Int. J. Dev. Neurosci.*, 5: 11–16.

Hauser, K.F., McLaughlin, P.J. and Zagon, I.S. (1987) Endogenous opioids regulate dendritic growth and spine formation in developing rat brain. *Brain Res.*, 416: 157–161.

Hays, S.E., Houston, H., Beinfeld, M.C. and Paul, S.M. (1981) Postnatal ontogeny of cholecystokinin receptors in rat brain. *Brain Res.*, 213: 237–241.

Hedge, G.A. and Huffman, L.J. (1987) Vasopressin and endocrine function. In D.M. Gash and G.J. Boer (Eds.), *Vasopressin, Principles and Properties*, Plenum Press, New York, pp. 435–476.

Herman, J.P., Thomas, G.J., Laycock, J.F., Gartside, I.B. and Gash, D.M. (1986) Behavioral variability within the Brattleboro and Long-Evans rat strains. *Physiol. Behav.*, 36: 713–721.

Inagaki, S., Shiosaka, S., Takatsuki, K., Iida, H., Sakanaka, H., Senba, E., Hara, Y., Matsuzaki, T., Kawai, Y. and Tohyama, M. (1982) Ontogeny of somatostatin-containing neuron system of the rat cerebellum including its fiber connections: an experimental and immunohistochemical analysis. *Dev. Brain Res.*, 3: 509–527.

Insel, I.R., Battaglia, G. and De Souza, E. (1987) Neuronal receptors in development. *Neuroendocrine Lett.*, 9: 136.

Kastin, A.J., Kostrzewa, R.M., Schally, A.V. and Coy, D.H. (1980) Neonatal administration of met-enkephalin facilitates maze performance of adult rats. *Pharmacol. Biochem. Behav.*, 13: 883–886.

Kirby, M.L. (1983) Changes in ^{3}H-naloxone binding in spinal cord of rats treated prenatally with morphine. *Neuropharmacology*, 22: 303–307.

Koch, B. and Lutz-Bucher, B. (1985) Specific receptors for vasopressin in the pituitary gland: evidence for down-regulation and desensitization of adrenocorticotropin-releasing factors. *Endocrinology*, 116: 671–676.

Lauson, H.D. (1974) Metabolism of neurohypophyseal hormones. In W.H. Sawyer and E. Knobil (Eds.), *Handbook of Physiology, Section 7, Vol. IV*, Am. Phys. Soc., Washington, pp. 287–293.

Lichtensteiger, W. and Schlumpf, M. (1985) Modification of early neuroendocrine development by drugs and endogenous peptides. In Parvez et al. (Eds.), *Progress in Neuroendocrinology, Vol. 1*, VNU Science Press, pp. 153–166.

McGregor, G.P., Woodmans, P.L., O'Shaughnessy, D.J., Ghatei, M.A., Polak, J.M. and Bloom, S.R. (1982) Developmental changes in bombesin, substance P, somatostatin and vasoactive intestinal polypeptide in the rat brain. *Neurosci. Lett.*, 28: 21–27.

Meriney, S.D., Gray, D.B. and Pilar, G. (1985) Morphine-induced delay of normal cell death in the avian ciliary ganglion. *Science*, 228: 1451–1453.

Meyerson, B.J. (1985) Influence of early β-endorphin treatment on the behavior and reaction to β-endorphin in the adult male rat. *Psychoneuroendocrinology*, 10: 135–147.

Moldow, R.L., Kastin, A.J., Hollander, C.S., Coy, D.H. and Sandman, C.A. (1981) Brain β-endorphin-like immunoreactivity in adult rats given β-endorphin neonatally. *Brain Res. Bull.*, 7: 683–686.

Moratella, R., Sanchez-Franco, F. and Del Rio, J. (1986) Long-term administration in rats induced by neonatal administration of vasopressin antiserum. *Life Sci.*, 38: 109–115.

Moratella, R., Borrell, J., Sanchez-Franco, F. and Del Rio, J. (1987) Neonatal administration of vasopressin antiserum induces long-term deficits on active and passive avoidance behaviour in rats. *Behav. Brain Res.*, 23: 231–237.

Nyakas, C. (1975) Influence of corticosterone and ACTH on the postnatal development of learning and memory functions. In K. Lissak (Ed.), *Hormones and Brain Function*, New York, Plenum Press, pp. 83–89.

Nyakas, C., Lévay, G., Viltsek, J. and Endrözci, E. (1981) Effects of neonatal ACTH[4–10] administration on adult adaptive behavior and brain tyrosine hydroxylase activity. *Dev. Neurosci.*, 4: 225–232.

Öney, T. and Kaulhausen, H. (1982) The value of the angiotensin sensitivity test in the early diagnosis of hypertensive disorders in pregnancy. *Am. J. Obstet. Gynecol.*, 142: 17–20.

Oosterbaan, G.P. (1986) Amniotic oxytocin and vasopressin in the human and the rat. Thesis, University of Amsterdam.

Oosterbaan, G.P., Swaab, D.F. and Boer, G.J. (1985a) Oxytocin and vasopressin in the rat do not readily pass from the mother to the amniotic fluid in late pregnancy. *J. Dev. Physiol.*, 7: 89–97.

Oosterbaan, G.P., Swaab, D.F. and Boer, G.J. (1985b) Increased amniotic vasopressin levels in experimentally growth-retarded rat fetuses. *J. Dev. Physiol.*, 7: 89–97.

Oyama, T., Matsuki, A., Taneichi, T., Ling, N. and Guillemin, R. (1980) β-endorphin in obstetric analgesia. *Am. J. Obstet. Gynecol.*, 137: 613–616.

Peruzović, M. and Miković, K. (1986) Prenatal ACTH and corticosteroids, development and behavior in rat. *Monogr. Neural Sci.*, 12: 103–111.

Petracca, F.M., Baskin, D.G., Diaz, J. and Dorsa, D.M. (1986) Ontogenic changes in vasopressin binding site distribution in rat brain: an autoradiographic study. *Dev. Brain Res.*, 28: 63–68.

Ravid, R., Swaab, D.F., Van der Woude, Tj.P. and Boer, G.J. (1986) Immunocytochemically-stained vasopressin binding sites in rat brain – ventricular application of vasopressin/Accurel in the Brattleboro rat. *J. Neurol. Sci.*, 76: 317–333.

Reubi, J.-C., Palacios, J.M. and Maurer, R. (1986) Specific LHRH receptors in the rat hippocampus and pituitary visualized with autoradiography. In E.E. Müller and R.M. MacLeod (Eds.), *Neuroendocrine Perspectives*, Elsevier Science Publishers, Amsterdam, pp. 341–346.

Rodier, P.M. (1977) Correlations between prenatally-induced alteration in CNS cell populations and postnatal function. *Teratology*, 16: 235–246.

Ruis, H., Rolland, R., Doesburg, W., Broeders, G. and Corbey, R. (1982) Oxytocin enhances onset of lactation among mothers delivering prematurely. *Br. Med. J.*, 283: 340–347.

Saint-Côme, C., Acker, G.R. and Strand, F.L. (1982) Peptide influences on the development and regulation of motor performances. *Peptides*, 3: 439–449.

Sandman, C.A., McGivern, R.F., Berka, C., Walker, J.M., Coy, D.H. and Kastin, A.J. (1979) Neonatal administration of β-endorphin produces 'chronic' intensity to thermal stimuli. *Life Sci.*, 25: 1755–1760.

Saunders, N.R. (1977) Ontogeny of the blood-brain barrier. *Exp. Eye Res. Suppl.*, pp. 523–550.

Seyler, L.E., Pomerlean, O.F., Fertig, J.B., Hunt, D. and Parker, K. (1986) Pituitary hormone response to cigarette smoking. *Pharmacol. Biochem. Behav.*, 24: 159–162.

Shewey, L.M. and Dorsa, D.M. (1986) Enhanced binding of ³H-arginine[8]-vasopressin in the Brattleboro rat. *Peptides*, 7: 701–704.

Slotkin, T.A., Whitmore, W.L., Salvaggio, M. and Seidler, F.J. (1979) Perinatal methadone addiction affects brain synaptic development of biogenic amine systems in the rat. *Life Sci.*, 24: 1223–1229.

Slotkin, T.A., Wiegel, S.J., Whitmore, W.L. and Seidler, F.J. (1982) Maternal methadone administration: deficit in development of alpha-noradrenergic responses in developing rat brain as assessed by norepinephrine stimulation of ³³Pi incorporation into phospholipids in vivo. *Biochem. Pharmacol.*, 31: 1899–1902.

Smith, P.J., Brook, C.G.D., Pringle, P.J., Rivier, J., Vale, W. and Thorner, M.O. (1986) The induction of growth hormone secretion following long term treatment of growth hormone deficient children with growth hormone releasing hormone 1–40. In E.E. Müller and R.M. MacLeod (Eds.), *Neuroendocrine Perspectives, Vol. 5*, Elsevier Science Publishers BV, Amsterdam, pp. 143–150.

Snijdewint, F.G.M. and Boer, G.J. (1986) Vasopressin and vasopressin-antagonists applied to neonatal Wistar rat: effects on body and brain development and water metabolism. *Neurobehav. Toxicol. Teratol.*, 8: 213–217.

262

Snijdewint, F.G.M. and Boer, G.J. (1988a) Neonatal treatment of Wistar rats with vasopressin-antagonist dP[Tyr(Me)^2]AVP inhibits body and brain development and induces polyuria. *Neurotoxicol. Teratol.*, submitted.

Snijdewint, F.G.M. and Boer, G.J. (1988b) Cell death is enhanced in the developing brain of the vasopressin-deficient Brattleboro rat. *Dev. Brain Res.*, submitted.

Snijdewint, F.G.M., Boer, G.J. and Swaab, D.F. (1985) Body and brain growth following continuous perinatal administration of arginine- and lysine-vasopressin to the homozygous Brattleboro rat. *Dev. Brain Res.*, 2: 269–277.

Snijdewint, F.G.M., Van Leeuwen, F.W., Pool, C.W. and Boer, G.J. (1987) Simultaneous localization and quantification of vasopressin and oxytocin binding sites in the developing Wistar and Brattleboro rat brain. *Neurosciences*, 22: Suppl. 701P.

Sonderegger, T., O'Shea, S. and Zimmerman, E. (1979) Progeny of male rats addicted neonatally to morphine. *Proc. West. Pharmacol. Soc.*, 22: 137–139.

Steele, W.J. and Johannesson, T. (1975) Effects of prenatally-administered morphine on brain development and resultant tolerance to the analgesic effect of morphine in offspring of morphine-treated rats. *Acta Pharmacol. Toxicol.*, 36: 243–256.

Strand, F.L. and Kung, T.T. (1980) ACTH accelerates recovery of neuromuscular function following crushing of peripheral nerve. *Peptides*, 1: 135–138.

Stratton, L.O., Gibson, C.A., Kolar, K.G. and Kastin, A.J. (1976) Neonatal treatment with TRH affects development, learning and emotionality in the rat. *Pharmacol. Biochem. Behav.*, 5: 65–67.

Swaab, D.F. (1980) Neuropeptides and brain development – a working hypothesis. In C. Di Benedetta et al. (Eds.), *Multidisciplinary Approach to Brain Development*, Elsevier/North-Holland Biomedical Press, Amsterdam, pp. 181–196.

Swaab, D.F. and Ter Borg, J.P. (1981) Development of peptidergic systems in the rat brain. Proc. Ciba Foundation Symp., 'The fetus and independent life', pp. 271–294.

Swaab, D.F., Visser, M. and Tilders, F.J.H. (1976) Stimulation of intrauterine growth in rat by α-MSH. *J. Endocrinol.*, 70: 445–449.

Swaab, D.F., Boer, G.J. and Visser, M. (1977) The fetal brain and intrauterine growth. *Postgrad. Med. J.*, 54 (Suppl. 1): 63–73.

Telegdy, G., Balázs, M. and Fekete, M. (1986) Effects of pre- and postnatal cholecystokinin treatment on brain development in rats. *Monogr. Neural Sci.*, 12: 153–160.

Tinius, T.P., Beckwith, B.E. and Preussler, D.W. (1987) Prenatal administration of arginine vasopressin impairs memory retrieval in adult rats. *Peptides*, 8: 01–07.

Tsang, D. and Ng, S.C. (1980) Effect of antenatal exposure to opiates on the development of opiate receptors in rat brain. *Brain Res.*, 188: 199–206.

Uphouse, L., Tilson, H. and Mitchell, C.L. (1983) Long-term effects of behavioral testing on serum hormones and brain weight. *Life Sci.*, 33: 1395–1400.

Van der Helm-Hylkema, H. (1973) Effecten van vroeg neonataal toegediend ACTH en aan ACTH verwante peptiden op de somatische en gedragsontwikkeling van de rat. Thesis, University of Utrecht, The Netherlands.

Van der Helm-Hylkema, H. and De Wied, D. (1976) Effect of neonatally injected ACTH and ACTH analogues on eye-opening of the rat. *Life Sci.*, 18: 1099–1104.

Van Haaren, F., Van de Poll, N.E. and Van Oyen, H.G. (1985) Age effects on passive avoidance behavior of vasopressin-deficient Brattleboros. *Physiol. Behav.*, 34: 115–117.

Van Wimersma Greidanus, T.B. (1982) Disturbed behavior and memory of the Brattleboro rat. *Ann. N.Y. Acad. Sci.*, 394: 655–662.

Veldhuis, H.D., Nyakas, C. and De Wied, D. (1985) Neuropeptides and functional recovery after brain damage. In B.E. Will, P. Schmitt and J.C. Dalzymple-Alford (Eds.), *Brain Plasticity, Learning and Memory*, Plenum Press, New York, pp. 26–32.

Versteeg, D.M., Tanaka, M. and De Kloet, E.R. (1978) Catecholamine concentration and turnover in discrete regions of the brain of the homozygous Brattleboro rat deficient in vasopressin. *Endocrinology*, 103: 1654–1661.

Vorhees, C.V. (1981) Effects of prenatal naloxone exposure on postnatal behavior development of rats. *Neurobehav. Toxicol. Teratol.*, 3: 295–301.

Warren, P.H. and Gash, D.M. (1983) Hyperreflexive behavior in Brattleboro rats. *Peptides*, 4: 421–424.

Weström, B.R., Ekman, R., Svendsen, L., Svendsen, J. and Karlsson, B.W. (1987a) Levels of immunoreactive insulin, neurotensin, and bombesin in porcine colostrum and milk. *J. Ped. Gastroent. Nutr.*, 6: 460–465.

Weström, B.R., Folkesson, H.G., Lundin, S. and Karlsson, B.W. (1987b) Intestinal transmission of the nonapeptide DDAVP in developing rats. Int. FIP Satellite Symp. 'Disposition and delivery of peptide drugs', Sept. 5–6, Leiden, The Netherlands, p. 10.

Whitnall, M.H., Key, S., Ben-Barak, Y., Ozato, K. and Gainer, H. (1985) Neurophysin in the hypothalamo-neurohypophysial system. II. Immunocytochemical studies of the ontogeny of oxytocinergic and vasopressinergic neurons. *J. Neurosci.*, 5: 98–109.

Wit, J.M., Hijman, R., Jolles, J., Wolters, W.H.G., Van Ree, J.M., Van den Brande, J.L. and De Wied, D. (1986) Effect of desglycinamide-arginine[8]-vasopressin (DGAVP) on cognitive functions in children with memory disorders. Symposium 'Neuropeptides and Brain Function', Utrecht, The Netherlands, May 28–30, abstr. P 55.

Wright, W.A. and Kutscher, C.L. (1977) Vasopressin administration in the first month of life: effects on growth and water metabolism in hypothalamic diabetes insipidus rats. *Pharmacol. Biochem. Behav.*, 6: 505–509.

Zadina, J. E. and Kastin, A. J. (1986) Neonatal peptides affect developing rats: β-endorphin alters nociception and opiate receptors, corticotropin-releasing factor alters cortico-sterone. *Dev. Brain Res.*, 29: 21–29.

Zadina, J. E., Kastin, A. J., Coy, D. H. and Adinoff, B. A. (1985) Developmental, behavioral, and opiate receptor changes after prenatal or postnatal β-endorphin, CRF, or Tyr-MIF-1. *Psychoneuroendocrinology*, 10: 367–383.

Zadina, J. E., Banks, W. A. and Kastin, A. J. (1986) Central nervous system effects of peptides, 1980–1985: a cross-listing of peptides and their central actions from the first six years of the journal Peptides. *Peptides*, 7: 497–537.

Zagon, I. S. and McLaughlin, P. J. (1982) Analgesia in young and adult rats perinatally exposed to methadone. *Neurobehav. Toxicol.*, 4: 455–457.

Zagon, I. S. and McLaughlin, P. J. (1983) Behavioral effects of prenatal exposure to opiates. *Monogr. Neural Sci.*, 9: 159–168.

Zagon, I. S. and McLaughlin, P. J. (1985) Naltrexone's influence on neurobehavioral development. *Pharmacol. Biochem. Behav.*, 22: 441–448.

Zagon, I. S. and McLaughlin, P. J. (1986) β-Funaltrexamine (β-FNA) and the regulation of body and brain development in rats. *Brain Res. Bull.*, 17: 5–9.

Zagon, I. S. and McLaughlin, P. J. (1987) Endogenous opioid systems regulate cell proliferation in the developing rat brain. *Brain Res.*, 412: 68–72.

Zagon, I. S., Rhodes, R. E. and McLaughlin, P. J. (1985) Distribution of enkephalin immunoreactivity in germinative cells of developing rat cerebellum. *Science*, 227: 1049–1051.

Discussion

R. Balazs: It is interesting that the negative effect of vasotocin on brain growth seems to be mediated through GABA, as it has been reported that in certain parts of neuron systems GABA has a trophic influence on nerve cells. This brings me to a more general point concerning trophic effects. These seem to be maturation-dependent, and therefore in vivo, when cells may be at different development stages, the effects can be easily masked.

G. J. Boer: Goldstein and Rodica (1986) describe their effects in terms of total brain weight and tissue parameters. So regional differences, which could be indicative for your point, were not reported.

E. R. De Kloet: Does your observation on the presence of the vasopressin (VP) and oxytocin (OT) mRNA as well as the presence of VP and OT immunoreactivity in the fetal brain imply that processing of the precursors for these peptides occurs in the same way as in the adult brain? In other words,

are VP and OT found in the brain already bioactive around birth?

G. J. Boer: There is no reason to believe that processing is different. However, there is evidence that the maturation of the processing process for the OT precursor is delayed. Immunocytochemistry revealed the fetal presence of both VP and OT precursor, as well as of VP, but OT staining is only visible around rat birth. VP is not only present very early in the cell nuclei of the hypothalamus, but is also present extrahypothalamically as well as in the pituitary. Moreover, it can be released from the fetal pituitary in vitro, and is present in serum of newborns (cf. Boer, 1987). It can, therefore, be bioactive if any binding site is at hand.

T. D. Yih: Were there abnormal fetuses obtained in the study in which the Brattleboro rat was treated with vasopressin (VP) during pregnancy? According to Jost (1951) vasopressin includes peculiar defects in rats, e.g. absence or reduction of digits of the extremities.

G. J. Boer: In these studies VP and lysine-VP were given in a dosage that cured the polyurea of the VP-deficient Brattleboro mothers, that is given as near-physiological levels. No abnormalities of the kind you mentioned were seen. However, we know from our own studies that 10 times higher dosage rates with VP in normal rat induce fetal growth reduction (Oosterbaan et al., 1985).

J. Del Rio: I would like to make a comment on the similar deficits in passive avoidance behavior found in rats after perinatal administration of either vasopressin or vasopressin antiserum. It is possible to think that vasopressin has a biphasic effect on memory processes and a facilitating or disrupting effect may depend on the dose. In the latter case, a high enough dose of vasopressin could perhaps induce a deleterious effect on specific receptors for this neuropeptide.

G. J. Boer: Although I immediately agree with a stage- and dose-dependency of the vasopressin effects, it does not explain why lasting behavioral changes occur in the same direction when neonatal occupation of vasopressin receptors was either low or high. However, one might speculate that the underlying neurochemical changes are different and that changes in other vasopressin-related central functions might reveal more about this.

References

Boer, G. J. (1987) Development of vasopressin systems and their functions. In D. M. Gash and G. J. Boer (Eds.), *Vasopressin, Principles and Properties*, Plenum Press, New York, pp. 117–175.

Goldstein, R. and Rodica, B. (1986) Pharmacological evidence that effects of vasotocin on brain maturation are mediated by GABA mechanisms. *Int. J. Dev. Neurosci.*, 4: 305–309.

Jost, A. (1951) Sur le rôle de la vasopressine et de la cortico-stimuline (A. C. T. H.) dans la production expérimentale de lésions des extrémités foetales (hémorragies, nécroses, amputations congénitales). *C R Séances Soc. Biol. Paris*, 145: 1805–1809.

Oosterbaan, H. P., Swaab, D. F. and Boer, G. J. (1985) Oxytocin and vasopressin in the rat do not readily pass from the mother to the amniotic fluid in late pregnancy. *J. Dev. Physiol.*, 7: 55–62.

G.J. Boer, M.G.P. Feenstra, M. Mirmiran, D.F. Swaab and F. Van Haaren
Progress in Brain Research, Vol. 73
© 1988 Elsevier Science Publishers B.V. (Biomedical Division)

CHAPTER 17

Perinatal exposure to methadone: how do early biochemical alterations cause neurofunctional disturbances?

Theodore A. Slotkin

Department of Pharmacology, Duke University Medical Center, Durham, NC 27710, USA

Introduction

As is often the case with neurobehavioral teratogenesis, the adverse effects of opiates on development were first noted in man and later extended to experimental animal models of drug abuse. Neurological and behavioral abnormalities in the offspring of opiate addicts have long been known (Zagon et al., 1982, 1984; Cooper et al., 1983; Zagon and McLaughlin, 1984). The introduction of synthetic opiates, particularly methadone, intended to suppress drug craving and illicit drug use, allowed the studies of opiate effects on development to be conducted with appropriate control for socio-economic factors, other drugs, perinatal nutrition and withdrawal stress (Cooper et al., 1983). Despite elimination of these confounding variables, neurobehavioral sequelae of perinatal opiate exposure were still observed. Subsequently, behavioral disturbances were duplicated in numerous animal models of opiate addiction (Zagon et al., 1982, 1984). By far the most popular species has been the rat, which has the advantage that major phases of nervous system development occur postnatally, thus aiding investigation. Studies conducted in our and other laboratories over the past 20 years have examined whether there is a biochemical basis for such behavioral effects, and this review summarizes progress made toward identifying the sequence of events occurring in the perinatal opiate syndrome.

Central catecholamine pathways

Catecholaminergic synapses, because of their ubiquity in both the central and the peripheral nervous system, have provided some of the most useful information concerning mechanisms of neurobehavioral teratology. If biochemical alterations underlie the deleterious effects of perinatal methadone exposure on neural performance, then a minimal assumption is that actions on synaptic development and/or function must be an immediate predecessor of the behavioral disturbances. Studies from several laboratories have confirmed that biogenic amine neurotransmitter levels are indeed altered in the offspring of perinatally addicted rats (McGinty and Ford, 1980; Slotkin et al., 1981; Slotkin, 1983). Typically, transmitter content is reduced; however, changes in transmitter levels do not indicate necessarily whether functional changes in synaptic development have occurred. Accordingly, it is important to examine several markers which delineate development of central catecholaminergic synapses (Fig. 1).

Development of function of a noradrenergic synapse requires a coordinated maturation of nerve terminals, their ability to synthesize, store and release transmitter, and post-synaptic ontogeny of receptors and appropriate linkages of the receptors to cellular processes (adenylate cyclase, phosphoinositide turnover, ion channels). In the rat, the majority of these events occur postnatally,

266

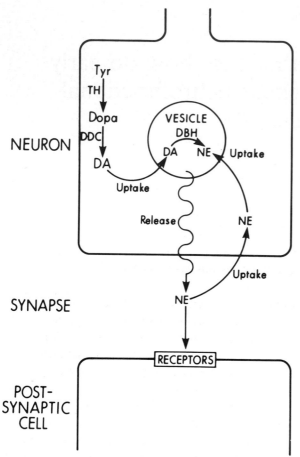

Fig. 1. Schematic representation of a noradrenergic synapse, showing biochemical markers of transmitter biosynthesis and storage, synaptic development, and postsynaptic action. Abbreviations: Tyr = tyrosine, TH = tyrosine hydroxylase, Dopa = dihydroxyphenylalanine, DDC = dopa decarboxylase, DA = dopamine, DBH = dopamine β-hydroxylase, NE = norepinephrine.

during the second to third weeks after birth (Slotkin and Thadani, 1980; Slotkin, 1986a,b). Development of noradrenergic nerve terminals can be monitored by the rise in synaptic uptake of norepinephrine into pinched-off nerve-ending preparations ('synaptosomal uptake'). Similarly, the ability of the terminals to manufacture norepinephrine can be evaluated through measurements of tyrosine hydroxylase activity, the rate-limiting factor in catecholamine bio-

synthesis. The final stage of presynaptic development appears to be the arrival in the nerve terminals of synaptic vesicles, which are necessary to convert dopamine to norepinephrine, to store the norepinephrine and to release it into the synapse upon appropriate stimulation. Vesicle maturation can be evaluated through measurements of uptake of norepinephrine into isolated vesicle preparations ('vesicular uptake'), and is a process separable from synaptosomal uptake. At the postsynaptic site, receptor development can be monitored directly through radioligand binding techniques, and responses elicited to specific agonists can be used to evaluate development of functional receptor-mediated responses. Although postsynaptic receptors are ordinarily present well before the development of presynaptic nerve terminals, a considerable degree of subsequent receptor maturation and sensitivity is dependent upon arrival of terminals at the appropriate developmental stage (Deskin et al., 1981; Friedhoff and Miller; 1983; Jones et al., 1985).

Using these biochemical indices of synaptogenesis and synaptic function, our group has shown that development of noradrenergic projec-

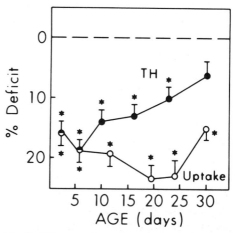

Fig. 2. Effects of maternal methadone administration (5 mg/kg daily to rats) on two CNS biochemical markers of presynaptic noradrenergic development in the offspring, i.e., tyrosine hydroxylase (TH) activity and synaptosomal uptake of [³H]norepinephrine. (Lau et al, 1977; Slotkin et al., 1979; Seidler et al., 1982).

tions in the CNS is slowed in offspring of pregnant rats receiving methadone (Lau et al., 1977; Slotkin et al., 1979; Slotkin and Thadani, 1980; Seidler et al., 1982). As shown in Fig 2, both tyrosine hydroxylase activity and synaptosomal uptake of norepinephrine are substantially below normal throughout postnatal development, suggesting a primary defect in transmitter biosynthesis and in the development of nerve terminals themselves. The relatively smaller effect on tyrosine hydroxylase suggests that some compensatory changes occur in transmitter synthesis to partially offset deficiencies in numbers of nerve terminals (synaptosomal uptake marker), and indeed the turnover of norepinephrine, an index of nerve activity, is not abnormally low in these animals (Slotkin et al., 1981). The same conclusions have been reached in studies of brain regions by McGinty and Ford (1980), who also found that the changes in uptake are largely reflective of altered numbers of terminals (change in uptake V_{max}).

In order to draw a parallel between these biochemical alterations and behavioral sequelae, however, it is necessary to show that delays in presynaptic terminal development are accompanied by functional alterations in transmitter

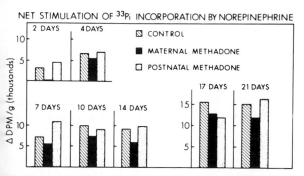

Fig. 3. Development of postsynaptic α_1-adrenergic receptor-mediated CNS phosphoinositide turnover in offspring of pregnant and nursing rats receiving methadone ('Maternal Methadone') and neonatal rats given methadone by direct injection ('Postnatal Methadone') (Slotkin et al., 1982). The response is significantly reduced in the maternally exposed group but not in the postnatally treated rats.

reactivity (Slotkin et al., 1982). Examination of the linkage of postsynaptic α_1-noradrenergic receptors to membrane phosphoinositide turnover indicated that these receptors are consistently hypofunctional in offspring of methadone-treated rats (Fig. 3). Recent studies have also indicated that opiate exposure during early development can compromise the ontogeny of adrenergic receptor sites themselves (Wang et al., 1986), a biochemical finding which could account for these functional changes. Interestingly, no such hypofunctionality is seen in rats given methadone by direct injection postnatally, indicating that a specific prenatal critical period exists in which opiates can perturb postsynaptic receptor-mediated functions.

A key question raised by these findings is whether adverse effects of opiate exposure on synaptogenesis are restricted to specific transmitter systems, or whether instead a general impairment of neuronal development occurs. Studies conducted on biochemical markers of development of other transmitter systems suggest that opiates do impair synaptogenesis in a widespread manner throughout the CNS (Fig. 4). Synaptosomal uptake of dopamine or serotonin is equally affected as for norepinephrine, and maturation of vesicular uptake systems appears to be a target as well. One potentially confounding factor is that opiates retard general body and brain growth. Nutritional or overall growth-related factors, however, do not appear to be responsible for the majority of the effects on synaptogenesis. This can be shown by a comparison of maternal methadone treatment vs. direct methadone injections to neonates. Although both groups show equivalent inhibition of body growth, and the directly injected pups show a greater inhibition of brain growth, the effects on presynaptic development are much more profound in the maternally exposed animals, a case similar to that seen for postsynaptic markers, described above. Additionally, unlike the situation with methadone, simple nutritional deprivation generally 'spares' brain development,

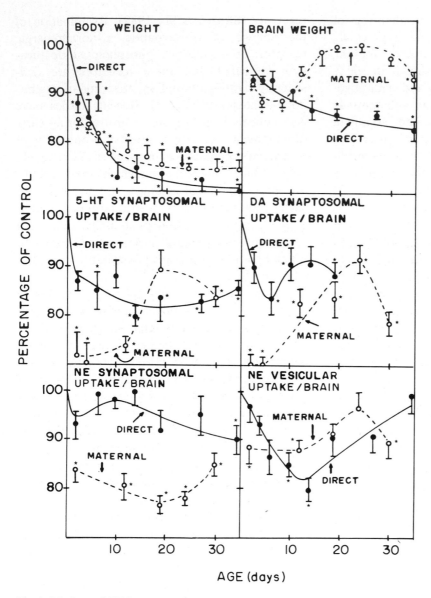

Fig. 4. Markers of CNS presynaptic development and tissue weight in rats exposed to methadone via maternal administration or by direct postnatal injections to neonates (Slotkin et al., 1979). Abbreviations: 5-HT = 5-hydroxytryptamine (serotonin), DA = dopamine, NE = norepinephrine.

resulting in essentially normal patterns of CNS synaptogenesis (Brazier, 1975; Dodge et al., 1975; Reinis and Goldman, 1980).

Control of cellular development

The finding of widespread deficits in synaptogenesis caused by prenatal methadone exposure indicates that early biochemical events mediating neuronal development may be a primary target for opioids. Recent work on intracellular control of macromolecule biosynthesis in developing neurons points to the ornithine decarboxylase (ODC)/polyamine system as a primary regulator of these events (Slotkin and Bartolome, 1986). The ODC/polyamine system has been shown to regulate neuronal cell replication, differentiation, migration and axonogenesis, and to provide an early index for perturbations in these processes caused by environmental insults (cf. Slotkin and Bartolome, 1986; Bell and Slotkin, Ch. 23 of this volume). Thus, studies have also conducted on the effects of perinatal exposure to drugs of abuse (Butler and Schanberg, 1975; Slotkin et al., 1976; Thadani et al., 1977; Slotkin and Thadani, 1980). Agents which delay general neuronal cellular maturation thus tend to cause a prolongation of the period in which ODC activity remains high. Examination of ODC in brains of rats whose mothers received methadone confirms that a delay in maturation is present (Fig. 5). The effects on ODC precede the known inhibitory actions of opiates on nucleic acid and protein synthesis in developing brain as well as those on synaptogenesis (Slotkin et al., 1976, 1979, 1980a, 1981, 1982; Lau et al., 1977; McGinty and Ford, 1980; Slotkin and Thadani, 1980; Seidler et al., 1982; Zagon and McLaughlin, 1982; Kornblum et al.,

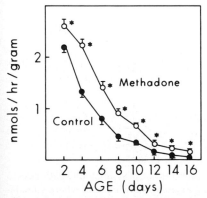

Fig. 5. Postnatal elevation in brain ornithine decarboxylase activity (ODC) in the offspring of rats given methadone (Slotkin et al., 1976, 1980a; Seidler et al., 1982).

1987), and thus may represent one of the early biochemical events which produce the later functional deficits. Because the ODC/polyamine system is basic to every developing tissue, it would be expected that such perturbations would lead to generalized actions in other tissues whose development is sensitive to opiates. In fact, examination of ODC in methadone-exposed neonates confirms that delayed developmental patterns occur prior to the appearance of growth deficits in all other tissues as well (Slotkin et al., 1976, 1980a; Seidler et al., 1982). The intimate relationships among ODC, axonogenesis/synaptogenesis and growth of the brain have been further demonstrated by the fact that when maternal methadone doses are adjusted downward to the point at which ODC is no longer affected, both brain growth and synaptogenesis are also spared (Slotkin et al., 1980a; Seidler et al., 1982).

The definitive studies which indicate a mechanistic, rather than just correlative, relationship between the ODC/polyamine system and effects of methadone on synaptic development, have been provided by experiments with α-difluoromethylornithine (DFMO). DFMO is a specific, irreversible inhibitor of ODC, has no opiate-like effects and, indeed, has no other known actions. Short-term inhibition of the enzyme by maternally administered DFMO results in a postnatal ODC/polyamine pattern very similar to that of methadone (Slotkin et al., 1983). The consequence of this ODC pattern is a delay in synaptogenesis nearly identical to that obtained with maternal methadone treatment (Fig. 6), characterized by reductions in tyrosine hydroxylase activity, synaptosomal uptake of norepinephrine and synaptosomal uptake of dopamine. As with methadone, a critical prenatal period exists in which adverse effects are maximized; postnatal DFMO treatment has a much smaller effect. These results are consistent with the view that a specific biochemical system which controls the timing of cellular maturation in the CNS is a primary target for opiate action, and that the subsequent effects on synaptogenesis, synap-

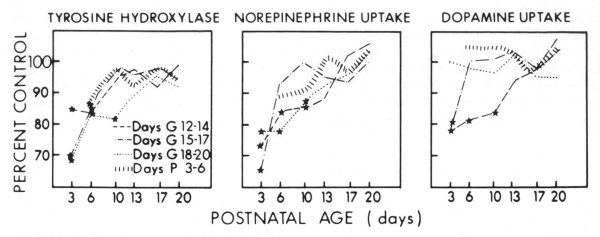

Fig. 6. Effects of short-term prenatal inhibition of ornithine decarboxylase by α-difluoromethylornithine (DFMO) on postnatal development of CNS presynaptic markers: tyrosine hydroxylase and synaptosomal uptake of norepinephrine and dopamine (Slotkin et al., 1983). DFMO was given during discrete 3-day periods during gestation (G) or postnatally (P).

tic function and behavior may thus represent the ultimate consequence of early perturbations of this system. Indeed, studies in tissue culture confirm that alterations of ODC may be directly elicited by stimulation of opiate receptors (Vernadakis et al., 1981), suggesting that primary maturational control could involve this pathway. Zagon and coworkers have further demonstrated that normal growth is modulated by endogenous opioid substances, and that interference with opiate receptor systems during early development can disrupt the program for cell acquisition, growth and synaptogenesis in the CNS (Zagon and McLaughlin, 1983). The adverse effects of methadone on neural development may therefore represent an inappropriate stimulation of a natural modulator of cellular development.

Peripheral sympathetic nervous system and neonatal survival

In view of the generalized effects of perinatal methadone on central synaptogenesis, it is particularly surprising that peripheral sympathetic synapses are not only spared the delay of development, but actually show precocious onset of function (Bareis and Slotkin, 1978, 1980; Slotkin et al., 1980b). It is thus worthwhile to examine the characteristics which delineate the onset of peripheral neuronal function and to determine why opiates may exert unique actions in these pathways. Ontogeny of sympathetic function can be divided into three specific developmental periods (Slotkin et al., 1980b) (Fig. 7):
(1) Even before birth, sympathetic target tissues, such as the heart and adrenal medulla, possess

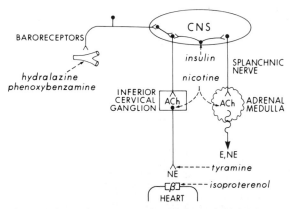

Fig. 7. Schematic representation of sympathetic pathways to the heart and adrenal medulla, showing sites where stimulatory drugs act. Abbreviations: CNS = central nervous system, ACh = acetylcholine, E = epinephrine, NE = norepinephrine, β = β-noradrenergic receptor.

postsynaptic receptors for norepinephrine (heart) and acetylcholine (adrenal medulla), and these receptors are linked to functional responses of the tissues. However, reflex stimuli, such as insulin-induced hypoglycemia or systemic hypotension, are unable to cause end-organ stimulation due to immaturity of central, ganglionic and post-ganglionic synapses.

(2) By the end of the first postnatal week, synaptogenesis occurs in ganglia and at post-ganglionic sites to permit transmission of efferent sympathetic signals, thus permitting responses to hypoglycemia. However, afferent sensory input from baroreceptors is not yet capable of eliciting responses.

(3) During the third to fourth weeks, baroreceptor regulation of sympathetic output first appears and matures, consequent on development of central mediation of sensory input–sympathetic output relationships. Tonic sympathetic activity becomes markedly elevated during this period, a process which appears to regulate the final adjustment of end-organ sensitivity to sympathetic stimulation and to play a role in end-organ cell differentiation.

It is thus of considerable interest that neonatal rats given methadone or the offspring of methadone-treated dams show a much earlier onset of reflex sympathetic capabilities than do normal rats. In the sympatho-adrenal axis, this can be demonstrated by premature development of catecholamine secretion elicited by insulin-induced hypoglycemia (Fig. 8). Ordinarily, newborn rats do not respond to hypoglycemia because of immaturity of splanchnic neuronal connections to the adrenal (Slotkin, 1973, 1986a; Bartolome et al., 1977; Bareis and Slotkin, 1978), and a full response is not obtained until the end of the first postnatal week. In contrast, responses are detectable at 2 days of age in neonatal rats given methadone and at 4 days of age in offspring of methadone-treated dams (Bareis and Slotkin, 1978; Slotkin et al., 1980b). Similar studies have confirmed a premature onset of synaptic function in the cardiac-sympathetic axis (Bareis and Slotkin, 1978; Slotkin et al., 1981), suggesting

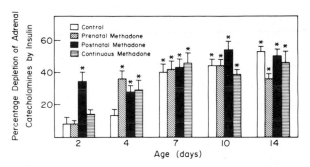

Fig. 8. Accelerated development of neuronal function in the sympatho-adrenal axis of rats exposed to methadone via prenatal, postnatal or continuous (prenatal + postnatal) administration to their dams (Bareis and Slotkin, 1978, 1980; Slotkin et al., 1980b). Reflex CNS-derived discharge of the splanchnic nerve was achieved through insulin-induced hypoglycemia.

that generalized actions on peripheral autonomic synaptogenesis have occurred. Examination of norepinephrine turnover rates suggest at least one mechanism by which these actions may be produced (Fig. 9). In contrast to the inhibition of transmitter levels and general lack of effect on turnover seen in the CNS of methadone-exposed neonates, cardiac norepinephrine turnover is consistently elevated (Slotkin et al., 1981). Since turnover is a reflection of neuronal impulse activity, and because neuronal outgrowth is thought to depend upon impulse flow (Black, 1978), this finding may explain why opiate exposure produces a facilitatory effect on synaptic development in peripheral sympathetic pathways. The absence of an increase in turnover in the brain suggests that impulse flow is not elevated in developing CNS cell populations, and hence synaptogenesis would not be accelerated at these sites. In the absence of an overriding effect of impulse flow, synapses associated with central catecholaminergic neurons are subjected to slowing of development due to the effects of methadone on cellular development, as outlined above, whereas those in the periphery are spared.

A key question is why impulse flow is elevated in sympathetic pathways of neonatal rats exposed

272

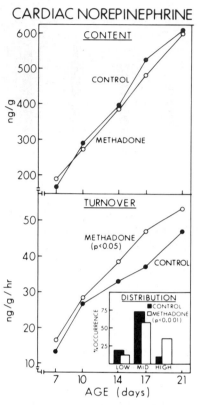

CARDIAC NOREPINEPHRINE

Fig. 9. Increased norepinephrine turnover in the cardiac-sympathetic axis of developing rats whose mothers received methadone (Slotkin et al., 1981).

perinatally to methadone. First, opiates have been shown to cause reflex activation of sympathetic pathways in mature rats (Anderson and Slotkin, 1975; Bareis and Slotkin, 1978). Additionally, recent studies have shown that opiates possess a special relationship to sympathetic tissues: opiate peptides are contained within the same cells as sympathetic transmitters, and structures such as the adrenal medulla contain high concentrations of opiate receptors (Viveros et al., 1979). Recent work from our laboratory (Chantry et al., 1982) has confirmed that endogenous opioids may serve to modulate catecholamine release in neonatal sympathetic tissues, a function which is not prominent in adulthood. Thus, it is likely that the effects of perinatal opiate exposure on sym-

pathetic development differ from those in the CNS because of these highly specific mechanisms. However, an additional role for opiate-induced stress cannot be ruled out as a contributing factor: studies in both animals and man indicate the presence of stress even during apparently well-maintained opiate addiction, as evidenced by increases in plasma corticosteroid levels in the period between injections (Cooper et al., 1983). The potentially adverse effects of maternal stress will be discussed later in this review.

Studies of opiate-induced alterations of sympathetic neuronal development also provide a unique opportunity to study the relationship between maturation of biochemical and physiological properties of synapses, and the impact of these events on whole animal physiology. The development of neuronal pathways represents not only the acquisition of mature, adult-like function, but also comprises the specific loss of specialized mechanisms designed for the survival of the neonate. The control of cardiovascular and respiratory status represents the 'behavioral' endpoint of autonomic mechanisms. One of the most important peripheral catecholamine actions is in aiding the adaptation of the newborn to extrauterine life. Both respiratory and cardiovascular status change drastically during the process of birth, and interference with these processes invariably compromises viability. Recent studies have shown birth is accompanied by a profound 'catecholamine surge,' wherein plasma levels of epinephrine and norepinephrine may total 50–200 nmol/liter, values which are an order of magnitude above typical adult concentrations (Lagercrantz and Slotkin, 1986; Slotkin, 1986a). The relatively high proportion of epinephrine indicates that the majority of the response involves the adrenal medulla, and studies from our and other laboratories suggest that the hypoxia associated with birth is an important trigger of adrenal reactivity (Seidler and Slotkin, 1985, 1986). As discussed above, the neonate does not normally possess functional splanchnic innervation of the adrenal medulla, and thus the

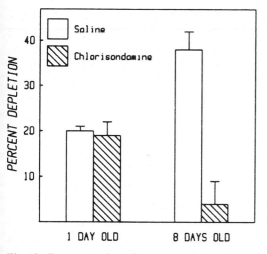 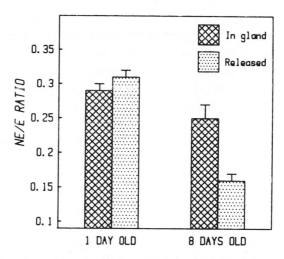

Fig. 10. Demonstration of non-neurogenic release of adrenal catecholamines by hypoxia (7% oxygen for 2 h) in neonatal rats (Seidler and Slotkin, 1985). Left panel: at 1 day of age, hypoxia causes release of catecholamines which cannot be blocked by chlorisondamine, a nicotinic antagonist. By 8 days of age, the response is purely neurogenic and is thus blocked by chlorisondamine. Right panel: the non-neurogenic secretion is not preferential for either norepinephrine (NE) or epinephrine (E), in that the proportion released is exactly the same as that in the adrenal; the neurogenic secretion at 8 days is preferential for epinephrine.

question arises as to how hypoxia-induced catecholamine secretion can take place without input from the CNS. As shown in Fig. 10, the neonatal adrenal has unique properties which enable it to release catecholamines in the absence of neural stimulation. In 1-day-old rats, hypoxia evokes catecholamine secretion and the response is not blocked by chlorisondamine, a drug which interrupts neural input to the adrenal. By 8 days of age, the response to hypoxia can still be obtained, but now is completely neurally-dependent. A further demonstration that secretion is non-neurogenic in the 1-day-old rat is that no preferential release of epinephrine vs. norepinephrine occurs; instead, the response involves secretion in exactly the same proportion as is present in the tissue. In older rats, the release is preferential for epinephrine because specific nerve fibers can be activated which innervate epinephrine-containing cells (Lewis, 1975; Seidler and Slotkin, 1985).

What is the function of the profound catecholamine release in the neonatal adrenal? We have been able to demonstrate that adrenomedullary

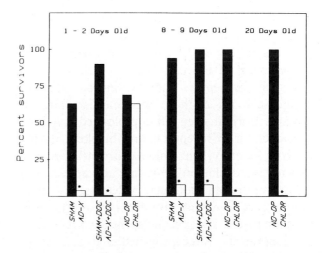

Fig. 11. Survival during hypoxia (5% oxygen, 90 min at 1–2 days of age, 37.5 min at 8–9 days, 15 min at 20 days) in animals adrenalectomized with or without corticosteroid (DOC) replacement, or in animals pretreated with a nicotinic antagonist (chlorisondamine, CHLOR) (Seidler and Slotkin, 1985). The importance of adrenal catecholamines is shown by the failure to survive in the adrenalectomized groups, regardless of DOC administration. CHLOR results in mortality during hypoxia only in the 8–9-day and 20-day-old rats, where neural input has become functional.

secretion is essential to surviving hypoxia of approximately the same degree as that experienced during birth (Seidler and Slotkin, 1985, 1986). Adrenalectomy, with or without steroid hormone replacement, results in loss of the ability of the newborn to tolerate hypoxic conditions (Fig. 11), a result which can be contrasted with the lack of effect of chlorisondamine, which blocks neural input. Although adrenomedullary catecholamines are still important in surviving hypoxia in older animals, the responses are completely neurally-mediated, as a similar hypoxia intolerance can be demonstrated with chlorisondamine treatment. Two classes of peripheral actions of the amines appear to be crucial: respiratory adjustments mediated primarily through β_2-receptors, and cardiovascular adjustments operating through α-receptors. The respiratory effects have been well-defined previously (surfactant release, increased lung compliance, lung liquid reabsorption; Lagercrantz and Slotkin, 1986), but the cardiovascular effects have only recently been elucidated (Seidler et al., 1987). The most important α-mediated neonatal action of catecholamines is on cardiac conduction. The myocardium of the newborn is particularly enriched in α-receptors and, so long as catecholamines can act at these sites, cardiac function remains normal even after prolonged hypoxia. However, if α-receptors are blocked during hypoxia (phenoxybenzamine treatment), there is a progressive decline in sinus rate and appearance of atrioventricular conduction defects, progressing to cardiac arrest. By the end of the first postnatal week, the special dependence of cardiac conduction on α-receptor-mediated actions of catecholamines disappears, and the respiratory dependence on β_2-receptor stimulation is no longer as important (Seidler and Slotkin, 1985; Seidler et al., 1987).

The disappearance of non-neurogenic adrenomedullary secretory mechanisms appears to result from the development of innervation and the arrival of CNS-derived signals at the end-organs. Early neonatal denervation of the adrenal results

in a prolongation of the period in which the specialized release process can be elicited, and acceleration of neuronal development causes the premature disappearance of this capability (Seidler and Slotkin, 1985, 1986). In dealing with the effects of neurobehavioral teratogens, then, particular importance must be ascribed to treatments, like methadone, which shift the timing of peripheral neuronal development. Two situations which have been well-studied are neonatal hyperthyroidism and late gestational maternal stress (Seidler and Slotkin, 1985). In both these cases, peripheral sympathetic synaptogenesis is accelerated, and consequently the specialized responses to hypoxia are lost. The functional consequence of this alteration is best illustrated in Fig. 12. Although hyperthyroid neonates or the offspring of stressed dams are capable of surviving hypoxia, their responses are similar to those of more mature animals and are dependent upon neural signals. Thus, administration of chlorisondamine leads to loss of hypoxia tolerance, whereas no

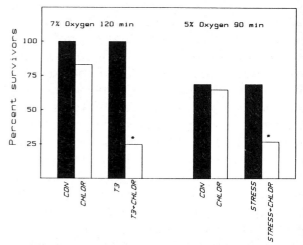

Fig. 12. Effects of neonatal hyperthyroidism and maternal stress on survival of 1–2-day-old rats exposed to hypoxia (Seidler and Slotkin, 1985). CON = control, T3 = tri-iodothyronine, CHLOR = chlorisondamine. Accelerated neuronal development in the sympatho-adrenal axis increases the dependence of survival on maintenance of neural function, as shown by the fact that CHLOR increases hypoxia-induced mortality in either the T3 or stress groups.

such neural dependence is evident in normal neonates. This may, however, represent a significant liability. If CNS development is at a sufficient level to process appropriate sensory input and stimulate the nerve supply to the adrenal and other sympathetic targets, then a problem might not necessarily exist. However, if for any reason CNS neural function or transmitter actions are compromised, then the neonate will be more vulnerable in situations where peripheral neural development has been accelerated. Hypoxia itself may be one of those cases, since prolonged oxygen deprivation results in failure of neural conduction. In the case of maternal methadone exposure, a particular vulnerability may be produced because peripheral neuronal development is accelerated whereas CNS development is slowed. Furthermore, because stimulation of opiate receptors interferes with neonatal adrenomedullary catecholamine secretion (Chantry et al., 1982), opiate-exposed fetuses will be inherently less responsive to hypoxia. Thus, maternal opiate use results in premature loss of non-neurogenic protective mechanisms, suppressed responsiveness, and insufficient CNS synaptic development to relay sensory input to sympathetic efferent neural pathways. The combination of these neural effects may contribute to the greater perinatal mortality and increased incidence of Sudden Infant Death noted in offspring of addicted women, as well as neonatal mortality in animal models of opiate abuse (Zagon et al.,1982; Cooper et al., 1983; Zagon and McLaughlin, 1984).

Catecholamines and development of non-neural tissues

The emergence of sympathetic neuronal function and the disappearance of the unique neonatal adrenomedullary secretory mechanism is accompanied by another phase of unusual peripheral responsiveness which peaks during the third postnatal week. This has been demonstrated biochemically through measurement of norepinephrine turnover and transmitter storage charac-

teristics, as well as by direct monitoring of neuronal impulse activity (Slotkin, 1973, 1986a,b; Seidler and Slotkin, 1981; Smith et al.,1982). Sympathetic tone may climb to twice or three times the adult level at this point, before declining toward the end of the first month postpartum (Fig.13). Once again, catecholamines play a functional role which is unique to the developing organism. First, the hyperactivity appears to mediate the final adjustments in the numbers of adrenergic receptors and their coupling to cellular function (Seidler and Slotkin, 1979; Lau and Slotkin, 1980; Slotkin, 1986a,b). In addition, the sympathetic neuronal signal may initiate the switchover of peripheral organs from growth by cell replication (dependence on DNA synthesis) to growth by cell enlargement (dependence on RNA and protein synthesis) (Claycomb, 1976; Slotkin, 1986b; Slotkin et al., 1987). In tissues such as the heart, the developmental decline in DNA synthesis coincides with the peak of sympathetic activity (Fig.13). Recently (Slotkin et al., 1987), we evaluated the relationship among the ontogeny of sympathetic projections to peripheral organs, the patterns of macromolecule synthesis in those organs, and the reactivity of synthetic

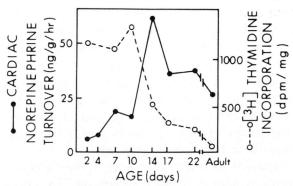

Fig. 13. Turnover of norepinephrine in sympathetic nerve terminals of the developing rat heart and comparison with DNA synthesis in the myocardium (Slotkin, 1986b). The results show the coincidence of the timing of sympathetic hyperactivity and the cessation of cardiac cell replication.

processes to β-adrenergic stimulation by isoproterenol. The major developmental rise in norepinephrine concentration and turnover, as well as in numbers of β-receptors, occurred during the second to fourth postnatal weeks in renal and lung sympathetic pathways, and slightly earlier in the cardiac-sympathetic axis. The developmental decline in DNA synthesis in heart, kidney and lung coincided with the maturation of sympathetic projections. Direct stimulation of β-receptors by the in vivo administration of isoproterenol caused acute reductions in DNA synthesis in an age-dependent manner. In the heart, isoproterenol was first able to suppress DNA synthesis at 5 days of age and a maximal effect was seen at 9 days; this early phase was characterized by a rapid time constant of coupling of β-receptors to the DNA effect (maximal effect at 6 h after isoproterenol). Reactivity was lessened by 12 days of age and thereafter displayed a longer time constant (maximal effect at 12-24 h). Reactivity of DNA synthesis to isoproterenol challenge was slightly different in kidney and lung (detectable by 2 days of age), but bore developmental characteristics similar to the pattern in the heart (peak of reactivity at 9 days and a decline in reactivity and lengthening of the time constant after 16 days). No such relationship was evident for the effects of isoproterenol on RNA or protein synthesis.

These results thus support the hypothesis that sympathetic input regulates cell replication patterns in developing peripheral organs. Because the coupling of β-receptors to termination of DNA synthesis disappears with the maturation of physiological responses to receptor stimulation, sympathetic suppression of cell replication is expressed only during the second critical period in development (i.e. the phase in which transient sympathetic hyperactivity appears).

Again, what is the importance of these mechanisms to neurobehavioral teratology? In situations where sympathetic tone is elevated or sympathetic neuronal connections are established prematurely, one would expect to see an eventual deficit in cell acquisition by non-neural tissues receiving catecholaminergic signals. As shown above, this is the case with perinatal opiate treatment, and the same property is shared by other perturbations which evoke similar peripheral neuronal alterations. In one case (methylmercury exposure), a direct test of this hypothesis has been conducted (Bartolome et al., 1984). Peripheral sympathetic denervation was able to prevent abnormalities of kidney growth, confirming that premature arrival of neuronal signals and/or elevated sympathetic activity during early development can disrupt the timing of cellular maturation in non-neural tissues.

Conclusions

The results reviewed here are consistent with the view that behavioral alterations caused by developmental insults have underlying biochemical causes which can be traced to teratological changes in the maturation and/or function of synapses in the CNS and periphery. Significantly, disjunct insults (drugs, physical factors, hormonal status) can cause similar biochemical and behavioral damage because events common to the developing nervous system are vulnerable during selective critical periods. Thus, any treatment which affects cell replication, differentiation, migration or synaptogenesis will share some functional end-points with apparently unrelated factors that influence the same cellular processes although differing in the primary mechanisms of action. The perinatal opiate syndrome illustrates these non-specific, as well as specific, features of neurobehavioral teratology. Disruption of cellular development in the CNS leads to delayed synaptogenesis and defects in presynaptic and postsynaptic biochemical elements which are the major determinants of synaptic activity. The CNS effect is widespread and not transmitter-specific. In contrast, effects of opiate exposure on peripheral sympathetic neuronal development display selective actions involving increased impulse activity, accelerated synaptogenesis and direct, opiate-receptor-mediated suppression of non-neurogenic neonatal adrenomedullary secretory responses. The combination of delayed synaptic development in the CNS, accelerated neuronal competence in the periphery and interference with specialized adrenal catecholamine mechanisms contributes to the greater risk of mortality in the perinatal opiate syndrome, and may also have a long-term impact on cellular development of non-neural structures.

Acknowledgement

This work was supported by grants USPHS HD-09713 and NS-06233.

References

Anderson, T. R. and Slotkin, T. A. (1975) Effects of morphine on the rat adrenal medulla. *Biochem. Pharmacol.*, 24: 671–679.

Bareis, D. L. and Slotkin, T. A. (1978) Responses of heart ornithine decarboxylase and adrenal catecholamines to methadone and sympathetic stimulants in developing and adult rats. *J. Pharmacol. Exp. Ther.*, 205: 164–174.

Bareis, D. L. and Slotkin, T. A. (1980) Maturation of sympathetic neurotransmission in the rat heart. I. Ontogeny of the synaptic vesicle uptake mechanism and correlation with development of synaptic function. Effects of neonatal methadone administration on development of synaptic vesicles. *J. Pharmacol. Exp. Ther.*, 212: 120–125.

Bartolome, J., Trepanier, P. A., Chait, E. A., Barnes, G. A., Lerea, L., Whitmore, W. L., Weigel, S. J. and Slotkin, T. A. (1984) Neonatal methylmercury poisoning in the rat: effects on development of peripheral sympathetic nervous system. Neuronal participation in methylmercury-induced cardiac and renal overgrowth. *Neurotoxicology*, 5: 45–54.

Black, I. B. (1978) Regulation of autonomic development. *Annu. Rev. Neurosci.*, 1: 183–214.

Brazier, M. A. (1975) *Growth and Development of the Brain: Nutritional, Genetic, and Environmental Factors*, Raven, New York, 399 pp.

Butler, S. R. and Schanberg, S. M. (1975) Effect of maternal morphine administration on neonatal rat brain ornithine decarboxylase (ODC). *Biochem. Pharmacol.*, 24: 1915–1918.

Chantry, C. J., Seidler, F. J. and Slotkin, T. A. (1982) Non-neurogenic mechanism for reserpine-induced release of catecholamines from the adrenal medulla of neonatal rats: possible modulation by opiate receptors. *Neuroscience*, 7: 673–678.

Claycomb, W. C. (1976) Biochemical aspects of cardiac muscle cell differentiation: possible control of deoxyribonucleic acid synthesis and cell differentiation by adrenergic innervation and cyclic adenosine 3':5'-monophosphate. *J. Biol. Chem.*, 251: 6082–6089.

Cooper, J. R., Altman, F., Brown, B. S. and Czechowicz, D. (1983) *Research on the Treatment of Narcotic Addiction: State of the Art*, U.S. Dept. of Health and Human Services Publication No. (ADM) 83–1281, Washington, 751 pp.

Deskin, R., Seidler, F. J., Whitmore, W. L. and Slotkin, T. A. (1981) Development of α-noradrenergic and dopaminergic receptor systems depends on maturation of their pre-synaptic nerve terminals in the rat brain. *J. Neurochem.*, 36: 1683–1690.

Dodge, P. R., Prensky, A. L. and Feigin, R. D. (1975) *Nutrition and the Developing Nervous System*, Mosby, St. Louis, 538 pp.

Friedhoff, A. J. and Miller, J. C. (1983) Prenatal psychotropic drug exposure and the development of central dopaminergic and cholinergic neurotransmitter systems. *Monogr. Neural Sci.*, 9: 91–98.

Jones, L. S., Gauger, L. L., Davis, J. N., Slotkin, T. A. and Bartolome, J. V. (1985) Postnatal development of brain alpha$_1$-adrenergic receptors: in vitro autoradiography with [^{125}I] HEAT in normal rats and rats treated with alpha-difluoromethylornithine, a specific, irreversible inhibitor of ornithine decarboxylase. *Neuroscience*, 15: 1195–1202.

Kornblum, H. I., Loughlin, S. E. and Leslie, F. M. (1987) Effects of morphine on DNA synthesis in neonatal rat brain. *Dev. Brain Res.*, 31: 45–52.

Lagercrantz, H. and Slotkin, T. A. (1986) The 'stress' of being born. *Sci. Am.*, 254(4): 100–107.

Lau, C., Bartolome, M. and Slotkin, T. A. (1977) Development of central and peripheral catecholaminergic systems in rats addicted perinatally to methadone. *Neuropharmacol.*, 16: 437–478.

Lau, C. and Slotkin, T. A. (1980) Maturation of sympathetic neurotransmission in the rat heart. II. Enhanced development of presynaptic and postsynaptic components of noradrenergic synapses as a result of neonatal hyperthyroidism. *J. Pharmacol. Exp. Ther.*, 212: 126–130.

Lewis, G. P. (1975) Physiological mechanisms controlling secretory activity of adrenal medulla. In S. R. Geiger (Ed.), *Handbook of Physiology, section 7, vol. VI*, American Physiological Society, Washington, pp. 309–319.

McAnulty, P. A., Yusuf, H. K. M., Dickerson, J. W. T., Hey, E. N. and Waterlow, J. C. (1977) Polyamines of the human brain during normal fetal and postnatal growth and during postnatal malnutrition. *J. Neurochem.*, 28: 1305–1310.

McGinty, J. F. and Ford, D. H. (1980) Effects of prenatal methadone on rat brain catecholamines. *Dev. Neurosci.*, 3: 224–234.

Morris, G., Nadler, J. V., Nemeroff, C. B. and Slotkin, T. A. (1985) Effects of neonatal treatment with 6-aminonicotinamide on basal and isoproterenol-stimulated ornithine decarboxylase activity in cerebellum of the developing rat. *Biochem. Pharmacol.*, 34: 3281–3284.

Reinis, S. and Goldman, J.M. (1980) *The Development of the Brain: Biological and Functional Perspectives*, Thomas, Springfield, 400 pp.

Seidler, F.J., Brown, K.K., Smith, P.G. and Slotkin, T.A. (1987) Toxic effects of hypoxia on neonatal cardiac function in the rat: α-adrenergic mechanisms. *Toxicol. Lett.*, in press.

Seidler, F.J. and Slotkin, T.A. (1979) Presynaptic and postsynaptic contributions to ontogeny of sympathetic control of heart rate in the preweanling rat. *Br. J. Pharmacol.*, 65: 531–534.

Seidler, F.J. and Slotkin, T.A. (1981) Development of central control of norepinephrine turnover and release in the rat heart: responses to tyramine, 2-deoxyglucose and hydralazine. *Neuroscience*, 6: 2081–2086.

Seidler, F.J. and Slotkin, T.A. (1985) Adrenomedullary function in the neonatal rat: Responses to acute hypoxia. *J. Physiol.*, 358: 1–16.

Seidler, F.J. and Slotkin, T.A. (1986) Ontogeny of adrenomedullary responses to hypoxia and hypoglycemia: role of splanchnic innervation. *Brain Res. Bull.*, 16: 11–14.

Seidler, F.J., Whitmore, W.L. and Slotkin, T.A. (1982) Delays in growth and biochemical development of rat brain caused by maternal methadone administration: are the alterations in synaptogenesis and cellular maturation independent of reduced maternal food intake? *Dev. Neurosci.*, 5: 13–18.

Slotkin, T.A. (1973) Maturation of the adrenal medulla. II. Content and properties of catecholamine storage vesicles of the rat. *Biochem. Pharmacol.*, 22: 2033–2044.

Slotkin, T.A. (1983) Effects of perinatal exposure to methadone on development of neurotransmission: biochemical bases for behavioral alterations. *Monogr. Neural Sci.*, 9: 153–158.

Slotkin, T.A. (1986a) Development of the sympathoadrenal axis. In P.M. Gootman (Ed.), *Developmental Neurobiology of the Autonomic Nervous System*, Humana, New Jersey, pp. 69–96.

Slotkin, T.A. (1986b) Endocrine control of synaptic development in the sympathetic nervous system: the cardiac sympathetic axis. In P.M. Gootman (Ed.), *Developmental Neurobiology of the Autonomic Nervous System*, Humana, New Jersey, pp. 97–133.

Slotkin, T.A. and Bartolome, J. (1986) Role of ornithine decarboxylase and the polyamines in nervous system development. *Brain Res. Bull.*, 17: 307–320.

Slotkin, T.A. and Thadani, P.V. (1980) Neurochemical teratology of drugs of abuse. In T.V.N. Persaud (Ed.), *Neural and Behavioural Teratology, Advances in the Study of Birth Defects, Vol. 4*, MTP, Lancaster, pp. 199–234.

Slotkin, T.A., Lau, C. and Bartolome, M. (1976) Effects of neonatal or maternal methadone administration on ornithine decarboxylase activity in brain and heart of developing rats. *J. Pharmacol. Exp. Ther.*, 199: 141–148.

Slotkin, T.A., Whitmore, W.L., Salvaggio, M. and Seidler, F.J. (1979) Perinatal methadone addiction affects brain synaptic development of biogenic amine systems in the rat. *Life Sci.*, 24: 1223–1229.

Slotkin, T.A., Seidler, F.J. and Whitmore, W.L. (1980a) Effects of maternal methadone administration on ornithine decarboxylase in brain and heart of the offspring: relationships of enzyme activity to dose and to growth impairment in the rat. *Life Sci.*, 26: 861–867.

Slotkin, T.A., Seidler, F.J. and Whitmore, W.L. (1980b) Precocious development of sympatho-adrenal function in rats whose mothers received methadone. *Life Sci.*, 26: 1657–1663.

Slotkin, T.A., Weigel, S.J., Barnes, G.A., Whitmore, W.L. and Seidler, F.J. (1981) Alterations in the development of catecholamine turnover induced by perinatal methadone: differences in central vs. peripheral sympathetic nervous systems. *Life Sci.*, 29: 2519–2525.

Slotkin, T.A., Weigel, S.J., Whitmore, W.L. and Seidler, F.J. (1982) Maternal methadone administration: deficit in development of alpha-noradrenergic responses in developing rat brain as assessed by norepinephrine stimulation of $^{33}P_i$ incorporation into phospholipids in vivo. *Biochem. Pharmacol.*, 31: 1899–1902.

Slotkin, T.A., Seidler, F.J., Whitmore, W.L., Weigel, S.J., Slepetis, R.J., Lerea, L., Trepanier, P.A. and Bartolome, J. (1983) Critical periods for the role of ornithine decarboxylase and the polyamines in growth and development of the rat: effects of exposure to α-difluoromethylornithine during discrete prenatal or postnatal intervals. *Int. J. Dev. Neurosci.*, 1: 113–127.

Slotkin, T.A., Whitmore, W.L., Orband-Miller, L., Queen, K.L. and Haim, K. (1987) β-Adrenergic control of macromolecule synthesis in neonatal rat heart, kidney and lung: relationship to sympathetic neuronal development. *J. Pharmacol. Exp. Ther.*, 243: 101–109.

Smith, P.G., Slotkin, T.A. and Mills E. (1982) Development of sympathetic ganglionic neurotransmission in the neonatal rat: pre- and postganglionic nerve response to asphyxia and 2-deoxyglucose. *Neuroscience*, 7: 501–507.

Thadani, P.V., Lau, C., Slotkin, T.A. and Schanberg, S.M. (1977) Effect of maternal ethanol ingestion on neonatal rat brain and heart ornithine decarboxylase. *Biochem. Pharmacol.*, 26: 523–527.

Vernadakis, A., Estin, C. and Gibson, A. (1981) Methadone effects on ODC activity in neuronal and glial cultures. *Trans. Am. Soc. Neurochem.*, 12: 266.

Viveros, O.H., Diliberto, E.J., Hazum, E. and Chang, K. (1979) Opiate-like materials in the adrenal medulla: evidence for storage and secretion with catecholamines. *Mol. Pharmacol.*, 16: 1101–1108.

Wang, C., Pasulka, P., Perry, B., Pizzi, W.J. and Schnoll, S.H. (1986) Effect of perinatal exposure to methadone on brain opioid and α_2-adrenergic receptors. *Neurobehav. Toxicol. Teratol.*, 8: 399–402.

Zagon, I.S. and McLaughlin, P.J. (1982) Comparative effects of postnatal undernutrition and methadone exposure on protein and nucleic acid contents of the brain and cerebellum in rats. *Dev. Neurosci.*, 5: 385–393.

Zagon, I.S. and McLaughlin, P.J. (1983) Naltrexone modulates growth in infant rats. *Life Sci.*, 33: 2449–2454.

Zagon, I.S. and McLaughlin, P.J. (1984) An overview of the neurobehavioral sequelae of perinatal opioid exposure. In J. Yanai (Ed.), *Neurobehavioral Teratology*, Elsevier, Amsterdam, pp. 197–234.

Zagon, I.S. and McLaughlin, P.J., Weaver, D.J. and Zagon, E. (1982) Opiates, endorphins and the developing organism: a comprehensive bibliography. *Neurosci. Biobehav. Rev.*, 6: 439–479.

Zagon, I.S. and McLaughlin, P.J. and Zagon, E. (1984) Opiates, endorphins and the developing organism: a comprehensive bibliography, 1982–1983. *Neuroscience Biobehav. Rev.*, 8: 387–403.

Discussion

M.A. Corner: How can one reconcile the stimulatory effect of chronic methadone in view of the reported depressant actions for acute treatment on spontaneous and reflex motility?

T.A. Slotkin: Increased nerve stimulation probably does accelerate the course of neural development as suggested by the work of Ira Black in the 1970s. However, early depolarization of neurons probably compresses the time course of neural differentiation (Patterson, 1978) and we invariably find an eventual functional deficit in these nerve pathways.

M.A. Corner: Could the augmented sympathetic outflow be a causal factor in the concomitant accelerated synaptogenesis?

T.A. Slotkin: Elliott (1912) first reported on sympathetic activation by morphine nearly 80 years ago. The specific effect of opiates on sympathetic neuronal development is probably a reflection of this selective stimulation.

G.J. Boer: Since at birth, next to a noradrenalin (NA) response, high endogenous β-endorphin serum levels are also obvious (Fachinetti et al., 1982), do you see any correlation between these responses?

T.A. Slotkin: At birth, there is a surge of β-endorphin, corticosteroids and a variety of peptides. It is unlikely that the peptides arise mainly from the adrenal, as the proportion of catecholamines secreted is much larger than that of the peptides. The current view is that most of the β-endorphin released at birth arises from the CNS and pituitary.

References

Black, I.B. (1978) Regulation of autonomic development. *Annu. Rev. Neurosci.*, 1: 183–214.

Elliott, T.R. (1912) Control of the suprarenal glands by the splanchnic nerves. *J. Physiol. (London)*, 44: 374–409.

Facchinetti, F., Bagnoli, F., Bracci, R. and Genazzani, A.R. (1982) Plasma opioids in the first hours of life. *Pediatr. Res.*, 16: 95–98.

Patterson, P.H. (1978) Environmental determination of autonomic neurotransmitter functions. *Annu. Rev. Neurosci.*, 1: 1–17.

SECTION IV

Food and Environmental Factors

G.J. Boer, M.G.P. Feenstra, M. Mirmiran, D.F. Swaab and F. Van Haaren
Progress in Brain Research, Vol. 73
© 1988 Elsevier Science Publishers B.V. (Biomedical Division)

CHAPTER 18

Excitotoxic food additives: functional teratological aspects

John W. Olney

Departments of Psychiatry and Pathology, Washington University School of Medicine, St. Louis, Missouri, USA

Introduction

The putative excitatory neurotransmitters, glutamate (Glu) and aspartate (Asp), and several of their structural analogues, comprise a family of excitotoxic compounds, which are so called because of their potential for destroying central neurons by excessive stimulation of postsynaptic excitatory membrane receptors. The ability of these agents, when administered systemically, to penetrate specialized regions of brain, including the endocrine hypothalamus, and either excite or destroy neurons in these regions, makes them useful tools for studying the neuroendocrine or other functional roles of such neurons. Since several excitotoxins are naturally contained in or artificially added to foods and since such agents have synergistic neurotoxic potential when administered orally in combination, they constitute a family of environmental neurotoxicants of interest from a public health standpoint. Despite evidence from animal studies that the immature nervous system is much more vulnerable than the adult to excitotoxin-induced damage, Glu and other excitotoxins are used quite heavily world-wide as additives to foods ingested by infants and children. Here I will review information pertaining to the potential teratological consequences of excitotoxin exposure in early life. I use the term 'teratological' in its broadest sense to include adverse effects on the organism at any preadult stage of development.

The nature of Glu/Asp neurotoxicity

In recent years, the excitatory amino acids (EAA), Glu and Asp, have become recognized both as neurotoxins and as the leading neurotransmitter candidates at the majority of excitatory synapses in the mammalian CNS (Watkins, 1978; Olney, 1978). The first evidence suggesting that Glu might have neurotoxic properties was reported by Lucas and Newhouse (1957), who found that subcutaneous administration of Glu to suckling mice caused acute degeneration of neurons in the inner portions of the developing retina. In studies confirming this observation (Olney, 1969a,b, 1971), it was further discovered that systemically administered Glu destroys neurons in circumventricular organ (CVO) regions of brain that lack blood-brain barriers. In subsequent studies (Olney and Ho, 1970; Olney et al., 1972, 1973a,b, 1980; Olney, 1974a) it was shown that this toxic effect could be induced by either oral or parenteral administration of Glu and that many species of experimental animals are susceptible. Moreover, if very large amounts of Glu are administered to the pregnant rhesus monkey late in gestation (Olney, 1974b) it results in damage to the fetal brain (Fig. 1).

In molecular specificity studies it was found (Olney et al., 1971) that specific structural analogues of Glu known to share the neuroexcitatory properties of Glu reproduce its neurotoxic effects, that these analogues have a

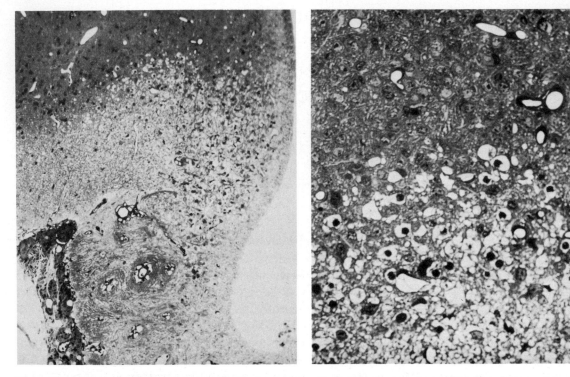

Fig. 1. These micrographs depict an acute lesion in the infundibular (arcuate) nucleus of the hypothalamus of a fetal rhesus monkey exposed to Glu in utero (Olney, 1974b). Glu was administered intravenously to the pregnant mother on the 152nd day of gestation and the fetus was removed by cesarian section 5 h later, anesthetized and perfused with fixative to permit evaluation of the brain by light and electron microscopy. Shown on the left is an overview of the lesion and on the right a magnified view at the margin of the lesion depicting acutely degenerating neurons below and normal tissue above. Each degenerating neuron has a dark pyknotic nucleus surrounded by a vacuous halo of edematous cytoplasm, which are the characteristics that typify acute Glu cytopathology in any animal species (panel on the left = ×75; on the right = ×220).

parallel order of potencies for their excitatory and toxic actions and that analogues lacking excitatory activity also lack neurotoxicity. In ultrastructural studies (Olney, 1969a, 1971; Olney et al., 1971, 1972) it was shown that Glu exerts its toxic action on dendrosomal portions of the neuron where Glu excitatory synaptic receptors are located. These and related observations gave rise to the excitotoxic hypothesis that an excitatory mechanism and Glu excitatory synaptic receptors mediate Glu neurotoxicity.

The excitotoxic hypothesis was confirmed in studies demonstrating that agents which antagonize the excitatory actions of potent Glu agonists (Watkins, 1978) also prevent such agonists from destroying CNS neurons in vivo (Olney et al., 1979, 1981). Subsequently, several subtypes of excitatory amino acid receptor have been described (Watkins, 1978), the N-methyl-D-aspartate receptor being the best-characterized and most abundant in mammalian brain (Monaghan and Cotman, 1985). Glu is considered a mixed agonist capable of acting at all excitatory amino acid receptor subtypes. It is now well established from both in vitro (Olney et al., 1986; Rothman and Olney, 1986, 1987) and in vivo (Olney et al., 1979, 1981) studies that agents which block the excitatory actions of a given EAA agonist also block its toxic action.

When the brain-damaging properties of Glu

were first discovered, the focus of attention was primarily on exogenous Glu, which, at the time, was being liberally added to baby foods. However, since Glu and Asp are found naturally in the CNS in very high concentration, it was also proposed that these endogenous excitotoxins might play a role in neurodegenerative diseases (Olney et al., 1971). Gradually, over the past decade, evidence implicating endogenous excitotoxins in several neurodegenerative conditions (reviewed in Olney, 1986) has been reported, the strongest evidence perhaps being that pertaining to brain damage associated with hypoxia-ischemia (Rothman and Olney, 1986). It has been shown (Benveniste et al., 1984) in rat brain that, under ischemic conditions, endogenous Glu and Asp are released by CNS cells and accumulate in high concentrations extracellularly where they can exert excitotoxic action at EAA receptors. Intense interest is currently being focused on the possibility that EAA antagonists might be effective in preventing hypoxic-ischemic neuronal degeneration in stroke, cardiac arrest, perinatal asphyxia, etc. (Rothman and Olney, 1986, 1987; Gil et al., 1987; McDonald et al., 1987). Thus, today we are witnessing an ironic situation; while knowledgeable neuroscientists are fervently attempting to develop methods for protecting CNS neurons against the neurotoxic potential of endogenous Glu and Asp, other elements of society are vigorously promoting the unlimited use of exogenous Glu and Asp as food additives.

Teratological considerations

The risk posed by exposing immature humans to exogenous excitotoxins will be discussed in terms of two different mechanisms.

Late-occurring sequelae of excitotoxin-induced brain damage

Because the arcuate hypothalamic nucleus (AH), a neuroendocrine regulatory center, is one of the CVO brain regions damaged by systemically administered Glu, animals treated with Glu in infancy manifest multiple neuroendocrine disturbances and have an abnormal body habitus in adulthood (Olney, 1969b; Kizer et al., 1978; Olney and Price, 1978, 1980). The fully developed syndrome (Fig. 2) includes obesity, skeletal stunting, reproductive failure and hypoplasia of the adenohypophysis and gonads, together with abnormally low hypothalamic, pituitary or plasma levels of luteinizing hormone (LH), growth hormone (GH) and prolactin (Prl). This syndrome has been reproduced in mice, rats and hamsters but has not been tested for reproducibility in other mammalian species. It is relevant to add that Asp is as effective as Glu in inducing this neuroendocrine deficiency state (Schainker and Olney, 1974; Pizzi et al., 1978).

Neuroendocrine perturbations from nontoxic doses

It has been shown that a subtoxic dose of Glu (about 25% of the dose required to damage AH neurons), administered subcutaneously to weanling or adult male rats, induces a rapid elevation of LH (Olney et al., 1976) and a depression of pulsatile output of GH (Terry et al., 1981). Moreover, several potent excitatory analogues of Glu, when administered subcutaneously in subtoxic doses, mimic the LH-releasing action of Glu, and have the same order of potencies for this Glu-mimetic activity as for their neuroexcitatory and neurotoxic activities (Price et al., 1978a). N-Methylaspartate (NMA), which Price et al. (1978b) considered the most satisfactory of the potent excitotoxins for use as an LH-releasing agent, is now being employed as a tool for studying gonadotrophin regulatory pathways (Schainker and Cicero, 1979; Olney and Price, 1980; Wilson and Knobil, 1982; Nemeroff, 1983; Gay and Plant, 1987). It has been shown that a subtoxic dose of NMA induces an acute release of LH, follicle-stimulating hormone and Prl in adult female rhesus monkeys (Wilson and Knobil, 1982) or prepubertal male rhesus monkeys (Gay and Plant, 1987). These effects are exerted at a suprapituitary level, since neither NMA nor Glu releases these hormones from in vitro monkey or

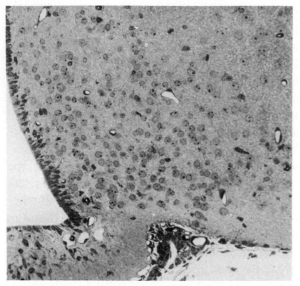

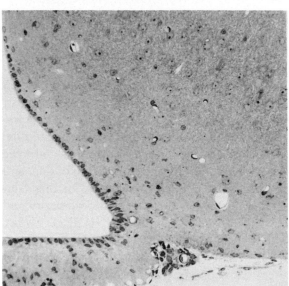

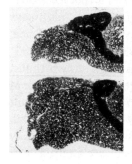
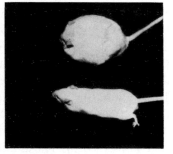

rat pituitary (Tal et al., 1983). The LH-releasing action of NMA is dependent on AH neurons, in that rats which have been treated with Glu in infancy to remove AH neurons do not respond to an NMA challenge with LH release (Olney and Price, 1980). It has been shown that specific antagonists of the excitatory action of NMA block both its neurotoxic action on AH neurons and its LH-releasing action (Olney and Price, 1980; Olney et al., 1981; Gay and Plant, 1987). Based on these findings, we propose that excitotoxins, in subtoxic doses, induce acute perturbations in hormonal parameters by penetrating CVO zones and activating certain neurons that regulate pituitary hormonal outputs. This kind of neuropathological mechanism, although more subtle than brain damage, warrants consideration in the safety evaluation of these agents, since repetitive perturbations in plasma hormone levels in pre-adult consumers could adversely influence growth and development.

Factors relevant to risk

Homergism among excitotoxins

Many years ago it was shown that Asp and Glu, when given orally by feeding tube to 10-day-old mice, add to one another's toxic action on hypothalamic neurons (Olney and Ho, 1970). More recently it was demonstrated that a similar

Fig. 2. The normal arcuate hypothalamic nucleus (AH) of an infant mouse is shown at the top with the same brain region of an infant mouse 4 days following subcutaneous Glu treatment depicted immediately below. In the AH of the Glu-treated animal, note the absence of neurons (the sparse cell bodies visible are mostly glia) and widening of the ventricle in compensation for the loss of neuronal mass. A short, fat adult mouse bearing an AH lesion from neonatal Glu treatment is depicted at the lower right with a normal litter mate control immediately below. Directly across from each mouse is his pituitary gland (one half of each gland is shown). In the absence of AH neurons, the adenohypophysis of the Glu-treated mouse has failed to develop to the normal size (Olney and Price, 1980).

additive mechanism is operative when solutions containing various combinations of Glu and Asp are voluntarily ingested by weanling mice (Olney et al., 1980). When other excitotoxins are tested in combination (Olney, 1974a), it is seen that each adds to the neurotoxicity of another in proportion to its own excitotoxic potency. The brain-damaging potential of protein hydrolysates (Olney et al., 1973a) stems from the fact that they contain substantial amounts of Glu, Asp and cysteic acid which act additively (homergistically) to destroy CVO neurons. The term 'homergism' was adopted from Goodman and Gilman (1970) as follows: 'If two drugs produce the same overt effect, they are termed homergic and… if the drugs are close congeners that act on the same receptors, doses of one drug should substitute for those of the other, in proportion to their relative potencies, over a wide range of combinations. Only drugs that exhibit this dose addition are properly described as additive.' In evaluating the safety of any given excitotoxin, the possibility that it will be consumed in combination with other environmentally encountered excitotoxins must be considered if a meaningful estimate of risk is to be obtained.

Multiple excitotoxins in foods

Excitotoxins, in addition to being found naturally in certain food sources, have biological properties which invite their use as food additives. The well-known flavor-enhancing properties of Glu, for example, stem from its excitatory (depolarizing) action on sensory taste receptors (Yamashita et al., 1973). The aspartate molecule, when combined with phenylalanine to form the dipeptide, Aspartame, also presumably interacts with taste receptors, the result being that a sweet flavor is perceived. After ingestion, the dipeptide is rapidly hydrolysed to release Asp, which is absorbed into the blood (Ranney and Oppermann, 1979). Hydrolysed vegetable protein (HVP) is added to many of the same foods that are seasoned with Glu. This product contains very high concentrations of both Glu and Asp and

sometimes cysteic acid. It is the free Glu content in HVP and the ability of Glu to depolarize taste receptors which provides the major rationale for using HVP as a flavor additive to foods. Sulfite, which has been used for years as a chemical additive by nearly all branches of the food industry (Synge, 1977), promotes rupture of cystine disulfide bonds and combines with the cysteine thus formed to produce the potent excitotoxin, cysteine-S-sulfonic acid (Olney et al., 1975). Whether the presence of this excitotoxin in foods poses a serious risk is not known because no effort has been made, thus far, to determine how much is present in processed foods or to establish how readily it is absorbed into the blood. For many years, Glu has been one of the most widely and heavily used food additives in existence. Since Aspartame (Nutrasweet, Equal) is rapidly becoming the most widely distributed sugar substitute in the world, it is an inescapable fact that two of the most widely consumed food additives in the world are excitotoxins which, when administered orally to experimental animals, destroy nerve cells in the brain. For a discussion of the amounts of various excitotoxins that are intentionally added to foods, see Olney (1980, 1984).

Certain brain regions lack blood-brain barriers

When Glu or Asp are administered orally or subcutaneously, they are prevented by blood-brain barriers from entering the brain (Perez and Olney, 1972) except in certain regions known collectively as circumventricular organs (CVO) which lack blood-brain barriers (Brightman and Broadwell, 1976). It is in these brain regions that systemically administered excitotoxins destroy neurons or, at lower doses, excite neurons and induce changes in hormonal parameters regulated by these neurons. That excitotoxins circulating in the blood have selective access to CVO neurons has been demonstrated autoradiographically (Inouye, 1976) and by quantitative regional microhistochemistry (Perez and Olney, 1972; Price et al., 1981, 1984). The peculiar permeability of

CVO blood vessels to various blood-borne substances, which presumably relates to their fenestrated endothelial walls, is demonstrable in animals of any age, just as excitotoxin-induced CVO damage is demonstrable in animals of any age.

Oral intake nearly as toxic as parenteral

While some neurotoxic agents are much more effective when administered parenterally than orally, this is not the case for either Glu or Asp. When administered in aqueous solution by feeding tube, these agents are about 75% as effective in damaging brain as when administered in aqueous solution subcutaneously. The several species in which brain damage following oral administration of Glu has been demonstrated are rats (Burde et al., 1971; Okaniwa et al., 1979), mice (Olney and Ho, 1970), guinea pigs (Olney et al., 1973b) and monkeys (Olney et al., 1972). There is good agreement among laboratories that Glu and Asp are effective in destroying CVO neurons in either infant mice or rats beginning at an oral dose of 0.5 g/kg (Okaniwa et al., 1979; Olney and Ho, 1970; Olney, 1976).

For many years it was argued that Glu and Asp are safe food additives because brain damage had never been shown from voluntary ingestion of these substances. It is true that in the oral studies demonstrating brain damage, Glu and Asp were administered in aqueous solution by feeding tube (gavage), the purpose of this approach being to maintain precise control over the amount and rate of oral intake. In response to this alleged flaw in research design, we offered aqueous solutions containing Glu, Asp or Glu + Asp to weanling mice that had been deprived of fluids overnight (12 h) and demonstrated (Olney et al., 1980) that they eagerly imbibed enough of the adulterated liquids to destroy CVO neurons (Fig. 3). This illustrates that voluntary ingestion of Glu and Asp by animals can cause brain damage and reinforces other evidence (Stegink et al., 1979b) suggesting that human ingestion of these substances in aqueous solution (for example, soups containing Glu and beverages containing Asp) might repre-

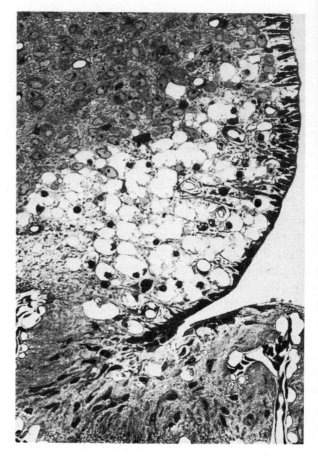

Fig. 3. A light micrograph depicting acutely necrotic neurons in the arcuate hypothalamic nucleus of a 21-day-old mouse 4 h following voluntary ingestion of 0.35 ml of a 10% aqueous Glu solution (× 220) (Olney et al., 1980).

sent optimal conditions for sustaining 'self-inflicted' brain damage.

Young are most vulnerable

Although adult animals are susceptible to excitotoxin-induced brain damage, they are substantially less vulnerable than infant animals, since it requires a four-fold higher dose of Glu or Asp, by either oral or subcutaneous administration, to destroy a given number of CVO neurons in adult compared to infant brain (Olney, 1976). The change in vulnerability from infancy to adulthood does not occur abruptly; when mice were studied at four ages (10, 21, 45 and 60 days) they were found to have a gradually increasing threshold for susceptibility to Glu-induced brain damage. The same has been demonstrated in rats dosed orally at various ages with Asp (Okaniwa, 1979). It is not clear whether this reflects primarily: (a) age-related differences in gastrointestinal absorption of acidic amino acids, (b) an age differential in the rate at which these amino acids are metabolically cleared from blood, or (c) an age-related increase in the efficiency of mechanisms operative in CVO brain tissue for terminating the excitotoxic activity of these agents. If vulnerability in the human varies similarly with age, it follows that humans of all ages are vulnerable but infants and young children are substantially more vulnerable than adults.

Species generality of Glu/Asp neurotoxicity

It has been demonstrated that systemically administered Glu destroys neurons in the central nervous system of mice, rats, rabbits, chicks, guinea pigs, hamsters, cats and monkeys (reviewed in Olney, 1980). It is not surprising that many species are vulnerable to the systemic neurotoxicity of Glu, since Glu excites neurons in the central nervous system of all vertebrate species tested, and absence of blood-brain barriers in CVO regions of brain is also a species-general phenomenon. On the other hand, species apparently do differ significantly in gastrointestinal absorption and/or metabolic clearance of Glu, since a given oral load of Glu produces much higher plasma Glu elevations in man than in monkey (see below).

Silent nature of excitotoxin lesion

It is sometimes argued that Glu and Asp are safe food additives because humans have been exposed to these compounds in one form or another for many years without sustaining apparent harm. This argument overlooks the fact that brain damage from Glu or Asp is a silent phenomenon. When infant animals are given brain-damaging doses of Glu or Asp, they fail to manifest overt signs of distress as CVO neurons are acutely degenerating; indeed, there are no obvious changes in the animal's appearance or behavior until he is approaching adulthood. Thus, if a human infant or child were to sustain hypothalamic damage from Glu or Asp, delayed sequelae such as obesity and subtle disturbances in the neuroendocrine status of the individual are the types of effects to be expected and it would not be until adolescence or perhaps early adulthood that such effect would become fully manifest. It would be very difficult to establish retrospectively that such effects are the consequences of Glu ingestion 20 years previously.

Gastrointestinal absorption of excitotoxins

Glu, the only excitotoxin for which extensive data are available, is absorbed from the gastrointestinal tract into blood more efficiently in humans than in any other species studied to date. Oral Glu tolerance tests have been conducted on both infant and adult mice and monkeys over a wide range of loading doses (100–2000 mg/kg) and on adult humans with the top loading dose restricted to 200 mg/kg (comparable data on human young are nonexistent). These findings (Himwich et al., 1954; Bizzi et al., 1977; Steglink et al., 1979a), which are summarized graphically in Fig. 4, reveal that each species has a separate and distinct dose–response profile, with monkeys and mice being more similar to one another than humans are to either. Mice are less tolerant than monkeys (higher plasma Glu values from a given load), infants of either species are less tolerant than adults, and the adult human is far less tolerant than either mice or monkeys of any age. Since an age differential is clearly evident for both mice and monkeys, with the infant animal consistently developing higher plasma Glu levels than the adult from any given load, it is reasonable to assume that a similar age differential might exist for the human, such that the slope of the response curve for the human infant would be steeper than for the human adult. In Fig. 4, a hypothetical dose–response curve is drawn for the human

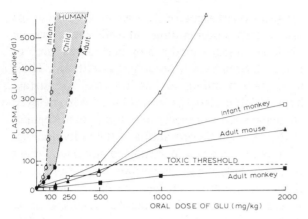

Fig. 4. Oral dose–response data for infant and adult monkeys or mice and adult humans with hypothetical data points (connected by dash lines) inserted for human infants and for higher doses than have been tested on human adults. The data for the mice and monkeys are from Stegink et al. (1979a). The data for adult humans at 60 mg/kg are from Bizzi et al. (1977), at 100 and 150 mg/kg from Stegink et al. (1979a) and at 200 mg/kg from Himwich et al. (1954). Hypothetical data points are entered for human infants, and the area between the curves for human infants and adults is stippled to indicate the zone in which data points for human children presumably would fall if test data for human young were available. It should be noted that the data points given for adult humans are means, and that there were striking individual variations noted in each human study. Thus, the curve for some individual humans would be steeper than is shown here. The oral dose (500 mg/kg) and plasma Glu concentration (60–100 μmol/dl) at which infant mice begin to sustain brain damage is indicated as the toxic threshold (dashed line).

infant, and the shaded area between the curves for the human infant and adult indicates where human children might be expected to fall. It should be mentioned (not shown in graph) that gastrointestinal absorption of Glu in human adults is characterized by extreme individual variation, with some individuals displaying much higher plasma Glu elevations that others following the same loading dose (Himwich et al., 1954; Stegink et al., 1979b). Since human children are often exposed to acute Glu intake loads in the range 100–150 mg/kg, it is instructive to note that this amount of Glu (150 mg/kg) results in a

20-fold mean plasma Glu elevation in adult humans compared to a 4-fold and 0-fold elevation in adult mice and monkeys, respectively.

Cultural factors

Increasing concern has been expressed in recent years over the indiscriminate use of Glu as a food additive in certain cultures where commercial promotion of this additive has been particulary successful and, in the absence of objective educational programs, the public has remained ignorant of its potential risks. For example, in a recent UNICEF-sponsored survey of eating practices in Korea (Citizens Alliance for Consumer Protection of Korea, 1987), it was learned that the average per capita consumption of this food additive among certain population segments is nearly 4 g/day, with individual daily intakes varying from 0 to 1719 mg/kg body wt. (the latter = 120 g for a 70 kg adult). Moreover, in restaurants it was found that up to 9.9 g were being added to single dishes, including certain soups. In addition, in the absence of an educational program, there has been no effort to limit the exposure of young children; indeed, young children sometimes consume the same gram amounts as their adult counterparts but, since they have a much smaller body mass to distribute it over, this represents a much higher dose. This is potentially a serious problem considering the greater vulnerability of the immature nervous system to the neurotoxic action of Glu.

Summary and concluding remarks

Here I have discussed the excitotoxic amino acids – glutamate, aspartate and certain of their structural analogues – some of which are neurotransmitter candidates and/or widely used food additives, and all of which have both neuroexitatory and neurotoxic activities. Evidence is presented for the excitotoxic concept which holds that an excitatory and synapse-related mechanism underlies the neurotoxicity of these compounds. When administered either orally or parenterally to experimental animals, these agents penetrate circumventricular organ (CVO) brain regions and either excite or destroy CVO neurons which have important neuroendocrine regulatory functions. Immature organisms are more sensitive than adults to the excitotoxic actions of these agents. Thus, the teratological potential of excitotoxins lies primarily in their ability to induce neuroendocrine dysfunction either by destroying neurons that mediate neuroendocrine regulation or by excessive stimulation of such neurons causing repetitive perturbations in hormonal parameters during growth and development. Ways in which the consumer may be exposed to these agents are considered and relevant mechanisms of risk are discussed.

References

Benveniste, H., Drejer, J., Schousboe, A. and Diemer, N.H. (1984) Elevation of the extracellular concentratins of glutamate and aspartate in rat hippocampus during transient cerebral ischemia monitored by intracerebral microdialysis. *J. Neurochem.*, 43: 1369–1374.

Bizzi, A., Veneroni, E., Salmona, M. and Garatinni, S. (1977) Kinetics of monosodium glutamate in relation to its neurotoxicity. *Toxicol. Lett.*, 1: 123–130.

Brightman, M.N. and Broadwell, R.D. (1976) The morphological approach to the study of normal and abnormal brain permeability. *Adv. Exp. Med. Biol.*, 69: 41.

Burde, R.M., Schainker, B. and Kayes, J. (1971) Monosodium glutamate: acute effect of oral and subcutaneous administration on the arcuate nucleus of the hypothalamus in mice and rats. *Nature*, 233: 58.

Citizens' Alliance for Consumer Protection of Korea (1986) A study of the use of MSG in Korea. United Nations Children's Fund (UNICEF), pp. 1–9.

Gay, V.L. and Plant, T.M. (1987) N-Methyl-D,L-aspartate elicits hypothalamic gonadotropin-releasing hormone release in prepubertal male rhesus monkeys (*Macaca mulatta*). *Endocrinology*, 120: 2289–2296.

Gill, R., Foster, A.C. and Woodruff, G.N. (1987) Systemic administration of MK-801 protects against ischemia-induced hippocampal neurodegeneration in the gerbil. *J. Neurosci.*, 3343–3349.

Goodman, L.S. and Gilman, A. (Eds.) (1970) *The Pharmacological Basis of Therapeutics*, 4th edn., Macmillan, New York, p. 25.

Himwich, W.A., Peterson, I.M. and Graves, I.P. (1954) Ingested sodium glutamate and plasma levels of glutamic acid. *J. Appl. Physiol.*, 7: 196–201.

Inouye, M. (1976) Selective distribution of radioactivity in the neonatal mouse brain following subcutaneous administration of ^{14}C-labeled monosodium glutamate. *Congenital Anomalies*, 16: 79–84.

Kizer, J.S., Nemeroff, C.B. and Youngblood, W.W. (1978) Neurotoxic amino acids and structurally related analogs. *Pharmacol. Rev.*, 29: 301–318.

Lucas, D.R. and Newhouse, J.P. (1957) The toxic effect of sodium L-glutamate on the inner layers of the retina. *AMA Arch. Ophthalmol.*, 58: 193.

McDonald, J., Silverstein, F.S. and Johnston, M.V. (1987) The glutamate antagonist MK-801 attenuates perinatal hypoxic-ischemic brain injury. *Ann. Neurol.*, 22: 407.

Monoghan, D.T. and Cotman, C.W. (1985) Distribution of N-methyl-D-aspartate sensitive L-^{3}H-glutamate-binding sites in rat brain. *J. Neurosci.*, 5, 2909–2919.

Nemeroff, C.B. (1983) Effects of neurotoxic excitatory amino acids on neuroendocrine regulation. In K. Fuxe, P. Roberts and R. Schwarcz (Eds.), *Excitotoxins*, Macmillan, London, pp. 295–307.

Okaniwa, A., Hori, M., Masuda, M., Takeshita, M., Hayaski, N. and Wada, I. (1979) Histopathological study on effects of potassium aspartate on the hypothalamus of rats. *J. Toxicol. Sci.*, 4: 31–46.

Olney, J.W. (1969a) Glutamate-induced retinal degeneration in neonatal mice. Electron microscopy of the acutely evolving lesion. *J. Neuropathol. Exp. Neurol.*, 28: 455–474.

Olney, J.W. (1969b) Brain lesions, obesity and other disturbances in mice treated with monosodium glutamate. *Science*, 164: 719–721.

Olney, J.W. (1971) Glutamate-induced neuronal necrosis in the infant mouse hypothalamus: an electron microscopic study. *J. Neuropathol. Exp. Neurol.*, 30: 75–90.

Olney, J.W. (1974a) Occult mechanisms of brain dysfunction. In A. Vernadakis and N. Weiner (Eds.), *Drugs and the Developing Brain*, Plenum, New York.

Olney, J.W. (1974b) Toxic effects of glutamate and related amino acids on the developing central nervous system. In W.N. Nyhan (Ed.), *Heritable Disorders of Amino Acid Metabolism*, John Wiley, New York.

Olney, J.W. (1976) Brain damage and oral intake of certain amino acids. In G. Levi, L. Battistin and A. Lajtha (Eds.), *Transport Phenomena in the Nervous System: Physiological and Pathological Aspects*, Plenum, New York.

Olney, J.W. (1978) Neurotoxicity of excitatory amino acids. In E. McGeer, J.W. Olney and P. McGeer (Eds.), *Kainic Acid as a Tool in Neurobiology*, Raven, New York.

Olney, J.W. (1980) Excitatory neurotoxins as food additives: an evaluation of risk. *Neurotoxicology*, 2: 163–192.

Olney, J.W. (1984) Excitotoxic food additives – relevance of animal studies to human safety. *Neurobehav. Toxicol. Teratol.* 6: 455–462.

Olney, J.W. (1986) Excitotoxic amino acids. *News Physiol. Sci. (NIPS)*, 1: 19–23.

Olney, J.W. and Ho, O.L. (1970) Brain damage in infant mice following oral intake of glutamate, aspartate or cysteine. *Nature*, 227: 609–610.

Olney, J.W. and Price, M.T. (1978) Excitotoxic amino acids as neuroendocrine probes. In E. McGeer, J.W. Olney and P. McGeer (Eds.), *Kainic Acid as a Tool in Neurobiology*, Raven, New York.

Olney, J.W. and Price, M.T. (1980) Neuroendocrine interactions of excitatory and inhibitory amino acids. *Brain Res. Bull.*, 5: Suppl. 2, 361–368.

Olney, J.W., Ho, O.L. and Rhee, V. (1971) Cytotoxic effects of acidic and sulphur-containing amino acids on the infant mouse central nervous system. *Exp. Brain Res.*, 14: 61–76.

Olney, J.W., Sharpe, L.G. and Feigin, R.D. (1972) Glutamate-induced brain damage in infant primates. *J. Neuropathol. Exp. Neurol.*, 31: 464–488.

Olney, J.W., Ho, O.L. and Rhee, V. (1973a) Brain damaging potential of protein hydrolysates. *N. Engl. J. Med.*, 289: 392–395.

Olney, J.W., Ho, O.L., Rhee, V. and deGubareff, T. (1973b) Neurotoxic effects of glutamate. *N. Engl. J. Med.*, 289: 1374–1375.

Olney, J.W., Misra, C.H. and deGubareff, F. (1975) Cysteine-S-sulfate: brain damaging metabolite in sulfite oxidase deficiency. *J. Neuropathol. Exp. Neurol.*, 34: 167–176.

Olney, J.W., Cicero, T.J., Meyer, E.R. and deGubareff, T. (1976) Acute glutamate-induced elevations in serum testosterone and luteinizing hormone. *Brain Res.*, 112: 420–424.

Olney, J.W., deGubareff, T. and Labruyere, J. (1979) α-Aminoadipate blocks the neurotoxic action of N-methyl-aspartate. *Life Sci.*, 25: 537–540.

Olney, J.W., Labruyere, J. and deGubareff, T. (1980) Brain damage in mice from voluntary ingestion of glutamate and aspartate. *Neurobehav. Toxicol.*, 2: 125–129.

Olney, J.W., Labruyere, J., Collins, J.F. and Curry, K. (1981) D-Aminophosphonovalerate is 100-fold more powerful than D-alpha-aminoadipate in blocking N-methylaspartate neurotoxicity. *Brain Res.*, 221: 207–210.

Olney, J.W., Price, M.T., Fuller, T.A., Labruyere, J., Samson, L., Carpenter, M. and Mahan, K. (1986) The anti-excitotoxic effects of certain anesthetics, analgesics and sedative-hypnotics. *Neurosci. Lett.*, 68: 29–34.

Perez, J.V. and Olney, J.W. (1972) Accumulation of glutamic acid in arcuate nucleus of infant mouse hypothalamus following subcutaneous administration of the amino acid. *J. Neurochem.*, 19: 1777–1781.

Pizzi, W.J., Tabor, J.M. and Barnhart, J.E. (1978) Somatic, behavioral and reproductive disturbances in mice following neonatal administration of sodium L-aspartate. *Pharmacol. Biochem. Behav.*, 9: 481–485.

Price, M.T., Olney, J.W. and Cicero, T.J. (1978a) Acute elevations of serum luteinizing hormone induced by kainic acid, N-methylaspartic acid or homocysteic acid. *Neuroendocrinology*, 26: 352–358.

Price, M.T., Olney, J.W., Mitchell, M.V., Fuller, T. and Cicero, T.J. (1978b) Luteinizing hormone releasing action of N-methylaspartate is blocked by GABA or taurine but not by dopamine antagonists. *Brain Res.*, 158: 461–465.

Price, M.T., Olney, J.W., Lowry, O.H. and Buchsbaum S. (1981) Uptake of exogenous glutamate and aspartate by circumventricular organs but not other regions of brain. *J. Neurochem.*, 36: 1774–1780.

Price, M.T., Pusateri, M.E., Crow, S.E., Buchsbaum, S., Olney, J.W. and Lowry, O.H. (1984) Uptake of exogenous aspartate into circumventricular organs but not other regions of adult mouse brain. *J. Neurochem.*, 42: 740–744.

Ranney, R.E. and Oppermann, J.A. (1979) A review of the metabolism of the aspartyl moiety of aspartame in experimental animals and man. *J. Environ. Pathol. Toxicol.*, 2: 979–985.

Rothman, S.M. and Olney, J.W. (1986) Glutamate and the pathophysiology of hypoxic-ischemic brain damage. *Ann. Neurol.*, 19: 105–111.

Rothman, S.M. and Olney, J.W. (1987) Excitotoxicity and the NMDA receptor. *Trends NeuroSci.*, 10: 299–302.

Schainker, B.A. and Cicero, T.J. (1979) Acute central stimulation of luteinizing hormone by parenterally administered N-methyl-DL-aspartic acid in the male rat. *Brain Res.*, 184: 425–437.

Schainker, B. and Olney, J.W. (1974) Glutamate-type hypothalamic-pituitary syndrome in mice treated with aspartate or cysteate in infancy. *J. Neural. Transm.*, 35: 207–215.

Steginck, L.D., Reynolds, W.A., Filer, Jr., L.J., et al. (1979a) Comparative metabolism of glutamate in the mouse, monkey and man. In L.J. Filer, Jr., S. Garattini, M.R. Kare, W.A. Reynolds and R.J. Wurtman (Eds.), *Glutamic Acid: Advances in Biochemistry and Physiology*, Raven, New York.

Steginck, L.D., Filer, Jr., L.J., Baker, G.L., Mueller, S.M. and Wu-Rideout, M.Y.-C. (1979b) Factors affecting plasma glutamate levels in normal adult subjects. In L.J. Filer, Jr., S. Garattini, M.R. Kare, W.A. Reynolds and R.J. Wurtman (Eds.), *Glutamic Acid: Advances in Biochemistry and Physiology*, Raven, New York, pp. 333–351.

Synge, R.L.M. (1977) The problems of assessing the safety of novel protein-rich foods. *Proc. Nutr. Soc.*, 36: 197.

Tal, J., Price, M.T. and Olney, J.W. (1983) Neuroactive amino acids influence gonadotrophin output by a suprapituitary mechanism in either rodents or primates. *Brain Res.*, 273: 179–182.

Terry, L.C., Epelbaum, J. and Martin, J.B. (1981) Monosodium glutamate: acute and chronic effects on rhythmic growth hormone and prolactin secretion, and somatostatin in the undisturbed male rat. *Brain Res.*, 217: 129–136.

Watkins, J.C. (1978) Excitatory amino acids. In E. McGeer,

J.W. Olney and P.L. McGeer (Eds.), *Kainic Acid as a Tool in Neurobiology*, Raven Press, New York.

Wilson, R.C. and Knobil, E. (1982) Acute effects of *N*-methyl-DL-aspartate on the release of pituitary gonadotrophins and prolactin in the adult female rhesus monkey. *Brain Res.*, 248: 177–179.

Yamashita, S., Ogawa, H. and Sato, M. (1973) The enhancing action of 5'-ribonucleotide on rat gustatory nerve fiber response to monosodium glutamate. *Jpn. J. Physiol.*, 23: 59–68.

Discussion

C.V. Kellogg: Considering some of the endocrine consequences of glutamate toxicity in the young animal, such as hyperinsulinemia, one might suspect changes in the balance of branched chain vs. aromatic amino acids. This then could alter the exchange transport of the neutral amino acids into the brain. Have you measured plasma amino acids?

J.W. Olney: These aspects have not been studied.

M.V. Johnston: Patients have been reported (Plaitakis et al., 1982) who are genetically 'intolerant' of glutamate (Glu) and develop unusually high serum Glu levels after oral Glu administration. Is it possible that there is a group of people who genetically might be especially susceptible to neurotoxic effects of Glu or aspartate or might expose a fetus to high levels during pregnancy?

J.W. Olney: I would expect that these 'intolerant' individuals would be a population at increased risk for circumventricular organ (CVO) brain damage, if exposed to exogenous Glu during infancy or childhood. A given oral load of Glu will then produce abnormally high blood levels of Glu, and CVO neurons will be flooded with high and potentially excitotoxic concentrations of Glu. Whether the fetus may be at increased risk due to the genetic defect in the mother would depend on whether the defect alters the ability of the placenta to regulate Glu transfer from the maternal to fetal circulation. Nothing is known about this. If both the mother and the fetus have the genetic defect, any excess of Glu transferred to the fetus (due to the maternal defect) would be compounded by the inability of the fetus to metabolize it. Nothing is known on this point either.

B. Weiss: I have been an admirer of your work for a long time, and also have been most sympathetic toward it because of my own experience with research on the behavioral effects of food colors (Weiss et al., 1980). Naturally, the work, which confirmed the hypothesis in principle, was attacked by some elements of the food industry. Among the more astonishing attacks was one by Frederich Stare of Harvard, who asserted that the problem was trivial because sensitivity was pronounced only in the youngest children. Your early work was also attacked on the basis of assertions about 'irrelevance' of various kinds, and I think it would be helpful for you to review for us some of that history.

J.W. Olney: That, unfortunately, is a very long history. I will just share with you a few vignettes.

Immediately after I published my original findings (Olney, 1969) describing Glu-induced brain damage and the neuroendocrine disturbances associated therewith, I came under fire from various directions and soon learned that my assailants had something in common – they were all affiliated in one way or another with the Glu and/or food industries. Glu was being added in large amounts to baby foods at the time and one group of industry apologists wrote an indignant letter to Science (Blood et al., 1969) denouncing my experiments on grounds that it is inappropriate to use baby animals to test the toxicity of Glu because their enzyme systems are immature. They saw nothing wrong with adding huge amounts of Glu to baby foods, however, as it did not even occur to them that immaturity of the human infant's enzyme systems might be a relevant concern.

In the late 1960s and early 70s, the Food and Drug Administration (FDA) in the USA had a practice of referring food regulatory issues to a quasi-governmental 'Food Protection Committee' and this is the forum they attempted to use to resolve the Glu/baby food issue. I presented evidence before this committee but they seemed more receptive to an industry spokesman who assured them that destruction of neurons in the arcuate nucleus of the hypothalamus was of no importance because these neurons are not known to have any functional significance. While this committee proceeded to declare Glu safe, I began looking into the background of the committee and learned that it was founded by, funded by and totally controlled by the food industry and that most of the members of the subcommittee appointed to investigate the Glu/baby food issue had strong financial ties with the Glu and/or food industries. The committee chairman was receiving money from both industries at the time of the committee deliberations. I described this appalling situation in testimony before the US Senate Nutrition Committee in 1972 which resulted in the Senate Committee pressing FDA until they agreed to adopt more objective referral channels.

Another way that the Glu industry wielded influence over the regulatory process (and still does) was to fund numerous studies purporting to investigate Glu neurotoxicity but carefully designed to avoid finding evidence for such toxicity. Then they published the evidence in toxicology journals editorially controlled by the very authors of the studies (or their cronies) and deluged FDA with such evidence. These studies were performed by fellow travellers of the food industry, not by experienced neuroscientists. Over the past 15 years, FDA Bureau of Foods has routinely accepted such evidence uncritically. I have observed repeatedly that the Bureau is content to weigh evidence by the pound. Not surprisingly, this usually leads them to conclude that the weight of evidence on contested food safety issues favors industry's position.

H.H. Swanson: I was surprised that aspartate elevates serum prolactin level, similar to LH and FSH, since the main influence of the hypothalamus on pituitary prolactin secretion is inhibitory rather than stimulatory.

J.W. Olney: I do not know the mechanism by which *N*-methylaspartate (NMA) induces an elevation of serum prolactin, but Dr. Knobil and his colleagues are very accomplished primate neuroendocrinologists so I am inclined to believe their findings (Wilson and Knobil, 1982). One possibility would be that the inhibitory tone maintained by hypothalamic neurons over prolactin secretion is disrupted or over-ridden by the excitatory action of NMA on these neurons, the net effect being a disinhibition of prolactin release.

H.H. Swanson: Whenever I travel to the US, I note the great number of very fat adults and children. Do you think this could be associated with glutamate in baby food?

J.W. Olney: I think it is quite possible that ingestion of Glu in childhood could contribute to subsequent obesity in certain individual cases but there are obviously other potential causes of obesity that must be considered. Whether obesity is truly more prevalent in the USA than in Europe would have to be established by objective criteria before your casual observation could be considered an established fact. Whether obese people, either in the USA or Europe, have had greater exposure to Glu than slim people in the same societies is also a relevant question but one for which a reliable answer is hard to obtain.

R. Ravid: How would you explain the distinct destructive effect of glutamate in both extremes of the lifespan: in infant and in aged animals and humans?

J.W. Olney: Exogenous Glu is more effective in destroying CNS neurons in infant than adult animals but it is capable of destroying neurons at both age extremes. I suspect that the greater vulnerability of immature animals derives from the immaturity of several systems, perhaps the most important of which is the Glu uptake system that is primarily responsible in the adult nervous system for inactivating the excitatory action of Glu.

D.F. Swaab: Is the placenta an effective barrier against monosodium glutamate or related compounds?

J.W. Olney: It has been demonstrated in rhesus monkeys that the placenta regulates the amount of Glu that is transferred from the maternal to fetal circulation and thereby provides a steady-state environment for the fetus. However, this homeostatic mechanism can be overwhelmed as we have shown (Olney et al., 1972) by administering a large dose of Glu intravenously to the pregnant rhesus monkey in late gestation. This resulted in the transfer of enough Glu across the placenta to cause a striking lesion in the fetal hypothalamus.

D.F. Swaab: Are those brain areas that are preferentially lesioned in the hypoxic neonate (e.g. Sommer's zone) indeed the areas that have the glutamate receptors?

J.W. Olney: The Sommer's zone of the hippocampus is very sensitive to seizure-mediated and hypoxic degeneration and the neurons in this zone have perhaps the highest density of Glu receptors in the brain. However, there are other regions of brain that are sensitive to hypoxic degeneration but do not have a high density of Glu receptors. The explanation for this is currently under investigation.

References

Blood, F., Oser, B. and White, P. (1969) Monosodium glutamate. *Science*, 165: 1028.

Olney, J.W. (1969) Brain lesions, obesity and other disturbances in mice treated with monosodium glutamate. *Science*, 164: 719–721.

Olney, J.W., Sharpe, L.G. and Feigin, R.D. (1972) Glutamate-induced brain damage in infant primates. *J. Neuropathol. Exp. Neurol.*, 31: 464–488.

Plaitakis, A., Berl, S. and Yahr, M.D. (1982) Abnormal glutamate metabolism in an adult-onset degenerative neurological disorder. *Science*, 216: 193–196.

Weiss, B., Williams, J.H., Margn, S., Abrams, B., Cian, B., Citron, L.J., Cox, C., McKibben, J., Ogar, D. and Schulz, S. (1980) Behavioral responses to artificial food colors. *Science*, 207: 1487–1488.

Wilson, R.C. and Knobil, E. (1982) Acute effects of *N*-methyl-DL-aspartate on the release of pituitary gonadotropins and prolactin in the adult female rhesus monkey. *Brain Res.*, 248: 177–179.

G.J. Boer, M.G.P. Feenstra, M. Mirmiran, D.F. Swaab and F. Van Haaren
Progress in Brain Research, Vol. 73
© 1988 Elsevier Science Publishers B.V. (Biomedical Division)

CHAPTER 19

Organometals and brain development

Zoltan Annau

The Johns Hopkins University, Department of Environmental Health Sciences, Baltimore, MD 21205, USA

The study of the mechanisms of neurotoxicity and their relationship to behavioral changes is intimately involved in the question of neurobiological function and behavioral expression. The field of neuroscience owes its rapid development to the fact that researchers have been willing to cross disciplinary lines to investigate the functions of the nervous system. The fields of neurotoxicology and behavioral toxicology, which have evolved during the past 20 years, also represent an attempt to extend the knowledge in neuroscience into an applied area dealing with the effects of toxic chemicals on nervous system function. Two reasons can be advanced for the rapid development of neurotoxicology: one is the pressing need to understand the mechanisms and expressions of toxicity of pharmaceutical agents and environmental chemicals, and the other, more familiar to basic neuroscience researchers, is that through the study of neurotoxic chemicals we often gain a better understanding of nervous system function, and sometimes can use experimental compounds to create models of human disease states that otherwise could not be modeled in animals. This latter approach has been largely successful because chemicals have been found that destroy specific neurochemical substrates without necessarily destroying fiber paths coursing in the vicinity of these substrates. The two most successful experimental approaches along these lines have been the use of kainic acid lesions to create an animal model of Huntingtons's chorea (Coyle et al., 1978), and the use of 1-methyl-4-phenyl-1,2,3,6-tetrahydropyridine (MPTP) to create a model of parkinsonism. The great interest in MPTP research comes from the fact that there was already evidence from drug abusers that the chemical was capable of inducing parkinsonism in humans that seemed indistiguishable from the idiopathic disease (Langston et al., 1984). Work with both of these chemicals has been successful because of the previous intensive investigations on the etiology of these diseases in the basic and clinical neurosciences.

In contrast to these well-recognized clinical problems, there have been few epidemics of environmental intoxication with neurotoxic chemicals and when these have occurred the causes were recognized relatively rapidly and the problems solved by eliminating or reducing the use of the chemical. The widespread exposure of large populations to chemicals such as lead and mercury has for the most part not been considered life-threatening and therefore has received limited attention from researchers. In addition, when these chemicals produce overt toxic symptoms at relatively large doses, the symptoms may be relatively diffuse, making the investigation of their mechanisms of action difficult.

In this paper we shall review some of the evidence on the neurotoxicity of the organometals methyl mercury, trimethyl tin and trimethyl lead. Organometals were chosen because they may represent the most toxic forms of the heavy metals and also because they either have or may become serious environmental hazards. Methyl mercury was selected because it is associated with the most important examples of human environmental intoxication and also because it exerts its maximum effect during the perinatal period, which may be the most sensitive period of the nervous system to the action of neurotoxic chemicals. In addition, we shall review some of the evidence regarding the toxicity of triethyl lead and trimethyl tin, which seem to exert their toxic action primarily on the limbic system and come somewhat closer to the experimental neurotoxicants such as kainic acid. These chemicals are found in the environment, but so far have not posed a serious health threat to populations.

Methyl mercury

The first important episode of methyl mercury (MM) intoxication occurred in 1953 in Minamata, Japan. One of the striking aspects of this outbreak of mercury poisoning was that asymptomatic mothers gave birth to severely mentally retarded children, who subsequently showed only slight recovery of function (Kojima and Fujita, 1973). Subsequent examination of some of the victims who died revealed that the mercury exposure had reduced the total brain mass by up to 40% (Harada, 1976), an effect also seen in primates (Fig. 1).

These striking effects of prenatal intoxication also raised the possibility that at lower doses of exposure, deterioration in mental performance could be observed, without the radical destruction of neuronal populations. In order to investigate this, animals were exposed to MM at various times during gestation. Spyker et al. (1972), using mice, showed that a single injection of MM given to the mother during the first trimester of gestation produced behavioral changes without overt signs of toxicity in either the mother or the offspring. This demonstration of 'behavioral' teratology confirmed the human data obtained in Minamata, and led other investigators to extend these findings through both behavioral and neurobiological studies. These investigations have recently been

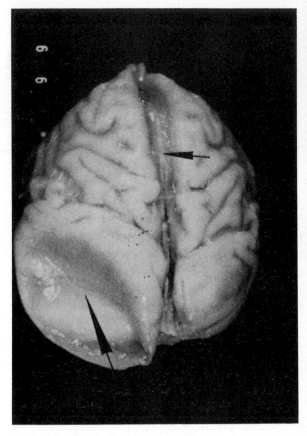

Fig. 1. Extensive hypotrophy of the brain of an infant monkey congenitally exposed to methyl mercury. Arrows point to loss of mass at visual cortex and widening of interhemispheric sulci. Taken from Mottet et al., 1987.

reviewed extensively (Eccles and Annau, 1987; Chang and Annau, 1984), and several interesting features of prenatal MM intoxication have emerged.

First, administration of MM postnatally has been shown to lead to mitotic arrest within 24 h and subsequent cell loss at 48 h in the cerebellum (Sager et al., 1982). Similar results, though somewhat less severe, were seen when the mercury was administered on day 12 of gestation in a subsequent study (Rodier et al., 1984). Khera (1973) had demonstrated in cats that prenatal exposure results in an incomplete granular layer in the cerebellum as well as alterations in the cytoarchitecture. Delayed myelination and delayed migration of the external granule cells were also described by Khera et al. (1974) and Khera and Tabacova (1973). The delayed migration of cells in the parietal cortex has also been described recently by Choi (1986). At the electron microscopic level, Chang (1987) has reported that in the early stages of intoxication there is an increase in neuronal lysosomes associated with the disintegration of the rough endoplasmic reticulum, followed by focal cytoplasmic degradation and neuronal vacuolation.

Behavioral studies in animals have confirmed the early observations on the human victims both in Minamata and later in Iraq (Amin-Zaki et al., 1976). Thus Eccles and Annau (1982a) showed that rats treated on gestational days 8 and 15 with either 5 or 8 mg/kg of MM showed altered development of motor activity in the pre-weaning period. This alteration was reflected in changes in the dopaminergic system (Cuomo et al., 1984). When tested as adults in a two-way avoidance-learning task, MM-exposed animals demonstrated a retardation not only in acquisition, but also in retention of this task. This latter effect was greatly increased when the mercury was injected on day 15 of gestation. An additional interesting finding reported by these investigators was the altered responsiveness of the mercury-treated animals to the psychoactive agent amphetamine (Eccles and Annau, 1982b). An earlier paper by Hughes and Sparber (1978) had reported similar results with amphetamine, and these authors suggested that one of the delayed effects of prenatal intoxication may be altered drug metabolism. It was not clear from the results of Hughes and Sparber, however, whether the altered behavioral sensitivity displayed by their rats was due to central or peripheral mechanisms. While the use of pharmacological challenges has become very popular in neurotoxicology (see Walsh and Tilson, 1986) as a way of determining the potential mechanism of neural injury, very little effort has been expended on determining the reason for the altered drug sensitivity. Hughes and Sparber reported that the effect they observed was only apparent in males, thus raising the possiblity that hormonal influences may play a role in this delayed expression of neurotoxicity.

In addition to the behavioral investigations of prenatal toxicity, both electrophysiological and neurochemical measurements have been made. These have been reviewed recently (Annau and Eccles, 1987; Komulainen and Tuomisto, 1987) and, while there seems to be no doubt that high doses of mercury will cause injury to the peripheral nervous system as well, the central nervous system is by far the most sensitive target. Using the visual evoked potential technique, Dyer et al. (1978) have shown that a single prenatal exposure to MM will alter the evoked potential recorded in the adult offspring. One of the interesting findings of this study was the shortening of the latencies of some of the components of the evoked potential, which the authors speculated could have been caused by the loss of small fibers because of the mercury treatment. In terms of neurochemical measurements following MM treatment, Komulainen and Tuomisto conclude that while the mercury does have potent inhibitory effects in vitro, in vivo the effects seem considerably less impressive.

Thus, perinatal administration of MM has been shown to (1) interfere with neuronal migration, (2) delay and reduce myelination, and (3) arrest mitosis and reduce the number of neurons. These effects are correlated with (1) transient alterations in the development of motor activity, (2) reduced ability to learn and retain complex tasks, and (3) altered responsiveness to pharmacological agents, as well as to altered neurophysiological responses in the visual system. These effects have been relatively well defined in many experimental models and have confirmed that this chemical even at very low doses can cause irreversible damage to the immature nervous system, as can be seen in recent literature reviews (Eccles and Annau, 1987).

298

Trimethyl tin

Interest in research on the neurotoxicity of trimethyl tin (TMT) started with a paper published in 1979 by Brown et al., who described the behavioral and pathological changes seen in rats following either single or repeated doses of this organotin. The behavioral symptoms consisted of increased aggressiveness, vocalizations, tremors, seizures and hyperreactivity. These symptoms persisted for approximately two to three weeks and then subsided. Neuropathological examination of the brains of the exposed animals showed severe damage to the hippocampus (Fig. 2) and lesser damage to other parts of the limbic system such as the pyriform cortex and amygdala. Because this organotin seemed such an ideal 'limbic system' poison, this research paper was followed by extensive studies on the nature and mechanisms of toxicity.

The observations of Brown et al. were confirmed and extended by subsequent studies (Dyer et al., 1982a). The dose–response function for this chemical was extremely steep for the rat, with the LD_{50} at about 7.3 mg/kg and the LD_{100} at 10 mg/kg. Following the injection of TMT, there was a mild hypothermia which persisted for about four days and was directly related to dose. Several behavioral alterations occurred within two days of injection. A fine tremor-at-rest was seen at the higher doses. Increased reactivity to handling which increased over time was also observed. Animals that showed this symptom also appeared to be likely to have seizures. The final behavioral morbidity appeared to be tail self-mutilation, with 50% of the animals showing this at the 7 mg/kg dose (Dyer et al., 1982b). Ruppert et al. (1983) showed that when placed in figure-eight maze, the animals dosed with 7 mg/kg became hyperactive after 24 h and remained so up 50 days after dosing.

Not surprisingly, given the significant destruction of hippocampal pyramidal cells, several measures of learning and retention showed major alterations following TMT administration. Animals exhibited retention deficits in a passive avoidance task which was evident at 5, 6 and 7 mg/kg and was not dose-related (Walsh et al., 1982a). At 7 mg/kg, rats were significantly impaired in a series of problem-solving tasks in the Hebb-Williams maze (Swartzwelder et al., 1982). The animals exhibited more errors, less error reduction over days and showed perseverative behavior that seemed characteristic of animals with hippocampal lesions. A further test of the hippocampal damage was also performed by

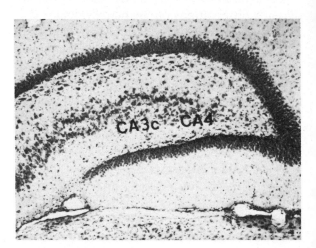

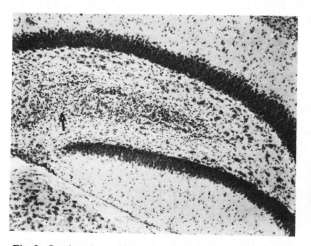

Fig. 2. Section through the hippocampus at normal rat (top) and rat exposed to 3 mg/kg of TMT once a week for 3 weeks. Note extensive loss of pyramidal cells in areas CA3 and CA4. Taken from Valdes et al., 1983.

Walsh et al. (1982b), who trained their animals in a radial-arm maze prior to TMT administration. Fifteen days after TMT dosing (6 mg/kg), the animals were retrained in the maze. There was a severe disruption of maze performance during retraining which persisted up to 70 days post-dosing.

Other measures of TMT-induced damage to the nervous system indicated that the pathology was not restricted to the limbic system. Dyer et al. (1982c) showed that when rats were implanted with chronic recording electrodes in the optic tract and the visual cortex, the TMT-treated rats exhibited an increase in latencies and decreases in amplitudes in the early peaks of the visual evoked potential at both electrode locations. These changes were suggestive of retinal damage. Other changes in the later components of the evoked potential were suggestive of altered arousal. A more detailed analysis of the seizure susceptibility of TMT-treated animals also showed that these animals were more susceptible to seizures induced by pentylenetetrazol, a general (not limbic-system-specific) convulsant, indicating that the early hypothesis of TMT being a specific limbic system or hippocampal toxicant was not confirmed (Dyer et al., 1982d).

Other areas of investigation included neurochemical studies of TMT-induced damage, as well as perinatal exposures. Valdes et al. (1983) showed that neurochemical alterations occured in intrinsic hippocampal neurotransmitters and not in extrinsic transmitters such as norepinephrine, and Ali et al. (1985) showed that there was a significant reduction in muscarinic cholinergic binding in whole brain and frontal cortex 2–7 days following treatment. In utero exposure, however, failed to show this neurochemical effect or the neuropathological pattern of adult TMT administration, suggesting that the immature nervous system was less sensitive to this toxicant than the fully developed nervous system (Paule et al., 1986). This was further confirmed by Lipscomb et al. (1986), who showed that the fetal brain concentration was identical to the maternal

brain concentration 96 h after exposure, although at 338 h the fetal brain levels were significantly lower than the maternal. Chang (1984) has also shown that administration of TMT up to post-natal day 4 causes relatively little pathology, but after that developmental day the pathology increases markedly, an observation also reported by Ruppert et al. (1983)

Thus, while the most severe damage induced by TMT in the adult animal is clearly in the hippocampus, as revealed by behavioral and pathological studies, it has also become clear that many other parts of the nervous system are also involved in the pathology (Chang et al., 1982). It is of great interest that, unlike methyl mercury, trimethyl tin seems to be less toxic in the fetal brain than the adult brain, although during the neonatal period, at least in the rat, this lack of sensitivity to toxicity diminishes rapidly.

Triethyl lead

The organo leads which have been used as gasoline additives in increasingly large quantities until recently (Grandjean and Nielsen, 1979) have been associated with many cases not only of accidental human intoxication (Beattie et al., 1972), but also of voluntary ingestion as 'sniffing' as an inexpensive drug of abuse (Valpey et al., 1978). The symptoms are clearly associated with central nervous system disorders and are characterized by disturbances of emotionality and memory as well as increased motor excitability, not unlike those seen after human TMT poisoning (Ross et al., 1981).

A recent review of the neurotoxicology of organo leads (Walsh and Tilson, 1984), in fact, makes a strong case for the similarity in the neurobehavioral pathology between TMT and triethyl lead (TEL), the toxic metabolite of tetraethyl lead, the gasoline additive. Not only are the pathological lesions seen in the adult animal following TEL administration concentrated in the limbic system, particularly the hippocampus, but also the behavioral effects are in accordance with the expectations of this type of lesion. More specifically, the animals show improved two-way avoidance learning, and impaired passive avoidance and spatial learning. Further, chemical analyses have shown that the hippocampus concentrates lead and that the concentrations of essential elements such as copper and zinc are decreased following TEL exposure (Niklowitz and Yeager, 1973). The neonatal brain again appears to be exquisitely sensitive to this neurotoxic agent (Booze et al., 1983). Konat (1984) has shown that administration of TEL to neonatal rats results in very significant hypomyelination because oligodendrocytes appear to be particularly targeted. This suggests that TEL, while having many similarities to TMT in its effect on the limbic system, may yet have its own unique toxicity, at least in the neonatal brain.

Mechanisms of toxicity

The biochemical and metabolic changes caused by methyl mercury administration have been reviewed recently by Chang (1987). Following mercury administration, the incorporation of amino acids into the nervous system is reduced significantly (Yoshimo et al., 1966) resulting in decreased protein synthesis. In addition, Verity et al. (1977) have suggested that a disruption of mitochondrial respiration may also inhibit synaptosomal protein synthesis, and further studies (Frenkel and Harrington, 1983) have shown that DNA and RNA synthesis in isolated mitochondria is inhibited. Finally, Sager et al. (1983) have reported microtubule disruption by methyl mercury. These studies indicate that mercury may disrupt all levels of the nervous system, particularly in the developing organism, and may explain the relative sensitivity of the organism to its toxicity.

In both triethyl lead and trimethyl tin intoxication protein synthesis inhibition seems to play a major role in the development of pathology. Recently Costa and Sulaiman (1986) have shown that following TMT administration protein synthesis is decreased significantly. Previous studies have shown that TMT inhibits oxidative phosphorylation (Aldridge and Street, 1971), and Costa and Sulaiman have suggested that this may indirectly account for the inhibition of protein synthesis. Konat (1986) has reviewed the triethyl lead toxicity literature and has indicated that this chemical also inhibits protein synthesis, not only at the neuronal level, but also at the level of myelin formation, where it inhibits proteins involved in membrane assembly.

It appears therefore that all of these organic metals have certain common properties that account for their toxicities. While the neuropathologies of TEL and TMT have certain similarities in the brain regions affected, the neuropathology of MM is clearly very different, suggesting that considerably more complex underlying biochemical mechanisms are involved in their individual toxicities.

Summary and conclusion

This brief review of the neurotoxicity of three organometals has shown that each metal seems to have its own pattern of toxicity which changes as a function of developmental stage of the brain. Methyl mercury in the fetal brain may be the most indiscriminately toxic compound because of its cytotoxicity. The nature of the neurotoxicity of prenatal exposure to TEL remains to be elucidated but in the neonatal period it may have both glial and neuronal targets. Finally, TMT at this time seems relatively non-toxic in the fetal period, but becomes extremely toxic to limbic system neurons in the neonatal period. The sensitivity of the hippocampus to a variety of environmental insults has puzzled investigators for many years, and even though, as has been pointed out above, there is some evidence that it concentrates lead (both organic and inorganic forms) this does not account for the total pathology seen.

The relationship between behavioral and neurobiological indices of toxicity is becoming closer as we learn to use our knowledge regarding brain lesions and behavioral effects and apply specific behavioral techniques derived from this literature to the testing of neurotoxicity of environmental chemicals (see Wenk and Olton, 1986). It is also quite evident that as we descend the dose-response curve of neurotoxic chemicals, we continue to uncover additional evidence of subtle alterations of nervous system dysfunction. These subtle, often 'latent' effects of perinatal intoxication have rarely been investigated in human populations. Needleman (1986) was one of the first to call attention, in the case of inorganic lead exposure, to such effects by developing the techniques to measure them. As we become more concerned with both the consequences of environmental hazards and widespread drug abuse we have to increase our efforts to establish the no-effect dose for all chemicals. It is our hope that through the continued investigations of animal models of perinatal neurotoxicity and concurrent human studies, we will ultimately be able to safeguard the health of human populations.

References

Aldridge, W.N. and Street, B.W. (1977) The relation between the specific binding of trimethyltin and triethyltin to mitochondria and their effects on various mitochondrial functions. *Biochem. J.*, 124: 221–234.

Ali, S.F., Slikker, W., Jr., Newport, G.D. and Goad, P.T. (1985) Cholinergic and monoaminergic alterations in the mouse central nervous system following acute trimethyltin exposure. *Acta Pharmacol. Toxicol.*, 59: 179–188.

Amin-Zaki, L., Ehassani, S., Majeed, M.A., Clarkson, T.W., Doherty, R.A., Greenwood, M.R. and Giovanoli-Jakubczak, T. (1976) Perinatal methyl mercury poisoning in Iraq. *Am. J. Dis. Child.*, 130: 1070–1076.

Annau, Z. and Eccles, C.U. (1987) Sensory deficits caused by exposure to methyl mercury. In C.U. Eccles and Z. Annau (Eds.), *The Toxicity of Methyl Mercury*, The Johns Hopkins University Press, Baltimore, pp. 104–113.

Beattie, A.D., Moore, M.R. and Goldberg, A. (1972) Tetraethyl lead poisoning. *Lancet*, ii: 12–15.

Booze, R.M., Tilson, H.A., Annau, Z. and Mactutus, C.F. (1983) Neonatal triethyl lead neurotoxicity in rat pups: Initial observations and quantification. *Neurobehav. Toxicol. Teratol.*, 5: 367–375.

Brown, A.W., Aldridge, W.N., Street, B.W. and Verschoyle, R.D. (1979) The behavioral and neuropathological sequelae of intoxication by trimethyltin compounds. *Am. J. Pathol.*, 104: 59–82.

Chang, L.W. (1984) Trimethyltin induced hippocampal lesions at various neonatal ages. *Bull. Environ. Contam. Toxicol.*, 33: 295–301.

Chang, L.W. (1987) The experimental neuropathology of methyl mercury. In C.U. Eccles and Z. Annau (Eds.), *The Toxicity of Methyl Mercury*, The Johns Hopkins University Press, Baltimore, pp. 54–72.

Chang, L.W. and Annau, Z. (1984) Developmental neuropathology and behavioral teratology of methyl mercury. In J. Yanai (Ed.), *Neurobehavioral Teratology*, Elsevier, Amsterdam, pp. 405–432.

Chang, L.W., Tiemeyer, T.M., Wenger, G.R., McMillan, D.E. and Reuhl, K.R. (1982) Neuropathology of trimethyltin intoxication. I. Light microscopy study. *Environ. Res.*, 29: 435–444.

Choi, B.H. (1986) Methylmercury poisoning of the developing nervous system: I. Pattern of neuronal migration in the cerebral cortex. *Neurotoxicology*, 7: 591–600.

Coyle, J.T., McGeer, E.G., McGeer, P.L. and Schwarz, R. (1978) Neostriatal injections: a model for Huntington's chorea. In E.G. McGeer, J.W. Olney and P.L. McGeer (Eds.), *Kainic Acid as a Tool in Neurobiology*, Raven Press, New York, pp. 139–159.

Costa, L.G. and Sulaiman, R. (1986) Inhibition of protein synthesis by trimethyltin. *Toxicol. Appl. Pharmacol.*, 86: 189–196.

Cuomo, V., Ambrosi, L., Annau, Z., Cagiano, R., Brunello, N. and Racagni, G. (1984) Behavioral and neurochemical changes in offspring of rats exposed to methyl mercury during gestation. *Neurobehav. Toxicol. Teratol.*, 6: 249–254.

Dyer, R.S., Eccles, C.U. and Annau, Z. (1978) Evoked potential alterations following prenatal methyl mercury exposure. *Pharmacol. Biochem. Behav.*, 8: 127–141.

Dyer, R.S., Walsh, T.J., Swartzwelder, H. and SandWayner, M.J. (Eds.) (1982a) The neurotoxicology of the alkyltins. *Neurobehav. Toxicol. Teratol.*, 4: 125–278.

Dyer, R.S., Walsh, T.J., Wonderlin, W.F. and Bercegeay, M. (1982b) The trimethyltin syndrome. *Neurobehav. Toxicol. Teratol.*, 4: 127–133.

Dyer, R.S., Howell, W.E. and Wonderlin, W.F. (1982c) Visual system dysfunction following acute trimethyltin exposure in rats. *Neurobehav. Toxicol. Teratol.*, 4: 191–196.

Dyer, R.S., Wonderlin, W.F. and Walsh, T.J. (1982d) Increased seizure susceptibility following trimethyltin administration in rats. *Neurobehav. Toxicol. Teratol.*, 4: 203–208.

Eccles, C.U. and Annau, Z. (1982a) Prenatal methyl mercury exposure: I. Alterations in neonatal activity. *Neurobehav. Toxicol. Teratol.*, 4: 371–376.

Eccles, C.U. and Annau, Z. (1982b) Prenatal methyl mercury exposure: II. Alterations in learning and psychotropic drug sensitivity in adult offspring. *Neurobehav. Toxicol. Teratol.*, 4: 377–382.

302

Eccles, C.U. and Annau, Z. (Eds.) (1987) *The Toxicity of Methyl Mercury*, The Johns Hopkins University Press, Baltimore.

Frenkel, G.D. and Harrington, L. (1983) Inhibition of mitochondrial nucleic acid synthesis by methyl mercury. *Biochem. Pharmacol.*, 32: 1454–1456.

Grandjean, P. and Nielsen, T. (1979) Organolead compounds: environmental health aspects. *Residue Rev.*, 72: 97–148.

Harada, M. (1976) Minamata disease. Chronology and medical report. *Bull. Inst. Constitut. Med. Kumamoto Univ.*, 25: Suppl. 1–60.

Hughes, J.A. and Sparber, S.B. (1978) d-Amphetamine unmasks postnatal consequences of exposure to methyl mercury. *Pharmacol. Biochem. Behav.*, 4: 385–301.

Khera, K.S. (1973) Teratogenic effects of methyl mercury in the cat: note on the use of this species as a model for teratogenicity studies. *Teratology*, 8: 293–303.

Khera, K.S. and Tabacova, S.A. (1973) Effects of methylmercuric chloride on the progeny of mice and rats treated before or during gestation. *Food Cosmet. Toxicol.* 11: 243–254.

Khera, K.S., Iverson, F., Hierlihy, L., Tanner, R. and Trivett, G. (1974) Toxicity of methyl mercury in neonatal cats. *Teratology*, 10: 69–76.

Kojima, K. and Fujita, M. (1973) Summary of recent studies in Japan on methyl mercury poisoning. *Toxicology*, 1: 43–62.

Komulainen, H. and Tuomisto, J. (1987) The neurochemical effects of methyl mercury in the brain. In C.U. Eccles and Z. Annau (Eds.), *The Toxicity of Methyl Mercury*, The Johns Hopkins University Press, Baltimore, pp. 172–189.

Konat, G. (1984) Triethyllead and cerebral development: an overview. *Neurotoxicology*, 5: 87–96.

Langston, J.W., Forno, L.S., Rebert, C.S. and Irwin, I. (1984) Selective nigral toxicity after systemic administration of l-methyl-4-pheny-1,2,5,6-tetrahydropyridine (MPTP) in the squirrel monkey. *Brain Res.*, 292: 390–394.

Lipscomb, J.C., Paule, M.G. and Slikker, Jr., W. (1986) Fetomaternal kinetics of ^{14}C-trimethyltin. *Neurotoxicology*, 7: 581–590.

Mottet, K.N., Shaw, C.-M. and Burbacher, T.M. (1987) The pathological lesions of methyl mercury intoxication in monkeys. In: C.E. Eccles and Z. Annau, (Eds.), *The Toxicity of Methyl Mercury*, The Johns Hopkins Press, Baltimore, pp. 73–103.

Needleman, H.L. (1986) Epidemiological studies. In Z. Annau (Ed.) *Neurobehavioral Toxicology*, The Johns Hopkins University Press, Baltimore, pp. 279–287.

Niklowitz, W.J. and Yeager, D.W. (1973) Interference of Pb with essential brain tissue Cu, Fe and Zn as main determinant in experimental tetraethyllead encephalopathy. *Life Sci.*, 13: 897–905.

Paule, M.G., Reuhl, K., Chen, J.J., Ali, S.F. and Slikker, Jr., W. (1986) Developmental toxicology of trimethyltin in the rat. *Toxicol. Appl. Pharmacol.*, 84: 412–417.

Rodier, P.M., Aschner, M. and Sager, P.R. (1984) Mitotic arrest in the developing CNS after prenatal exposure to methyl mercury. *Neurobehav. Toxicol. Teratol.*, 6: 379–386.

Ross, W.D., Emmett, E.A., Steiner, J. and Tureen, R. (1981) Neurotoxic effects of occupational exposure to organotins. *Am. J. Psychiatry*, 138: 1092–1095.

Ruppert, P.H., Dean, K.R. and Reiter, L.W. (1983) Developmental and behavioral toxicity following acute postnatal exposure of rat pups to trimethyltin. *Neurobehav. Toxicol. Teratol.*, 5: 421–429.

Ruppert, P.H., Walsh, T.J., Reiter, L.W. and Dyer, R.S. (1982) Trimethyltin-induced hyperactivity: time course and pattern. *Neurobehav. Toxicol. Teratol.*, 4: 135–140.

Sager, P.R., Doherty, R.A. and Olmsted, J.B. (1983) Interaction of methylmercury with microtubles in cultured cells and in vitro. *Exp. Cell Res.*, 146: 127–137.

Sager, P.R., Doherty, R.A. and Rodier, P.M. (1982) Effects of methyl mercury on developing mouse cerebellar cortex. *Exp. Neurol.*, 77: 179–193.

Spyker, J.M., Sparber, S.B. and Goldberg, A.M. (1972) Subtle consequences of methylmercury exposure: behavioral deviations in offspring of treated mothers. *Science*, 177: 621–623.

Swartzwelder, H.S., Hepler, J., Holahan., W., King, S.E., Leverenz, H.A., Miller, P.A. and Myers, R.D. (1982) Impaired maze performance in the rat caused by trimethyltin treatment: problem-solving deficits and preservation. *Neurobehav. Toxicol. Teratol.*, 4: 169–176.

Valdes, J.J., Mactutus, C.F., Santos-Anderson, R., Dawson, Jr., R. and Annau Z. (1983) Selective neurochemical and histological lesions in rat hippocampus following chronic trimethyltin exposure. *Neurobehav. Toxicol. Teratol.*, 5: 357–361.

Valpey, R., Sumi, S.M., Dopass, M.K. and Goble, G.J. (1978) Acute and chronic progressive encephalopathy due to gasoline sniffing. *Neurology*, 28: 345–350.

Verity, M.A., Brown, W.J., Cheung, M. and Czer, G. (1977) Methyl mercury inhibition of synaptosome and brain slice protein synthesis: in vivo and in vitro studies. *J. Neurochem.*, 29: 673–679.

Walsh, T.J. and Tilson, H.A. (1984) Neurobehavioral toxicology of organoleads. *Neurotoxicology*, 5: 67–86.

Walsh, T.J. and Tilson, H.A. (1986) The use of pharmacological challenges. In Z. Annau (Ed.), *Neurobehavioral Toxicology*, The Johns Hopkins University Press, Baltimore, pp. 244–267.

Walsh, T., Gallagher, M., Bostock, E. and Dyer, R.S. (1982a) Trimethyltin impairs retention of a passive avoidance. *Neurobehav. Toxicol. Teratol.*, 4: 163–168.

Walsh, T.J., Miller, D.B. and Dyer, R.S. (1982b) Trimethyltin, a selective limbic system toxicant, impairs radial-arm maze performance. *Neurobehav. Toxicol. Teratol.*, 4: 177–184.

Wenk, G. L. and Olton, D. S. (1986) Lesion analysis. In Z. Annau (Ed.), *Neurobehavioral Toxicology*, The Johns Hopkins University Press, Baltimore, pp. 268–278.

Yoshino, Y., Mozai, T. and Nakao, K. (1966) Distribution of mercury in the brain and its subcellular units in experimental organic mercury poisoning. *J. Neurochem.*, 13: 397–406.

Discussion

C. V. Vorhees: You raised an important issue about the possible changes in effects over time and the need for longitudinal analyses. Have you examined your methylmercury animals to see if the same animals that show altered activity were the same ones that showed the most disrupted avoidance performance?

Z. Annau: Unfortunately at the time we performed these experiments we did not keep track of the animals over the entire period and therefore this type of analysis was not available.

H. J. Romijn: Is tin as a metal just as toxic as its organic compound? If not, why have you chosen the organic compound in your studies?

Z. Annau: Tin as a metal is not considered very toxic. We chose trimethyl tin because it is a widely used chemical (in anti-fouling paints on boats, and as plasticizers in the plastics industry) and because of several human accidental exposures that showed this form of tin to be extremely neurotoxic.

B. E. Leonard: Trimethyl tin is suggested to be a limbic toxin. Bernadette Easton in my laboratory has recently shown that, following a single dose of this, there is a dose-dependent change in choline acetyltransferase and muscarinic receptor density in many regions outside the limbic areas. Regarding the behavioral defects after trimethyl tin, a major abnormality occurs in spatial learning at doses that have little effect on most other behavioral parameters. Would you like to comment on these points?

Z. Annau: It is clear from the recent trimethyl tin studies that it is not a specific limbic system poison, but that it also causes lesions in many other parts of the brain. Given its effects on the cholinergic system and the input of that system into septal-hippocampal pathways, it is not too surprising that you see spatial learning task deficits.

G. J. Boer: Is there any idea at what neurochemical level the organometals are acting to exert their deleterious effects?

Z. Annau: This in one of the areas of research that has not been exploited fully. Of course, each metal has a different mechanism of toxicity, and seems to interfere at several neurotransmitter systems.

T. A. Slotkin: How do you interpret changes in postsynaptic receptors and receptor-mediated responses without evaluating presynaptic function? Receptor up-regulation might represent a compensation for presynaptic hypofunction, thus producing a synapse wich operates normally.

Z. Annau: I agree that, based on our data, it is impossible to determine the exact location of the alteration, but that the postsynaptic alteration may be one such possible mechanism.

P. M. Rodier (comment): We have been able to measure Hg in all our experiments and I agree with you that much (probably most) of the variance we see in response to methyl mercury is due to differences in kinetics from animal to animal. We are constantly surprised at the difference in brain levels from the same dose!

G.J. Boer, M.G.P. Feenstra, M. Mirmiran, D.F. Swaab and F. Van Haaren
Progress in Brain Research, Vol. 73
© 1988 Elsevier Science Publishers B.V. (Biomedical Division)

CHAPTER 20

Alcohol as a social teratogen

Brian E. Leonard

Pharmacology Department, University College, Galway, Republic of Ireland

Introduction

Although the teratogenic effects of alcohol have been suspected since antiquity, it is only since the late 18th century that the possible detrimental effects of heavy alcohol consumption during pregnancy has received attention (Warner and Rosett, 1975). Sedgewick (1725, quoted by Warner and Rosett, 1975) was one of the first clinicians to suggest a link between the uncontrolled sale of gin in Britain and high rates of infant mortality but the general attitude of the medical profession at that time was ambiguous. Indeed, it was only fairly recently that the detrimental effects of alcohol exposure in utero on the subsequent development of the child was fully realized. Thus Lamache (1967) surveyed over 3000 children born in Western France with mental and physical defects and found that over 30% of the mothers were alcoholic. Subsequent studies in other European countries and in the United States of America confirmed the teratogenic potential of alcohol and the term foetal alcohol syndrome was introduced in the 1970s to describe the mental and physical abnormalities occurring in children born to alcoholic mothers (Jones et al., 1973; Clarren and Smith, 1978). Abel (1985a) has estimated the incidence of this syndrome as 1.1 per 1000 live births but as high as 25/1000 in children born to alcoholic women. The foetal alcohol syndrome is characterized by a combination of central nervous system dysfunction, growth deficiency and abnormal foetal characteristics.

In common with other birth defects, affected children show considerable individual variation regarding the severity of the damage. The term foetal alcohol effects has recently been suggested by Streissguth and Martin (1983) to describe the less extreme changes. Despite the wide recognition of the existence of the foetal alcohol syndrome, controversy exists regarding the importance of alcohol exposure as the sole factor causing the syndrome. Several studies have suggested that alcohol interacts with chronic malnutrition, smoking, drug abuse and inadequate ante-natal care (Aase, 1981; Streissguth et al., 1980; Lipson et al., 1983). While there is no satisfactory prospective data on the role of these factors in the foetal alcohol syndrome, studies in the United Kingdom by Wright et al. (1983) show that cigarette smoking increases the adverse effects of moderate alcohol consumption on foetal weight; heavy cigarette consumption is more frequent in the lower socio-economic groups who also have a higher incidence of the foetal alcohol syndrome. Another aspect which throws doubt on the view that this syndrome is only caused by alcohol exposure arises from the prevalence rates amongst the offspring of alcoholic women; this has been estimated to vary from 20 to 30% for the complete syndrome (Streissguth et al., 1973) and to 50 to 70% for the foetal alcohol effects (Sokol et al., 1980). The variation in the rate of metabolism of the toxic metabolite acetaldehyde (Majewski, 1981), genetic factors modifying the teratogenicity of alcohol (Abel, 1982) and the resistance of the foetus to the harmful effects of alcohol (Christoffel and Salofsky, 1975) could also play a role. Nevertheless, it seems reasonable to conclude that the presence of alcohol throughout the main stages of pre-natal development is the main factor predisposing the child to the foetal alcohol syndrome.

Rodent models of alcoholism

In an attempt to investigate the effects of pre-natal exposure to ethanol on the subsequent development of the offspring, it is necessary to ensure that the method used to administer the drug to the pregnant rat has a minimal adverse effect on either the animal or her foetus (Leonard and Duffy, 1987). Intubation methods of ethanol administration, as described by Cannon et al. (1974) and Majchrowicz (1975) are invariably stressful and cause irritation of the gastrointestinal tract which compound the effect of ethanol on the malabsorption of essential nutrients. Methods, such as those described by Cicero (1980), in which an aqueous solution of ethanol is the sole source of fluid available to the animals, only leads to the development of a mild degree of tolerance and dependence, while the inhalation technique, whereby ethanol saturated air is passed at a constant rate through the cage containing the rodents (Mullin and Fenko, 1983), produces a wide variation in blood alcohol concentrations and is associated with a high death rate. An additional complication of the inhalation method arises when pyrazole is administered concurrently with the ethanol exposure to inhibit liver alcohol dehydrogenase activity and thereby maintain a constant blood alcohol concentration. Pyrazole is known to be hepatotoxic, while its direct effects on the developing foetus are uncertain. For these reasons it would seem inadvisable to use such a method to develop a rodent model of the foetal alcohol syndrome. Perhaps the most appropriate method for administering ethanol to the pregnant rat involves the use of a nutritionally balanced liquid diet to which the drug is administered in increasing concentrations.

Such methods have been developed by Freund (1980) and Lieber and De Carli (1982) and have the advantage that the nutritional value of the diet can be adjusted to ensure that gross weight loss and malnutrition, often associated with ethanol administered by other methods, is minimal. Specially prepared nutritionally balanced liquid diets are now commercially available but these are invariably expensive. For the past 5 years we have been using a commercially available calf-milk replacer which is vitamin enriched and relatively inexpensive. The growth rate and general physical status of rats consuming such a liquid diet, together with rat chow, is indistinguishable from those animals fed the standard diet of rat chow and water (Keane and Leonard, 1983; Corbett and Leonard, 1984).

Rodent models of the foetal alcohol syndrome

Some of the first studies on the effects of pre-natal exposure to ethanol in animals dates back nearly one hundred years (Combemale, 1888) and has been reviewed by Wallgren and Barry (1970) and Green (1974). These early studies revealed that prenatal ethanol exposure resulted in a decreased litter size, decreased birth weight and increased post-natal death of the neonates. However, many of these and subsequent studies omitted vehicle treated or pair-fed control groups and thereby precluded the effects of trauma due to the ethanol injection and maternal malnutrition. More recent studies have attempted to control for such factors and have shown that malformation of the foetus and the neonate are associated with in utero exposure to ethanol (Chernoff, 1975; Randall, 1977; Leichter and Lee, 1979). Most of these studies however concentrated on the effects of relatively high concentrations of ethanol (> 10 g/kg/day) and the effect of lower doses, which would be more compatible with the clinical situation, has not been studied in the same detail. Abel (1978), using the intubation method to administer relatively low doses of ethanol to pregnant rats (1.0 and 2.0 mg/kg/day), found that such treatment reduced food and fluid consumption and attenuated the gain in body weight relative to untreated controls. Similar changes were found, however, in a pair fed control group; there was no evidence of gross malformations in any of the offspring. It therefore appears that the effects of low doses of ethanol are primarily due to a reduction in maternal calorie intake than a direct effect of the drug per se. Furthermore, Abel (1978) could find no evidence of behavioural teratogenesis, as shown by a learning decrement in a number of tests, comparable to those reported for higher doses of ethanol. Hollstedt et al. (1977) critically assessed the similarities and differences between the foetal alcohol syndrome and the detrimental effects of the drug on the developing rodent. They concluded that the metabolic capacity to remove ethanol changes with age, with a maximum at adolescence. By contrast, the ability of ethanol to cause hypoglycaemia is more pronounced in the younger mammal and becomes less significant with age. In the view of these findings, the possibilities of extrapolation between experimental animals and man are rather limited.

An important question arises from the studies cited regarding the method used to administer ethanol. Vorhees and Butcher (1982) compared the effects of administration of ethanol to rodents by gavage with the results of administering the same quantity of the drug by liquid diet; significant reductions in the maternal body weight occurred after the drug was administered by gavage and this could have an adverse effect on foetal development that was unrelated to the direct effect of ethanol. Other studies have shown that a significant reduction in the foetal weight on the 20th day of gestation only occurs if ethanol is administered in the drinking water but no difference was found if ethanol forms part of a nutritionally balanced liquid diet (Samson, 1981).

Another factor frequently raised by investigators regarding the treatment of the neonate born to ethanol-dependent mothers, concerns the need for cross fostering. Shaywitz et al. (1979) using a cross-fostering procedure, suggested that there

may be a maternal contribution from dams exposed to ethanol before parturition on the behaviour of their offspring. Hill and Means (1982) reported that the maternal behaviour of ethanol-treated dams towards their pups was essentially normal despite a greater variability in litter size and a large number of deaths occurring during the weaning period. These studies clearly suggest that the prenatal effects of ethanol on post-natal behaviour may be mediated both by direct exposure of the foetus to the drug and also the post-natal effects of the mother's behaviour. Whereas cross-fostering may help to eliminate any ethanol induced abnormality in the mother's behaviour on her ethanol exposed pups, it will not eliminate changes induced in the foster mother which may result from ethanol-induced abnormalities in the behaviour of the foster pups. This fact does not seem to have been fully considered by those investigators who insist that a cross-fostering technique be applied before any meaningful conclusions may be reached concerning the teratogenic effects of ethanol.

Behavioural and biochemical effects of pre-natal exposure to alcohol in rodents

In recent years, we have attempted to develop a rodent model of the foetal alcohol syndrome which eliminates many of the criticisms levelled at previous rodent models. In essence, ethanol was given in increasing concentrations in a nutritionally enriched liquid mild diet to pregnant rats, the controls receiving an isocaloric milk diet under otherwise identical conditions. Those animals receiving ethanol during the post-natal period consumed approximately 15 g/kg/day. In order to separate the pre- and post-natal effects of ethanol on growth rate and behaviour, half of the animals exposed pre-natally to the drug were given the isocaloric control milk diet at birth while half of the animals not exposed to ethanol during the pre-natal period were exposed to the drug post-natally. Behavioural observations were made periodically during the weaning period and immediately following this period.

In the initial study, no marked differences were found in the growth rates of any of the treatment groups nor were any changes found in the activities of the serum enzymes commonly used as an index of the integrity of heart and liver tissue, despite the relatively high ethanol exposure throughout the critical periods of development (Moloney and Leonard, 1984a). On reaching maturity, there was an increase in the exploratory behaviour of the ethanol-exposed rats, however, and this effect appeared to depend primarily on the exposure of the animals to the drug during the post-natal period. The reason for this is uncertain. It is unlikely to be due to the presence of alcohol as the animals had not received the drug for at least 30 days before their exploratory activity was assessed. From these studies, it would appear that ethanol can act as a behavioural teratogen under conditions in which no adverse effects could be shown on the litter size, growth rate or maternal behaviour.

More recently we have extended this investigation to study the various stages of development during the immediate post-natal period and to assess the effects of pre- and post-natal ethanol exposure on exploratory behaviour in stressful

('open field' apparatus) and relatively non-stressful ('hole board' apparatus) novel environments. The stressful nature of the open field apparatus has been investigated by Levine et al. (1967) and fully evaluated more recently by Roth and Katz (1979). The experimental protocol used was essentially similar to that described by Moloney and Leonard (1984a).

The results of these studies show that the effects of pre-natal exposure to alcohol are subtle; there was no evidence of any gross abnormality in physical development and no difference was found between the body weights of pups which had been exposed in utero to alcohol and those which were not exposed to the drug. At the end of the first post-natal week, the mean weight of the alcohol-exposed offspring was 14.4 g while the weight of the controls was 14.2 g (Fig. 1). Furthermore, there was no evidence of any gross change in the maternal behaviour in the dams treated with alcohol following the birth of the pups, e.g., in the pup retrieving time. The only developmental differences in behaviour between the alcohol-exposed and control groups was found on hair development (controls, day 9; and experimental, day 11) and eye-opening (controls, day 16; and experimental, day 17). These observations are substantially similar to those reported by Osborne et al. (1980).

Following the weaning period (approximately 80 days), the behaviour of the rats in the open field and on the hole board apparatus were assessed. The results are summarized in Table 1 where it can be seen that, in the open field, both pre- and/or post-natal alcohol exposure is associated with a rise in the ambulation score; the changes in the rearing scores were less marked. Qualitative differences were found between the male and female offspring of the various treatment groups. Thus pre- and/or post-natal exposure of the female offspring to ethanol resulted in an elevation of the ambulation scores, whereas an increase in the ambulation score only occurred in the male offspring following pre- and post-natal exposure to the drug. Pre- and/or post-natal exposure to

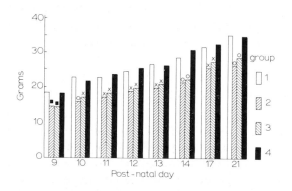

Fig. 1. Changes in body weights of rats exposed pre- and/or post-natally to alcohol. Group 1, controls (no alcohol given); group 2, alcohol administered during post-natal period only; group 3, alcohol administered pre- and post-natally; group 4, alcohol administered during pre-natal period only. ■, $P < 0.05$; ×, $P < 0.01$; ○, $P < 0.001$.

TABLE 1

Effects of pre- and post-natal ethanol exposure on the behaviour of rats in the 'open field' apparatus

Treatment group	Ambulation		Rearing	
	Female	Male	Female	Male
Controls	30 ± 10	49 ± 9	2.5 ± 0.9	7.0 ± 2.0
Group 1	85 ± 14[a]	64 ± 14	6.7 ± 2.7	8.9 ± 3.0
Group 2	69 ± 19	80 ± 7[a]	7.2 ± 2.6	6.3 ± 1.7
Group 3	68 ± 11[b]	67 ± 13	11.8 ± 4.1[a]	5.1 ± 1.3

In this experiment, Groups 1, 2 and 3 received the following treatments. Group 1, exposed to ethanol during weaning period only; Group 2, exposed to ethanol throughout the pre- and post-natal period until animals were weaned; Group 3, exposed to ethanol during the pre-natal period only. See Moloney and Leonard (1984a) for details. Results expressed as Mean ± S.E.M. Ambulation and rearing scores assessed for 3 min period.

[a] $P < 0.05$.

[b] $P < 0.025$ vs. controls.

alcohol also resulted in increased rearing behaviour in the female offspring, whereas in the male offspring rearing behaviour was hardly affected by the drug. From this study it would appear that the changes in behaviour in the female offspring were more consistent than in the males.

The effects of pre- and/or post-natal exposure to alcohol in the behaviour of rats placed on the relatively non-stressful novel environment of the hole board apparatus differed considerably from those changes seen in the open field, no changes being found in the ambulation score of any of the experimental groups. It must be stressed that alcohol was not administered to any of the rats after they had been weaned, i.e., approximately 30 days before the open field and exploratory behaviours were determined.

In addition to slight impairments in sensory-motor development, other authors have reported delays in the righting reflex, the emergence of hearing (as assessed by the startle response) and in the righting response to a brief blast of air (Hard

et al., 1985). These impairments due to pre-natal ethanol exposure were however of brief duration. Further studies of emotional development by these authors showed that pre-natal exposure to the drug is associated with a decreased frequency of ultrasonic vocalization during the first 6 post-natal days compared to the controls. Ultrasonic vocalization is a means whereby the pups attract the attention of the mother and thereby activate her maternal behaviour (Noirot, 1972). As the development of ultrasonic vocalization appears to be retarded in ethanol-exposed neonates, it may be assumed that the behaviour of the mother would also appear to be abnormal. This further serves to emphasize the limitations of cross-fostering when attempts are made to differentiate between the effects of ethanol on the mother and her offspring.

Changes in locomotor activity in rats exposed to ethanol in utero have been reported by several investigators (Bond and Di Giusto, 1976; Shaywitz et al., 1979; Osborne et al. 1980) as well as ourselves (Moloney and Leonard, 1984a). However, this effect would appear to depend on the age at which the animals are tested. Thus Bond and Di Giusto (1977) reported that the offspring were more active at 28 and 56 days of age but not at 112 days of age; Abel (1985a) reported that the age-dependent hyperactivity was also related to the concentration of ethanol in the maternal diet. As these studies were used on surrogate mothers, it would appear that pre-natal ethanol exposure alone is sufficient to induce hyperactivity in the offspring. The behaviour of rats in the T-Maze and Shuttle Box is also impaired following in utero ethanol exposure (Shaywitz et al., 1979). Hyperactivity, poor attenuation span, impaired habituation and abnormalities in cognitive and perceptual development have been described as part of the symptom complex in children of alcoholic mothers, referred to as attention deficit disorder (Shaywitz et al., 1987). It would therefore appear that the rodent model of the foetal alcohol syndrome replicates at least some of the major behavioural changes reported to occur in man. It is also of interest to note that hyperactivity in childhood may pre-dispose an individual to alcoholism in adulthood (Goodwin et al. 1975; Cantwell, 1972). Studies in rodents by Bond and Di Giusto (1976) demon-strated that the offspring of rats treated with ethanol during pregnancy were both hyperactive and showed enhanced preference for ethanol on reaching maturity when compared with the appro-priate controls. At present it is unclear whether it is the hyperactivity which predisposes the animal to alcoholism or the pre-natal alcohol exposure which predispose to both alcoholism and hyper-activity!

There is general agreement that rats prenatally exposed to ethanol are hyperactive and show deficiencies in passive and active avoidance (Bond and Di Giusto, 1977, 1978; Lochry and Riley, 1980). The effects of pre-natal ethanol exposure on the behavioural development of rodents has been reviewed by Bond (1981). These effects of pre-natal ethanol exposure would appear to be dependent on the daily dose of ethanol administered to the pregnant animal and only appear to become apparent following the administration of high doses of the drug which often leads to a reduction in maternal weight and calorie intake (Abel, 1978). Such factors do not always appear to have been considered by investi-gators.

Although pre-natal alcohol exposure can pro-duce gross neuropathological changes throughout the brain, behavioural and neuroanatomical in-vestigators have identified the hippocampus as a primary site of action of the drug. While some behavioural impairments seen during the early stages of post-natal development decrease with the maturity of the animal (Riley et al., 1979), other behavioural anomalies appear to be per-sistent. It is presently uncertain whether the alcohol-induced structural damage to the hip-pocampus is a consequence of the exposure of this region of the brain to the drug at a specific stage of foetal development or occurs independently of the time of exposure during the pre-natal period.

TABLE 2

Similarities between pre-natal alcohol exposure and hip-pocampal dysfunction on the behaviour of the rat (after Abel, 1985b)

Type of behaviour	Pre-natal alcohol exposure	Hippocampal dysfunction
Passive avoidance	–	–
Maze learning	–	–
Reversal learning	–	–
Spontaneous alteration	–	–
Schedule-controlled behaviour		
CRF	0	0
DRL	–	–
Extinction	–	–
Locomotor activity	+	+

–, impaired; +, increased; 0, no change in performance. CRF, continuous reinforcement; DRL, differential reinforce-ment of low rates.

Abel (1985b) has summarized the changes in various types of behaviour found in rats following pre-natal exposure to alcohol and shown how they resemble qualitatively those behavioural changes that result from hippocampal lesions produced by other methods. The similarities between pre-natal alcohol exposure and hippo-campal dysfunction are summarized in Table 2.

How can ethanol act as a behavioural teratogen?

It is well established that severe structural damage to the brain occurs in infants who have been exposed to high doses of ethanol during the pre-natal period. Pre- and post-natal dystrophy, development delay and microcephaly are typical features of children with the foetal alcohol syn-drome. These effects may result from the action of ethanol on all developmental stages of the CNS, especially in the period of organogenesis and histogenesis during early pregnancy (Clarren et al., 1978). It is evident however that ethanol can also interfere with the 'brain growth spurt' which

311

occurs late in CNS development and is an important factor in the aetiology of the foetal alcohol syndrome; mental retardation and persistent behavioural deficits may arise as a consequence of this action and in the absence of malformations (Streissguth and Martin, 1983).

In contrast to the human brain, the final vulnerable stage of the growth spurt in rats occurs in the first 2 or 3 post-natal weeks and a peak growth velocity and myelination at post-natal days 6 to 9 (Dobbing and Sands, 1971). Several studies in rats have shown that pre- and post-natal exposure produces a significant reduction in total brain weight, especially in the cerebellum (Abel, 1978; Diaz and Samson, 1980), selective loss of Purkinje cells (Phillips and Cragg, 1983), impaired maturation of Purkinje cells and retarded synaptic development (Volk et al., 1981). Detailed histological changes have been noted also in dendritic spine distribution in pyrimidal cells (Stoltenburg-Didinger and Spohr, 1983), deficits in dendritic structure in the hippocampus (Abel et al., 1983) and a reduction in pyramidal neurons in the hippocampus (Barnes and Walker, 1981). Bauer-Moffett and Altman (1975) have also shown that the alcohol-induced reduction of cerebellar neurons differs from those changes produced by infantile malnutrition.

West and Hodges-Savola (1983), in a detailed study of the histological changes occurring in the hippocampus of rats exposed pre-natally to alcohol, have shown that alcohol exposure results in significant alterations in the topographical organization of the zinc-rich mossy fibre system of the rat hippocampus. The abnormal terminal field that resulted from such an alcohol-induced derangement existed for at least 9 months after birth and shows that alcohol exposure in utero, during the period of brain development roughly equivalent to the first and second trimesters in the human, can produce permanent alterations in brain circuitry.

The mechanisms whereby ethanol can produce these detrimental effects on brain structure are numerous, but two actions of ethanol deserve particular attention because they may help to unify the apparently disparate effects of the drug on brain development. The first action of interest concerns the effects of ethanol on the pre-natal formation of neural cell adhesion molecules (N-CAM). These molecules are essentially gangliosides that are bound to the cell surface. Their complex and highly varied oligosaccharide units, rich in sialic acid, seem to be involved in many basic membrane-related events such as cellular migration, recognition and adhesion (Greig and Jones, 1977). In addition, these molecules are also constituents of a number of receptors and enzymes (McLawhon et al., 1981). Stibler et al. (1983) have shown that ethanol exposure in utero results in a reduction in the incorporation of sialic acid into membrane-bound sialoglyco-conjugates and that this effect occurs in the nerve terminals. It may therefore be hypothesized that a reduction in N-CAM could lead to an inhibition of neuronal migration at a critical stage of development with a consequent premature aggregation and adhesion of the neurons leading to the structural damage characteristic of the foetal alcohol syndrome. Such effects are undoubtedly complicated by a reduction in the placental transport of amino acids, glucose and other nutrients which could arise as a consequence of hypoxia (Abel, 1985).

Another possible site of action of ethanol on foetal brain development, an effect which has been investigated in detail in adult animals (Littleton and John, 1977; Chin and Goldstein, 1981; Goldstein, 1984), relates to the changes in lipid composition of the neuronal membrane resulting from the inhibition of the synthesis of polyunsaturated fatty acids which play a vital role in the maintenance of neuronal membrane fluidity. The various mechanisms whereby ethanol can produce these effects on membrane lipid composition has been briefly reviewed by Leonard (1984). The effect of ethanol on the lipid composition of the cell membrane could contribute to changes in the activities of membrane bound enzymes, transport sites for neurotransmitters and ions, receptor sites located on nerve terminals and cell bodies, etc. Several studies have reported that the activities of membrane bound ATPases from the brains of rats exposed to ethanol during the pre-natal period are reduced (Rangaraj and Kalant, 1980; Guerri and Grisolia, 1982; Moloney and Leonard, 1984b). While such an effect may lead to a change in amino acid, electrolyte and neurotransmitter transport across the neuronal membrane (Fisher et al., 1986), it would be premature to conclude that this could account for the numerous structural and functional changes in brain development seen in animals and man following pre-natal exposure.

Changes in neurotransmitters following pre-natal exposure to alcohol

This brief review of the effects of alcohol on brain development would be incomplete without a discussion of its effects on central neurotransmission. Our own studies have shown that the male offspring of alcohol-treated dams show little change in the cortical concentrations of noradrenaline, dopamine, serotonin or GABA (Duffy and Leonard, 1988). However, significant effects were observed in the female offspring of alcohol-treated dams, the concentrations of GABA, dopamine, serotonin and its major metabolite 5-hydroxyindoleacetic acid being significantly reduced; post-natal exposure of the female offspring resulted in slight (but non-significant) increases in the concentration of GABA, noradrenaline and dopamine. These results are summarized in Table 3. Such differences between the sexes would not appear to be associated with differences in brain weight, body weight or caloric intake. However, it is possible that such changes may be causally related to the enhanced hyperactivity of the female offspring when placed in the stressful novel environment of the open field apparatus.

Lucchi et al. (1983) studied the effect of pre- and post-natal alcohol exposure on dopamine

TABLE 3

Effect of pre- and post-natal ethanol exposure on the concentrations of some neurotransmitters in the amygdaloid cortex

Pre-natal treatment:		No ethanol	No ethanol	Ethanol	Ethanol
Post-natal treatment:		No ethanol	Ethanol	Ethanol	No ethanol
Neurotransmitter					
GABA	female ($n = 30$)	100 ± 6	127 ± 4^a	27 ± 15^b	70 ± 12
	male ($n = 30$)	100 ± 11	115 ± 20	109 ± 18	149 ± 6^b
5-HT	female	100 ± 8	98 ± 17	25 ± 22	33 ± 12^b
	male	100 ± 37	94 ± 26	92 ± 20	181 ± 17^a
5-HIAA	female	100 ± 7	117 ± 6	56 ± 18^b	62 ± 11^a
	male	100 ± 9	102 ± 18	121 ± 18	91 ± 15

Results expressed as percentage of control group. No ethanol = $100 \pm$ S.E.M. Absolute values for this group were: GABA: female, 658 ± 42; male, 258 ± 29. 5-HT: female, 0.177 ± 0.02; male, 0.161 ± 0.006. 5-HIAA: female, 0.10 ± 0.007; male, 0.22 ± 0.02. All values expressed as $\mu g/g$ wet weight. A slight rise also occurred in the dopamine concentrations of the rats in the group treated with ethanol during the post-natal period only; there was a 27% increase in the dopamine concentration of this group which was significantly greater ($P < 0.05$) than the non-ethanol treated group. The absolute concentration of the control group was $0.272 \pm 0.02 \mu g/g$.
[a] $P < 0.01$; [b] $P < 0.001$.

metabolism and receptor density in rats. These investigators showed long-lasting modifications of dopaminergic functions occur after pre-natal exposure; dopamine receptor function was shown to be decreased, while the turnover of the amine was concurrently increased. These effects were ascribed to a selective action of alcohol and not due to nutritionally related foetal defects. Unlike our findings, these investigators found a decrease in the spontaneous locomotor activity of male rats exposed to alcohol in utero.

Other investigators have provided evidence that pre-natal exposure to alcohol results in a reduction in the concentration of dopamine in the striatum, but these investigators also reported a significant reduction in the noradrenaline concentrations in the hypothalamus. They concluded that the primary neurotransmitter defect resulting from pre-natal exposure to alcohol was on the noradrenergic system (Detering et al., 1980a). These investigators have also shown that the pre-natal exposure of the rat to alcohol results in dissimilar changes in the activities of those enzymes involved in catecholamine synthesis and that this could account for the selective effect of the drug on noradrenaline concentrations in different brain regions (Detering et al., 1980b).

Maternal alcohol intake may produce different effects, or have no effect on dopaminergic function in the foetal central nervous system of the rat according to the stage of pregnancy at which the dam receives the drug (Lucchi et al., 1984). It is also well established that the effects of alcohol on central neurotransmitter metabolism depend on whether the drug is administered acutely or chronically (Kuriyama et al., 1971; Mena and Herrera, 1980) and on the dosage and route of administration (Pohorecky et al., 1974).

Mena et al. (1986) investigated the possible differences in the effects of alcohol on pregnant versus virgin female rats as any differences in the effects of alcohol, or its metabolite acetaldehyde, might be crucially important in explaining the neurotoxicity of the drug on the developing foetal brain. Their results showed that changes in basal neurotransmitter concentrations did not differ and, furthermore, that alcohol produces a similar degree of hypoglycaemia in both groups of un-fasted animals. When the monoamine and metabolite concentrations in the 21-day-old rat foetuses were determined following an acute dose of alcohol to the dams, no changes in neurotransmitter concentrations were detected; this finding contrasts with the effects of chronic alcohol intake (Mena et al., 1984) which suggests that at a later gestation period the foetal rat brain is less vulnerable to the effects of maternal alcohol intake than at the earlier stages of brain development. This view is supported by the findings of Lucchi et al. (1984) who described permanent changes in brain dopaminergic transmission in rat offspring of dams to whom alcohol had been administered on the 4th day of gestation only. It would appear that acetaldehyde production by the foetus is negligible, as evidenced by the low blood concentration of the metabolite in the foetal blood compared to that found in the dams (Mena et al., 1986) which reflects the low alcohol dehydro-genase activity found in the foetal liver at a late stage of gestation (Sjoblom et al., 1978). In view of the well-established effects of acetaldehyde on central neurotransmitter metabolism (Sippel and Kesaniemi, 1975; Sjoblom et al., 1978), it may be concluded that the incapacity of the foetal liver to form acetaldehyde, and of the placenta to oxidize this metabolite when formed by the dam, may protect the foetus against the maternal alcohol intake during the late gestation period.

Summary and Conclusion

In this short review of the effect of alcohol on the behavioural and neurochemical aspects of mammalian development evidence is presented to suggest that the behavioural changes seen in the rat following pre-natal exposure to the drug may bear some similarity to those seen in children suffering from the foetal alcohol syndrome. Providing care is taken to minimize non-specific changes which may arise due to maternal malnutrition, weight loss, etc., the rodent model may prove to be of value in elucidating the mechanisms whereby alcohol causes its neurotoxic effects which underlie its behavioural teratogenicity. The effects of alcohol on the lipid compositon of the neuronal membranes, and on the function of neural cell adhesion molecules (N-CAM) during critical stages of neuro-ontogenesis, are probably of primary importance in determining the selective neurotoxicity of alcohol. The changes in the activities of the biogenic amine neurotransmitter systems, and in the GABA-ergic system, which have been reported in rodents following pre-natal exposure to alcohol, are possibly secondary to the changes in the neuronal structure.

Acknowledgement

Some of the studies reported in this review were supported by a grant from the Medical Research Council of Ireland.

References

Aase, J.M. (1981) The fetal alcohol syndrome in American Indians – a high risk group. *Neurobehav. Toxicol. Teratol.*, 3: 153–156.

Abel, E.L. (1978) Effects of ethanol on pregnant rats and their offspring. *Psychopharmacology*, 57: 5–10.

Abel, E.L. (1982) Characteristics of mothers of fetal alcohol syndrome children. *Neurobehav. Toxicol. Teratol.*, 4: 3–6.

Abel, E. L., Jacobsen, S. and Sherwin, B. J. (1983) In utero exposure: functional and structural brain damage. *Neurobehav. Toxicol. Teratol.*, 5: 139–146.

Abel, E. L. (1985a) Pre-natal effects of alcohol on growth: a brief review. *Fed. Proc.*, 44: 2318–2322.

Abel, E. L. (1985b) Late sequelae of fetal alcohol syndrome. In U. Rydberg, C. Alling, J. Engel, B. Pernow, L.A., Pellborn and S. Rossner (Eds.), *Alcohol and the Developing Brain*, Raven Press, New York, pp. 125–133.

Barnes, D.A. and Walker, D.W. (1981) Pre-natal ethanol exposure permanently reduces the number of pyramidal neurons in rat hippocampus. *Dev. Brain Res.*, 1: 333–340.

Bauer-Moffett, C. and Altman, J. (1975) Ethanol induced reductions in cerebellar growth of infant rats. *Exp. Neurol.*, 48: 378–382.

Bond, N.W. and Di Giusto, E.L. (1976) Effect of pre-natal alcohol consumption on 'open field' behaviour and alcohol preference in rats. *Psychopharmacologia* (Berlin), 46: 163–165.

Bond, N.W. and Di Giusto, E.L. (1977) Pre-natal alcohol consumption and 'open field' behaviour in rats: effects of age at time of testing. *Psychopharmacology*, 52: 331–312.

Bond, N.W. and Di Giusto, E.L. (1978) Avoidance conditioning and Hebb-Williams maze performance in rats prenatally with alcohol. *Psychopharmacology*, 8: 69–71.

Bond, N.W. (1981) Pre-natal alcohol exposure in rodents: review of its effects on offspring activity and learning ability. *Aust. J. Psychol.*, 33, 331–344.

Cannon, D.S., Baker, T.B., Berman, R.F. and Atkinson, C.A. (1974) A rapid technique for producing ethanol dependence in the rat. *Pharmacol. Biochem. Behav.*, 9: 831–834.

Cantwell, D.P. (1972) Psychiatric illness in families of hyperactive children. *Arch. Gen. Psychiat.*, 27: 414–417.

Chernoff, G.A. (1975) A mouse model of the foetal alcohol syndrome. *Teratology*, 11: 14.

Chin, J.H. and Goldstein, D.B. (1981) Effects of low concentrations of ethanol on the fluidity of spin-labelled erythrocyte and brain membranes. *Mol. Pharmacol.*, 13: 435–441.

Christoffel, K.K. and Salofsky, I. (1975) Fetal alcohol syndrome in dizygotic twins. *J. Pediatr.*, 87: 963–967.

Cicero, T.J. (1980) Alcohol self-administration, tolerance and withdrawal in humans and animals: theoretical and methodological issues. In H. Rigter and J.C. Crabbe (Eds.), *Alcohol Tolerance and Dependence*. Elsevier, Amsterdam.

Clarren, S.K., Alvord, E.C., Sumi, S.M., Streissguth, A.P. and Smith, D.W. (1978) Brain malformation related to prenatal exposure to ethanol. *J. Pediatr.*, 92: 64–67.

Clarren, S.K. and Smith, D.W. (1978) The fetal alcohol syndrome. *New Engl. J. Med.*, 292: 1063–1067.

Combemale, F. (1988) La descendance des alcooliques. *Misc. Nerv. Syst.*, 82: 14–213.

Corbett, R. and Leonard, B.E. (1984) Effects of carnitine on changes caused by chronic administration of alcohol. *Neuropharmacology*, 23: 269–271.

Detering, N., Collins., R.M., Hawkins, R.L., Pozand, P.J. and Karahasan, A. (1980a) Comparative effects of ethanol and malnutrition on the development of catecholaine neurons: Changes in neurotransmitter levels. *J. Neurochem.*, 4: 1587–1596.

Detering, N., Edwards, E., Ozard, P. and Karahasan, A. (1980b) Comparative effects of ethanol and malnutrition on the development of catecholamine neurons: changes in specific activities of enzymes. *J. Neurochem.*, 34: 297–304.

Diaz, J. and Samson, H.H. (1980) Impaired brain growth in neonatal rats exposed to ethanol. *Science*, 208: 751–753.

Dobbing, J. and Sands, J. (1971) Vulnerability of developing brain. *Biol. Neonate*, 19: 363–378.

Duffy, O. and Leonard, B.E. (1988) Changes in behaviour and brain neurotransmitter following pre- and post-natal exposure of rats to ethanol: a rodent model of the foetal alcohol syndrome. *Submitted for publication.*

Fischer, S. E., Duffy, L. and Atkinson, M. (1986) Selective fetal malnutrition, effect of acute and chronic ethanol exposure upon rat placental Na, K-ATP'ase activity. *Alcoholism Clin. Exp. Res.*, 10: 284–292.

Freund, G. (1980) Comparison of alcohol dependence, withdrawal and hangover in humans and animals. In E. Eriksson, J. Sinclair and V. Kiianmaa (Eds.), *Animal Models of Alcohol Research*, Academic Press, New York.

Goodwin, D. W., Schulsinger, F., Hermansen, L., Gaze, S. R. (1975) Alcoholism and the hyperactive child sydrome. *J. Nerv. Ment. Dis.* 160: 349–353.

Goldstein, D. B. (1984) The effect of drugs on membrane fluidity. *Ann. Rev. Pharmacol. Toxicol.*, 241: 43–64.

Green, H. G. (1974) Infants of alcoholic mothers. *Am. J. Obst. Gynaecol.*, 118: 713–716.

Greig, R. and Jones, M. (1977) Mechanisms of intracellular adhesion. *Biosystems*, 9: 43–55.

Guerri, C. and Grisolia, S. (1982) Effects of pre-natal and post-natal exposure of rats to alcohol: changes in (Na + K)ATP'ase. *Pharmacol. Biochem. Behav.*, 17: 927–932.

Hard, E., Dahlgren, I. L., Engel, J., Larsson, K., Lindh, A. S. and Musi, B. (1985) Impairment of reproductive behaviour in prenatally ethanol-exposed rats. In U. Rydberg, C. Alling, J. Engel, B. Pernow, L. A. Pellborn and S. Rossner (Eds.) *Alcohol and the Developing Brain*, Raven Press, New York, pp. 93–108.

Hill, L. J. and Means, L. W. (1982) Effects of alcohol consumption during pregnancy on subsequent maternal behaviour in rats. *Pharmacol. Biochem. Behav.*, 17: 125–130.

Hollstedt, C., OIlsson, O. and Rydberg, U. (1977). The effect of alcohol on the developing organisms. *Med. Biol.* 55: 1–14.

Jones, K. L., Smith, D. W., Ulleland, C. N. and Steissguth, A. P. (1973) Pattern of malformation in offspring of chronic alcoholic mothers. *Lancet*, i: 1267–1271.

Keane, B. and Leonard, B. E. (1983) Changes in 'open field' behaviour and in some membrane bound enzymes following the chronic administration of ethanol in the rat. *Neuropharmacology*, 22: 555–557.

Kuriyama, K., Rauscher, G. E. and Sze, P. Y. (1971) Effect of acute and chronic administration of ethanol on the 5-hydroxytryptamine turnover and tryptophan hydroxylase activity of the mouse brain. *Brain Res.*, 26: 450–454.

Lamache, A. N. (1967) Reflexions sur la descendance des alcooliques. *Bull. Acad. Natl. Med.*, 155: 517–524.

Leichter, J. and Lee, M. (1979) Effect of maternal ethanol administration on physical growth of the offspring of rats. *Growth*, 43: 288–297.

Leonard, B. E. (1984) Possible relationships between thiamine, carnitine, polyunsaturated fatty acids and the neurotoxicity of alcohol. *Alcohol Alcoholism*, 19: 97–99.

Leonard, B. E. and Duffy, O. (1987) Behavioural consequences on in utero exposure to ethanol: a rodent model

of the foetal alcohol syndrome? In J. Fujii and P. M. Adams (Eds.) *Functional Teratogenesis*, Teikyo University Press, pp. 89–100.

Levine, S., Haltmeyer, G. C., Kavas, G. G. and Denenberg, V. H. (1967) Physiological and behavioural effects of infantile stimulation. *Physiol. Behav.*, 2:

Lieber, C. S. and De Carli, L. M. (1982) The feeding of alcohol in liquid diets: two decades of applications and 1982 update. *Alcohol Clin. Exp. Res.*, 6: 523–530.

Littleton, J. M. and John, G. (1977) Synaptosomal membrane lipids of mice during continuous exposure to ethanol. *J. Pharm. Pharmacol.*, 29: 579–580.

Lipson, A. H., Walsh, D. A. and Webster, W. S. (1983) Fetal alcohol syndrome – a great pediatric imitation. *Med. J. Aust.*, 1: 266–267.

Lochry, E. A. and Riley, E. P. (1980) Retention of passive avoidance and T-maze escape in rats exposed to alcohol pre-natally. *Neurobehav. Toxicol. Teratol.*, 2: 107–115.

Lucchi, L., Covelli, V., Petkov, V. V., Spano, P. F. and Trabucchi, M. (1983) Effects of ethanol, given during pregnancy, on the offspring dopaminergic system. *Pharmacol. Biochem. Behav.*, 19: 567–570.

Lucchi, L., Covelli, V., Spano, P. F. and Trabucchi, M. (1984) Acute ethanol administration during pregnancy: effects on central dopaminergic transmission in rat offspring. *Neurobehav. Toxicol. Teratol.*, 6: 19–21.

Majchrowicz, E. (1975) Introduction of physical dependence upon ethanol and the associated behavioural changes in rats. *Psychopharmacology*, 43: 245–254.

Majewski, F. (1981) Alcoholembryopathy: some facts and speculations about pathogenesis. *Neurobehav. Toxicol. Teratol.*, 3: 129–135.

Mena, M. A. and Herreva, E. (1980) Monoamine metabolism in rat brain regions following long-term alcohol treatment. *J. Neural. Transm.*, 47: 227–236.

Mena, M. A., Martin del Rio, R. and Herreva, E. (1984) The effect of long-term ethanol maternal ingestion and withdrawal on brain regional monoamine and amino acid precursors in 15 day old rats. *Gen. Pharmacol.*, 15: 151–154.

Mena, M. A., Zorzano, A. and Herreva, E. (1986) Acute effects of ethanol on brain, plasma and adrenal monoamine concentrations in virgin and pregnant rats and their foetuses. *Neurochem. Int.*, 9: 371–378.

McLawhon, P., Schoon, G. and Dawson, G. (1981) Glycolipids and opiate action. *Eur. Cell. Biol.* 25: 353–358.

Moloney, B. and Leonard, B. E. (1984a) Pre-natal and post-natal effects of alcohol on the rat. I. Changes in body weight and exploratory activity. *Alcohol Alcoholism.*, 19: 131–136.

Moloney, B. and Leonard, B. E. (1984b) Pre-natal and post-natal effects of alcohol on the rat. II. Changes in γ-aminobutyric acid concentration and adenosine triphosphatase activity in the brain. *Alcohol Alcoholism*, 19: 137–140.

Mullins, M.J. and Fenko A.P. (1983) Alterations in dopaminergic function after subacute ethanol administration.
J. Pharmacol. Exp. Ther., 225: 694–698.

Noirot, E. (1972) Ultrasounds and maternal behaviour in
small rodents. *Dev. Psychobiol.*, 5: 371–378.

Osborne, G.L., Caul, W.F. and Fernandez, K. (1980) Behavioural effects of pre-natal ethanol exposure and differential early experience in rats. *Pharmacol. Biochem.
Behav.*, 12: 393–401.

Phillips, S.C. and Cragg, B.G. (1983) Chronic consumption
of alcohol by adult mice: effect on hippocampal cells and
synapses. *Exp. Neurol.* 80: 218–226.

Pohorecky, L.A., Jaffe, L.S. and Berkelly, H.A. (1974)
Effects of ethanol on serotonergic neurons in the rat brain.
Res. Commun. Chem. Pathol. Pharmacol., 8: 1–11.

Randall, C.L. (1977) Teratogenic effects of in utero ethanol
exposure. In K. Blum, (Ed.), *Alcohol and Opiates: Neurochemical and Behavioural Mechanisms.*, Academic Press,
New York.

Rangaraj, N. and Kalant, A. (1980) Acute and chronic
catecholamine-ethanol interaction on rat brain (Na$^+$ +
K$^+$)-ATP'ase. *Pharmacol. Biochem. Behav.*, 13 (Supp. 1):
183–189.

Riley, E.P., Lochry, E.A., Shapiro, N.R. and Baldwin, J.
(1979) Response perseveration in rats exposed to alcohol
prenatally. *Pharmacol. Biochem. Behav.*, 10: 255–259.

Roth, K.A. and Katz, R.J. (1979) Stress, behavioral arousal
and 'open field' activity – a reexamination of emotionality
in the rat. *Neurosci. Biobehav. Rev.*, 3: 247–263.

Samson, H.H. (1981) Maternal ethanol consumption and
fetal development in the rat: a comparison of ethanol
exposure techniques. *Alcohol Clin. Exp. Res.*, 5: 67–74.

Shaywitz, S.E., Cohen, D.J. and Shaywitz, B.A. (1980)
Behaviour and learning difficulties in children of normal
intelligence born to alcoholic mothers. *J. Pediatr.*, 96: 978.

Shaywitz, S.E., Cohen, D.J. and Shaywitz, B.A. (1987) The
expanded foetal alcohol syndrome (EFAS). Behavioural
and learning deficits in children with normal intelligence.
Pediatr. Res. 12, 375.

Shaywitz, B.A., Griffieth, G.G. and Warshaw, J.B. (1979)
Hyperactivity and cognitive deficits in developing rat pups
born to alcoholic mothers. *Neurbehav. Toxicol. Teratol.*, 1:
113–122.

Sippel, H.W. and Kesaniemi, Y.A. (1975) Placental and
foetal metabolism of acetaldehyde in the isolated placenta
and foetus. *Acta Pharmacol. Toxicol.*, 37: 49–55.

Sjoblom, M., Pilstrom, L. and Morland, J. (1978) Activity of
alcohol dehydrogenase and acetaldehyde dehydrogenases
in the liver and placenta during development of the rat.
Enzyme, 23: 108–115.

Sokol, R.J., Miller, R.B. and Reed, G. (1980) Alcohol abuse
during pregnancy: an epidemiologic study. *Alcoholism (NY)*,
4: 135–145.

Stibler, H., Burns, E., Kruckeberg, T., Gaetano, P., Cerven,
E., Borg, S. and Tabakoff, B. (1983) Effect of ethanol on
synaptosomal sialic acid metabolism in developing rat
brain. *J. Neurol. Sci.*, 59: 21–35.

Stoltenburg-Didinger, G. and Spohre, H.L. (1983) Fetal
alcohol syndrome and mental retardation: spine distribution of pyrimidal cells in prenatal alcohol exposed rat
cerebral cortex. *Dev. Brain Res.*, 11: 119–123.

Streissguth, A.P. Jones, K.L., Smith, D.W. and Ulleland,
C.N. (1973) Patterns of malformation in offspring of
chronic alcoholic mothers. *Lancet*, i: 1267–1271.

Streissguth, A.P., Landesman-Dwyer, S., Martin, J.C. and
Smith, D.W. (1980) Teratogenic effects of alcohol in
humans and laboratory animals. *Science*, 209: 353–361.

Streissguth, A.P. and Martin, J.C. (1983) Prenatal effects of
abuse in humans and laboratory animals. In B.V. Kissin
and H. Begleiter (Eds.) *The Pathogenesis of Alcoholism.*
Plenum Press, New York.

Volk, B., Maletz, M., Tiedemann, M., Mall, G., Klein, C. and
Berler, H.H. (1981) Impaired maturation of Purkinje cells
in the fetal alcohol syndrome of the rat. *Acta Neuropathol.*,
54: 19–29.

Vorhees, C.V. and Butcher, R.E. (1982) Behavioural teratogenicity. In K. Snell (Ed.), *Developmental Toxicity*,
Croom-Helm, London, pp. 249–297.

Wallgren, H. and Barry, H. (1970) *Actions of Alcohol*. Elsevier,
Amsterdam.

Warner, R.H. and Rosett, H.L. (1975) The effects of drinking
on offspring. An historical survey of the American and
British literature. *J. Stud. Alcohol*, 36: 1395–1420.

West, J.R. and Hodges-Savola, C.A. (1983) Permanent hippocampal mossy fiber hyperdevelopment following prenatal ethanol exposure. *Neurobehav. Toxicol. Teratol.*, 5:
139–150.

Wright, J.T., Waterson, J., Barrison, I.G., Toplis, P., Lewis,
I.G., Gordon, M., MacRae, K.D., Marnis, N.F. and
Murray, I.M. (1983) Alcohol consumption, pregnancy and
low birth rate. *Lancet*, i: 663–665.

Discussion

J.F. Orlebeke: Can your results not be (partly) explained by
vitamin B deficiency since the calf milk replacer did not
contain vitamin B at all?

B.E. Leonard: I think this is unlikely as the animals have
access to standard rat chow throughout the experiment.
Nevertheless, it is possible that alcohol could induce a subclinical deficiency of thiamine although we never found any
pathological evidence to suggest this.

E. Fride: There are a number of perinatal treatments which
result in deficiencies, reminiscent of hippocampal dysfunction. Therefore, do you think that the abnormalities,
similar to hippocampal dysfunction after perinatal alcohol

administration, is due to a specific alcohol-hippocampus interaction, or due to the temporal relation between hippocampal development and perinatal treatment?

B. E. Leonard: I can only speculate that the effect of alcohol in causing hippocampal malfunction is due to a direct effect of the drug. There is evidence from studies of the chronic effect of alcohol on the adult rat that the hippocampus is particularly sensitive to changes in neurotransmitter function and lipid composition (Leonard, 1987). Such findings help to support the view that the hippocampus of the neonate may be particularly vulnerable to the actions of alcohol.

C. V. Vorhees: Could you comment on the fact that you see females as being less active in the open field, while most find females to be more active? Also, you stated that the open-field test is more stressful than the hole-board. Could you explain your basis for this comment?

B. E. Leonard: In answer to your first point, this observation may be related to the age of the rats when tested. I agree with you that most studies have shown that female rats are more active than males. Regarding your second point, we have measured plasma corticosterone levels in rats exposed to mild footshock, the open field apparatus illuminated by bright light and the hole board apparatus illuminated by red light (O'Connor and Leonard, unpublished observations). The latter exposure only resulted in a marginal rise in corticosterone whereas the former situations resulted in the corticosterone level being at least double that observed in resting, unstressed rats.

Reference

Leonard, B. E. (1987) Ethanol as a neurotoxin. *Biochem. Pharmacol.* 36: 2055–2059.

G.J. Boer, M.G.P. Feenstra, M. Mirmiran, D.F. Swaab and F. Van Haaren
Progress in Brain Research, Vol. 73
© 1988 Elsevier Science Publishers B.V. (Biomedical Division)

CHAPTER 21

Prenatal stress effects on functional development of the offspring

Marta Weinstock, Ester Fride and Raya Hertzberg

Department of Pharmacology, The Hebrew University-Hadassah Medical School, Jerusalem, Israel

Introduction

In the past few decades it has become increasingly clear that the development and later behaviour of an immature organism is not only determined by genetic factors and the postnatal environment, but also by the maternal environment during gestation (Joffe, 1969). This in turn is influenced by drugs, disease, nutrition and stressful life events (Joffe, 1978; Swaab and Mirmiran, 1984). This review is concerned with the effects of maternal psychological stress on the development and behaviour of the offspring. The term 'psychological stress' is used to denote situations which, although not physically harmful in terms of causing direct tissue damage, evoke behavioural and physiological responses which are characteristic of the 'stress' response (Selye, 1955). These include new, intense or rapidly changing environmental conditions, sudden or unexpected events, as well as those from which there is no escape or over which the organism has no control (Appley and Trumbell, 1967).

Early reports that prenatal psychological stress in human subjects may influence the behaviour of the offspring prompted a large number of studies in experimental animals in an attempt to provide more precise information about the nature of the changes induced by such stress and their underlying mechanisms. Many of the methodological problems inherent in the design of these early

experiments are discussed in an excellent review by Archer and Blackman (1971). Although the conclusion from this review is that gestational stress of different types is likely to have an influence on offspring behaviour, its nature and direction are inconsistent. From these and later studies it became clear that the irreproducibility of the findings was often due to failure to control for the litter variable (Chapman and Stern, 1979) and of a number of other important factors in the experimental design. These include the type of behavioural test on the offspring, which in turn should be dictated by the nature of the changes expected; the maternal environment at the time of stress; the intensity of stress; its timing and frequency throughout gestation, in relation to critical stages of foetal development; the reaction of the hippocampo-hypothalamo-hypophyseal-adrenal (HPA) systems of the mother and foetus to the stressor. In the absence of any direct neural connections between the mother and foetus it has been postulated that hormones (e.g., glucocorticoids, adrenaline) transported from the maternal blood to the placenta are the most likely mediators (Joffe, 1978).

Several more recent clinical studies on pre- and perinatal stress have indicated that a number of fairly consistent abnormalities occur in the children. Even allowing for the differences in the development patterns and behavioural complexities in human and rodent species, the design of experiments on the latter could be more closely modelled on the clinical findings than they have been in the past.

The influence of prenatal stress on human development and behaviour

All these studies have of necessity been retrospective in nature, thereby posing their own methodological and interpretational difficulties. We have chosen three different approaches to the problem, in which some attempt has been made to control for other factors that could influence the findings. In none of them however can postnatal factors be excluded.

The first of these types of prenatal stress is the effect of unpredictable noise, such as that experienced by residence in close proximity to an airport. Unlike traffic noise, habituation does not usually occur to this disturbance because of its irregular and unforseeable nature. It thus provides a continuous irritation, accompanied by physiological and endocrinological reactions (Battig et al., 1980). The psychological effects of this stressor have been demonstrated in reports of feelings of helplessness. This includes a decrease in motivation to initiate new responses and an increase in aggression and irritability (Cohen et al., 1980).

Noise has been shown to increase the incidence of low birth weight, congenital malformations and sleep disturbances in the infants (Jones and Tauscher, 1978; Knipschild et al., 1981; Schell, 1981). Since the infants usually continued to live and develop in this environment, one cannot conclude whether any subsequent behavioural abnormalities that have been reported, such as social apprehension, anxiety in the face of threatened peer aggression and fear of novelty (Sontag, 1970) are due only to gestational factors. A direct effect of noise on the developing foetus can also not be ruled out (Sontag, 1970).

A different approach, described by Stott (1973), was to assess infant morbidity in a randomly selected population and relate this to pregnancy conditions, without prior preconceptions. This study demonstrated a highly significant correlation between infant morbidity and maternal stress in the form of interpersonal tensions and discord, usually with the husband and or close family members. The psychological stress induced was described as "continuous or liable to disrupt at any time and incapable of resolution either by action or adjusting to it". Infant morbidity included eczema, bronchitis and other respiratory problems, poor growth, pale colour, swallowing difficulties, late physical development, e.g. walking, and speech defects. There was also a higher incidence of early behavioural problems in these infants who were described as restless, clinging, hyperactive and exhibiting habit disorders, such as prolonged incontinence. This particular study did not investigate the behaviour in older childhood or adolescence of these infants, but another study by this author showed the incidence of behavioural disturbance to be 2.5–3-times higher in mentally retarded children in whom there was clear evidence of prenatal stress (Stott, 1959).

The third study, compared the early development and childhood behaviour of boys born to mothers who were pregnant during the threat and occurrence of the 6-Day Arab-Israeli War in 1967, with those born in a similar socioeconomic background, 1–2 years later (Meier, 1985). As in the previous studies, the author found significant delays in development, walking, speech and toilet training and several behavioural differences. The prenatally stressed children were described as antisocial, tense, regressive, easily irritated and inconsiderate to their peers.

In each of these three studies, the mothers were in aversive situations from which there was no escape or over which they had no control. Adaptation of the organism is much less likely to occur under such conditions (Quirce et al., 1981; Swenson and Vogel, 1983; Muir and Pfister, 1986) and, as such, they may be expected to be potentially more harmful. The most consistent effects of these and other prenatal stressors on the children was found to be a reduction in birth weight and development rate and in the potential adaptability to the demands of the environment.

Experimental maternal stressors in rodents

The original study of Thompson (1957) subjected the rat dam to an almost pure form of psychological stress. The rat was given a warning stimulus which it had previously learned to associate with impending electric shock but from which it could not escape. This situation is reminiscent of those described earlier in the clinical studies. Moreover, clear physiological signs of anxiety, pilo-erection and excessive defecation were present during testing. This type of gestational stress, in which both the conditioned and unconditioned stimulus were present either before or during pregnancy, or both, has been employed in many later studies (Archer and Blackman, 1971; Masterpasqua et al., 1976; Pollard, 1984).

Another form of prenatal stress often used is crowding of the pregnant dams, either by placing many of them together in a cage (Keeley, 1962) or alone with a number of aggressive males (Dahloff et al., 1977, 1978; Moore and Power, 1986). The latter is considered a more stressful condition since it resulted in severe disruption in maternal behaviour (Archer and Blackman, 1971). This in itself can strongly influence the development and behaviour of the offspring.

A more severe form of stress (as judged by the intensity of the reaction of the dam) from which there is also no escape and which has often been used, is restraint, usually at elevated external temperatures (Barlow et al., 1978; Chapman and Stern, 1979; Ward and Weisz, 1984; Kinsley and Svare, 1986). Although this form of stress has been shown to produce physical changes in the rats (e.g., marked weight loss) its effects will be considered in this review in comparison to those induced by the other stressors.

In all of these experiments the dam was removed from the home cage in order to inflict the stress. Hutchings and Gibbon (1970) suggested that this may be a crucial variable in prenatal stress studies as it disrupts the contact of the mother with her nesting site. Since they found no difference in the behaviour of the offspring from mothers who were only handled (removed to another cage) and those given conditioned avoidance training with electric shocks, they suggested that any subsequent treatment after the removal of the dam is probably irrelevant.

In our experiments we attempted to overcome this difficulty by allowing the pregnant dams to remain in their home cages throughout stress application. In order to confirm that it was the unpredictability of aircraft noise that was the major disruptive element in human prenatal stress, we compared the effects of noise (90–100 db) applied randomly in an irregular manner throughout pregnancy with that given an equal number of times on a regular daily basis during the last trimester (Fride and Weinstock, 1984).

Many of the differences in the influence of prenatal stress on the offspring behaviour, particularly in the earlier studies could probably be accounted for by failure to control for the litter variable. In the majority of them all the pups from three to five stressed and control dams were used, thereby constricting the error variance and substantially increasing their degrees of freedom (Abbey and Howard, 1973). This is well illustrated in a study by Chapman and Stern (1979), who found that the significant effect on open field behaviour in prenatally stressed rats was no longer present when the litter variable was controlled.

In an attempt to determine whether the effects of gestational stress are mediated prenatally or are due to different rearing by a previously stressed mother, several investigators have used a fostering design. Although in many studies it could be demonstrated that most of the effect on the pup was due to prenatal factors (Archer and Blackman, 1971; Barlow et al., 1978; Fride et al., 1986) there were some differences if the prenatally-stressed pups were reared by control or stressed mothers (Joffe, 1969; Thompson and Grusec,

1970; Fride et al., 1986) and vice versa. Dams stressed while pregnant gave more attention to their pups (Muir and Pfister, 1984), and prenatally stressed pups elicited less stimulation (anogenital licking) from unstressed foster dams than did control pups (Moore and Power, 1986). Therefore it appears that cross-fostering does not eliminate the possibility that altered maternal stimulation may mediate some prenatal stress effects.

Effect of prenatal stress on maternal glucocorticoid release

In the majority of previous studies, stress was applied either daily throughout pregnancy, or only during the last trimester (Archer and Blackman, 1971; Peters, 1986). In one study, it was given for shorter periods during each trimester but always on at least three consecutive days (Barlow et al., 1978). Each of the stressors described above including handling, has been shown to cause a release of glucocorticoids when the animal is first subjected to it (Seggie and Brown, 1975; Smith and Gala, 1977; Hennessy and Levine, 1978; Armario et al., 1986). Corticosterone readily reaches the foetal circulation from the maternal blood (Zarrow et al., 1970) and can interact with specific receptors in the developing brain, lung and liver, (Giannopoulos, 1975; de Kloet, 1984). The ability of a given tissue to respond to glucocorticoids may be present long before the normal ontogenic response occurs. Moreover, the biological end-point of the response may differ at different stages of maturation (Giannopoulos, 1975). For example, glucocorticoids can retard foetal lung development if given before a critical day (Torday et al., 1986) but stimulate it when given at a later date or vice versa depending upon the species (Liggins and Howie, 1972; Anderson et al., 1981).

It is known that adaptation of the HPA axis occurs to some forms of stress, particularly when this occurs in a regular manner in non-pregnant animals (Pfister and King, 1976; File, 1982), but not to others (Wong et al., 1982; Kant et al.,

1983; Gamallo et al., 1986). It is therefore possible that maternal hormone release may no longer occur in response to some stressors after repetition. If such adaptation of the maternal HPA axis has taken place before a critical phase of foetal organ maturation occurs, one may not see any alteration in physical development or behaviour. This possibility has not been systematically studied and only a few investigators have measured plasma hormonal levels in pregnant dams and their foetuses during the last week of gestation after repeated application of the stressor.

Plasma corticosterone (CORT) levels were still very high on the last day of pregnancy in two studies in which restraint stress was applied to the dam daily, either from day 14 of gestation (Ward and Weisz, 1984) or from day 18 (Barlow et al., 1978), and on day 19, after the rats had been handled and injected with saline from the first day of pregnancy (Peters, 1986). These findings indicated that adaptation to these stressors had not occurred.

However, when noise stress (90–100 db) (Fride and Weinstock, 1984) was given on a regular daily basis from day 15 of gestation (daily late pregnancy stress, DLS) the rats appeared to have become completely habituated by the third exposure as plasma CORT did not rise above control values. In contrast, when the same

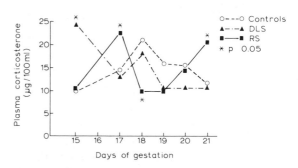

Fig. 1 Plasma corticosterone levels in pregnant dams subjected to noise stress on a daily or random basis throughout pregnancy. (O‒‒O) Controls. (▲‒·‒▲) Daily stress from day 14–21. (■‒■) Random stress from days 1–12. *$P < 0.05$ vs control. Values represent the mean ± S.E.M. from six to ten dams for each treatment per day.

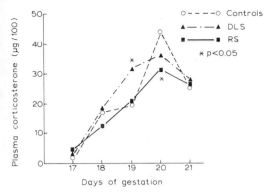

Fig. 2 Plasma corticosterone levels in foetuses of pregnant dams subjected to noise stress on a random or daily basis throughout pregnancy. For legends see Fig. 1. *P < 0.05 vs control. Values represent mean ± S.E.M. from six to ten litters for each treatment per day.

stressor was applied an equal number of times but on a random, unpredictable basis, three times weekly throughout pregnancy (random stress, RS), a completely different pattern of maternal plasma CORT levels emerged during the last week of pregnancy (see Fig. 1). Corticosterone was significantly elevated on days 17 and 21 but abnormally low on day 18 of gestation.

The two noise stress schedules also produced different patterns in foetal plasma CORT (see Fig. 2). As in previous studies (Milkovic et al., 1973; Chatelain et al., 1980) levels rose sharply from day 17 to a peak on day 20 and then declined. In DLS foetuses CORT levels appeared to peak one day earlier than in controls, while those in RS foetuses showed a more gradual rise, reaching somewhat lower peak levels on day 20. These findings demonstrate that the maternal and foetal response to gestational stress differed according to the nature of the stress, the timing of its application and whether it was given regularly or on a random basis.

Effect of prenatal stress on early physical development

In spite of the fact that several studies on the effects of prenatal stress in humans have shown a reduction in the birth weights and early physical development of the children, few investigators have looked for changes in the later parameter in experimental animals. The results of some of these studies are summarized in Table 1. In five different experiments in which the dam was restrained or immobilized, the weight of the pups was reduced at birth or at day 7 of age. In all these studies a significant reduction also occurred in maternal body weight and food intake. Offspring body weight was not reduced by a variety of other stress procedures, including a milder form of restraint (Rojo et al., 1985) or chronic maternal ACTH administration and was even increased after maternal crowding (Dahlof et al., 1978).

Significant delays in ear opening and in the development of the auditory startle response occurred after restraint of the dam for 9 hours daily on days 12–14, 15–17 or 18–20, and motor function was also retarded, particularly after stress on the later days of pregnancy (Barlow et al., 1978).

Fride and Weinstock (1984) compared the effects of noise and light stress applied either daily throughout pregnancy (DS), randomly, three times weekly throughout pregnancy (RS) or daily, from day 14–21 (DLS) on the development of a number of dynamic postural adjustments during the first 2 weeks of life. Pups from RS mothers showed an overall delay in the appearance of motor activities such as the righting reflex, cliff avoidance and walking on an inclined plane, compared to pups from control mothers. In contrast, DLS pups developed more quickly in all these tests, while the DS pups did not differ significantly from controls. The maturation of more complex co-ordination as assessed by swimming ability (Schapiro et al., 1970) was also delayed in RS pups and accelerated in DLS pups. These findings demonstrate that, as in humans, a form of unpredictable stress from which the rat dam could not escape resulted in significant delays in physical and motor development. They also show that the same type of maternal stress can either increase or delay the rate of maturation of early

TABLE 1

Effect of prenatal stress on early development

Authors	Stressor	Timing (days)	Body wt. of pup	Development of male sexual organs	Motor development
Anderson, 1985	restraint	14–21	↓[a]	↓	–
Barlow, 1978	restraint	15–17	↓[a]	–	↓
Barlow, 1978	restraint	18–20	↓[a]	–	↓
Kinsley and Svare, 1986	restraint	13–18	↓[a]	–	–
Chapman and Stern, 1979	restraint (+)	14–21	0	–	–
Dahloff et al., 1978	restraint	14–21	↓	↓	–
Moore and Power, 1986	crowding (+)	1–21	0	↓	–
Dahloff et al., 1978	crowding	14–21	↑	↓	–
Fride and Weinstock, 1984	noise (+)	14–21	0	–	↑
Fride and Weinstock, 1988	noise (+)	1–21	0	–	↓

[a] Weight of mother decreased by stress. +, controlled for litter variable; ↓ decreased; ↑ increased; 0 unchanged; – not measured.

motor behaviour of the offspring according to the timing of its application. More severe stressors, such as restraint, retard growth rate and physical development, possibly due to a marked reduction in maternal food intake (Kinsley and Svare, 1986).

The development of male sexual organs and activity was delayed or impaired by several forms of maternal stress. Restraint from days 14–21 caused a significant reduction in the testes weight and anogenital distance at birth (Dahloff et al., 1978), while crowding only decreased anogenital distance (Dahloff et al., 1978; Moore and Power, 1986). Restraint stress also reduced by about 50% the area of the sexual dimorphic nucleus in the preoptic area of the hypothalamus (SDA-POA) in male but not female offspring (Anderson, 1985). This form of stress has been found to feminize male sexual behaviour at adulthood (Ward, 1972, 1984). Similar abnormalities in male sexual development and behaviour can be induced by maternal treatment with opiates (Badway et al., 1981; Ward et al., 1983), suggesting that they may be mediated by excess foetal opiodergic activity induced by stress (Lim and Funder,

1983). Evidence in favour of such a suggestion has recently been provided by Ward et al. (1986) who found that maternal treatment with naltrexone, an opioid receptor antagonist, during the last week of gestation, could prevent the adverse effects of prenatal stress on male sexual development and behaviour. Since many of the physical parameters described above were measured at birth or soon after, it is likely that they were mediated by prenatal factors.

The effect of prenatal stress on open field behaviour of offspring

In the vast majority of studies in rodents, investigators tested offspring for ambulatory activity in some form of open field apparatus (Archer and Blackman, 1971; Joffe, 1978). Less frequently the number of faecal pellets deposited or the incidence of defecation was also recorded. Together, these measures have been accepted as denoting an alteration in emotionality (Hall, 1934; Archer, 1973). If locomotor activity is decreased and defecation increased, the animal is considered to be more 'emotional' than the control.

Table 2

The effect of prenatal stress on open field behaviour

Authors	Stressor	Strain of rat	Timing in days	Open field measures	
				Ambulation	Defecation
Thompson, 1957	conditioned avoidance training	LE	1–21	↓	↑
Thompson et al., 1962	conditioned avoidance training	LE	1–21	↓	↑
Thompson et al., 1982	conditioned avoidance training	SD	1–21	↑	↓
Hutchings and Gibbon, 1970	conditioned avoidance training	SD	14–20	↑	↓
Hutchings and Gibbon, 1970	conditioned avoidance training	SD	7–13	↑	↓
Masterpasqua et al., 1976	conditioned avoidance training	SD	5–21	↑	↓
Moore and Power, 1986	overcrowding (+)	LE	1–21	0	0
Meisel et al., 1979	restraint	SD	14–21	0	0
Chapman and Stern, 1979	restraint (+)	SD		0	0
Rojo et al., 1985	mild restraint (+)	W	1–21	0	0
Peters, 1982	handling	SD	1–21	↑	↓
Hutchings and Gibbon, 1970	handling	SD	14–20	↑	↓
Ader and Plaut, 1968	handling	CR	1–21	0	↓

↓ decreased; ↑ increased; 0 unchanged; + controlled for litter variable; LE, Long Evans; SD, Sprague-Dawley; CR, Charles Rivers; W, Wistar.

Table 2 summarizes some examples of the influence of different gestational stressors in various rat strains on open field behaviour. Emotionality was increased in the offspring in two studies by Thompson et al. (1962) using the stress paradigm of conditioned avoidance previously described in Long-Evans rats but not in Sprague-Dawleys. In most other experiments there was either no change or an increase in ambulation, particularly in the male offspring. There are several possible reasons for these discrepancies. Estimates of the total amount of locomotion in the open field can encompass different types of functionally unrelated activities such as exploration or rapid movement induced by fear (Archer and Blackman, 1971). In general, females display greater locomotion and less defecation than males (Blizzard et al., 1975). Several forms of prenatal stress, restraint (Ward, 1972; Meisel et al., 1979), crowding and conditioned avoidance testing (Dahlof et al., 1977; Masterpasqua et al., 1976) have all been found to decrease sexual activity in males, often inducing feminine (lordotic) be-

haviour. An inverse correlation was found between the decrease in male sexual activity and the degree of locomotion in the open field (Masterpasqua et al., 1976). Thus an increase in open field locomotion may also represent an alteration to a more feminine pattern of behaviour.

Reactivity of the hypothalamic-hypophyseal-adrenal axis of prenatally stressed rats

It is possible that maternal pituitary-adrenal hormones reaching the foetal hippocampus at a critical time during development can cause permanent alterations in the reactivity of the HPA axis (Sapolsky et al., 1984). This in turn may result in changes in behaviour, particularly under stressful conditions.

In a few studies, the response of the HPA-axis in adult prenatally stressed offspring to stress has been assessed by measuring the rise in plasma CORT. No consistent effect of gestational stress has emerged from these studies. Daily conditioned avoidance training (Pollard, 1984) or handling of the pregnant dams (Ader and Plaut, 1968) resulted in smaller increases in plasma CORT levels in the offspring of both sexes or in females only when subjected to mild forms of stress. When combined with saline injections, handling of the dams produced a greater response in the offspring after stress than in controls (Peters, 1982).

The noise stress procedure resulted in either an exaggerated or diminished response of the offspring HPA system to stress according to the timing of its application to the dam (Fig. 3). The male offspring of rats stressed randomly throughout pregnancy (RS) responded with a greater increase in plasma CORT after the first and subsequent eight exposures to the open field than controls, and there was no indication of adaptation as CORT levels remained at peak levels throughout. Offspring of both sexes of daily stressed dams (DLS) (females not shown) showed smaller increases in CORT levels than the control and a more rapid adaptation to the novelty stress (Sadeh, 1986).

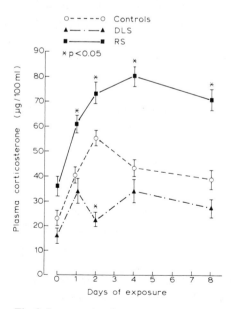

Fig. 3 Increase in plasma corticosterone in response to repeated open field exposure in prenatally stressed male offspring. For legends see Fig. 1. *$P < 0.05$ vs control. Values represent mean $\pm$ S.E.M. from six to ten pups from different litters for each exposure.

The hippocampus plays a major role in habituation to novelty and the regulation of the response to stressful stimuli (Isaacson, 1974). Both neonatal cortisol injection (Douglas, 1975) and the random stress paradigm resulted in a significant delay in the development of spontaneous alternation (SA) behaviour (Fride et al., 1986) which has been linked to hippocampal function. In contrast, pups of DLS mothers showed normal development of SA behaviour (Fride, 1986). The impaired response of the HPA system of RS offspring to novelty stress and its poor adaptation may be an expression of a permanent alteration in hippocampal function caused by exposure in utero to high levels of maternal corticosterone during a critical period, e.g., days 17 or 21 of gestation (Fig. 1). High levels of glucocorticoids in the developing foetus or neonate may be able to reduce the number of specific steroid binding sites in the hippocampus (Turner and Taylor, 1976; Sapolsky et al., 1984; Wood and Rudolph, 1984). If such an effect lasts into adulthood it may impair the negative feedback regulation by glucocorticoids on the hippocampus.

Coping behaviour of prenatally stressed rats

Examination of the clinical findings among children of prenatally stressed mothers revealed signs of maladaptation to novelty, poor social interaction, impaired ability to perform routine problems and heightened anxiety in the face of potential aggression (Meier, 1985; Sontag, 1970). In the majority of studies on the behaviour of prenatally stressed animals, the open field (novelty stress) has been the test employed to assess reactivity or emotionality. In order to increase the anxiety of water maze learning, Thompson et al. (1962) applied electric shocks to the offspring of prenatally stressed and control rats and found that the learning rate was significantly slower in the former. It is interesting to note that these same rats showed increased locomotor activity and normal defecation in the open field, further illustrating the lack of specificity of the latter test. In our studies, using the noise-stress paradigm of daily or random application, we have used a number of behavioural measures which were specifically designed to determine whether prenatally stressed rats are less able to cope with normal life-sustaining behaviours if these are performed in anxiety-provoking situations.

The first of these involved the assessment of maternal behaviour (pup retrieval) in the female offspring of prenatally stressed rats. Under normal conditions, in which the dam had to return her pups to the home cage after passing through a 60 cm alley, both DLS and RS females performed as controls. However, when an airstream (mildly aversive for rats) was directed onto the alley, almost 50% of RS females failed to return their pups and the rest took significantly longer than the controls to do so (Fride et al., 1985). In contrast, DLS mothers all returned their pups like the controls, in spite of the presence of the airstream (Sadeh, 1986).

In another experiment, male and female offspring of RS mothers were trained to run down an alley for food reward. Following acquisition, the animals were given punishment trials in which shocks (0.3 mA, 0.5 ms) was delivered to the floor of the goal section in addition to the food reward. The experimental animals of both sexes inhibited their food seeking response more quickly than controls in the face of punishment (Fride et al., 1986).

Because of the lack of a clear interpretation of the open field behaviour, we used a more selective test of timidity, based on the natural aversion of rodents for open spaces (Briley et al., 1985; Pellow and File, 1986). When 6 months of age RS and DLS offspring and their respective controls were placed for 10 min in a 'plus maze'. This consisted of two arms which were enclosed by 40 cm high walls and two perpendicular arms without walls. The time spent in open arms has been shown to be inversely proportional to the level of anxiety and is selectively increased by antianxiety agents (Pellow and File, 1986). The results of this experiment are shown in Fig. 4.

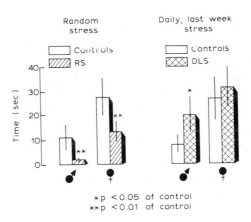

Fig. 4 Time spent by prenatally stressed pups in open arms of plus maze.

Both male and female RS offspring spent significantly less time than controls in the open arms, while the DLS males spent more time there. This showed that the random stress paradigm increased fearfulness in the face of novelty, while the daily stress decreased it. These experiments taken together with those described in the preceding sections demonstrate unequivocally that gestational stress can significantly alter the ability of the offspring to cope with anxiety-provoking situations at adulthood.

Further experiments are required to determine whether other forms of prenatal psychological stress are able to alter the coping behaviour of the offspring in this way and whether the outcome is so critically dependent on the timing of the stress.

Conclusions

The nature of the effect of prenatal stress on early physical development and later behaviour appears to depend upon genetic factors, the severity of the stress and its timing. These in turn determine whether abnormal maternal and foetal hormonal and neuronal activity will occur at a critical period of foetal development. Severe forms of gestational stress, e.g., restraint, result in a significant maternal and foetal weight loss. Physical development in both sexes is slowed and sexual activity in males is impaired. This is associated with decreased testosterone levels which may result from excess foetal opioid activity.

Milder forms of stress, handling, crowding or noise, presented from day 14 of gestation or earlier, either have no effect on physical development or accelerate it; adaptation of HPA response to stress occurs more rapidly and timidity or emotionality in novel environments is reduced. In contrast, the same stress presented in an unpredictable manner, retards physical and hippocampal development. At adulthood, stress adaptation is slowed and life sustaining behaviours are easily disrupted under conflict conditions.

References

Abbey, H. and Howard, E. (1973) Statistical procedure in developmental studies on species and multiple offspring. *Dev. Psychobiol.*, 6: 329–335.

Ader, R. and Plaut, S.M. (1968) Effects of prenatal maternal handling and differential housing on offspring emotionality, plasma corticosterone levels and susceptibility to gastric erosion. *Psychosom. Med.*, 30: 277–286.

Anderson, D.K. (1985) Effects of prenatal stress on the differentiation of the sexually dimorphic nucleus of the preoptic area (SDN-POA) of the rat brain. *Brain Res.*, 332: 113–118.

Anderson, G.C., Lamden, M.P., Cidlowski, J.A. and Ashikaga (1981) Comparative pulmonary surfactant-inducing effect of three corticosteroids in the near term infant. *Am. J. Obstet. Gynec.*, 139: 562–564.

Appley, M.H. and Trumbull, R. (1967) On the concept of psychological stress. In M.H. Apply and R. Trumbull (Eds.) *Psychological Stress: Issues in Research*. Appleton-Century Crofts, New York, pp. 1–14.

Archer, J.E. (1973) Tests for emotionality in rats and mice: A review. *Anim. Behav.*, 21: 205–235.

Archer, J.E. and Blackman, D.E. (1971) Prenatal psychological stress and offspring behavior in rats and mice. *Develop. Psychobiol.*, 4: 193–248.

Armario, A., Montero, J.L. and Balasch, J. (1986) Sensitivity of corticosterone and some metabolic variables to graded levels of low intensity stresses in adult male rats. *Physiol. Behav.*, 37: 559–561.

Badway, D., Orth, J. and Weisz, J. (1981) Effect of morphine on $\Delta^5 3\beta$-OL steroid dehydrogenase (3βOHD) in Leydig cells of fetal rats: a quantitative cytochemical study. *Anat. Rec.*, 199: 15a.

Barlow, S.M., Knight, A.F. and Sullivan, F.M. (1978) Delay in postnatal growth and development of offspring produced by maternal restraint stress during pregnancy in the rat. *Teratology*, 18: 211–218.

Battig, K., Zeier, H., Muller, R. and Buzzi, R. (1980) A field study on vegetative effects of aircraft noise. *Arch. Environ. Hlth.*, 35: 228–235.

Blizzard, D.A., Lippman, H.R. and Chen, J.J. (1975) Sex differences in open-field behavior in the rat: the inductive and activational role of gonadal hormones. *Physiol. Behav.*, 14: 601–608.

Briley, M., Chopin, P., File, S.E. and Pellow, S. (1985) Validation of a test of anxiety in the rat based on exploratory activity in a plus-maze. *Br. J. Pharmacol.*, 86: 456P.

Chapman, R.H. and Stern, J.M. (1979) Failure of severe maternal stress or ACTH during pregnancy to affect emotionality of male rat offspring. Implications of litter effects for prenatal studies. *Dev. Psychobiol.*, 12: 255–267.

Chatelain, A., Dupouy, J.P. and Allaume, P. (1980) Fetal-maternal adrenocorticotropin and corticosterone relationships in the rat: effects of maternal adrenalectomy. *Endocrinology*, 106: 1297–1303.

Cohen, S., Evans, G.W., Krantz, D.S. and Stokols, D. (1980) Physiological, motivational and cognitive effects of aircraft noise on children. *Am. Psychologist*, 35: 231–243.

Dahlof, L.-G., Hard, E. and Larsson, K. (1977) Influence of maternal stress on offspring sexual behaviour. *Anim. Behav.*, 25: 958–963.

Dahlof, L.-G., Hard, E. and Larsson, K. (1978) Influence of maternal stress on the development of the fetal genital system. *Physiol. Behav.*, 20: 193–195.

Douglas, R.J. (1975) The development of hippocampal function. In R.L. Isaacson (Ed.) *The Hippocampus, Vol. 1*, Plenum Press, New York, pp. 327–361.

File, S.E. (1982) The rat corticosterone response: habituation and modification by chlordiazepoxide. *Physiol. Behav.*, 29: 91–95.

Fride, E. (1986) Effects of prenatal noise and light stress on behavioural and neurochemical functions during development and at adulthood in the rat. Ph.D. Thesis. Hebrew University, Jerusalem, Israel.

Fride, E., Dan, Y., Feldon, J., Halevy, G. and Weinstock, M. (1986) Effects of prenatal stress in prepubertal and adult rats. *Physiol. Behav.*, 37: 681–687.

Fride, E., Dan, Y., Gavish, M. and Weinstock, M. (1985) Prenatal stress impairs maternal behaviour in a conflict situation and reduces hippocampal benzodiazepine receptors. *Life Sci.*, 36: 2103–2109.

Fride, E., Soreq, H. and Weinstock, M. (1986b) Are the effects of gestational stress on motor development and cerebellar cholinesterase activity mediated prenatally? *Int. J. Dev. Neuroscience*, 4: 407–413.

Fride, E. and Weinstock, M. (1984) The effects of prenatal exposure to predictable or unpredictable stress on early development in the rat. *Dev. Psychobiol.*, 17: 651–660.

Gamallo, A., Villanua, A., Trancho, G. and Fraile, A. (1986) Stress adaptation and adrenal activity in isolated and crowded rats. *Physiol. Behav.*, 36: 217–221.

Giannopoulos, G. (1975) Early events in the action of glucocorticoids in developing tissues. *J. Steroid Biochem.*, 6: 623–631.

Hall, C. S. (1934) Emotional behavior in the rat. I. Defecation and urination as measures of individual differences in emotionality. *J. Comp. Psychol.*, 18: 385–403.

Hennessy, M. B. and Levine, S. (1978) Sensitive pituitary-adrenal responsiveness to varying intensities of psychological stimulation. *Physiol. Behav.*, 21: 295–297.

Hutchings, D. E. and Gibbon, J. (1970) Preliminary study of behavioral and teratogenic effects of two stress procedures administered during different periods of gestation in the rat. *Psychol. Rep.*, 26: 239–246.

Isaacson, R. L. (1974) The hippocampus. In: *The Limbic System*. New York, Plenum Press, pp. 161–218.

Joffe, J. M. (1969) *Prenatal Determinants of Behaviour*. Oxford, Pergamon Press.

Joffe, J. M. (1978) Hormonal mediation of the effects of prenatal stress on offspring behavior. In G. Gottlieb (Ed.), *Studies on the Development of Behavior and the Nervous System: Early Influences, Vol. 4*, Acad. Press, New York, pp. 108–144.

Jones, F. N. and Tauscher, J. (1978) Residence under an airport landing pattern as a factor in teratism. *Arch. Environ. Health*, 33: 10–12.

Kant, G. J., Bunnell, B. N., Mougey, E. H., Pennington, L. L. and Meyerhoff, J. L. (1983) Effects of repeated stress on pituitary cyclic AMP, and plasma prolactin, corticosterone and growth hormone in male rats. *Pharmacol. Biochem. Behav.*, 18: 967–971.

Keeley, K. (1962) Prenatal influence on behaviour of offspring of crowded mice. *Science*, 135: 44–45.

Kinsley, C. and Svare, B. (1986) Prenatal stress effects: are they mediated by reductions in maternal food and water intake and by body weight gain? *Physiol. Behav.*, 37: 191–193.

de Kloet, E. R. (1984) Adrenal steroids as modulators of nerve cell function. *J. Steroid Biochem.*, 20: 175–181.

Knipschild, P., Meier, H. and Salle, H. (1981) Aircraft noise and birth weight. *Int. Arch. Occup. Environ. Health*, 48: 131–136.

Liggins, G. C. and Howie, R. N. (1972) A controlled trial of antepartum glucocorticoid treatment for prevention of the respiratory distress syndrome in premature infants. *Pediatrics*, 50: 515–525.

Lim, A. T. W. and Funder, J. W. (1983) Stress-induced changes in plasma, pituitary and hypothalamic immunoreactive β-endorphin: Effects of diurnal variation, adrenalectomy corticosteroids and opiate agonists and antagonists. *Neuroendocrinology*, 36: 225–234.

Masterpasqua, F., Chapman, R. H. and Lore, R. K. (1976) The effects of prenatal psychological stress on the sexual behavior and reactivity of male rats. *Dev. Psychobiol.*, 9: 403–411.

Meier, A. (1985) Child psychiatric sequelae of maternal war stress. *Acta Psychiatr. Scand.*, 72: 505–511.

Meisel, R. L., Dohanich, G. P. and Ward, I. (1979) Effects of prenatal stress of avoidance acquisition on open field performance and lordotic behaviour in male rats. *Physiol. Behav.*, 22: 527–531.

Milkovic, S., Milkovic, K. and Pannovic, J. (1973) The initiation of fetal adrenocorticotrophic activity in the rat. *Endocrinology*, 92: 380–384.

Moore, C. L. and Power, K. L. (1986) Prenatal stress affects mother-infant interaction in Norway rats. *Dev. Psychobiol.*, 19: 235–245.

Muir, J. L. and Pfister, H. P. (1984) Effects of prenatal stress and postnatal enrichment on mother-infant interactions and problem-solving ability in rats. Presented at *Int. Soc. for Develop. Psychobiol.*, Oct. 1984. Baltimore, MD USA.

Muir, J. L. and Pfister, H. P. (1986) Corticosterone and prolactin responses to predictable and unpredictable novelty stress in rats. *Physiol. Behav.*, 37: 285–288.

Pellow, S. and File, S. E. (1986) Anxiolytic and anxiogenic drug effects on exploratory activity in an elevated plus-maze: a novel test of anxiety in the rat. *Pharmacol. Biochem. Behav.*, 24: 525–529.

Peters, D. A. V. (1982) Prenatal stress: effects on brain biogenic amine and plasma corticosterone levels. *Pharmacol. Biochem. Behav.*, 17: 721–725.

Peters, D. A. V. (1986) Prenatal stress: Effect on development of rat brain serotoninergic neurones. *Pharmacol. Biochem. Behav.*, 24: 1377–1382.

Pfister, H. P. and King, M. G. (1976) Adaptation of glucocorticosterone response to novelty. *Physiol. Behav.*, 17: 43–46.

Pollard, I. (1984) Effects of stress administered during pregnancy on reproductive capacity and subsequent development of the offspring of rats: prolonged effects on the litter of a second pregnancy. *J. Endocrinol.*, 100: 301–306.

Quirce, C. M., Odio, M. and Solano, J. M. (1981) The effects of predictable and unpredictable schedules of physical restraint upon rats. *Life Sci.*, 28: 1897–1902.

Rojo, M., Marin, B. and Menendez-Patterson, A. (1985) Effects of low stress during pregnancy on certain parameters of the offspring. *Physiol. Behav.*, 34: 895–899.

Sadeh, M. (1986) The influence of gestational stress of the rat on behaviour of its offspring at adulthood. M. Sc. Thesis. Hebrew University, Jerusalem, Israel.

Sapolsky, R. M., Krey, L. C. and McEwen, B. S. (1984) Stress down-regulates corticosterone receptors in a site specific manner in the brain. *Endocrinology*, 114: 287–292.

Shapiro, S., Salas, M. and Vukovich, K. (1970) Hormonal effects on ontogeny of swimming ability in the rat: assessment of central nervous system development. *Science*, 168: 147–150.

330

Schell, L.M. (1981) Environmental noise and human pre-natal growth. *Am. J. Physiol. Anthropol.*, 56: 63–70.

Seggie, J.A. and Brown, G.M. (1975) Stress response patterns of plasma corticosterone, prolactin, and growth hormone in the rat, following handling or exposure to a novel environment. *Can. J. Physiol. Pharmacol.*, 53: 629–637.

Seyle, H. (1955) Stress and disease. *Science*, 122: 625–631.

Smith, W.W. and Gala, R.R. (1972) Influence of restraint on plasma prolactin and corticosterone in female rats. *J. Endocrinol.*, 74: 303–314.

Sontag, L.W. (1970) Effect of noise during pregnancy upon foetal and subsequent adult behaviour. In B.L. Welch and A.S. Welch (Eds.), *Physiological Effects of Noise*, Plenum Press, New York, pp. 131–141.

Stott, D.N. (1959) Evidence for prenatal impairment of temperament in mentally-retarded children. *Vita Humana*, 2: 125–148.

Stott, D.N. (1973) Follow-up study from birth of the effects of prenatal stress. *Dev. Med. Child Neurol.*, 15: 770–787.

Swaab, D.F. and Mirmiran, M. (1984) Possible mechanisms underlying the teratogenic effects of medicines on the developing brain. In J. Yanai (Ed.), *Neurobehavioural Toxicology*, Elsevier, Amsterdam, pp. 55–71.

Swenson, R.M. and Vogel, W.H. (1983) Plasma catecholamine and corticosterone as well as brain catecholamine changes during coping in rats exposed to stressful footshock. *Pharmacol. Biochem. Behav.*, 18: 689–693.

Thompson, W.R. (1957) Influence of prenatal maternal anxiety on emotionality in young rats. *Science*, 15: 698–699.

Thompson, W.R., Watson, J. and Charlesworth, W.K. (1962) The effects of prenatal maternal stress on offspring behavior in rats. *Psychol. Med. Monogr.*, 76: 1–26.

Thompson, W.R. and Grusec, J. (1970) Studies of early experience. In P.H. Mussen (Ed.), *Carmichael's Manual of Child Psychology, Third Edn., Vol. 1*, Wiley, New York, pp. 565–654.

Torday, J.S., Zinman, A.M. and Nielsen, H.C. (1986) Glucocorticoid regulation of DNA, protein and surfactant phospholipid in developing lung. *Dev. Pharmacol. Ther.*, 9: 124–131.

Turner, B.B. and Newman Taylor, A. (1976) Persistent alteration of pituitary-adrenal function in the rat by pre-pubertal corticosterone treatment. *Endocrinology*, 98: 1–9.

Ward, I. (1972) Prenatal stress feminizes and demasculinizes the behaviour of males. *Science*, 175: 82–84.

Ward, I. (1984) The prenatal stress syndrome: Current status. *Psychoneuroendocrinology*, 9: 3–11.

Ward, O.B., Orth, J.M. and Weisz, J. (1983) A possible role of opiates in modifying sexual differentiation. In M. Schlumpf and W. Lichtensteiger (Eds.), *Monographs in Neural Sciences. 9. Drugs and Hormones in Brain Development*. S. Karger, Basel, pp. 194–200.

Ward, I.L. and Weisz, J. (1984) Differential effects of maternal stress on circulating levels of corticosterone, progesterone and testosterone in male and female rat fetuses and their mothers. *Endocrinology*, 84: 1145–1635.

Ward, O.B., Monaghan, E.P. and Ward, I. (1986) Naltrexone blocks the effects of prenatal stress on sexual behaviour differentiation in male rats. *Pharmacol. Biochem. Behav.*, 25: 573–576.

Wong, C.C., Dohler, K.D. and Muhlen, A. (1982) Stress-induced hormone release in rats does not adapt to repeated stress exposure. *Neurosci. Lett., Suppl. 7*: S471.

Wood, C.E. and Rudolph, A.M. (1984) Can maternal stress alter fetal adrenocorticotrophin secretion? *Endocrinology*, 115: 298–301.

Zarrow, M.O., Philpott, J. and Denenberg, V. (1970) Passage of ^{14}C-corticosterone from the rat mother to the foetus and neonate. *Nature*, 226: 1058–1059.

Discussion

J.F. Orlebeke: How do you know that prenatal stress is the causal factor and not postnatal maternal behavior (which is different too)?

M. Weinstock: I cannot be sure in my studies, neither can the authors of the clinical reports. However, cross-fostering of prenatally stressed pups does not remove the developmental or behavioral alteration both in our studies and in others.

B.S. McEwen: Can you tell us how random and regular prenatal stress affects spontaneous alternation behavior later in life?

M. Weinstock: Random noise stress delays the development of this behavior significantly on days 21 and 24 of postnatal life, while daily stress (14–21) does not.

D.F. Swaab: What exactly is the evidence that corticosteroids are central in the mechanism of the stress effects on the fetus? One other possibility might be that uterine activity is changed (e.g., due to catecholamines). A change in uterine activity might alter fetal brain development in various ways (affecting sleep stages, blood flow, etc.). If corticosteroids would not be central in the mechanism, their levels might not be representative for the severity of the stressor.

M. Weinstock: There is no direct evidence. Maternal corticosterone levels were essentially normal in daily stressed rats in our experiments after three exposures and their offspring showed normal development, while those of randomly stressed mothers were abnormally elevated especially on day 21. I also showed that other stress paradigms which had resulted in behavioral abnormalities all had high maternal corticosterone levels during the last days of gestation. Moreover, injection of corticosterone to 1-day-old pups produces similar delays in the maturation of early motor activities, spontaneous alternation and some later behaviors to those occurring after prenatal stress. Lastly, if stress resulted in alterations in uterine contractability in response to raised levels of plasma catecholamines, one might have expected to see more developmental damage in the offspring whose mothers were regularly subjected to the stress than inter-mittently, unless, of course, the adrenal medulla and sympa-thetic system adapts as readily to the stress as does the hypothalamo-pituitary adrenal (HPA) system. However, I have no direct evidence for this adaptation.

P.M. Rodier: Your conclusions state that stress led to delay or impairment of hippocampal development, but you did not measure hippocampal development, did you?

M. Weinstock: This was not a conclusion but a hypothesis. The only data we have relating to a possible interference with hippocampal function in the offspring of randomly stressed rats is the delay in the development of spontaneous alterna-tion behavior. We would like to measure corticosterone binding sites in the hippocampus of the offspring of dams receiving the two different stress schedules when we have overcome some technical difficulties inherent in the tech-nique.

C.V. Vorhees: I was wondering if the older epidemiological studies you reviewed on stress controlled or stratified for variables such as maternal alcohol consumption or smoking?

M. Weinstock: No mention is made in the studies by Meier (1985) or Stott (1973) of maternal alcohol consumption or smoking.

M. Mirmiran: There were obvious differences between maternal and fetal cortisone response to stress, i.e., enhanced maternal cortisone and depression of fetal cortisone. Since cortisone ought to be enhanced as a function of stress, could I conclude from your data that the observed decreased fetal cortisone is a result of increased maternal cortisone produc-tion (inhibiting fetal cortisone) rather than a direct response of the fetus to stress?

M. Weinstock: Our data do not enable us to answer this question. We can only say that the pattern of response of the mothers given the stress at different time schedules differs from each other and from the controls. The same is true for the fetuses.

M. Mirmiran: Would you comment on the casual report (Dörner, 1986) indicating a higher risk of homosexuality in children born during the second world war?

M. Weinstock: Dörner (1986) reported a significantly higher incidence of homosexual males born to mothers who were pregnant in Germany during the latter part of the Second World War. Several experimental studies in rats have shown that severe forms of maternal stress, such as restraint or overcrowding can impair the development of male sexual organs, reduce the size of the sexual dimorphic nucleus in the hypothalamus and feminize sexual behavior (Anderson, 1985; Ward, 1972). These effects may be mediated by opioid peptides since they can be mimicked by opiate administration to the pregnant dam and prevented by naltrexone given daily to the stressed rat (Ward et al., 1986). There may therefore be some support for the suggestion that gestational stress can predispose towards male homosexuality.

References

Anderson, D.K. (1985) Effects of prenatal stress on the dif-ferentiation of the sexually dimorphic nucleus of the pre-optic area (SDN-POA) of the rat brain. *Brain Res.*, 332: 113–118.

Dörner (1986) Hormone-dependent brain development and preventive medicine. In G. Dörner, S.M. McCann and L. Martini (Eds.), *Systemic Hormones, Neurotransmitters and Brain Development. Monogr. Neural Sci., Vol. 12*, pp. 17–27.

Meier, A. (1985) Child psychiatric sequelae of maternal war stress. *Acta Psychiatr. Scand.* 72: 505–511.

Stott, D.H. (1973) Follow-up study from birth of the effects of prenatal stress. *Dev. Med. Child Neurol.*, 15: 770–787.

Ward, I. (1972) Prenatal stress feminizes and demasculinizes the behaviour of males. *Science*, 175: 82–84.

Ward, O.B., Monaghan, E.P. and Ward, I. (1986) Naltrexone blocks the effects of prenatal stress on sexual behaviour differentiation in male rats. *Pharmacol. Biochem. Behav.*,

SECTION V

Neurochemical Mechanisms

G.J. Boer, M.G.P. Feenstra, M. Mirmiran, D.F. Swaab and F. Van Haaren
Progress in Brain Research, Vol. 73
© 1988 Elsevier Science Publishers B.V. (Biomedical Division)

CHAPTER 22

Structural–functional relationships in experimentally induced brain damage

Patricia M. Rodier

Department of Obstetrics and Gynecology, School of Medicine and Dentistry, University of Rochester, Rochester, NY, USA

The purpose of this chapter is to introduce some of the themes of neuroteratology by tracing its historical connections to the study of somatic malformations. This is most easily done by discussing studies of general teratogens, that is, ones which affect all cells. Antimitotic agents are a classic example of teratogens with general effects. Of course, there are neuroteratogens with much more specific actions and much more restricted effects – diazepam acts at the benzodiazepine receptor (Simmons et al., 1984) and monosodium glutamate is toxic only to cells with glutamate receptors (Olney, 1969) – but the effects of general teratogens can include rather discrete brain lesions as well, and studies of these form a bridge to teratology as a whole. It was from studies of this class of agents that we first recognized that early disruption of brain structure would result in lasting behavioral changes. In this chapter, we shall also consider the possibility that structural–functional relationships are not necessarily unidirectional. That is, recent studies suggest that some of the somatic structural changes noted in teratology may actually reflect malfunctions of the brain systems controlling growth and development.

Correspondence: P.M. Rodier, Ph.D., OB/GYN Box 668, University of Rochester, 601 Elmwood Ave., Rochester, NY, 14642, USA.

Structural changes during development lead to lasting functional abnormalities

In 1954, Wilson revolutionized the field of teratology by demonstrating that a single agent, X-irradiation, could cause many different malformations if it was delivered at different stages of development. Because X-ray interfered with cells in the mitotic cycle, and all cells are mitotic at some point in development, it led to injury to the palate at one stage, to the heart at another, and to the brain at another. This seems obvious today, but the literature prior to Wilson's report consisted mainly of studies attempting to link each birth defect with a cause. The studies of X-ray changed the way people thought about congenital malformations. They focussed attention on critical periods and they showed that specific malformations could arise from the most general sorts of injuries.

At the same time, Hicks (1954) described how X-ray exposure at different periods of gestation and postnatal life altered the developing brain. While Wilson (1954) had looked for gross malformations, Hicks was observing more subtle alterations – not only exencephaly, but thinning of the cortex, changes in laminar patterns, and so forth. Further, Hicks was seeing these effects after exposures at stages of development later than those associated with most gross malformations,

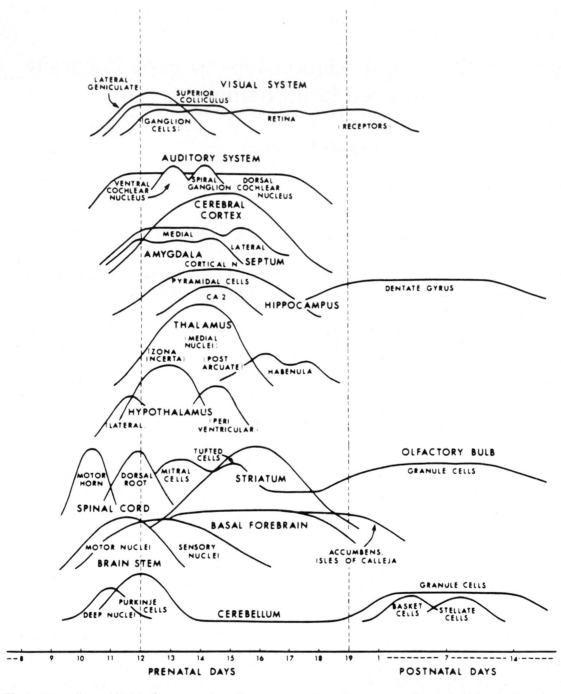

Fig. 1. Autoradiographic data from many investigators demonstrate the sequence of neuron production in various regions of the mouse CNS. Curves represent the bursts of proliferation for a cell type. The area under the curves is not representative of the number of cells formed and the position of cell groups on the *y* axis is arbitrary. Dotted vertical lines indicate the last day when gross malformations are induced by interference with mitosis (embryonic day 12) and the day of birth (Rodier, 1980).

demonstrating that brain damage could occur in individuals of normal appearance, as we know it does in human cases.

By the late 50s, other groups were documenting the behavioral effects of early X-irradiation (Furchtgott and Echols, 1958; Furchtgott et al., 1958; Werboff et al., 1961). The behavioral effects, like the anatomical ones, were dependent on the time of exposure, and some of the behavioral studies demonstrated effects at doses well below those that had been investigated anatomically.

The growing use of [^{3}H]thymidine autoradiography by many investigators eventually resulted in an outline of the birthdates of many neuronal populations (reviewed by Rodier, 1980). With this

information in hand, it became possible to interfere with neuron production, measure the cell loss, and compare the injury to that predicted by the time of exposure. Fig. 1 shows a summary of times of neuron production in the mouse, and Fig. 2 displays the significant changes in dimensions of the CNS associated with insults to proliferation at several stages of gestation. It is possible to map the sites of cell loss by linear measures of matched sections because early cell loss is reflected in tissue volume, rather than cell density. While reductions were produced by treatment at each stage of development investigated, the locations of the reductions differed from one treatment time to another. As can be seen by

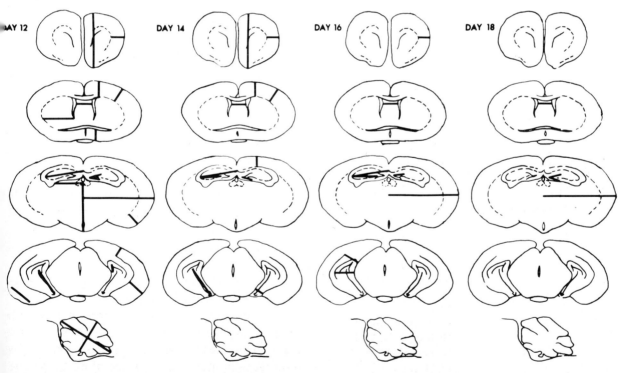

Fig. 2. Measures significantly reduced by azacytidine treatment at four different prenatal exposure times are compared in this display. Each line represents a measurement which differed from control values at P < .02. To judge the size of various brain structures, treated and control brains were cut coronally to produce views of four matched levels of the CNS for comparisons of cortex, thalamus, hippocampus, etc. The cerebellum was cut sagittally. The sets of matched sections were then measured under the microscope at about 30 points, using an ocular grid. Groups of about 15 animals were evaluated for each condition, and each treated group was compared to the controls by analysis of variance. Both the number and location of reductions changed as treatment time was varied (Rodier, 1984).

comparing Figs. 1 and 2, the sites reduced by treatment with 5-azacytidine, a cancer chemotherapeutic drug with antimitotic properties, agree well with those predicted by autoradiography. For example, note how the size of the cerebellum is reduced only by treatment on embryonic day 12 (E12), the only day in this set when cerebellar cells are produced. The cerebral cortex forms posterior to anterior and medial to lateral, a pattern that is repeated in the regions affected by treatment.

In the series of experiments from which these morphologic measures were drawn, the same animals were studied behaviorally (Rodier et al., 1975; Rodier, 1977; Rodier and Reynolds, 1977; Rodier et al., 1979; Rodier and Gramann, 1979). As in the X-ray studies, the results of behavioral testing were dependent on the time of treatment. For example, early treatment (E12) led to hypoactivity in adulthood, while treatments in the middle of brain development led to hyperactivity, and later treatment (E18) led to hypoactivity. Thus, as in the morphologic studies, time of treatment determined not only the degree of abnormality, but the quality of the abnormality as well. That this is a characteristic typical of injuries to mitotic cells of the CNS can be seen in Table 1, where activity data for several agents are summarized. The pattern of activity effects varies with time of treatment in the same way with the different teratogens. It is not a characteristic of azacytidine, but a characteristic of the particular brain damage induced at different treatment times. The simplest description of the structural–functional relationship for these data is that injuries to the hippocampus and cerebral cortex lead to hyperactivity, while injuries to the cerebellum lead to hypoactivity. The morphology of X-ray and methylazoxymethanol (MAM)-exposed brains agrees with this hypothesis (for a comparison of neuroanatomical effects of X-ray, MAM and azacytidine, see Rodier, 1986). While this description is surely an oversimplification, it reinforces the point that there is nothing surprising in data suggesting different behavioral effects from the same agent delivered at different times, because the location of the brain injuries differs just as dramatically as the behavioral results.

Not all behavioral effects vary so neatly with time of exposure. For example, several motor tasks have been observed to be affected by teratogens at almost every stage of development. In this case, the earliest and latest treatment times seem to give more consistently abnormal results, while treatment in the middle period yields some positive and some negative effects (Table 2). Considering that many parts of the brain are involved in the performance of most of the behaviors tested

TABLE 1

Lists of studies show that significant effects on general activity of adult animals exposed to antimitotic agents during development can be segregated by exposure time and direction of effect. While occasional studies find no significant effect, time of exposure is the critical variable in determining whether the offspring are hyperactive or hypoactive. Such results occur because the location of brain lesions is dependent on the time of treatment.

Hypoactivity	Hyperactivity
Early antimitotic treatment	
– X-ray (Werboff et al., 1962)	
– Azacytidine (Rodier et al., 1979)	
Middle-period antimitotic treatment	
	– X-ray (Werboff et al., 1962; Fowler et al., 1962; Furchtgott and Echols, 1958)
	– Azacytidine (Rodier et al., 1975; Rodier et al., 1979)
	– MAM (Rabe and Haddad, 1972; Vorhees, et al., 1984; Kabat et al., 1985)
Late antimitotic treatment	
– X-ray (Furchtgott and Echols, 1958; Wallace and Altman, 1970a,b; Nash, 1973)	
– Azacytidine (Rodier et al., 1975)	
– MAM (Kabat et al., 1985)	

TABLE 2

Lists of studies of motor effects caused by antimitotic agents administered during brain development show that these effects are less clearly time-dependent than those for activity. Most motor testing has been carried out in postnatally-exposed animals, in which antimitotic action almost invariably alters coordination or motor development. The results from early and middle prenatal exposures are less consistent, but the number of studies is relatively small.

Positive effects	Negative effects
Early antimitotic treatment	
– X-ray (Werboff et al., 1961)	
– Hydroxyurea (Butcher et al., 1975)	
– Azacytidine (Rodier et al., 1979)	
Midde-period antimitotic treatment	
– X-ray (Furchtgott et al., 1958; Hicks et al., 1959; Werboff et al., 1961; Sikov et al., 1962)	– Azacytidine (Rodier et al., 1975, 1979)
– Azacytidine (Rodier et al., 1975)	– MAM (Haddad et al., 1977; Giurgea et al., 1982)
– MAM (Ciofolo et al., 1971)	
Late antimitotic treatment	
– X-ray (Furchtgott and Echols, 1958; Hicks et al., 1959; Yamazaki et al., 1960; Sikov et al., 1962; Wallace and Altman, 1970a,b; Brunner and Altman, 1973)	
– Azacytidine (Rodier et al., 1975)	
– MAM (Shimada and Langman, 1970; Haddad et al., 1977; Kabat et al., 1985)	

thus far, such mixed results are not surprising.

Occasionally, it has been possible to examine structural–functional relationships in more detail. For example, in one of the azacytidine studies a particular treatment time yielded great variance in behavioral and morphologic outcomes (Rodier and Reynolds, 1977). Therefore, it was possible to ask how the morphologic effects correlated with the behavior effects *within* the treated group. Table 3 shows that the animals with the most extreme behavioral effects (hyperactivity, increased active avoidance, and decreased passive avoidance) shared only one brain reduction – a diminution of the CA3 and 4 regions of the hippocampus. While several other measures were reduced in the treated group compared to controls, they were not correlated with the behavioral effects. Body weight and brain weight were significantly correlated with behavior, but were not significantly correlated with the size of CA3 and 4. Thus, it appears that this region is related to the behavioral effects in some way other than just reflecting the overall degree of damage. Perhaps more importantly, many of the affected areas appear to be unrelated to the behavioral effects.

TABLE 3

Correlations (r tet) of deviant behavior with regional brain size and weight measures within a group of adults treated with azacytidine on embryonic day 16 show that not all morphologic measures affected by treatment are correlated with deviant behavior. In this experiment, the size of CA3 + CA4 was the only brain measure (determined as indicated in Fig. 2) significantly related to deviant behavior.

Measure	r tet
Brain weight	+ 0.76[a]
Body weight	+ 1.00[a]
CA1 + CA2	+ 0.16
CA3 + CA4	+ 0.76[a]
Dorsal limb of dentate gyrus	+ 0.53
Ventral limb of dentate gyrus	+ 0.16
Frontal cortex	+ 0.16
Whole width of brain	+ 0.16
Septum	− 0.27
Thickness of hippocampus	+ 0.16

[a] $P = <0.02$.

While we cannot say that the changes in CA3 and 4 caused the behaviors observed, we can certainly interpret a lack of correlation to indicate that cell loss in the other areas is unlikely to be relevant to the outcome. In fact, the result in this study – an association between one measure of the hippocampus and the behaviors investigated – is exactly what would be predicted from the lesion literature, which includes many demonstrations of the disruption of avoidance learning and the induction of hyperactivity by hippocampal lesions (reviewed by Nadel et al., 1975).

In other studies, other behavioral characteristics of animals with hippocampal lesions have been demonstrated in animals treated to interfere with hippocampal development. For example, spatial memory, as tested in radial mazes, is disrupted by experimental lesions of the structure in adults (Olton, 1977), or by azacytidine exposure on E14, but not on E12 (Rodier et al., 1979). By noting the similar behavioral effects of developmentally induced lesions of a given structure and surgical lesions of the same structure, we do not intend to suggest that such lesions can be equated. Obviously, the physical differences in the two lesions, alone, would predict some differences in behavioral outcomes, and it should be easy to demonstrate that there are differences as well as similarities in the behavioral effects. Such a demonstration would require behavioral tests directed at a variety of functions. The tests described above were selected to focus on deficits that would be expected to arise from the morphologic injuries *common* to both types of lesion, rather than from injuries which differ between them. Thus, the similarities in behavioral effects only confirm that early and late lesions of the same structure often have the same functional effects, a point that had been demonstrated previously for neonatal vs. adult lesions of the hippocampus (Isaacson et al., 1968). If this were not the case, neuroteratologists would have had no way to guess what behaviors to test, even when they knew the neuroanatomical effects of their treatments. Just as in these early experiments,

neuroteratologists continue to be dependent on the researchers who have described the functional effects of anatomical or biochemical lesions, and on those who provide hypotheses or evidence as to the action of the teratogen on the CNS. Without both kinds of information, the array of functions to be tested makes our power to detect neurofunctional deficits low, unless we can afford to evaluate many aspects of function.

The teratology studies described above involved very general methods for screening behavior and morphology under many treatment conditions. Other work has produced more detailed descriptions of the effects of early interference with cell proliferation. For example, Cheema and Lauder (1984) have examined the distribution of connections between cell groups mismatched in number. Johnston and Coyle (1979) have described the transmitter biochemistry of cerebral cortex after MAM-induced loss of intrinsic neurons with sparing of projections to the missing cells. Recent research has also increased the list of agents with antimitotic action in the developing brain. Methylmercury (Sager et al., 1982) and nitrous oxide (Rodier et al., 1986) are now known to have at least part of their neuroteratogenic effects by way of interference with cell proliferation.

Can alteration of brain function lead to structural terata?

Because the effects of general teratogens on the nervous system could be related to somatic effects of the same agents, the data formed a bridge between the study of gross malformations and the study of brain damage, with its manifestations in behavior. However, the brain controls many functions not so obviously reflected in behavior. The use of the term 'functional neuroteratology' in the title of this conference acknowleges this. It is, of course, well known that neuroactive substances delivered during development can alter adult physiology, as in the effects of sex hormones (see Chapter 9, for example), but such effects have not been investigated after exposure to general teratogens. It is important to know whether general teratogens, such as antimitotic agents, can mimic such specific effects, because these agents are so widespread in the environment that the implication would be that such functional effects may occur with some frequency in clinical populations. Also, because these agents are known to cause damage to structures outside the CNS, it would be possible to mistake indirect effects mediated by brain damage, for direct effects of the teratogens on somatic tissue. In fact, not only physiological changes, but even somatic structural changes could be created by some patterns of brain damage. For example, many teratogens reduce body size or weight, but whether they do this directly, or by interference with subsequent growth, is rarely investigated.

Several lines of evidence suggest that the size or weight deficits commonly associated with birth defects could be secondary to brain damage. Growth deficiencies can arise in many ways, but most patients respond to growth hormone. This suggests a deficit in the production or release of the hormone from the somatotropes of the anterior pituitary. Such deficits can result from anomalies of the somatotropes themselves, or from anomalies of the growth hormone releasing factor cells of the hypothalamus, which act to stimulate the somatotropes. Either of these cell types could be reduced in number by a teratogenic insult, and there are indications that such injuries do occur. For example, in human populations, children with congenital defects of the facial midline have a greatly increased incidence of growth hormone deficiency (Rudman et al., 1978). That is, their short stature is not a direct result of the same injury which caused the midline abnormality. Instead, the midline injury is associated with some abnormality of growth hormone levels, and it is this functional deficit which leads to short stature.

The pattern of growth in the absence of growth hormone is distinctive. In humans growth rates do not depend on the hormone until some time after the age of two (reviewed by Cryer and Daughaday, 1977). In the mouse and rat, growth-hormone-deficient animals begin to diverge from normal animals after about two weeks of postnatal life, as seen in mutants such as the dwarf mouse, which lacks somatotropes (Snell, 1929; Smith and MacDowell, 1930). One teratological syndrome which appears to exhibit this pattern of growth is fetal alcohol syndrome (FAS). These children are born small, but their bone growth slows down at about two and a half years, so that they become smaller and smaller in comparison with controls (Streissguth et al., 1985). This pattern fits the hypothesis that *in utero* alcohol exposure results in a malfunction of the hypothalamic-pituitary axis. The initial injury must affect size directly, to explain the low birth weight of FAS children, but the later shift in growth rate could be attributed to a deficit in growth hormone. This would explain why a change in growth rate occurs at the time when the role of growth hormone becomes critical. It would be valuable to test this hypothesis in children with fetal alcohol syndrome for, unlike most teratological effects, growth hormone deficiency is treatable and, since we know little about its role aside from the stimu-

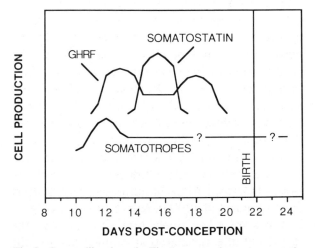

Fig. 3. Curves like those in Fig. 1 are used to represent the time of cell production for three sets of growth-controlling cells. Timing of production for growth hormone releasing factor (GHRF) cells and somatotropes is based on indirect evidence.

lation of growth, treatment might improve the status of the patient in unexpected ways.

In rodents, we know something about the timing of cell production for the various parts of the growth-controlling system, and we have data which suggest that exposure to general teratogens can alter the system. Fig. 3 shows a tentative outline of the production of the somatotropes, the growth hormone releasing factor (GHRF) cells of the arcuate nucleus, and the periventricular somatostatin cells, which inhibit growth hormone release. The estimate of timing of the appearance of somatotropes is based on the fact that gross defects of the pituitary can be induced by X-ray soon after closure of the neural tube (Hicks, 1954), and the cells in question are thought to be among the first of the trophic cells to form (Goodyer, 1981). What is more mysterious is how long their production period lasts, for mitosis in the pituitary continues at a low rate even in adults (e.g. Mastro and Hymer, 1973). Such a pattern of production might make the pituitary more resistant to permanent injury than neuron populations with very short production periods. The arcuate nucleus of the rat hypothalamus forms between about E13 and 19, according to Altman and Bayer (1978), with the anterior cells born before the posterior ones. These cell groups appear in the graph as two peaks, but the dip between them may be filled by the production of cells located in between the two sets for which birthdays are known. Whether the GHRF cells represent a subset of these clusters, with a slightly different proliferative period, is not known, but their time of production must fall sometime between E13 and 19. The period of production of the somatostatin cells inhibitory to the somatotropes is known from an autoradiographic study by Hoffman et al. (1980). As can be seen in Fig. 3, that period is extremely brief, and falls in the middle of the proliferation of neurons for the arcuate nucleus. This outline of cell production, if it is correct, suggests that growth deficiencies could be induced by insults to the developing rat hypothalamic-pituitary axis occurring at many

times during gestation, and possibly even after birth, but that growth excess, if it occurs at all, would be induced only during a very short interval at E15–17.

To determine whether a weight effect after exposure to a teratogen represents an effect on growth, as opposed to a direct effect on size, it is necessary to have weight data from several ages. Many teratology studies do not provide this information, but a few with results suggesting growth deficiency have been reported. The most striking is that of Fischer et al. (1972), in which rats were exposed to MAM at many stages of prenatal development. Rats exposed to MAM at some stages were the same size as controls at birth, but failed to grow at the same rate. Therefore, the body weights of treated animals became significantly different from those of controls only after several weeks of postnatal life. This was even more obvious in the authors' measures of organ weights, which were collected only for rats killed on post-natal day 14 or 35. Fig. 4 compares one of these measures (liver weight) to brain weight. The latter differed at birth, at 14 days after birth and at 35 days, but all other organs were normal

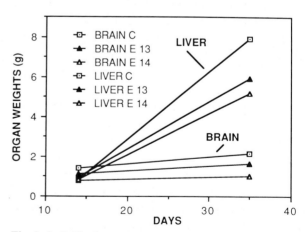

Fig. 4. Individual organ weights after E13 or E14 MAM exposure confirm that the brain was reduced in weight at the time of treatment, but somatic structures such as the liver were normal until their growth rate decreased postnatally (drawn from data of Fischer et al., 1972).

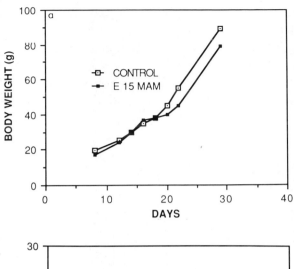

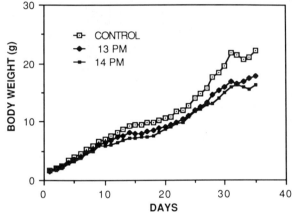

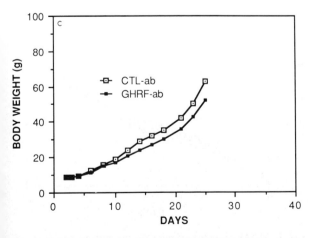

at 14 days, then failed to grow. This is strong evidence for initial brain damage with a subsequent effect on growth of the rest of the body. In two more recent studies, which included frequent sampling of weight, body weights after prenatal MAM are seen to diverge from control weights some time in the second week of rodent life. In the first instance, rats were treated on the morning of E15 (Kabat et al., 1985), while in the second (Rodier, study in progress) mice were treated on the evening of E13 or the evening of E14. These data are shown in Fig. 5a and b. The results suggest that the weight deficit typical of MAM-exposed subjects is not produced directly at the time of injury. Instead, it appears considerably later, as would be expected if the initial injury led to growth hormone deficiency. Fig. 5c shows the pattern of abnormal growth produced by blocking GHRF with the antibody to the hormone (Wehrenberg, 1986). This graph is virtually identical to the MAM growth deficit as seen in rats and mice (Fig. 5a and b). Whether the growth deficit following prenatal treatment results from injury to somatotropes or GHRF cells (or from some other cause) is not known, but the time of exposure in the cited studies is most compatible with an injury to the hypothalamus (cf. Fig. 3).

Have early brain injuries ever led to excessive growth? Johnston and Coyle (1979) demonstrated a significant increase in rat body weight after exposure to MAM late on E15 – precisely the time when rat somatostatin cells should be most vulnerable. Although the cause of that weight increase was not investigated, our pilot studies indicate that somatostatin cell numbers can be

Fig. 5. (a) Data from another MAM study in rats show the timing of the growth deficiency after exposure on E15 (redrawn from a graph by Kabat et al., 1985). (b) MAM treatment of fetal mice on the evening of E13 or E14 also reduced body weight in our recent study. As in rats, the effect appears postnatally, after a shift in the rate of growth. (c) Daily treatment with anti-GHRF vs. a control antiserum leads to a growth pattern similar to prenatal exposure to MAM, supporting the hypothesis that the teratological growth deficit could result from a growth hormone deficiency (redrawn from a graph by Wehrenberg, 1986).

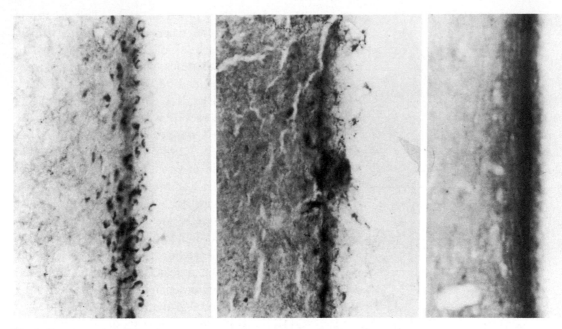

Fig. 6. Somatostatin cell numbers were reduced by about 50% by two azacytidine exposures (evening of embryological day 13 and morning of embryological day 14) in a pilot study in mice (Weisman, Hoffman and Rodier, unpublished data). ICC for somatostatin in animals killed at postnatal day 30 shows, from left to right, the periventricular region in a control, an azacytidine-treated animal, and a control animal stained with pre-absorbed serum (ICC control).

decreased by azacytidine treatment at an analogous stage of development in the mouse (Weisman et al, unpublished data; see Fig. 6), and MAM treatment at that stage (the morning of E14) failed to induce any significant decrease in weight, even though exposure 12 h before or after does reduce it significantly. Fig. 7 shows this group, added to the graph of groups with retarded growth, from the same study. Thus, it appears that damage to the hypothalamic-pituitary axis can alter body weight in either direction. Weight, of course, is not the best indicator of growth hormone activity, and studies now in progress will measure bone growth and growth hormone release directly, in animals treated to cause prenatal injuries to growth-controlling systems.

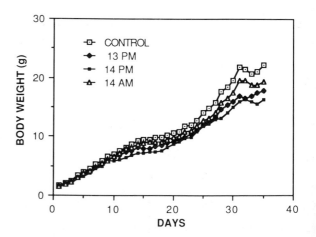

Fig. 7. MAM exposure of mice on the morning of embryologic day 14 did not lead to a significant reduction in body weight, as compared to controls, but earlier or later treatment did. The dose was 20 mg/kg in each case (Rodier, 1987, study in progress).

Summary and concluding remarks

We have chosen to concentrate on growth as an example of a function under brain control because the parts of the system are amenable to study. The availability of antisera to growth hormone, GHRF and somatostatin, the fact that the feedback loops of this system do not automatically adjust hormone levels to normal, and the fact that the target tissue includes most or all parts of the body (Russell and Spencer, 1984), making the target tissue an unlikely candidate for injury by an acute exposure to a teratogen, are features that make the system easy to investigate. However, this example of a neuroendocrine function subject to disruption by general teratogens is probably only one of many which deserve investigation.

While work on this subject is still in a very preliminary stage, it seems a most appropriate topic for this conference, because it allows us to view the relationship between somatic malformations and brain damage in a different way. Neuroteratologists tend to be most intrigued by disturbances of brain function occurring in the absence of somatic effects, because 'isolated' brain damage is common in humans, and is ignored by most standard safety testing. We wish to emphasize that injuries to developing brain may sometimes affect the structure and function of other organ systems, because it is probable that such combinations of effects are also common. From a safety point of view, this may make hazardous agents easier to detect in the laboratory, but from a medical point of view it makes description and recognition of brain damage syndromes even more complicated. We need more information on how brain damage is expressed. Otherwise, syndromes induced during development but expressed later in life are not likely to be recognized as teratological in origin, even if they have structural components.

Acknowledgement

Support for some of the studies came from NIH-NS 24287.

References

Altman, J. and Bayer, S.A. (1978) Development of the diencephalon in the rat: Autoradiographic study of the time of origin and settling patterns of neurons in the hypothalamus. *J. Comp. Neurol.*, 182: 945–972.

Brunner, R.L. and Altman, J. (1973) Locomotor deficits in adult rats with moderate to massive retardation of cerebellar development during infancy. *Behav. Biol.*, 9: 169–188.

Butcher, R.E., Hawver, K., Kazmaier, K. and Scott, W.J. (1975) Postnatal behavioral effects from prenatal exposure to teratogens. In P.L. Morselli, S. Garattini and F. Sereni (Eds.), *Basic and Therapeuric Aspects of Perinatal Pharmacology*, Raven, New York.

Cheema, S.S. and Lauder, J.M. (1984) Infrapyramidal mossy fibers in the hippocampus of methylazoxymethanol acetate induced micrencephalic rats. *Dev. Brain Res.*, 9: 411–415.

Ciofalo, V.B., Latranyi, M. and Taber, R.I. (1971) Effect of prenatal treatment of methylazoxymethanol acetate on motor perfomance, exploratory activity, and maze learning in rats. *Comm. Behav. Biol.*, 6: 223–226.

Cryer, P.E. and Daughaday, W.H. (1977) Growth hormone. IV. Disordered growth hormone secretion. In L. Martini and G.M. Besser (Eds.), *Clinical Endocrinology*, Academic Press, New York, pp. 258–271.

Fischer, M.H., Welker, C. and Waisman, H.A. (1972) Generalized growth retardation in rats induced by prenatal exposure to methylazoxymethanol acetate. *Teratology*, 5: 223–232.

Fowler, H., Hicks, S.P., D'Amato, CA. and Beach, F. (1962) Effects of fetal irradiation on behavior in the albino rat. *J. Comp. Physiol. Psychol.*, 55: 309–314.

Furchtgott, E. and Echols, M. (1958) Activity and emotionality in pre- and neonatally x-irradiated rats. *J. Comp. Physiol. Psychol.*, 51: 541–545.

Furchtgott, E., Echols, M. and Openshaw, J.W. (1958) Maze learning in pre- and neonatally x-irradiated rats. *J. Comp. Physiol. Psychol.*, 51: 178–180.

Giurgea, C., Greindl, M.G., Preat, S. and Puigdevall, J. (1982) Piracetam compensation of MAM-induced behavioral deficit in rats. In S. Corkin et al. (Eds.), *Alzheimer's disease: A Report in Progress*, Raven Press, New York, pp. 281–286.

Goodyer, C.C. (1981) Ontogeny of pituitary hormone secretion. In R. Collu et al. (Eds.), *Pediatric Endocrinology*, Academic Press, New York, pp. 99–147.

Haddad, R.K., Rabe, A., Dumas, R., Shek, J. and Valsamis, M.P. (1977) Transplacental induction of cerebellar ataxia in ferrets. *Teratology*, 15: 33.

Hicks, S.P. (1954) Mechanism of radiation anecephaly, anophthalmia, and pituitary anomalies. *Arch. Path.*, 57: 363–378.

Hicks, S.P., D'Amato, C.A. and Lowe, M.J. (1959) The development of the mammalian nervous system. *J. Comp. Neurol.*, 113: 435–469.

Hoffman, G.E., Dick, L.B. and Gash, D.M. (1980) Development of somatostatin: examination by the technique of combined autoradiography and immunocytochemistry. *Peptides*, 1, Suppl. 1: 79–83.

Isaacson, R.L., Nonneman, A.J. and Schmalz, L.W. (1968) Behavioral and anatomical sequelae of damage to the infant limbic system. In R.L. Isaacson (Ed.), *The Neuropsychology of Development*, Wiley, New York.

Johnston, M.V. and Coyle, J.T. (1979) Histological and neurochemical effects of fetal treatment with methylazoxymethanol on rat neocortex in adulthood. *Brain Res.*, 170: 135–155.

Kabat, K., Buterbaugh, G.B. and Echols, C.U. (1985) Methylazoxymethanol as a developmental model of neurotoxicity. *Neurobehav. Toxicol. Teratol.*, 7: 519–525.

Mastro, A. and Hymer, W.C. (1973) The effect of age and oltrone treatment on DNA polymerase activity in anterior pituitary glands of male rats. *J. Endocrinol.*, 59: 107–119.

Nadel, L., O'Keefe, J. and Black, A. (1975) Slam on the brakes: a critique of Altman Brunner and Bayer's response-inhibition model of hippocampal function. *Behav. Biol.*, 14: 151–162.

Nash, D.J. (1973) Influence of genotype and neonatal irradiation on open field locomotion and elimination in mice. *J. Comp. Physiol. Psychol.*, 83: 458–464.

Olney, J.W. (1969) Brain lesions, obesity, and other disturbances in mice treated with monosodium glutamate. *Science*, 164: 719–721.

Olton, D. (1977) Spatial memory. *Sci. Am.*, 236: 82–98.

Rabe, A. and Haddad, R.K. (1972) Methylazoxymethanol-induced microencephaly in rats: behavioral studies. *Fed. Proc.*, 31: 1536–1539.

Rodier, P.M. (1977) Correlations between prenatally-induced alterations in CNS cell populations and postnatal function. *Teratology*, 16: 235–246.

Rodier, P.M. (1980) Chronology of neuron development: animal studies and their clinical implications. *Dev. Med. Child Neurol.*, 22: 525–545.

Rodier, P.M. (1984) Exogenous sources of malformations in development: CNS malformations and developmental repair processes. In E. Gollin (Ed.), *Malformations of Development: Biological and Psychological Sources and Consequences*, Academic Press, New York, pp. 287–313.

Rodier, P.M. (1986) Behavioral effects of antimitotic agents administered during neurogenesis. In E.P. Riley and C.V. Vorhees (Eds.), *Handbook of Behavioral Teratology*, Plenum, New York, pp. 185–209.

Rodier, P.M. and Gramann, W.J. (1979) Morphological effects of interference with cell proliferation in the early fetal period. *Neurobehav. Toxicol.*, 1: 129–135.

Rodier, P.M. and Reynolds, S.S. (1977) Morphological cor-relates of behavioral abnormalities in experimental congenital brain damage. *Exp. Neurol.*, 57: 81–93.

Rodier, P.M., Webster, W.S. and Langman, J. (1975) Morphological and behavioral consequences of chemically-induced lesions of the CNS. In N. Ellis (Ed.), *Aberrant Development in Human Infancy: Human and Animal Studies*, Erlbaum, Hillsdale, New Jersey, pp. 177–185.

Rodier, P.M., Reynolds, S.S. and Roberts, W.N. (1979) Behavioral consequences of interference with CNS development in the early fetal period. *Teratology*, 29: 327–336.

Rodier, P.M., Aschner, M., Lewis, L.S. and Koeter, H.B.W.M. (1986) Cell proliferation in developing brain after brief exposure to inhalant anesthetics. *Anesthesiology*, 64: 680–687.

Rudman, D., Davis, T., Priest, J.H., Patterson, J.H., Kutner, M.H., Heymsfield, S.B. and Bethel, R.A. (1978) Prevalence of growth hormone deficiency in children with cleft lip or palate. *J. Pediatr.*, 93: 378–382.

Russell, S.M. and Spencer, E.M. (1985) Local injections of human or rat growth hormone or of purified human somatomedin-C stimulate unilateral tibial epiphysial growth in hypophysectomized rats. *Endocrinology*, 116: 2563–2567.

Sager, P.R., Doherty, R.A. and Rodier, P.M. (1982) Effects of methylmercury on developing mouse cerebellar cortex. *Exp. Neurol.*, 77: 179–193.

Shimada, M. and Langman, J. (1970) Repair of the external granular layer of the hamster cerebellum after prenatal and postnatal administration of methylazoxymethanol. *Teratology*, 3: 119–134.

Sikov, M.R., Resta, C.F., Lofstrom, J.E. and Meyer, J.S. (1962) Neurological deficits in the rat resulting from x-irradiation in utero. *Exp. Neurol.*, 5: 131–138.

Simmons, R.D., Kellogg, C.K. and Miller, R.K. (1984) Prenatal diazepam exposure in rats: long-lasting, receptor-mediated effects on hypothalamic norepinephrine-containing neurons. *Brain Res.*, 293: 73–83.

Smith, P.E. and MacDowell, E.C. (1930) A hereditary anterior-pituitary deficiency in the mouse. *Anat. Rec.*, 46: 249–257.

Snell, G.D. (1929) Dwarf, a new mendelian recessive character of the house mouse. *Proc. Natl. Acad. Sci. USA*, 15: 733–734.

Streissguth, A.P., Clarren, S.K. and Jones, K.L. (1985) Natural history of the fetal alcohol syndrome. *Lancet*, ii: 85–91.

Vorhees, C.V., Fernandez, K., Dumas, R.M. and Haddad, R.K. (1984) Pervasive hyperactivity and long-term learning impairments in rats with induced microencephaly from prenatal exposure to methylazoxymethanol. *Dev. Brain Res.*, 15: 1–10.

Wallace, R.B. and Altman, J. (1970) Behavioral effects of neonatal irradiation of the cerebellum: I. Qualitative observations in infant and adolescent rats. *Dev. Psychobiol.*, 2: 257–265.

Wallace R.B. and Altman, J. (1970) Behavioral effects of neonatal irradiation of the cerebellum: II. Quantitative studies in young-adult and adult rats. *Dev. Psychobiol.*, 2: 266–272.

Wehrenberg, W.H. (1986) The role of growth releasing factor and somatostatin on somatic growth in rats. *Endocrinology*, 118: 489–494.

Werboff, J., Goodman, I., Havlena, J. and Sikov, M.R. (1961) Effects of prenatal x-irradiation on motor performance in the rat. *Am. J. Physiol.*, 201: 703–706.

Werboff, J., Havlena, J. and Sikov, M.R. (1961) Effects of prenatal x-irradiation on activity emotionality, and maze-learning ability in the rat. *Radiat. Res.*, 16: 441–452.

Wilson, J.G. (1954) Differentiation and the reaction of rat embryos to radiation. *J. Cell. Comp. Physiol.*, Suppl. 1, 43: 11–38.

Yamazaki, J.N., Bennett, L.R., McFall, R.A. and Clemente, C.D. (1960) Brain radiation in newborn rats and differential effects of increased age. *Neurology*, 10: 530–536.

Discussions

J.M. Lauder: It seems important to also consider the possibility of rebound proliferation of cells when an antimitotic insult is presented for a short period of time and the agent produces a reversible effect on cell proliferation, for example methylazoxymethanol (MAM) and glucocorticoids. Do you have any comments on this?

P.M. Rodier: We have quantified such rebounds with a number of agents, by counting the number of mitotic figures over time during and after an insult (Andreoli et al., 1973; Rodier et al., 1986). In our studies, these rebounds of proliferation were never sufficient to bring cell numbers back to normal. However, I assume that a rebound could overshoot the appropriate number if the timing, degree of injury, etc., were just right. Obviously, to demonstrate such an effect, one would have to count the final cell number. I expect that such effects are much rarer than reductions of cell numbers.

T.D. Yih: Is the difference in effect observed after dosing on embryonic day 14 (E14) a.m. or p.m. a general feature or specific for the action of the drug and/or target organ? This is important in view of the fact that generally in teratogenicity testing, compounds are delivered in the morning (certainly in rat segment II and III studies; cf. Chapter 5 in this volume).

P.M. Rodier: Your question is indeed important. I am actually startled that I know the answer, because we have so little work completed on these studies. Fortunately, in our mouse study, E13 p.m. and E14 p.m. treatments with antimitogen gave weight reductions, while E14 a.m. did not (Rodier, work in progress). In the rat study of Johnston and Coyle (1979), in which rats exposed to MAM became oversized, the treatment occurred in the afternoon, while the

studies with weight reductions involved morning treatments (Fischer et al., 1972; Kabat et al., 1985). Thus, unless there is a complicated difference between mice and rats, it seems likely that the timing effects relate only to the time when growth-controlling cells form in the two species.

J. Sweeney: Are there drugs that effect neurogenesis in rat before postnatal day 10 and subsequently result in reduced progenitors and hypocellularity in the brain in general and not necessarily in specific regions?

P.M. Rodier: There are reports of agents delivered before day 10 affecting cell numbers. For example, a study by Sulik et al. (1981) indicates deficits in some parts of the CNS after ethanol exposure on day 7. As for the agents reducing the whole brain in a uniform fashion, I am not aware of such a teratological effect. Since many of us suspect that it is the mismatching of cells, rather than reduced numbers per se, that disrupts function, such an injury would be interesting to study. Of course, there are some chronic conditions, such as hypothyroidism (e.g. Balazs et al., 1971), which reduce neuron proliferation in general, but I do not know whether the effects are uniform, and I do not know whether they can occur over the whole course of neuron production, or only at later stages of development.

V.R. Sara: Your data remind me of the hypophysectomized rat where organ growth retardation begins to appear around 15–20 days postnatally, since this is the time when growth hormone (GH) begins to regulate insulin-like growth factor 1 (IGF-1) production (an early insult may have altered the sensitivity of the GH/IGF-1 system). Have you examined GH or IGF-1 in these animals?

P.M. Rodier: It was the similarity of teratologically induced growth deficits to those in the congenitally hypophysectomized rodent that interested us in this problem. We do, indeed, plan to measure GH levels. At this point, we do not have plans to study IGF-1. First, there is no indication from the clinical literature that IGF-1 is directly affected in cases of growth deficiency, except in several rare genetic syndromes (e.g. Laron et al., 1971) in which the somatic receptors for growth hormone appear to be defective. Perhaps such syndromes occur, and have been missed, but the present data suggest that if growth deficiency is teratological, the insult is more central. Second, the presence of multiple tissue sites for receptors for GH, for IGF-1 production, and for receptors for IGF-1 makes it unlikely that a brief, general teratogenic insult could affect all parts of the system simultaneously. Remember that the study by Fischer et al. (1972) showed postnatal growth deficiencies in all organs measured, except the brain, which was reduced from the time of MAM injury. It is easier to imagine an injury to the pituitary or the hypothalamus having effects on all these tissues, with their different times of development, than to hypothesize multiple peripheral injuries. Of course, if we find no effects on GH or GH releasing factor, we will have to study the peripheral parts of the system. Third, since IGF-1 influences growth in early development, a deficit in its production or in receptors for it would not account for postnatally appearing deficits in growth, like the ones I have reviewed. Of course, if our hypothesis of a central injury is correct, and treated animals are deficient in GH, the receptors for GH may be hypersensitive but that would be a side-effect of the functional problem, rather than an explanation of the growth deficiency.

D. F. Swaab: You made an important methodological point, stating that in affected brains cell density is not changed, but rather the size of the structures.This holds also for cell loss in aging (Swaab and Uylings, 1988). Did you also measure total cellular numbers for the somatostatin alterations?

P. M. Rodier: In the studies I described, it would be fairer to say that tissue volume is affected first, and cell density only when cell loss is extreme. We have seen changes in density with azacytidine when the loss was as high as 25 or 30%. Volume changes are more easily measured in some tissues than others (e.g. measures of layered structures, such as cerebral cortex, seem to pick up even very small changes in cell numbers). Therefore, I would not want to suggest that volume is a more sensitive measure in every case. Fortunately, in the case of somatostatin cells, we can count all the cells directly, because they are so few in number – only around 500 on each side of the ventricle – so we need not try to estimate a volume, which would be difficult with cells in this configuration.

References

Andreoli, J., Rodier, P.M. and Langman, J. (1973) The influence of a prenatal trauma on formation of Purkinje cells. *Am. J. Anat.*, 137: 87–102.

Balazs, R., Cocks, W.A., Eayrs, J.T. and Kovacs, S. (1971) Biochemical effects of thyroid hormones on the developing brain. In M. Hamburgh and E.J.W. Barrington (Eds.), *Hormones in Development*, Appleton Century Crofts, New York, pp. 357–379.

Fischer, M.H., Welker, C. and Waisman, H.A. (1972) Generalized growth retardation in rats induced by prenatal exposure to methylazoxymethanol acetate. *Teratology*, 5: 223–232.

Johnston, M.V. and Coyle, J.T. (1979) Histological and neurochemical effects of fetal treatment with methylazoxymethanol on rat neocortex in adulthood. *Brain Res.*, 170: 135–155.

Kabat, K., Buterbaugh, G.B. and Echols, C.U. (1985) Methylazoxymethanol as a devolpmental model of neurotoxicity. *Neurobehav. Toxicol. Teratol.*, 7: 519–525.

Laron, Z., Pertzelan, A., Karp, M., Kowadlo-Silbergeld, A. and Daughaday, W.H. (1971) Administration of growth hormone to patients with familial dwarfism with high plasma immunoreactive growth hormone: measurement of sulfation factor, metabolic and linear growth responses. *J. Clin. Endocrinol. Metab.*, 33: 332–342.

Rodier, P.M., Aschner, M., Lewis, L.S. and Koeter, H.B.W.M. (1986) Cell proliferation in developing brain after brief exposure to inhalant anesthetics. *Anesthesiology*, 64: 680–687.

Sulik, K.K., Johnston, M.C. and Webb, M.A. (1981) Fetal alcohol syndrome: Embryogenesis in a mouse model. *Science*, 214: 936–938.

Swaab, D.F. and Uylings, H.B.M. (1988) Comments on review by Coleman and Flood. Neuron numbers and dendritic extent in normal aging and Alzheimer's disease. Density measures: parameters to avoid. *Neurobiol. Aging*, in press.

G.J. Boer, M.G.P. Feenstra, M. Mirmiran, D.F. Swaab and F. Van Haaren
Progress in Brain Research, Vol. 73
© 1988 Elsevier Science Publishers B.V. (Biomedical Division)

CHAPTER 23

Coordination of cell development by the ornithine decarboxylase (ODC)/polyamine pathway as an underlying mechanism in developmental neurotoxic events

Joanne M. Bell and Theodore A. Slotkin

Department of Pharmacology, Duke University Medical Center, Durham, NC 27710, USA

Introduction

The appearance of alterations in behavioral function caused by a teratogen must have, as its basis, a primary action on cellular mechanisms. Teratological changes confined to behavioral (or biochemical) function can be as damaging as obvious gross skeletal or morphological abnormalities: subtle deficits may go unnoticed at birth and lead to a cascade of alterations in neurobehavioral functioning as the animal matures that make it progressively difficult to determine underlying primary alterations induced by the teratogen. Thus, early examination of the limited repertoire of physical skills in the very young animal may potentially provide more useful indices of primary neural alterations than long-term behavioral assessments at maturity. After the elucidation of early changes in behavior, the question of how these effects are initially induced is more readily approached. The finding that many diverse agents such as neurotoxins, food additives, nicotine, ethanol and opiates lead to similar behavioral and biochemical changes also raises the possibility that general interference with cellular development of neural tissues is a com-

mon feature of behavioral teratogenesis, and consequently the timetable of cell maturation and age of exposure may play a role as important as that of the teratogen itself. This chapter will discuss the ornithine decarboxylase (ODC)/polyamine pathway as a potential underlying biochemical mechanism of functional teratogenesis. Through study of its direct inhibition, this pathway is now known to regulate nucleic acid and protein synthesis in developing tissues, and thus may act as the common target for neurobehavioral, synaptogenic, morphological as well as cellular deficits in response to a diverse spectrum of developmental insults.

Effects of dietary food additives

It has been known for years that alterations in the maternal diet can have a deleterious effect on the offspring development (Winick and Noble, 1967). Of particular relevance is that during the pre-weaning period, the central nervous system of the offspring is rapidly undergoing cellular proliferation, differentiation and growth and is, therefore, particularly sensitive to a wide variety of perturbations (Dobbing and Smart, 1974). We

---

Correspondence: Dr. J.M. Bell, Dept. of Pharmacology, Duke Univ. Medical Center, Durham, NC 27710, USA.

have shown that perinatal dietary manipulations, by supplementation with common US/FDA-approved food additives have far-ranging consequences for offspring neurobehavioral and biochemical development.

In the past few years, the use of dietary lecithin supplements has received public attention due to the potential use of such agents in treating memory dysfunction (Bartus et al., 1982), as well as in reducing circulating cholesterol (Assman and Brewer, 1974). Lecithin is also found in varying amounts in many prepared foods because of its emulsifying properties (Wurtman, 1979). The favorable classification of lecithin by the GRAS commission in 1973 has led to widespread over-the-counter sale of these dietary supplements. However, soy lecithin preparations (SLPs), prepared from soy beans, contain a variety of phospholipids along with lecithin (which possesses a choline moiety). Nonsupervised intake of these impure SLPs by subsets of the lay population, such as pregnant women or women of childbearing age, may be potentially harmful to their offspring. Phospholipids are rapidly incorporated into developing brain, either as membrane constituents (Davidson and Dobbing, 1960) or acetylcholine (Atterwill and Prince, 1978), or both; thus, when fed to pregnant or lactating dams, SLPs could act in either fashion to influence maturation of cells in the central nervous system. In our experiments, we first fed rat dams an AIN 76 standard pelleted lab chow or the same lab chow supplemented with 5% soy lecithin from the 7th day of gestation until parturition with the offspring maintained on the same diet throughout the preweaning period (Bell and Lundberg, 1984). In order to first establish that perinatal SLP exposure has functional effects, we administered a modification of the Cincinnati neonatal test battery, selected for sensitivity to detect neurobehavioral toxicity in rats (Vorhees et al., 1979; Brunner et al., 1979). This battery consisted of tests of reflex righting, negative geotaxis, pivoting, swimming development, open field ambulation and morphine analgesia. Ani-

mals exposed to SLP during the perinatal period showed an initial decrease in latency to right on the first two postnatal days of life, indicating an acceleration of the maturation of this response; by postnatal (PN) day 4, however, these animals took longer to right than did controls. The same animals also showed a decreased latency for negative geotaxis, a response which undergoes its maturational development slightly later. To examine whether behavioral effects of SLP exposure extended beyond the immediate postnatal period, morphine analgesia was assessed in adulthood and again showed a decreased nociceptivity in the treated animals (Bell and Slotkin, 1985).

If these early-appearing behavioral abnormalities associated with perinatal exposure to SLP reflect actions at the cellular level, then changes in synaptogenesis or synaptic function should be occurring. SLP enrichment was found to elevate choline acetyltransferase (CAT) activity during early life, although such increases were not sustained beyond sexual maturity. Although these results suggested that ACh precursor-loading (choline moiety of SLP) could accelerate normal maturation of this enzyme system (Tucek, 1978), we also assessed postsynaptic reactivity of central cholinergic mechanisms by utilizing the ability of an intracisternally injected cholinergic agonist to stimulate ^{33}Pi incorporation into phospholipids, an effect known to be mediated by post-junctional muscarinic receptors (Friedel and Schanberg, 1972). Results obtained in this study (Bell et al., 1986b) provided direct evidence that perinatal SLP exposure produces perturbations of the sensitivity of developing central synapses to cholinergic stimuli: the reactivity of phospholipid incorporation of ^{33}Pi to carbachol was lowered in the whole brains of SLP exposed pups (Fig. 1). This effect was selective for the cholinergic system, as stimulation with another transmitter (dopamine) was not suppressed. However, SLP exposure also affected basal (unstimulated) membrane phospholipid incorporation (Fig. 2), indicating that abnormalities at the membrane level, associated

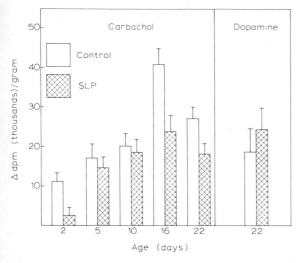

Fig. 1 Effects of dietary SLP exposure on stimulation of ^{33}Pi incorporation evoked by carbachol or dopamine. Data were expressed as differences between stimulated rats (agonist administration) and basal values. ANOVA indicated a significant increase in carbachol-induced stimulation with age as well as a significant overall reduction in stimulation caused by SLP (Bell et al., 1986b).

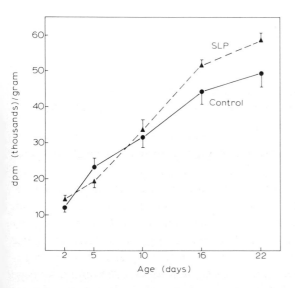

Fig. 2 Development of basal (unstimulated) ^{33}Pi incorporation into membrane phospholipids in brains of control and SLP-enriched rats. ANOVA indicated a significant age-related increase in corporation as well as an overall elevation caused by exposure to SLP (Bell et al., 1986b).

with the lipid moiety of SLP may also be present. Indeed, others (Brenneman and Rutledge, 1979) have shown that when young rats are fed experimental diets with abnormal lipid components, neuronal membrane properties and transmitter activities can be altered.

Since these data indicated that SLP-induced changes in synaptic populations could occur in pathways other than cholinergic, we examined the developmental characteristics of the catecholamines in discrete brain regions. Although transmitter levels of norepinephrine (NE) and dopamine (DA) were unaffected, the utilization rates (turnover) of both catecholamines as measured by α-methyl-p-tyrosine (AMPT) administration 2 h before sacrifice, were profoundly disturbed in an age-dependent, regionally-selective manner (Fig. 3). Values for utilization were generally lowered during the preweaning stage but showed a postweaning elevation which was most persistent in the midbrain + brainstem, shorter-lasting but more intense in the cerebellum and virtually non-existent in the cerebral cortex. Utilization rate can be affected by the efficiency of presynaptic recapture of released transmitter, since reuptake reduces the apparent amount of transmitter turned over: in order for alterations of uptake to produce their observed effects on utilization, uptake capabilities would have to be reduced at the ages at which utilization was found to be elevated, and increased when utilization was reduced. The SLP diet did have a significant effect on the development of uptake in the cerebellum, as well as producing a tendency toward altered uptake in the midbrain + brainstem (Fig. 4). However, utilization rates were often increased in the face of increased synaptosomal uptake (postweaning), indicating that the actual rate of transmitter utilization in the synaptic terminal was probably even higher than that measured.

Since recovery of transmitter from the synapse (primarily governed by synaptic uptake) could not directly account for the alterations of intraneuronal transmitter utilization, we evaluated another major component which could also play a

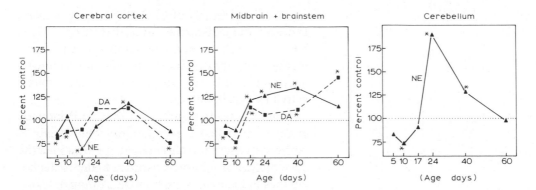

Fig. 3 Effects of SLP-enriched diet on utilization rates of norepinephrine (NE) and dopamine (DA) in brain regions. Catecholamine utilization rate (turnover) was assessed by administration of α-methyl-*p*-tyrosine methyl ester HC1 (AMPT, 300 mg/kg, i.p.) 2 h before sacrifice. AMPT inhibits tyrosine hydroxylase, the rate limiting step in catecholamine biosynthesis, and the disappearance of endogenous catecholamines after AMPT estimates the utilization rates. Asterisks denote individual age points at which differences were significant between dietary groups, assessed by Duncan's multiple range test (Bell et al., 1986c).

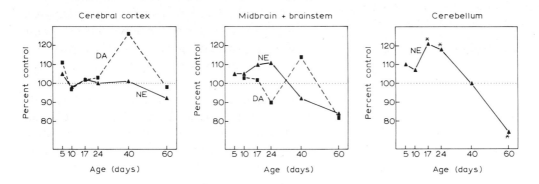

Fig. 4 Effects of SLP-enriched diet on synaptosomal uptake of [³H]norepinephrine (NE) and [³H]dopamine (DA) in brain regions. Asterisks denote individual age points at which differences were significant between two dietary groups, assessed by Duncan's multiple range test only where ANOVA indicated a significant overall effect or interaction (Bell et al., 1986c).

contributory influence to these functional alterations: release of transmitter into the synapse (primarily governed by impulse activity). Impulse activity-related release of transmitter into the synapse could than influence the overall net synaptic activity. One index of the degree of neuronal stimulation occurring during brain development is tyrosine hydroxylase, the rate-limiting enzyme in catecholamine biosynthesis (Brodie et al., 1966; Udenfriend, 1966). Examination of midbrain + brainstem confirmed that the postweaning period in which NE utilization was elevated in the SLP group was also associated

with significant elevations of tyrosine hydroxylase activity (Fig. 5). It should be noted, however, that enzyme levels were also elevated in midbrain + brainstem before weaning, a point at which utilization rates for NE (and DA) were generally reduced. This finding suggested that this earlier phase may also induce alterations in intraneuronal factors, such as catecholamine storage and degradation. Tyrosine hydroxylase was reduced in the cerebral cortex during the postweaning period, a pattern opposite to that seen in the midbrain + brainstem. Taken together, these data indicate that impulse activity was altered in

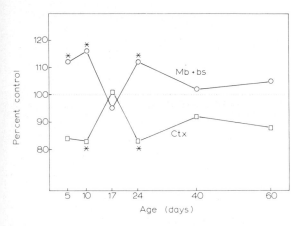

Fig. 5 Effects of SLP-enriched diet on tyrosine hydroxylase activity in cerebral cortex (Ctx) and midbrain + brainstem (Mb + bs). Asterisks denote individual age points at which differences were significant between the two dietary groups (Bell et al., 1986c).

a regionally selective, age-dependent manner in developing catecholaminergic systems (Bell et al., 1986c).

The observations that alterations caused by SLP extend beyond cholinergic systems, and that other dietary manipulations aimed at other transmitter systems can produce the same behavioral changes (Brunner et al., 1979), and that alterations of the amount of dietary saturated fats result in similar neurotransmitter abnormalities (Brenneman and Rutledge, 1979), suggest that common changes in underlying brain cell matura-

tional events may be shared by dissimilar substances. In order to assess the likelihood that SLP-exposure alters the development and activity of synaptic populations through a general interference with brain cell maturation, we examined standard indices of cell growth (nucleic acids and proteins) in brain regions of animals given SLP perinatally (Bell and Slotkin, 1985). As illustrated in Fig. 6, DNA content of the cerebellum was increased by SLP transiently at weaning, with a subsequent return toward normal values as the animals entered adulthood; RNA and protein levels were reduced. The effects of SLP on brain maturation appeared to be regionally specific. DNA in cerebral cortex were completely different from those in the cerebellum. Cortical DNA content was significantly subnormal, a difference which persisted into adulthood and which appeared permanent. Since DNA per cell is constant (Winick and Noble, 1965), this biochemical finding indicated a long lasting deficit in the number of cortical cells. There was also a compensatory hypertrophy of remaining cortical cells (elevated RNA and protein). The question left unanswered, however, was whether these events were predictable based upon early regulation of macromolecule synthesis.

One biochemical tool which has proven useful in the early evaluation of general growth and development is the activity of the enzyme ornithine decarboxylase (ODC). ODC catalyses the con-

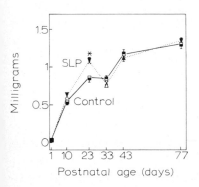
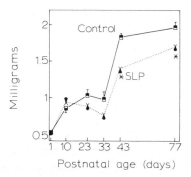

Fig. 6 DNA content of developing cerebellum (left) and cerebral cortex (right panel) in control rats and rats exposed to SLP-enriched diet. Asterisks denote individual age points at which differences were statistically significant (Bell and Slotkin, 1985).

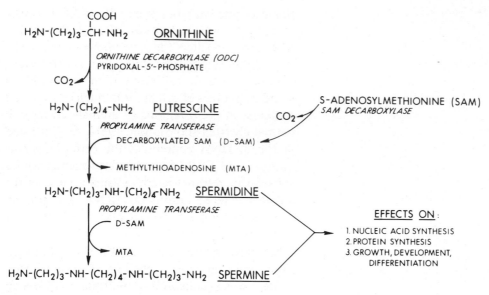

Fig. 7 Biosynthesis of the polyamines.

version of ornithine to putrescine, the first and probably rate-limiting step in the synthesis of the polyamines, a set of molecules which appears to be intimately associated with growth and differentiation (Russell and Durie, 1978; Tabor and Tabor, 1983) (Fig. 7). Polyamines have been shown to regulate DNA, RNA and protein synthesis in many growing systems, ranging from bacteria to mammals (Bachrach, 1973). Similarly, ODC activity is always highest when growth is

stimulated, and declines as growth ceases (Bartolome et al., 1980, 1982b). Evaluation of the roles of ODC and the polyamines in the developing mammalian nervous system indicate that the highest levels of these molecules are paralleled in each brain region by periods of most rapid cellular growth and replication (Anderson and Schanberg, 1972), and recent work has confirmed the direct control of macromolecule synthesis by the ODC/polyamine pathway (Slotkin

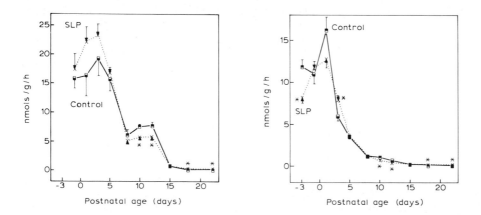

Fig. 8 ODC activity in developing cerebellum and cerebral cortex in control rats and rats exposed to SLP-enriched diet. Asterisks denote individual age points at which differences were statistically significant (Bell and Slotkin, 1985).

and Bartolome, 1986). Each developing region displays an unique developmental pattern of ODC activity. Because ODC possesses an extremely short turnover time of 10–20 min (Slotkin et al., 1983), its activity is exquisitely sensitive to detection of perturbations of brain development introduced by changes in the perinatal environment occurring at that time. Since SLP was administered during the period of rapid brain growth, changes in the patterns of ODC activity should have been able to predict the consequent alterations of cell growth and development in exposed offspring. Such was the case: ODC in the cerebellum of SLP-exposed rats was elevated in the immediate pre- and postnatal period and was prematurely lowered thereafter (Fig. 8). The 'compression' of the time course of ODC, i.e., initial promotion and premature decline, signalled the corresponding initial elevation of DNA followed by a persistent shortfall in the cellular content of other macromolecules. ODC patterns in an earlier maturing region, the cortex, were also changed. In that region, the ODC developmental pattern corresponded to a delayed maturational profile, i.e., initial suppression of activity followed by compensatory elevations. As predicted by this enzymatic marker, cortical DNA was permanently lowered. The regional differences between cerebellar and cortical ODC patterns

also raised the possibility that the ODC/polyamine system does not participate uniformly in the growth of these regions, but rather that there may be critical periods in which neural maturation is particularly sensitive to changes in ODC.

Effects of direct interference with the ODC/polyamine pathway

If disturbances of cell development are a potential underlying mechanism for later alterations in neuronal structure or function, direct suppression of the ODC/polyamine pathway with a specific, irreversible inhibitor, α-difluoromethylornithine (DFMO), should cause anomalies common to SLP as well as other neuroactive substances. DFMO has been shown to inhibit the growth of a variety of tumor and cell lines and arrests early embryogenesis of mammalian species (Raina and Janne, 1975). Prolonged administration of large doses of DFMO to pregnant rats causes fetal death and resorption if the drug is begun early in gestation (Fozard et al., 1980) or reduced neonatal vitality if begun later (Slotkin et al., 1983). However, when the dose or duration of treatment with DFMO is reduced or treatment begun postnatally, specific brain growth deficits do become apparent without effects on mortality or morbidity. This evidence supports the view that the

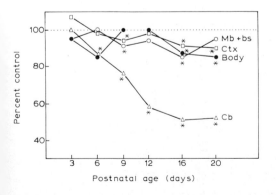 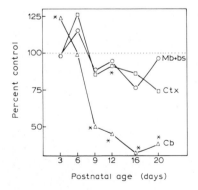

Fig. 9 Regional selectivity of the effect of postnatal DFMO administration (500 mg/kg once daily, begun the day after birth until weaning on PN day 21) on growth (left) and DNA content (right panel) in neonatal rat brain. Cb, cerebellum; Ctx, cerebral cortex; Mb + bs, midbrain + brainstem (Bell et al., 1986d).

ODC/polyamine system directly participates in brain development, but that selective actions of ODC inhibition with DFMO should become apparent when appropriate periods are selected for drug administration. In order to test this premise, we administered DFMO, utilizing treatment regimens which spanned different critical periods of development either postnatally (PN days 1–21) or during gestation (days G15–17) (Bell et al., 1986d).

Daily administration of DFMO begun at birth had a small, but significant effect on body growth as well as on growth of the cerebral cortex and midbrain + brainstem (Fig. 9). In contrast, a profound deficit was seen for growth of the cerebellum, where weights became reduced as early as six days postnatally and were 50% subnormal by the end of the third postnatal week. The regional selectivity of effects of postnatal DFMO on growth were mirrored by those on the content of DNA: by 16–20 days after birth, the DFMO group was missing two-thirds of its cerebellar DNA. In contrast, effects on DNA in the cortex and midbrain + brainstem tended to be transient and relatively minor. Postnatal DFMO administration also influenced cerebellar RNA and protein in a pattern similar to that seen for DNA, and again the effects in the other two regions were of small magnitude. Thus, postnatal DFMO clearly exerted its major actions on the cerebellum, the region in which activity is highest after birth (Bell et al., 1986d).

If sensitivity to DFMO involves cell populations specifically undergoing replication, then administration of the drug during different critical developmental periods should shift the regional selectivity of effect. A comparison of DFMO given prenatally on gestational days 15–17 with postnatal DFMO readily illustrates this concept: body weights of offspring receiving prenatal DFMO revealed significant deficits of greater magnitude than was seen with postnatal DFMO, but in this case, regional selectivity for brain growth was only slight (Fig. 10). Unlike the severe effects of postnatal DFMO on cerebellar DNA levels, prenatal DFMO treatment resulted in much smaller changes in DNA content in this region, with early reductions followed by a complete recovery by PN day 16. The most intense and persistent effect was seen in the cerebral cortex where there were initial elevations of DNA content, but a subsequent and permanent deficit. Cortical RNA was less affected, but altered in a similar pattern. Prenatal DFMO also had selective effects on cortical protein levels: the content was significantly and persistently reduced. Thus, despite the fact that short-term prenatal DFMO produced even more body growth retardation than did long-term postnatal DFMO, cerebellar growth was affected no more so than any other

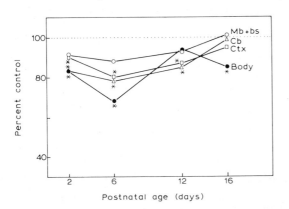
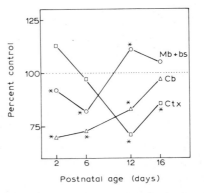

Fig. 10 Regional selectivity of the effect of prenatal DFMO administration (500 mg/kg twice daily to dams on gestational days 15–17) on growth (left) and DNA content (right panel) in neonatal rat brain. Cb, cerebellum; Ctx, cerebral cortex; Mb + bs, midbrain + brainstem (Bell et al., 1986d).

region. What is particularly noteworthy is that a degree of specificity toward a different brain region (cerebral cortex) was apparent in the prenatal group. Cerebral cortex ODC peaks earlier than in the cerebellum, with highest activity in the immediate antenatal period (Bell and Slotkin, 1985). Prenatal DFMO administration caused an eventual shortfall of both RNA and protein in cerebral cortex which was of greater magnitude than in either of the other two regions studied. This pattern is grossly similar to that caused by SLP exposure.

The biochemical studies support the view that the ODC/polyamine system participates in brain development particularly during periods of rapid cellular replication. Those structures which are undergoing proliferation at the time of DFMO administration are more severely affected than those structures that have either completed differentiation or have not yet begun: postnatal DFMO exerts major effects on cerebellar growth, while prenatal DFMO shifted these effects away from the cerebellum, and toward the cerebral cortex. Since we were able to demonstrate the need for maintenance of the ODC/polyamine system for growth, there should be structural correlates of interference with this system. Interestingly, the morphological studies indicate post-mitotic involvement of ODC in architectural development of brain regions, along with the expected selectivity for replicating cells. Because the cerebellum is a specific target during postnatal development, we have used this brain region to examine the impact of DFMO on laminar organization and cell migration, processes which, like synaptogenesis, represent post-mitotic events of major functional significance.

During postnatal maturation, the granule cells proliferate in the external granule cells layer and migrate to the internal layer, such that by the end of the third postnatal week the architectural organization of the cerebellar cortex is fairly complete (Altman, 1966). Animals given DFMO postnatally displayed aberrations which represented a combination of anti-mitotic actions and interfer-

ence with these post-mitotic events (Bartolome et al., 1985). In the case of the former, granule cell populations showed a progressive shortfall in number, in direct contrast to a lack of impact on Purkinje cells which have undergone their major divisions prior to initiation of DFMO treatment. With regard to post-mitotic events, at least two of the characteristics of the immature cerebellum persisted past weaning in the DFMO group: (1) although the total number of Purkinje cells was not altered, soma size was reduced and cells did not line up in the normally occurring discrete monolayer; and (2) the external granule cell layer remained detectable, and the internal granule cell layer was thinly populated with a proportion of granule cells becoming trapped in the molecular layer.

These findings suggested that DFMO could be used as a more selective tool for studying development than X-irradiation or cytotoxic drugs (Altman and Anderson, 1969; Singh and Champlain, 1972). With selection of appropriate doses and ages, the actions of DFMO on development can be targeted toward specific cell populations in a developing nervous system, while sparing postmitotic cells. To this end, we determined that the granule cells of the dorsal cochlear nucleus (DCN) of the hamster were similarly vulnerable to DFMO treatment (Schweitzer et al., 1987). Indeed, the granule cells of the DCN share many of the morphological attributes with the cerebellar cortex of the rat: neurons continue to proliferate after birth, and their postreplicative migration patterns make them both particularly vulnerable to depletion by DFMO. Administration of DFMO to hamsters after birth permitted selective depletion of granule cells, with an indirect reduction of fusiform cells (by virtue of its major input to these cells). More specifically, as with the cerebellum, DFMO administration resulted in a reduction in the density of cells in both the superficial and deep granule cell layers of the DCN (Fig. 11). These series of effects suggested that granule cells located in the superficial layer that would have migrated into the deep dorsal

358

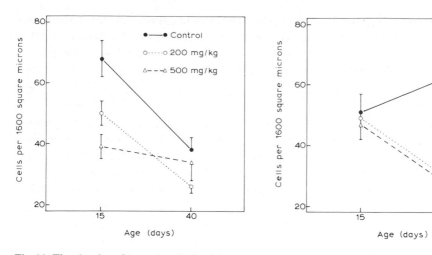

Fig. 11 The density of granule cells in the superficial (left) and deep dorsal cochlear nucleus (DCN) (right panel) following postnatal administration of DFMO from birth through weaning. Data indicate both treatments caused significant decreases in the density of granule cells in both the superficial and deep DCN (Schweitzer et al., 1987).

cochlear nucleus had either failed to develop or did not arrive at their final location. Thus, the use of DFMO allowed for the finding that in the DCN of the hamster, as well as the cerebellar cortex of rat, migrating cells from the superficial proliferative zone into deeper layers are dependent upon the ODC/polyamine pathway for these processes. As an additional note, our group has identified ODC in specific lamina of the developing cerebellum of the 9-day-old rat, using labelled DFMO and autoradiographic techniques (Morris et al., 1986). In keeping with the predominance of enzymatic activity in this specific region at this age as determined by biochemical measurements, ODC was detectable throughout the cerebellum, with labelling in both granule cell layers, as well as heavy labelling in the molecular layer. The morphological evidence as well as the structural localization of ODC supports not only a major association of enzyme activity with proliferative events, but a maintenance of this activity well into differentiation and later development.

If post-proliferative events are dependent upon the ODC/polyamine system, administration of DFMO during the first two postnatal weeks of life, the period marked by axogenesis and synap-

togenesis, should result in attenuation of synaptic maturation. Furthermore, if the behavioral and biochemical anomalies common to neuroactive substances have, as their basis, alterations of the ODC/polyamine system, the changes in synaptic maturation following such exposure should again be obtainable by the direct inhibition of ODC by DFMO. Daily postnatal administration of DFMO to neonatal rats did indeed result in a slowing of development of central catecholaminergic synapses (Slotkin et al., 1982). Fundamental alterations in brain membrane metabolism also could be detected through measurements of phospholipid incorporation of ^{33}Pi; DFMO suppressed the developmental increments in phospholipid synthesis normally accompanying synaptic outgrowth. Although the content of NE and DA in whole brain was unchanged by DFMO, the drug did cause initial reductions, and subsequent elevations, in catecholamine turnover. Similarly, if the DFMO treatment regimen was most effective during periods of rapid neuronal development, one would expect to see changes in the peripheral nervous system as well, since the postnatal development of noradrenergic nerve terminals and function in the periphery occurs even earlier than in the brain. Such was the case: examination of the levels and turnover of NE in cardiac sympathetic nerves indicated significant deficits in transmitter levels even at 1 week of postnatal age. As in the brain, some evidence of compensatory stimulation or recovery from inhibition of development was evidenced in cardiac sympathetic neurons, as the turnover rate became elevated by 21 days of age. These results indicate that the role of polyamines in nervous system development extends beyond phases of cell replication and into the period of architectural modelling and synaptic connection.

The studies of DFMO reviewed thus far have demonstrated the direct relationship between the ODC/polyamine system and control of nervous system development: we have shown that polyamines play a pivotal role in macromolecular synthesis, architectural organization and synaptic maturation. To illustrate that these types of structural and biochemical alterations are of functional significance, it should also be demonstrated that polyamines play a vital role in acquisition of behavioral competence. We have shown that the behavioral effects of DFMO are specifically dependent upon its actions during the same defined stages as have been identified for actions on cell replication and migration, axogenesis and synaptogenesis (Bell et al., 1986a). Administration of DFMO during gestation has its greatest adverse effects on early-appearing sensorimotor behaviors, such as reflex righting and negative geotaxis; on the other hand, postnatal DFMO treatment does not affect early measures of motor coordination (righting) and has a smaller impact on negative geotaxis than does prenatal DFMO. The predominance of prenatal DFMO-induced anomalies of early behaviors occurs despite the fact that the ODC/polyamine system has recovered from the effects of prenatal drug administration during the behavioral assessment period. Both this study and that of others (Genedani et al., 1985) were able to rule out a direct (i.e., not polyamine-related) effect of DFMO on behavioral development. Such evidence suggested that polyamine depletion during critical periods of prenatal brain growth results in permanent alterations in early-maturing regions with consequences which extend beyond the period in which polyamines are depleted. In contrast to the results obtained with prenatal inhibition of ODC, postnatal administration of DFMO beginning at birth and continuing up until weaning exerts it greatest effect on later-developing, more integrated forms of behavior. One such example was swimming development which involves a coordinated series of reflex responses (righting, vestibular, extensor-flexor). The progressive tendency toward coordinated movements, assessed by nose position and forelimb inhibition, was most severely delayed in animals given DFMO postnatally. In the same vein, both horizontal and vertical components of open field activity were lowered by postnatal DFMO, indicating a marked degree of hypoactivity, whereas prenatal DFMO resulted in only a reduction in vertical activity. It should be noted that the higher degree of integration of motor coordination required for swimming and open field activity is dependent, in large part, on development of competence of the cerebellum, the brain region which is the specific target for postnatal DFMO. The severe alterations in the biochemistry and morphological development of the cerebellum occurred at precisely the time at which functional behavioral deficits became evident.

Results of these behavioral studies confirm the crucial role played by the ODC/polyamine pathway in brain development. Inhibition of ODC by DFMO resulted in patterns of alterations which were dependent upon the period in which drug exposure occurred and the functional consequences of polyamine depletion during critical developmental periods could thus appear far beyond the point at which ODC and polyamine levels have returned to normal. The selectivity of behavioral effects of DFMO exposure for these periods paralleled the regional selectivity generated by the biochemical and anatomical timetable of maturation of each brain region.

Conclusions

From the experimental evidence described in this chapter, it is clear that the ODC/polyamine system plays a pivotal role in biochemical, morphological and behavioral responses to a diverse spectrum of insults. We have shown that direct inhibition of this pathway with DFMO produces a variety of deficits similar to those found with a neuroactive substance, in this case, dietary SLP. Indeed, work by our group on a number of neurotoxins, trophic agents and drugs of abuse, has determined that, following initial changes in ODC, alterations in macromolecular synthesis and synaptogenesis are predictable. Among the agents examined were corticosteroids and thyroid hormone (Anderson and Schanberg, 1975), nicotine (Slotkin et al., 1986b), methadone (Slotkin et al., 1976), food additives (Bell et al., 1985), methylmercury (Bartolome et al., 1982a) and hypoxia (Slotkin et al., 1986a). These findings provide support for the view that the ODC/polyamine pathway represents a common regulatory mechanism whose disruption leads to the subsequent observable patterns of neurobehavioral alterations. In this regard, a source of future work lies in the manipulation of ODC/polyamine levels to prevent or offset the consequences of teratogen exposure or environmentally induced perturbations. Indeed, a recently published study (Agnati et al., 1985) suggests that the polyamines may have a role as trophic factors in the brain following discrete lesions, and that the palliative effects of GM1 ganglioside acts through eliciting elevations of polyamines to prevent retrograde degeneration.

Finally, the development of specific treatments which affect polyamine levels, such as DFMO, in combination with the understanding of the timetables for replication and differentiation of specific cell types, will allow study of the functional consequences of selective developmental lesions. For instance, the use of DFMO as a probe to elucidate the functional importance of specific cell types (as we have shown with the DCN of the hamster) has provided valuable information in the field of auditory anatomy. It is therefore clear that further work on the ODC/polyamine system in brain development will be of significant interest not only for its relationship to neuroteratology but to an understanding of the relationships between neurochemical development and behavior.

Acknowledgments

This work was supported by USPHS HD-09713.

References

Agnati, L.F., Fuxe, K., Zini, I., Davalli, P., Corti, A., Calza, L., Toffano, G., Zoli, M., Piccini, G. and Goldstein, M. (1985) Effects of lesions and ganglioside GM1 treatment on striatal polyamine levels and nigral DA neurons. A role of putrescine in the neurotropic activity of gangliosides. *Acta Physiol. Sand.*, 124: 499–506.

Altman, J. (1966) Autoradiographic and histological studies of postnatal neurogenesis. II. A longitudinal investigation of the kinetics, migration and transformation of cells incorporating tritiated thymidine in infant rats, with special reference to postnatal neurogenesis in some brain regions. *J. Comp. Neurol.*, 128: 431–474.

Altman, J. and Anderson, W.J. (1969) Early effects of X-irradiation of the cerebellum in infant rats: decimation and reconstitution of the external granule layer. *Exp. Neurol.*, 24: 196–216.

Anderson, T.R. and Schanberg, S.M. (1972) Ornithine decarboxylase activity in developing brain. *J. Neurochem.*, 19: 1471–1481.

Anderson, R.R. and Schanberg, S.M. (1975) Effect of thyroxine and cortisol on brain ornithine decarboxylase and swimming behavior in developing rat. *Biochem. Pharmacol.*, 24: 495–501.

Assman, G. and Brewer, H. (1974) A molecular model of high density lipoproteins. *Proc. Natl. Acad. Sci. USA*, 71: 1534–1538.

Atterwill, C. and Prince, A. (1978) Multiple forms of choline acetyltransferase and the high affinity uptake of choline in brain of developing and adult rats. *J. Neurochem.*, 31: 719–725.

Bachrach, U. (1973) Function of Naturally Occurring Polyamines, Academic Press, New York.

Bartolome, J., Huguenard, J. and Slotkin, T.A. (1980) Role of ornithine decarboxylase in cardiac growth and hypertrophy. *Science*, 210: 793–794.

Bartolome, J., Chait, E.A., Trepanier, P., Whitmore, W., Weigel, S. and Slotkin, T.A. (1982a) Organ specificity of neonatal methylmercury hydroxide poisoning in the rat: Effects on ornithine decarboxylase activity in developing tissues. *Toxicol. Lett.*, 13: 267–276.

Bartolome, J., Trepanier, P., Chait, E.A. and Slotkin, T.A. (1982b) Role of polyamines in isoproterenol-induced cardiac hypertrophy: Effects of α-difluoromethylornithine, an irreversible inhibitor of ornithine decarboxylase. *J. Mol. Cell. Cardiol.*, 14: 461–466.

Bartolome, J., Schweitzer, L., Slotkin, T.A. and Nadler, J.V. (1985) Impaired development of cerebellar cortex in rats treated postnatally with α-difluoromethylornithine. *Neuroscience*, 15: 203–213.

Bartus, R., Dean, R., Beir, B. and Lippa, A. (1982) The cholinergic hypothesis of geriatric memory dysfunction. *Science*, 217: 408–417.

Bell, J.M. and Lundberg, P.K. (1985) Effects of a commercial soy lecithin preparation on development of sensorimotor behavior and brain biochemistry in the rat. *Dev. Psychobiol.*, 18: 59–66.

Bell, J.M., Slotkin, T.A. (1985) Perinatal dietary supplementation with a commercial soy lecithin preparation: Effects on behavior and brain biochemistry in the developing rat. *Dev. Psychobiol.*, 18: 383–394.

Bell, J.M., Madwed, D.S. and Slotkin, T.A. (1986a) Critical development periods for inhibition of ornithine decarboxylase by α-difluoromethylornithine: Effects on ontogeny of sensorimotor behavior. *Neuroscience*, 19: 457–464.

Bell, J.M., Whitmore, W.L., Barnes, G., Seidler, F.J. and Slotkin, T.A. (1986b) Perinatal dietary exposure to soy lecithin: Altered sensitivity to central catecholaminergic stimulation. *Int. J. Dev. Neurosci.*, 4: 497–501.

Bell, J.M., Whitmore, W.L., Cowdery, T. and Slotkin, T.A. (1986c) Perinatal dietary supplementation with a soy lecithin preparation: Effects on development of central catecholaminergic neurotransmitter system. *Brain Res. Bull.*, 17: 189–195.

Bell, J.M., Whitmore, W.L. and Slotkin, T.A. (1986d) Effects of α-difluoromethylornithine, a specific irreversible inhibitor of ornithine decarboxylase, on nucleic acids and proteins in developing rat brain: Critical perinatal periods for regional selectivity. *Neuroscience*, 17: 399–407.

Brenneman, D.E. and Rutledge, C.O. (1979) Alteration of catecholamine uptake in cerebral cortex from rats fed a saturated fat diet. *Brain Res.*, 179: 295–301.

Brodie, B.B., Costa, E., Dlabac, A., Neff, N.H. and Smookler, H.H. (1966) Application of steadystate kinetics to the estimation of synthesis rate and turnover time of tissue catecholamines. *J. Pharmacol. Exp. Ther.*, 154: 493–498.

Brunner, R.L., Vorhees, C.V., Kinney, L. and Butcher, R.E. (1979) Aspartame: Assessment of developmental psychotoxicity of a new artificial sweetener. *Neurobehav. Toxicol.*, 1: 79–86.

Davidson, A. and Dobbing, J. (1960) Phospholipid metabolism in nervous tissue: Metabolic stability. *Biochem. J.*, 75: 565–570.

Dobbing, J. and Smart, J. (1974) Vulnerability of developing brain and behavior. *Br. Med. Bull.*, 30: 164–168.

Fozard, J.R., Part, M.-L., Prakash, N.J., Grove, J., Schechter, P.J., Sjoerdsma, A. and Koch-Weser, J. (1980) l-Ornithine decarboxylase: An essential role in early mammalian embryogenesis. *Science*, 208: 505–508.

Friedel, P.O. and Schanberg, S.M. (1972) Effects of carbamylcholine and atropine on incorporation in vivo of [33]Pi into phospholipids of rat brain. *J. Pharmacol. Exp. Ther.*, 183: 326–332.

Genedani, S., Bernardi, M. and Bertolini, A. (1985) Developmental and behavioral outcomes of perinatal inhibition of ornithine decarboxylase. *Neurobehav. Toxicol. Teratol.*, 7: 57–65.

Morris, G., Nadler, J.V. and Slotkin, T.A. (1986) Autographic localization of ornithine decarboxylase in cerebellar cortex of the developing rat with (^{3}H)α-difluoromethylornithine. *Neuroscience*, 17: 183–188.

Raina, A. and Janne, J. (1975) Physiology of the natural polyamines putrescine, spermidine and spermine. *Med. Biol.*, 53: 121–147.

Russell, D. and Durie, B. (1978) Progress in Cancer Research and Therapy, Vol. 8. Polyamines as Biochemical Markers of Normal and Malignant Growth. Raven Press, New York.

Schweitzer, L., Bell, J.M. and Slotkin, T.A. (1987) Impaired morphological development of the dorsal cochlear nucleus in hamsters treated postnatally with α-difluoromethylornithine. *Int. J. Dev. Neurosci.*, in press.

Singh, B. and Champlain, J. (1972) Altered ontogeny of central noradrenergic neurons following neonatal treatment with 6-hydroxydopamine. *Brain Res.*, 48: 432–437.

Slotkin, T.A. and Bartolome, J. (1986) Role of ornithine decarboxylase and the polyamines in nervous system development: A review. *Brain Res. Bull.*, 17: 307–320.

Slotkin, T.A., Cowdery, T., Orband, L., Pachman, S. and Whitmore, W.L. (1986a) Effects of neonatal hypoxia on brain development in the rat: Immediate and long-term biochemical alterations in discrete regions. *Brain Res.*, 374: 63–74.

Slotkin, T.A., Greer, N., Faust, J., Cho, H. and Seidler, F.J. (1986b) Effects of maternal nicotine injections on brain development in the rat: Ornithine decarboxylase activity, nucleic acids and proteins in discrete brain regions. *Brain Res. Bull.*, 17: 41–50.

Slotkin, T.A., Gringolo, A., Whitmore, W.L., Lerea, L., Trepanier, P.A., Barnes, G.A., Weigel, S.J., Seidler, F.J. and Bartolome, J. (1982) Impaired development of central and peripheral catecholamine neurotransmitter systems in preweaning rats treated with α-difluoromethylornithine, a specific irreversible inhibitor of ornithine decarboxylase, *J. Pharmacol. Exp. Ther.*, 222: 746–751.

Slotkin, T.A., Lau, C. and Bartolome, J. (1976) Effects of neonatal or maternal methadone administration on ornithine decarboxylase activity in brain and heart of developing rats. *J. Pharmacol. Exp. Ther.*, 199: 141–148.

Slotkin, T.A., Seidler, F.J., Whitmore, W.L., Weigel, S.J., Slepetis, R.J., Lerea, L., Trepanier, P. and Bartolome, J. (1983) Critical periods for the role of ornithine decarboxylase and the polyamines in growth and development of the rat: Effects of exposure to α-difluoromethylornithine during a discrete prenatal or postnatal interval. *Int. J. Dev. Neurosci.*, 1: 113–127.

Tabor, H. and Tabor, C.W. (1983) Polyamines. Methods in Enzymology, Vol. 94. Academic Press, New York.

Tucek, S. (1978) Acetylcholine Synthesis in Neurons. Wiley, New York.

Udenfriend, S. (1966) Tyrosine hydroxylase. *Pharmacol. Rev.*, 18: 43–51.

Vorhees, C.V., Butcher, R., Brunner, R.L. and Sobotka, T. (1979) A developmental test battery for neurobehavioral toxicity in rats: A preliminary analysis using monosodium glutamate, calcium carageenan and hydroxyurea. *Toxicol. Appl. Pharmacol.*, 50: 267–282.

Winick, M. and Noble, A. (1965) Quantitative changes in DNA, RNA and protein during prenatal and postnatal growth in the rat. *Dev. Biol.*, 12: 451–466.

Winick, M. and Noble, A. (1967) Cellular response in rats during malnutrition at various ages. *J. Nutr.*, 89: 300–306.

Wurtman, R. (1979) Precursor control of transmitter synthesis. In A. Barbeau, J. Growdon and R. Wurtman (Eds.), Nutrition and the Brain, Vol. 5, New York, Raven Press.

Discussion

W. Lichtensteiger: If activity of ornithine decarboxylase (ODC) were influenced by various neurotransmitter systems, could you get indirect effects through drug action in these systems?

J.M. Bell: We measured ODC activity in developing brain, primarily in the first two postnatal weeks of life. At this time, neurotransmitter systems are still developing, and as yet show little functional response to drug treatments (Bell et al., 1986). In all treatments that we have presented here, ODC alterations preceded any change in developing neurotransmitter systems: such evidence suggests that it is the ODC/polyamine system which is first affected by the treatments, and then these changes predict macromolecular alterations which have consequences directly relevant to neurotransmitter systems.

R. Balazs: It is interesting that α-difluoromethylornithine (DFMO) interfered severely with the development of cerebellar granule cells, but not with that of the granule cells in the fascia dentata, although their generation occurs more or less during the same postnatal period. I wonder whether you have studied the development of the Bergmann glia in the cerebellum, since a specific defect may cause a selective effect in the cerebellum.

J.M. Bell: DFMO treatment did not seem to alter either the number of dentate granule cells or the lamination of the fascia dentata. Presumably either dentate granule cells do not require ODC activity postnatally to synthesize sufficient polyamines to support their replication and differentiation, or else they carry out these processes quite normally with reduced amounts of polyamines. In this respect, dentate granule cells differ from cerebellar granule cells. However, the severe effects of DFMO on developing granule cells suggest, firstly, that granule cell division requires the conversion of ornithine to polyamines and that the drug may also be affecting the number or orientation of Bergmann glia, along which the granule cells migrate. At this time, we have not directly assessed DFMO's effects on the Bergmann glia.

E. Fride: Schanberg et al. (1984) have shown that maternal deprivation causes a transient decrease in ODC activity. Could the mechanism underlying the effects of such acute environmental insult be similar to that involved in direct inhibition of ODC activity?

J.M. Bell: The mechanism of inactivation of ODC by DFMO is both highly specific and irreversible, and occurs at the active site of the enzyme. Following DFMO treatment, polyamine levels, particularly putrescine, are greatly reduced (Slotkin et al., 1982), indicating a shutdown in this conversion process. It is likely that environmental perturbations, whether by maternal deprivation or neuroactive substances, also act at this site, as the conversion process from ornithine to putrescine by ODC is the rate-limiting step in the synthesis of the polyamines.

G.J. Boer: Is there any evidence for a direct effect of any neuroactive compound on the ODC enzyme activity?

J.M. Bell: While our laboratory has investigated a number of indirect effects on ODC activity (such as that with cardiac beta-receptor stimulation by isoproterenol; Bartolome et al., 1982), we have not studied any directly acting neuroactive substances in this system. However, others (Lewis et al., 1978) have found that nanogram amounts of nerve growth factor can indeed induce a marked increase in enzyme activity.

M. Mirmiran: You have concluded that polyamines play a role in a variety of insults to the CNS. I should like to know your view on their possible role in CNS plasticity.

J.M. Bell: Like their synthesizing enzyme, ODC, putrescine and spermidine are acutely responsive to a large number of developmental perturbations, some of which we have mentioned today. They indeed are relatively plastic in the sense that following withdrawal of the insult or drug, rebound elevations can occur. However, despite their recovery, changes in macromolecular synthesis are still likely to result if the insult or drug was present during critical phases of cell differentiation. In the adult it also appears that polyamines are a requirement for recovery following lesions. Agnati et al. (1985) have found that the ganglioside GM1 requires the permissive action of putrescine to exert its protective effects against retrograde degeneration of nigral dopamine nerve cells following a partial hemitransection. Gilad and Gilad (1983) have also shown that an early increase in polyamine biosynthesis is an obligatory step for the survival of sympathetic neurons after axonal injury.

P.M. Rodier: Many of the effects you have reported could also be due to a loss of cells, rather than a specific effect on macromolecular synthesis. For example, you showed increasing difference in DNA between treated and control animals after DNA synthesis should have ended, suggesting that the treatment kills previously formed cells. Are you sure that cell numbers are not changing?

J.M. Bell: In an unpublished study, we pulse-labelled untreated and SLP (soy lecithin preparation)-treated and animals with tritiated thymidine on postnatal day 10, and measured retention of the label 2 weeks later. Results indicated no alterations in normally occurring cell death in the SLP-exposed animals. Additional evidence arguing against increases in cell death following treatment comes from the result that there were regionally different effects of the diet: while midbrain and cerebellum DNA content was unaffected (even transiently elevated in the case of the cerebellum), only the cerebral cortex showed large reductions in DNA levels. If SLP was indeed causing cell death, it would be likely that we would have seen reductions in DNA levels across all regions.

References

Agnati, L.F., Fuxe, K., Zini, I., Davalli, P., Corti, A., Calza, L., Toffano, G., Zoli, M., Piccini, G. and Goldstein, M. (1985) Effects of lesions and ganglioside GM1 treatment on striatal polyamine levels and nigral DA neurons. A role of putrescine in the neurotropic activity of gangliosides. *Acta Physiol. Scand.*, 124: 499–506.

Bartolome, J., Trepanier, P., Chait, E.A. and Slotkin, T.A. (1982) Role of polyamines in isoproterenol-induced cardiac hypertrophy: Effects of alpha-difluoromethylornithine, an irreversible inhibitor of ornithine decarboxylase. *J. Mol. Cell. Cardiol.*, 14: 461–466.

Bell, J.M., Whitmore, W.L., Cowdery, T. and Slotkin, T.A. (1986) Perinatal dietary supplementation with a soy lecithin preparation: Effects on development of central catecholaminergic neurotransmitter systems. *Brain Res. Bull.*, 17: 189–195.

Gilad, G.M. and Gilad, V.H. (1983) Polyamine biosynthesis is required for survival of sympathetic neurons after axonal injury. *Brain Res.*, 273: 191–194.

Lewis, M.E., Lakshmanan, J., Nagaiah, K., MacDonnell, P.C. and Guroff, G. (1978) Nerve growth factor increases activity of ornithine decarboxylase in rat brain. *Proc. Natl. Acad. Sci. USA*, 75(2): 1021–1023.

Schanberg, S.M., Evoniuk, G. and Kuhn, C. (1984) Tactile and nutritional aspects of maternal care: Specific regulators of neuroendocrine functions and cellular development. *Proc. Soc. Exp. Biol. Med.*, 175: 135–146.

Slotkin, T.A., Seidler, F.J., Trepanier, P., Whitmore, W.L., Lerea, L., Barnes, G.A., Weigel, S.J. and Bartolome, J. (1982) Ornithine decarboxylase and polyamines in tissues of the neonatal rat: Effects of alpha-difluoromethylornithine, a specific irreversible inhibitor of ornithine decarboxylase. *J. Pharm. Exp. Ther.*, 222: 741–745.

G.J. Boer, M.G.P. Feenstra, M. Mirmiran, D.F. Swaab and F. Van Haaren
Progress in Brain Research, Vol. 73
© 1988 Elsevier Science Publishers B.V. (Biomedical Division)

CHAPTER 24

Neurotransmitters as morphogens

Jean M. Lauder

Department of Anatomy, University of North Carolina, School of Medicine, Chapel Hill, NC 27514, USA

Introduction

The importance of morphogenetic cell movements for the shaping and patterning of the embryo has been known since Vogt first traced the complex movements of cells during gastrulation using his fate mapping technique (Vogt, 1929), and Spemann and Mangold (1924) discovered the importance of movement of the dorsal lip of the blastopore beneath the overlying ectoderm for induction of the nervous system. Since that time, numerous studies have emphasized the critical role played by cell movements and other morphogenetic processes in embryonic development (see Holtfreter and Hamburger, 1955; Gustafson and Toneby, 1963; Holtfreter, 1968), yet little is known of the motive forces controlling these dynamic processes.

In the adult nervous system, neurotransmitters are discrete intercellular signalling devices which mediate communication between cells in complex neural circuitries. However, they may have evolved to this specialized role from more general humoral functions in primitive organisms where they were used as both intra- and intercellular signalling devices (McMahon, 1974; Tomkins, 1975; Buznikov, 1980; Roth et al., 1982). These phylogenetically old functions appear to be reiterated in the embryo (Harris, 1981), where neurotransmitters play important roles in fundamental morphogenetic events such as cleavage and gastrulation, neurulation, and the formation of certain tissues, as outlined in this review. In addi-

tion, during the formation of neuronal circuits, when their adult function as mediators of neurotransmission is unfolding, neurotransmitters may be released from the tips of growing axons and sculpt the morphology of neighboring axons and target cells (Handa et al., 1986; Kater and Haydon, 1987; Lankford, 1987). Thus, during development, neurotransmitters can be considered as morphogenetic signals, a function which may reflect their evolutionary history.

The term 'morphogen' was originally coined by Turing (1952) in his mathematical model of morphogenesis, although the concept of gradients of diffusible morphogenetic substances ('formative stimuli', 'evocators') originated much earlier (Herbst, 1901; Morgan, 1901; Driesch, 1908; Child, 1915; Waddington, 1940) and provided the basis for theories of pattern formation in embryogenesis (Child, 1941; Waddington, 1962; Wolpert, 1969). 'Morphogen' has been operationally defined as a signalling or inducing substance which is emitted from a source or center from which it diffuses over a distance towards a 'sink', so that it is present in different concentrations along this route, i.e. it exists as a 'diffusion gradient' (Crick, 1970). It presumably exerts particular effects on cells exposed to it due to the different concentrations found along such a gradient (Child, 1941). This term has been used to describe substances involved in pattern formation in both vertebrate and invertebrate embryos (Wolpert, 1978; Marek and Kubicek, 1981; Bard and French, 1984; Eichele et al., 1985; Slack,

1987a,b; Slack et al., 1987; Smith, 1987; Thaller and Eichele, 1987) and in primitive organisms such as hydra and slime molds (Muller et al., 1977; Meinhardt, 1978; Schaller et al., 1979; Muller, 1984; Morris et al., 1987; Slack, 1987a; Williams et al., 1987).

Use of the term 'morphogen' in the context of neurotransmitters acting as regulators of morphogenetic processes gives it a more general meaning than its previous usage has suggested, although Turing (1952) originally defined it in a rather broad sense, even including hormones as possible morphogens. Moreover, since it so graphically depicts many of the roles neurotransmitters are proposed to play in development, and has already been used to describe the specific effects of serotonin on growth cone motility (Kater and Haydon, 1987), it would seem reasonable to propose it as a term to denote the morphogenetic functions of neurotransmitters generally.

Neurotransmitters in primitive organisms and early embryos

Neurotransmitter substances, including the catecholamines, serotonin (5-hydroxytryptamine, 5-HT), acetylcholine and γ-aminobutyric acid (GABA), have been found in a variety of primitive organisms and early invertebrate embryos in which no nervous system is present. In such cases, these substances appear to act as both intra- and intercellular signals involved in the control of cell proliferation, ciliary activity, motility, cell shape changes and morphogenetic cell movements.

The monoamines (norepinephrine, epinephrine, dopamine, 5-HT) and acetylcholine have been found in many protozoans (see Buznikov, 1984, for review). In *Tetrahymena*, intracellular concentrations of these substances have been reported to fluctuate during the cell division cycle (Sullivan and Sullivan, 1964; Iwata and Kariya, 1973). Moreover, the levels of 5-HT and dopamine vary inversely relative to each other during the stationary and log phases of growth in these

cells (Blum, 1970; Goldman et al., 1981). Since these transmitters are also released into the extracellular environment during particular phases of growth, it has been suggested that they may also act as intercellular signalling devices (Rodriguez and Renaud, 1980; Goldman et al., 1981). In addition, benzodiazepines have been shown to stimulate growth in *Tetrahymena*, suggesting that GABA may also play a role in controlling growth of these organisms (Darvas et al., 1985).

Other primitive organisms such as flatworms and planktonic abalone larvae also seem to use neurotransmitters as regulatory molecules. In planaria, regenerative processes, RNA and DNA synthesis, and Ca^{2+}-dependent protein kinase and adenylate cyclase activities are all stimulated by the catecholamines and 5-HT (Franquinet, 1979; Franquinet and Martelly, 1981). In the parasitic trematodes and cestodes, 5-HT from the host stimulates cell motility by acting through specific receptors linked to a highly responsive adenylate cyclase (Kasschau and Mansour, 1982; Mansour, 1983). This function appears similar to the effects of GABA on planktonic abalone, where it influences their motility, settling ability and metamorphosis (Morse et al., 1979). Choline acetyltransferase-deficient mutants of nematodes have also been identified which exhibit severe defects in growth (Rand and Russell, 1984), an effect which appears to be similar to the consequences of a mutation in *Drosophila* which affects the enzymes of acetylcholine metabolism, producing lethal growth-related defects in homozygotes and marked neuroanatomical abnormalities in heterozygotes (Hall et al., 1979). In hydra, one of the major morphogens, the 'head activator', is a neuropeptide (Schaller, 1973) which is also found in rat brain (Schaller, 1975). Moreover, both acetylcholine and 5-HT affect regional morphogenesis in the organism (Muller et al., 1977), although it is not known whether these effects are direct or occur through interactions with substances already identified as morphogens (Schaller et al., 1979). Thus, neurotransmitters appear to have effects on a number of different processes in primitive organisms, including growth, regeneration, motility, metamorphosis, and morphogenesis of specific body parts.

Early invertebrate embryos also appear to use neurotransmitters for the regulation of basic developmental functions. Following fertilization, cell division begins with cleavage of the egg into blastomeres. This process continues until a hollow sphere of cells is formed, the blastula. In certain embryos, among them sea urchins and fish, the blastula then hatches and swims freely through the use of cilia, which seems to be a prerequisite for initiation of gastrulation. Neurotransmitters such as the monoamines and acetylcholine have been implicated in both cleavage and gastrulation in the sea urchin, starfish and fish embryo based on their timely presence and the ability of related pharmacological agents to interfere with the normal progression of these developmental events (see Buznikov, 1980, 1984; Buznikov and Shmukler, 1981; and Toneby, 1977a for reviews).

Acetylcholine, 5-HT, dopamine and 5-HT-like substances such as tryptamine and 5-methoxytryptamine (5-MT) have been measured during cleavage of sea urchin blastomeres and found to occur in varying amounts depending on the number of the cleavage division and the phase of the cell cycle (Buznikov et al., 1964, 1968; Manukhin et al., 1981; Renaud et al., 1983; Buznikov, 1984; Markova et al., 1985). In the case of 5-HT and 5-MT, it appears that the levels of these two substances fluctuate in an inverse fashion during the first cleavage division, so that the amount of 5-HT decreases, while the level of 5-MT increases, a trend which continues throughout the blastula stage (Renaud et al., 1983).

Treatment of cleaving sea urchin or starfish embryos with 5-HT, tryptamine, dopamine, acetylcholine or their receptor antagonists produces defects primarily in the duration of cleavage itself, with few changes in the other phases of the cell cycle, which suggests that these substances interfere with the cleavage stimulus (Buznikov et al., 1970, 1981, 1984). In the case of 5-HT

antagonists, such as metergoline, these effects are accompanied by a decrease in intracellular cAMP and an increase in Ca^{2+} efflux, suggesting that this effect may involve 5-HT receptors linked to a Ca^{2+}-dependent adenylate cyclase (Renaud et al., 1983). It has been claimed that 5-HT (or 5-MT) is concentrated in the cleavage furrow (Emanuelsson, 1974), where 5-HT receptors may also be concentrated (Renaud et al., 1983). The defects produced by acetylcholine, 5-HT or dopamine receptor antagonists can be reversed by addition of the neurotransmitter substance itself (Buznikov et al., 1970), indicating that these are specific, receptor-mediated events. Blastomeres are also capable of taking up these substances, binding them with high affinity, and releasing them into their surround (Buznikov et al., 1975; Rakic et al., 1978a, b; Volina et al., 1983), which has led to the suggestion that they might also be used as intercellular signalling devices (Buznikov, 1984). Thus, neurotransmitter substances such as 5-HT, the catecholamines and acetylcholine appear to be important for the regulation of cleavage divisions in the sea urchin embryo, perhaps via specific intracellular receptors linked to Ca^{2+}-dependent adenylate cyclases. It is interesting to note that these same neurotransmitters have been implicated in cell proliferation occurring during brain development in rodents (Lauder and Krebs, 1978; Lauder et al., 1982; Patel et al., 1983; reviewed by Lauder and Krebs, 1984).

Stimulation of ciliary activity in sea urchin blastulae has been reported to occur in response to 5-HT, dopamine, acetylcholine and GABA. These effects also appear to be mediated by specific receptors and, in the case of the monoamines, to involve changes in intracellular Ca^{2+} and adenylate cyclase activity (Sherif, 1983). Moreover, the 'hatching enzyme', which is required for production of free-swimming blastulae, also appears to be under the control of 5-HT or related substances, since addition of 5-HT to the growth medium causes an inhibition of hatching in the sea urchin (Deeb, 1972). Dopamine has also been implicated in hatching of fish embryos, which appears to involve specific dopamine receptors (Schoots et al., 1983). Of related interest is the finding that both the fertilization of sea urchin eggs and sperm motility are inhibited by the 5-HT receptor antagonist metergoline (Parisi et al., 1984), suggesting that 5-HT may play a role in one or more aspects of the fertilization process.

Hatching of the echinoderm blastula is followed by the process of gastrulation, during which the ectoderm invaginates through the blastopore into the internal cavity of the blastula, thus forming the archenteron or primitive gut. Preceding the invagination process, primary mesenchyme cells migrate from the region of the blastopore into the blastocoel. These cells later differentiate into elements of the primitive skeleton (Gustafson and Toneby, 1971). These two phases of gastrulation, migration of the primary mesenchyme and invagination, are differentially sensitive to 5-HT and acetylcholine (Gustafson and Toneby, 1970, 1971). The main site of action of 5-HT appears to be the migrating primary mesenchyme, since treatment of gastrulating embryos inhibits the migration of these cells and leads to defective formation of the skeleton (Toneby, 1977a). Acetylcholine and its analogues, on the other hand, affect the invagination of the archenteron, leading to malformations of the gut. It has been proposed that 5-HT, located in the region of the blastopore, initiates gastrulation, whereas acetylcholine from the ectoderm controls invagination of the archenteron (Gustafson and Toneby, 1970; Toneby, 1977b). The primary intracellular site of action of 5-HT and related substances may be the cytoskeleton (Emanuelsson, 1974).

Monoamines and neurulation in birds and amphibians

Neurotransmitters such as the catecholamines and 5-HT are also present during early phases of vertebrate embryogenesis (see Baker, 1965, and reviews by Baker and Quay, 1969; Lauder, 1987; Lauder and Krebs, 1984) and have been suggested to influence the development of the nervous system and associated structures.

During gastrulation in the chick embryo, formation of the primitive streak is the equivalent of invagination of the archenteron in sea urchins and other invertebrate embryos. In the chick, 5-HT has been measured biochemically as early as 1 day of incubation, even before primitive streak formation (Ignarro and Shideman, 1968a,b). In addition, 5-HT has been localized by electron microscopic autoradiography in cells of the primitive streak following incubation with the radiolabelled precursor 5-hydroxytryptophan (5-HTP), where it was seen in association with yolk granules and elements of the cytoskeleton (Emanuelsson, 1976).

During neurulation, when the neural plate is transformed into the neural tube, both the neural tube and underlying notochord of chick and amphibian embryos have the ability to take up 5-HT or catecholamines at specific sites along their rostrocaudal extent (Allan and Newgreen, 1977; Godin, 1986; Godin and Gipouloux, 1986; Kirby and Gilmore, 1972; Lawrence and Burden, 1973; Newgreen et al., 1981; Rais et al., 1981; Sako et al., 1986; Sims, 1977, Wallace, 1982). Characteristically, sites for catecholamine uptake are located in the neural folds, notochord or floorplate region, whereas 5-HT uptake sites are seen in the floorplate and notochord. These sites are located in regions which are non-overlapping with those where catecholamine uptake is found, suggesting that these substances occupy mutually exclusive domains along the neuraxis (Wallace, 1979, 1982). The 5-HT uptake sites seem to have some of the characteristics of neuronal uptake in terms of concentration range and the ability of neuronal uptake inhibitors to block the appearance of these sites (Newgreen et al., 1981; Wallace, 1982; Wallace et al., 1985). It is not yet clear whether this is also true for the catecholaminergic sites.

The notochord may be a site of synthesis for both the catecholamines and 5-HT in birds and amphibians, since endogenous levels of these substances have been biochemically measured in this structure in the chick (Strudel, 1977a,b), isolated notochords from normal or exogastrulated frog embryos have been shown to contain detectable amounts of endogenous catecholamine histo-fluorescence (Godin, 1986; Godin and Gipouloux, 1986), and 5-HT immunoreactivity has been demonstrated in the notochord following incubation of chick embryos with either of its precursors, L-tryptophan or 5-HTP (Wallace, 1982; Wallace et al., 1985). All of these sites of neurotransmitter localization in the neural tube and notochord are transient, and their expression is temporally correlated with neural tube closure, suggesting that they may play some role in regulation of this morphogenetic event.

A number of neurochemicals, all of which interfere with 5-HT, catecholamine or acetyl-choline-related mechanisms, have been found to be teratogenic in the chick embryo, as have these neurotransmitters themselves or their precursors (Lawrence and Burden, 1973; Landauer, 1975, 1976; Palen et al., 1979). Defects caused by these substances include: abnormalities in growth and spreading of the blastoderm, primitive streak for-

TABLE 1

Morphogenetic disturbances provoked by serotonin, Catron®, diethyldithiocarbamate, 5-methyltryptamine and promethazine in chick embryos cultivated in vitro according to the beaker cultivation method (From Palen et al., 1979)

Substance	Age of embryos at onset of treatment (h of incubation	Number of embryos	% Abnormal embryos	Disturbances affecting[a]					
				Blasto-dermal expansion	Primitive streak formation	Brain formation	Neural tube closure	Somite formation	Heart formation
Serotonin (5 mM)	4	29	100	+	+	+ +	+ +	+ +	0
	12	21	100	+	+	+ +	+ +	+	+
	24	32	100	+		+	+ +	−	−
	30	19	90	+		+	+	−	−
Catron® (0.3 mM)	4	17	95	−	+	+ +	+ +	0	0
	12	19	85	−	−	+ +	+ +	+ +	+
	24	17	75	−		+ +	+ +	+	−
	30	19	75	−		+	+	−	−
Diethyldithio-carbamate (5 mM)	4	21	100	+	0	0	0	0	0
	12	16	100	+	0	0	0	0	0
	24	21	90	+		+ +	+ +	+	+
	30	17	65	+		+	+	−	−
5-Methyl-tryptamine (0.5 mM)	4	15	80	+	+	+ +	+ +	+ +	0
	12	19	85	+	+	+ +	+ +	+	0
	24	23	55	+		+ +	+ +	+	−
	30	16	45	+		+	+	−	−
Promethazine (0.1 mM)	4	18	80	−	+	+ +	+ +	+ +	+
	12	17	70	−	−	+ +	+	+	−
	24	22	55	−		+ +	+	+	−
	30	17	40	−		+	+	−	−

[a] The disturbances are graded as follows. For blastoderm expansion: +, depressed; −, normal. In all other cases: 0, development totally inhibited; + +, severe disturbances; +, modest disturbances; −, normal development.

mation, somitogenesis, torsion and flexure of the embryo, as well as malformations of the brain and spinal cord (Table 1). In the case of serotonergic analogues or precursors (e.g., L-tryptophan), their effectiveness in causing malformations seems to be related to their ability to interfere with degradation of yolk granules, which are taken up into the neural tube during closure and have the ability to synthesize and store 5-HT (Emanuelsson and Palen, 1975; Emanuelsson, 1976; Santander and Cuadrado, 1976; Palen et al., 1979). Thus, sites of 5-HT and catecholamine uptake and synthesis could be important in regulating morphogenetic cell movements during neurulation in the chick and frog embryo, a function which could be perturbed by exposure to psychoactive drugs acting through these neurotransmitter mechanisms.

Neurotransmitters and palate morphogenesis in the mouse

Neurotransmitters have also been implicated in the regulation of morphogenetic cell movements during palate development. For example, changes in levels of serotonin, catecholamines and GABA have been found in the mouse palate during different phases of palate formation (Zimmerman et al., 1981; Pisano and Greene, 1985; Wee et al., 1986). Moreover, when these neurotransmitters were added to the medium in whole embryo or tissue cultures, they produced different biochemical, cellular and morphological responses. The catecholamines and related drugs (e.g., norepinephrine, isoproterenol) stimulated adenylate cyclase (Waterman et al., 1976; Schreiner et al., 1986), apparently through a β-adrenergic receptor mechanism (Garbarino and Greene, 1984), and suppressed the growth of mesenchymal cells in culture (Pisano et al., 1986), whereas 5-HT stimulated cyclic GMP levels and protein carboxymethylase activity, while inhibiting cyclic AMP levels in the same system (Zimmerman et al., 1983). There is also evidence that these neurotransmitters may directly influence palatal morphogenesis, since 5-HT and acetylcholine have

been shown to stimulate palatal shelf reorientation in whole embryo culture, whereas GABA exerted an inhibitory effect, and norepinephrine and dopamine had no effect at all. Moreover, the GABA-related drug diazepam also partially inhibited palatal shelf reorientation in tissue culture and produced cleft palate in offspring when administered to pregnant mice (Wee et al., 1979, 1980; Wee and Zimmerman, 1983, 1985: Zimmerman and Wee, 1984). The effect of 5-HT on motility of cells has also been examined in palatal cultures, where it exerted a stimulatory effect on migration of mesenchymal cells from explants of palatal shelves (Venkatasubramanian and Zimmerman, 1983), and stimulated migration of dissociated mesenchymal cells toward a chemotactic stimulus (Zimmerman et al., 1983).

As discussed below, we have recently demonstrated that the epithelial covering of the murine palatal shelves has a specific uptake system for 5-HT, which is transiently expressed during the period of palatal morphogenesis (Lauder and Zimmerman, 1988; Zimmerman and Lauder, 1987). This epithelium is immediately adjacent to the underlying mesenchyme which interfaces with it through a meshwork of cellular processes (the 'cell process meshwork'; Sulik et al., 1979). Interactions between this epithelium and mesenchyme are thought to be important for morphogenesis of the palatal shelves (Brinkley, 1986). Together with the findings described above indicating that 5-HT can stimulate the growth and motility of palatal mesenchyme cells, possibly via receptor-mediated mechanisms, our finding of 5-HT uptake sites in the adjacent palatal epithelium raises the possibility that 5-HT could be concentrated in this epithelium, followed by release onto the subadjacent mesenchyme, where it might influence the growth and/or motility of these cells.

Neurotransmitters and morphogenesis of the neural tube, heart and craniofacial region in the mouse embryo

Until recently, little information has been available concerning neurotransmitter uptake or synthesis in regions of morphogenesis in the mammalian embryo, although Burden and Lawrence (1973) reported that in the rat ovum, zygote and 2–4-cell-stage embryo, endogenous fluorescence for catecholamines and 5-HT was present, which could be intensified by incubation in these substances, suggesting the presence of uptake mechanisms. Pienkowski (1977) reported that norepinephrine stimulated the first and inhibited the second cleavage division in the fertilized mouse ovum in vitro, suggesting that the monoamines could play a role in cleavage divisions in mammalian as well as sea urchin embryos. In addition, Schlumpf and Lichtensteiger (1979) demonstrated that the visceral yolk sac of the rat embryo could synthesize catecholamines.

That neurotransmitters may be important for regulating mammalian embryogenesis is indicated by the results of several pharmacological studies which have shown that 5-HT, L-tryptophan or tricyclic antidepressants (particularly those which act through serotonergic mechansims) can cause malformations of the skull, brain, spinal cord or vertebral column in rodents and humans (Guram et al., 1980, 1982; Idanpaan-Heikkila and Saxen, 1973; Jurand, 1980; van Cauteren et al., 1986). These findings indicate that the monoamines may be involved in morphogenesis of the nervous system and some components of the skeletal system in the mammalian embryo.

Recently, we have undertaken studies to determine whether 5-HT may act to regulate morphogenesis in the mouse embryo during neurulation and craniofacial development (Lauder et al., 1987, 1988; Lauder and Zimmerman 1988; Zimmerman and Lauder, 1987). For this purpose, the method of whole embryo culture was employed (Sadler, 1979), together with immunocytochemistry using a specific 5-HT antiserum (Wallace et al., 1982), to analyse sites of uptake and/or synthesis of 5-HT in mouse embryos grown in the presence of 5-HT or its precursors. In addition, a specific antiserum to purified serotonin binding protein (SBP, 45 KDa form; Kirschgessner et al., 1987; Liu et al., 1985, 1987; Tamir, 1983) was used to study possible sites of 5-HT binding in these embryos. In the adult, SBP binds 5-HT with high affinity (Tamir and Huang, 1974), acts as a storage protein for 5-HT in synaptic vesicles (Gershon et al., 1983; Tamir and Gershon, 1979), and is released along with 5-HT during exocytosis of such vesicles (Jonakait et al., 1979). Once in the extracellular milieu, 5-HT dissociates from SBP, an event which can be modulated by ions and gangliosides (Tamir and Liu, 1982; Tamir et al., 1980). We have also determined the teratogenicity of 5-HT and related compounds for embryos grown in their presence during critical phases of morphogenesis.

In mouse embryos at the headfold stage (embryonic day 9, E9), when the neural tube is still closing in the head and tail regions, we have observed sites of 5-HT uptake in the hindgut and heart (Fig. 1) following incubation of embryos with 5-HT and processing them for anti-5-HT immunocytochemistry. In the chick and frog embryo, 5-HT uptake sites are located in the floorplate of the neural tube and underlying notochord (Wallace, 1982; Wallace et al., 1985; Godin, 1986; Godin and Gipoloux, 1986), as discussed above. No such sites have yet been found in the neural tube or notochord of the mouse embryo, but prominent sites of 5-HT immunoreactivity (IR) were observed in the mouse foregut and hindgut adjacent to the neural tube in a configuration similar to that of the notochord in the chick and frog (Lauder, Thomas and Sadler, in preparation). Thus, considering the small size of the notochord in the mouse, and the juxtaposition of the foregut and hindgut to the neural tube, it is possible that with regard to 5-HT the gut performs a function analogous to that of the large notochord in the chick and frog embryo.

In terms of possible sites of 5-HT synthesis in

372

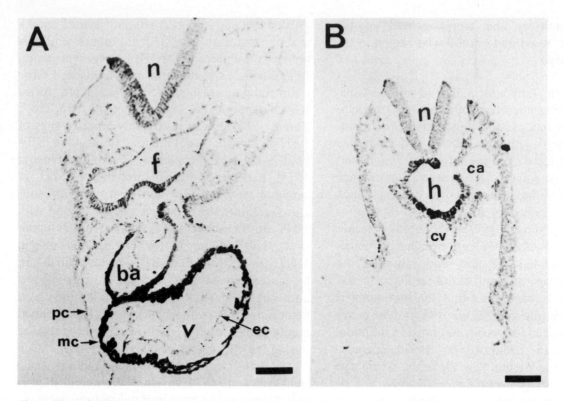

Fig. 1. Sites of 5-HT immunoreactivity in the heart, foregut (A) and hindgut (B) of the E9 (headfold stage) mouse embryo following 3 h incubation in medium containing 5-HT (10^{-5} M) plus nialamide and L-cysteine (cf. Table 2). A, anterior neuropore; B, caudal neuropore. n, neural tube; f, foregut; h, hindgut; ba, bulbus arteriosus; v, ventricle; ec, endocardium; pc, pericardium; mc, myocardium; ca, caudal artery; cv, caudal vein. Tranverse sections. Bars = 100 μm. (From Lauder, Thomas and Sadler, in preparation.)

the head-fold stage mouse embryo, the heart represents a good possibility, since 5-HT IR can be seen following incubation of embryos in L-tryptophan (L-TRP), the initial precursor for 5-HT synthesis. However, further experiments must be performed to verify the conclusion that the heart is a true site of 5-HT synthesis, including studies with L-TRP given together with an inhibitor of 5-HT uptake, as discussed below. In any case, the finding of a major site of 5-HT uptake (and possibly synthesis) in the embryonic mouse heart raises the possibility that some congenital heart malformations could have a drug-related etiology, if correlated with the use of serotonergic drugs during pregnancy.

The possible involvement of 5-HT in morphogenesis of the craniofacial region in the mouse embryo has also been investigated using the method of whole embryo culture with older embryos (Lauder et al. 1987, 1988; Lauder and Zimmerman 1987; Zimmerman and Lauder, 1987). In these experiments, day 12–14 embryos were exposed to 5-HT or related compounds for a short incubaton period (3–4 h), followed by processing for 5-HT immunocytochemistry, or for longer periods (1–2 days) followed by processing for scanning electron microscopy (SEM) or 1 μm plastic sections (Lauder, Thomas and Sadler, in preparation). When embryos were incubated for a short period in medium containing 5-HT plus the

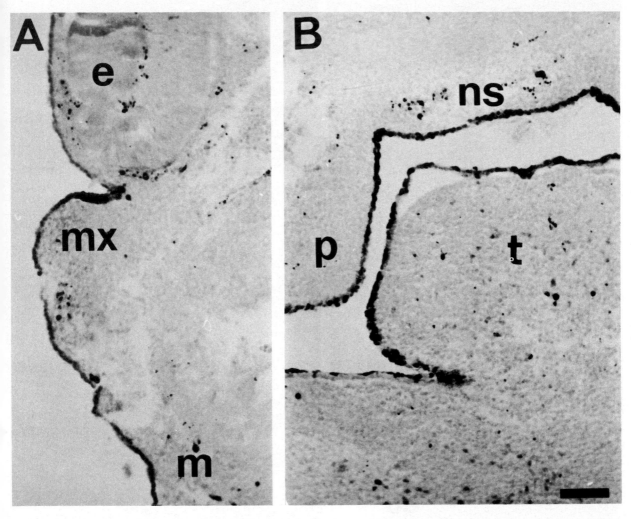

Fig. 2. Sites of 5-HT immunoreactivity in epithelia of the face, palate and oral cavity of the E12 mouse embryo following 3 h incubation in medium containing 5-HT (10^{-5} M) plus nialamide and L-cysteine (cf. Table 2). The same sites were seen with 10^{-7} M 5-HT, 10^{-5} M L-TRP, or with nialamide and L-cysteine alone. Culture medium consisted of 10% fetal calf serum and DMEM. Arrows indicate staining in the epithelial lining of the palatal shelves (p), tongue (t), nasal septum (ns), maxillary process (mx) and mandibular prominence (m). Some staining was also present in the epithelial covering of the eye (e). Transverse sections. Bar = 50 μm. (From Lauder and Zimmerman, 1988.)

monoamine oxidase (MAO) inhibitor nialamide (N) and the antioxidant L-cysteine (C), sites of 5-HT immunoreactivity (IR) were found in a number of locations in tissues of the head and neck. These sites included the surface epithelia of the head, face, nasal prominences, branchial arches, palate, oral cavity and associated nasal epithelium, the epithelium covering the eye, parts of the optic vesicle (Figs. 2 and 3A,C,E,G; Tables 2 and 3), and, in the brain, the epiphysis and roof of the diencephalon. It is noteworthy that all of these sites, except those in the brain, were

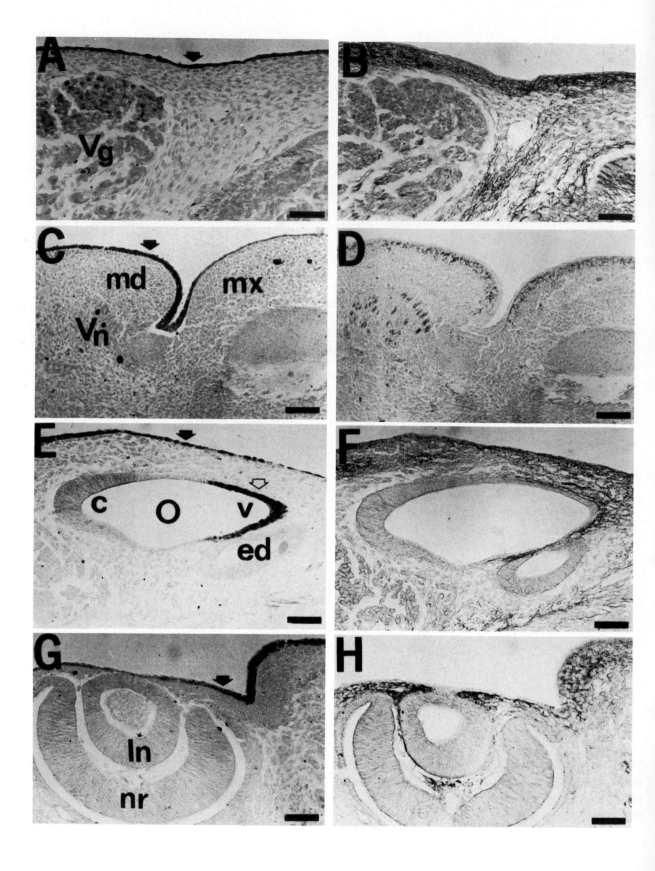

TABLE 2

Non-neuronal sites of 5-HT uptake in the day-12 mouse embryo following culture in the presence of 5-HT or related substances

Treatment (concentration of 5-HT in culture medium)	Location and relative intensity of immunoreactivity						n
	Epithelia					Brain: roof diencephalon epiphysis	
	Head	Face/arches	Oral cav.	Eye	Otocyst		
5-HT + NC ($10^{-5}/10^{-7}$ M)	+ +/+	+ +/+	+ +/+	+	+ +/+	+ +/0	14
5-HTP + NC ($10^{-5}/10^{-7}$ M)	+ +/+	+ +/+	+ +/+	(+)	+ +/+	0	12
L-TRP + NC ($10^{-5}/10^{-6}$ M)	+	+	+	(+)	+	0	6
NC	+	+	+	(+)	+	0	8
C	0	0	0	0	0	0	3
–	0	0	0	0	0	0	3
5-HT + C (10^{-5} M)	0	0	0	0	0	0	5
5-HTP + C (10^{-5} M)	0	0	0	0	0	0	4
L-TRP + C (10^{-5} M)	0	0	0	0	0	0	4
5-HT + NC + F (10^{-5} M)	0	0	0	0	0	0	3
5-HTP + NC + F (10^{-5} M)	0	0	0	0	0	0	4
L-TRP + NC + F (10^{-5} M)	0	0	0	0	0	0	4
NC + F	0	0	0	0	0	0	3

Uptake measured during 3 h with pretreatment periods of 1 h. Culture medium consisted of 75% heat-inactivated rat serum and 25% Tyrode's solution.
NC = nialamide + L-cysteine (10^{-5} M each) 1 h prior to treatment; L-TRP = L-tryptophan; 5-HTP = 5-hydroxytryptophan; F = fluoxetine (10^{-5} M) 1 h prior to treatment; Oral cav. = oral cavity and parts of nasal epithelium; face/arches = face and branchial arches 1 and 2.
Intensity of immunoreactivity was rated on a relative scale of 0 (none) to + + (very intense), (+) = less intense than + (seen at 10^{-5} M). From Lauder et al., 1988.

located in epithelia derived from the non-neural ectoderm (that part of the ectoderm not induced by the chordamesoderm, Vogt, 1929).

Using a specific antiserum to SBP, discussed above, we observed distinct regions of SBP IR in the mesenchyme of the head and face located immediately adjacent to most of the epithelial and brain sites of 5-HT uptake (Fig. 3B,D,F,H). This mesenchyme is formed from the neural crest (Johnston and Hazelton, 1972; Johnston, 1974;

Fig. 3. Sites of 5-HT immunoreactivity (arrows) in the epithelia of the head, jaw, otocyst and eye (left panels) of the E12 mouse embryo following 3 h incubation in 5-HT (10^{-5} M) plus nialamide and L-cysteine (cf. Table 2) compared to the distribution of immunoreactivity for serotonin binding protein (SBP) in nearby mesenchyme on adjacent sections (right panels). Culture medium consisted of heat-inactivated rat serum and Tyrode's solution. A, B: Head at the level of the trigeminal ganglion (5th cranial nerve; Vg); bars = 180 μm. C, D: Jaw (md, mandibular arch; mx, maxillary process; Vn, trigeminal nerve, 5th cranial nerve); bars = 280 μm. E,F: Ear (otocyst); solid arrow, 5-HT staining in the surface epithelium of head; clear arrow, 5-HT staining in the vestibular portion (v) of the otocyst (O); c, cochlear portion of otocyst; ed, endolymphatic duct; bars = 180 μm. G, H: Eye (ln, lens ventricle; nr, neural retina); arrow, 5-HT immune reaction in the surface epithelium of head; bar = 180 μm. Note the co-distribution of 5-HT staining in epithelial sites and SBP staining in adjacent mesenchyme. All sections are in the transverse plane. (From Lauder et al., 1988.)

TABLE 3

Sites of 5-HT immunoreactivity (IR) in epithelia of the palate, oral cavity and face following incubation of mouse embryos in media to which 5-HT or related substances were added

Age	Treatment	Location and relative amount of 5-HT IR				n
		Palate	Tongue	NS	MX/M	
E12–13	5-HT + NC (10^{-5} M)	+ + +	+ + +	+ + +	+ + +	3
	5-HT + NC (10^{-7} M)	+ + +	+ +	+ +	+ +	4
	L-TRP + NC	+ + +	+ + +	+ +	+ + +	4
	NC	+ + +	+ +	+ +	+ +	3
	5-HT + NC + F (10^{-7} M)	0	0	0	0	3
E14	5-HT + NC (10^{-5} M)	+ +	+	+	0	3
	5-HT + NC (10^{-7} M)	+	+	+	0	3
	L-TRP + NC	+ +	+	+	0	3
	NC	+	+	+	0	4
	5-HT + NC + F (10^{-7} M)	+	+	0	0	3

See legend to Table 2. Culture medium consisted of 10% fetal calf serum and 90% Dulbecco's minimal essential medium (DMEM).
MX/M = maxillary process and mandibular prominence; NS = nasal septum.
Amount of immunoreactivity was rated semi-quantitatively on a relative scale of 0 (none) to + + + (greatest). From Lauder and Zimmerman (1988).

LeLievre and LeDouarin, 1975; Nichols, 1986; Noden, 1984; Tan and Morriss-Kay, 1985) which is of neurectodermal origin (from the induced neural plate; Holtfreter and Hamburger, 1955), and is thus termed 'ectomesenchyme'.

Exceptions to the correlation between sites of 5-HT uptake and adjacent mesenchymal SBP IR were found, particularly with respect to the 5-HT uptake sites in the internal structures of the developing nose and mouth (e.g., the nasal epithelium, palate and oral cavity), where no SBP IR was seen in the surrounding mesenchyme. Since the neural-crest-derived 'ectomesenchyme' is usually considered to be in more superficial locations (Noden, 1984), it is likely that the internal mesenchyme of the nose and mouth is derived from the paraxial mesoderm. Thus, it is possible that the expression of SBP IR is specific to 'ectomesenchyme'.

Sites of SBP IR were also observed in a num-ber of locations which were not in association with sites of 5-HT uptake, including (1) the region between the surface epithelium and the somites in the tail region, (2) the perinotochordal sheath and adjacent mesenchyme surrounding the noto-chord, and (3) the meninges, especially those covering the hindbrain and fourth ventricle (Fig. 5A–C). It is possible that these also represent 'ectomesenchyme' derivatives, but this remains to be established. It should be noted that the noto-chord of the day 12–14 rat embryo also contains the enzyme aromatic L-amino acid decarboxylase (DDC; Teitelman et al., 1983), which is involved in the synthesis of 5-HT from 5-hydroxytrypta-mine (5-HTP), and of dopamine from L-dopa. However, we have found no evidence of noto-chordal synthesis of 5-HT in the mouse embryo, as yet, although it clearly exists in the chick and frog, as discussed above.

As far as can be ascertained from light micro-

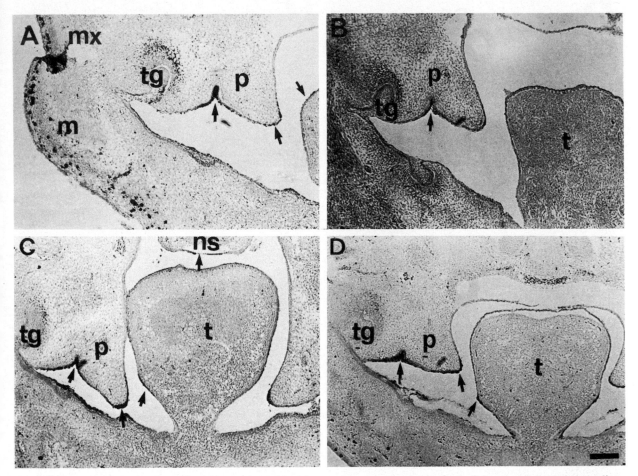

Fig. 4. Sites of 5-HT immunoreactivity in the palate and oral cavity of the E14 mouse embryo incubated for 3 h in medium containing 5-HT (A, 10^{-5} M; B, 10^{-7} M) preceded by nialamide and L-cysteine (cf. Table 2) or (C) medium containing the latter compounds alone. D: Embryos cultured without additives. Culture medium consisted of 10% fetal calf serum and DMEM. Arrows indicate immune reaction in the epithelial lining of the palatal shelves (p), tongue (t) and nasal septum(ns). Note the presence of immune reaction in the ectomesenchyme of the tooth germ (tg; A, B, C). The 5-HT staining present in the epithelia of the maxillary process (mx) and mandibular prominence (m) at E12 has disappeared. Transverse sections. Bars = 125 μm. (From Lauder and Zimmerman, 1988.)

scopic analysis of the mesenchymal SBR IR, it appears that this molecule is located on the outside of mesenchyme cells, filling the spaces between them (see Fig. 3). If present in such a location (which must be established by electron microscopy), it could be associated with components of the extracellular matrix and/or with cell adhesion molecules. This interpretation is supported by the finding that 5-HT binding to

SBP can be modulated by gangliosides (Tamir et al., 1980), as discussed above.

The sites of 5-HT uptake and mesenchymal SBP IR present in the E12 mouse embryo are transient, so that by E14 most of them have disappeared, except in the anterior palate, where a site of 5-HT uptake persists (Fig. 4; Lauder and Zimmerman, 1988). However, new sites of SBP IR have appeared by this time, particularly in

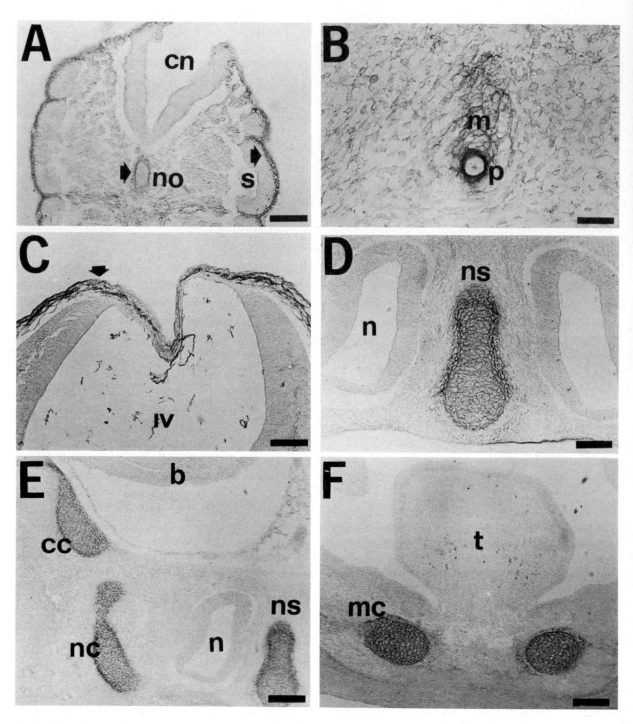

Fig. 5. Sites of serotonin binding protein (SBP) immunoreactivity in the E12 (A–C) and E14 (D–F) mouse embryo not associated with sites of 5-HT uptake. Embryos were cultured for 3 h in medium containing 5-HT (10^{-5} M) + nialamide and L-cysteine (cf. Table 2). A: Region of the caudal neuropore (cn). Arrows indicate SBP surrounding the notochord (no) adjacent to the brainstem showing SBP in the perinotochordal sheath (p) and mesenchyme (m); bar = 120 μm. C: Region of the 4th ventricle (iv); arrow, SBP in the meninges. Note IR floccular material in ventricle; bar = 280 μm. D–F: SBP of chondrogenesis sites in the nasal septum (ns), nasal capsule (nc), chondrocranium (cc) and jaw (mc: Meckel's cartilage); n, nasal cavity; b, brain; t, tongue; bars = 180 μm. All sections are in the transverse plane. (From Lauder et al., 1988.)

regions of chondrogenesis in the head, face and jaw (Fig. 5D–F; Lauder et al., 1988). As discussed above, all of the epithelial sites of 5-HT uptake are derived from the non-neural ectoderm, whereas the adjacent mesenchyme which expresses SBP IR is derived from the neural ectoderm. This mesenchyme gives rise primarily to skeletal elements and connective tissues in the head and first two branchial arches (Ciment and Weston, 1985; Noden, 1983) as a result of reciprocal interactions (Grobstein, 1967) with adjacent epithelia of the head and face (Bee and Thorogood, 1980; Tyler and Hall, 1977), the same epithelia where we have found sites of 5-HT uptake. The presence of SBP IR in neural-crest-derived 'ectomesenchyme' in E12 mouse embryos, and in chondrogenesis sites at later ages, suggests that SBP could be involved in the differentiation of these mesenchyme cells into skeletal elements in the craniofacial region, an event which may require interactions with epithelia which contain sites of 5-HT uptake. This possibility is supported by the report of Van Cauteren et al. (1986) that 5-HT administered to the pregnant rat at 9–11 days of gestation causes major malformations of the skull, including acrania, encephalocoele, cheiloschisis and ethmocephaly.

We have characterized the epithelial and brain sites of 5-HT uptake, described above, in terms of the presence of endogenous 5-HT, and their capacity for synthesis of 5-HT from precursors using two different whole embryo culture systems (see Tables 2 and 3; Lauder et al., 1987, 1988; Lauder and Zimmerman, 1988; Zimmerman and Lauder, 1987). For this purpose E12–14 embryos were incubated for 3–4 h in medium containing one of the 5-HT precursors L-TRP or 5-HTP in the presence of nialamide and L-cysteine (NC) or NC alone followed by 5-HT immunocytochemistry. In some experiments fluoxetine, an inhibitor of 5-HT uptake (Wong et al., 1974), was also added. All of the epithelial sites exhibited 5-HT IR following incubation in medium containing either L-TRP or 5-HTP, whereas the brain sites were not seen after these treatments. Like-

wise, the epithelial but not the brain sites were seen following incubation in medium containing NC alone, suggesting that they may contain endogenous stores of 5-HT (or take up 5-HT from some endogenous source). The appearance of 5-HT sites after incubation in medium containing 5-HT precursors and/or NC was blocked by fluoxetine in E12 embryos (Lauder et al., 1987, 1988; Lauder and Zimmerman 1988; Zimmerman and Lauder, 1987). Thus, we conclude that these sites are only able to take up 5-HT, which is normally synthesized elsewhere. However, in one of our studies (Table 3; Lauder and Zimmerman, 1988), those sites which still remained at E14 (mainly in the palate, Fig. 4) were not blocked by fluoxetine following treatment with 5-HT or L-TRP plus NC, although they were blocked by this drug in animals treated with NC alone (Table 3; Lauder and Zimmerman, 1988). Thus it is possible that those sites remaining at E14 have some limited capacity for 5-HT synthesis, but this interpretation must be made with caution because of the culture medium used in this study, which contained fetal calf serum and DMEM, which are themselves sources of 5-HT and L-TRP. Another characteristic of this system is the apparent ability to rapidly metabolize 5-HT, since in one of our studies (Table 2; Lauder et al., 1988) no detectable 5-HT IR could be seen at any of the epithelial or brain sites without an MAO inhibitor present in the medium, even when embryos were exposed to 5-HT. This suggests a high level of MAO activity in either the culture medium or embryo.

In current studies, we have begun to address the issue of whether 5-HT plays a functional role in neurulation and craniofacial development in the mouse embryo (Lauder, Thomas and Sadler, in preparation). For this purpose, we have grown mouse embryos for several days in the presence of 5-HT or pharmacological agents which inhibit its uptake or metabolism, followed by morphological assessment using SEM or 1 μm plastic sections. Embryos were cultured beginning at the headfold stage (E9) for 24 or 48 h in medium containing

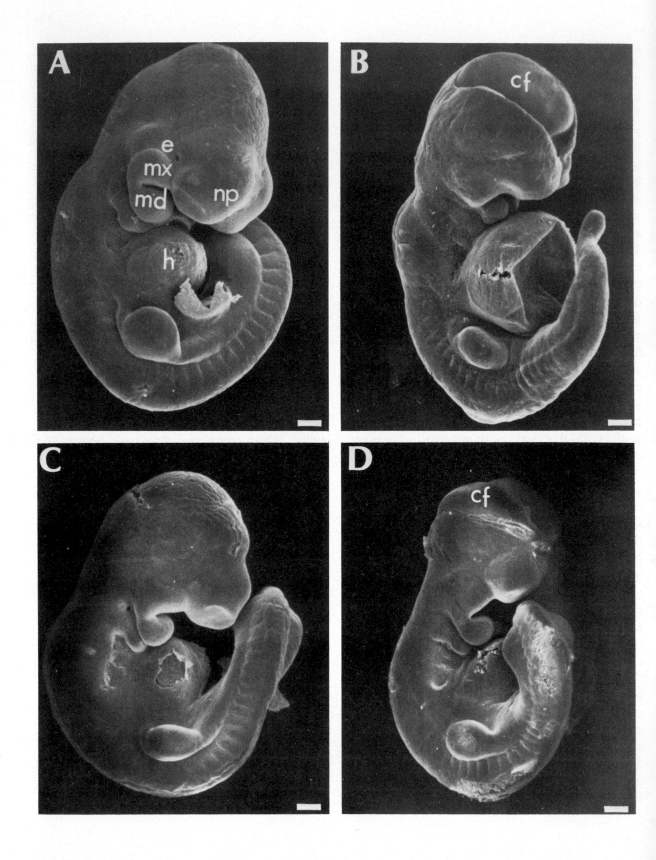

5-HT plus NC (Fig. 6C,D), fluoxetine (Fig. 6B) or just NC, and compared to embryos cultured in control media (containing only C; Fig. 6A). In embryos grown in the presence of 5-HT or fluoxetine, a number of defects were observed, including deficiencies in the head mesenchyme (not shown), hypoplastic maxillary processes and mandibular arches (Fig. 6C,D), hypoplastic fore-brains or open cranial neural folds (Fig. 6B,D), and abnormal eyes (Figs. 6B–D). The most dramatic and rapidly occurring defects were seen with fluoxetine (Fig. 6B). Much more minor, but related, defects were seen with NC alone (not shown).

Although further studies are required to assess the specificity of these effects, when taken to-gether with our previous immunocytochemical observations these results raise the possibility that uptake of 5-HT by epithelia and the expression of its binding protein in adjacent mesenchyme could play an important role in morphogenesis of the craniofacial region in the mouse embryo, especially the skeletal elements of the head, face and jaw which require epithelial-mesenchyme in-teractions for their development.

It should be noted that the malformations seen after treatment of embryos with 5-HT or fluoxetine are similar to those observed in whole embryo culture following exposure of rat or mouse embryos to 13-*cis*-retinoic acid (Accutane®). This drug, which is used clinically for the treatment of severe acne, is related to vitamin A (retinoic acid), a known teratogen, and itself a possible 'mor-phogen' (Thaller and Eichell, 1987). The cranio-facial abnormalities caused by this drug also seem to be related to interference with developing neural-crest-derived mesenchyme, particularly its migration and/or proliferation (Goulding and Pratt, 1986; Webster et al., 1986; Sulik et al., 1987).

Conclusions

This review has presented considerable evidence for morphogenetic functions of neurotransmitters during embryonic development, a role which may derive from their appearance early in evolution, still evidenced today by their presence in primitive organisms. These functions may be basic to both the initiation and orchestration of fundamental morphogenetic events at both the cellular and tissue levels of organization. In the light of such functions, use of the term 'morphogen' would seem appropriate to characterize these important regulatory molecules.

It is now important to investigate the cellular and molecular mechanisms underlying the mor-phogenetic roles of neurotransmitters in develop-ment. It will be of great interest to ascertain whether these mechanisms are as diverse as the functions they underlie, or whether they constitute a small set of basic events common to all cells and tissues where neurotransmitters exert their influence on morphogenetic processes.

In attributing such basic ontogenetic functions to neurotransmitters, we must also be cognizant of the issues this raises regarding the use of psychoactive drugs in pregnancy, particularly during the first trimester, since these compounds exert their effects on adult brain function via the

Fig. 6. Malformations in mouse embryos cultured in medium containing fluoxetine (B, 10^{-5} M) or 5-HT (C, 10^{-5} M; D, 10^{-4} M). Culture medium consisted of heat-inactivated rat serum and Tyrode's solution. Treatments were for 48 h beginning on E9 in medium containing nialamide and L-cysteine (10^{-5} M each). A: control (medium contained L-cysteine only). Note the hypoplastic maxillary process (mx), mandibular (md; 1st branchial arch) and nasal (np) prominences in embryos treated with 5-HT (C, D), which is more pronounced with increasing dose. Note also the open cranial folds in embryos treated with fluoxetine (B) or a high concentration of 5-HT (D). An enlarged heart (h) is also apparent in the fluoxetine-treated embryo (B). Embryos treated only with NC appeared intermediate between those shown in C and D. Eye rudiments (e) are hypoplastic or missing in all of the treated embryos (B–D). Bars = 250 μm. (From Lauder, Thomas and Sadler, in preparation.)

same neurotransmitter-related mechanisms which are now considered to be important for morphogenesis in the embryo.

Acknowledgements

This work was supported by NIH grant HD 22052. The author would like to thank Drs. Thomas Sadler, Ernest Zimmerman and Hadassah Tamir for their collaboration on the whole embryo culture studies, Drs. Katheleen Sulik and Malcolm Johnston for helpful discussions, and Robin Thomas and Robin Wynn for technical assistance.

References

Allan, I. J. and Newgreen, D. F. (1977) Catecholamine accumulation in neural crest cells and the primary sympathetic chain. *Am. J. Anat.*, 149: 413–421.

Baker, P. C. (1965) Changing serotonin levels in developing *Xenopus laevis. Acta Embryol. Morph. Exp.*, 8: 197–204.

Baker, P. C. and Quay, W. B. (1969) 5-hydroxytryptamine metabolism in early embryogenesis, and the development of brain and retinal tissues. *Brain Res.*, 12: 273–295.

Bard, J. B. L. and French, V. (1984) Butterfly wing patterns: How good a determining mechanism is the simple diffusion of a single morphogen? *J. Embryol. Exp. Morph.*, 84: 255–274.

Bee, J. and Thorogood, P. (1980) The role of tissue interactions in the skeletogenic differentiation of avian neural crest cells. *Dev. Biol.*, 78: 47–62.

Blum, J. J. (1970) Biogenic amines and metabolic control in Tetrahymena. In J. J. Blum (Ed.), *Biogenic Amines as Physiologic Regulators*, Prentice-Hall, Engelwood Cliffs, pp. 95–118.

Brinkley, L. (1986) Changes in mesenchymal cell-basal lamina relationships preceding palatal shelf reorientation in the mouse. *Am. J. Anat.*, 176: 367–378.

Burden, R. W. and Lawrence, I. E. (1973) Presence of biogenic amines in early rat development. *Am. J. Anat.*, 136: 251–257.

Buznikov, G. A. (1980) Biogenic monoamines and acetylcholine in protozoa and metazoan embryos. In J. Salanki and T. M. Turpaev (Eds.), *Neurotransmitters, Comparative Aspects*, Akademiai Kiado, Budapest, pp. 7–29.

Buznikov, G. A. (1984) The action of neurotransmitters and related substances on early embryogenesis. *Pharmac. Ther.* 25: 23–59.

Buznikov, G. A., Chudakova, I. V., Berysheva, L. V. and Vyazmina, N. M. (1968) The role of neurohumors in early embryogenesis. II. Acetylcholine and catecholamine content in developing embryos of sea urchin. *J. Embryol. Exp. Morph.*, 20: 119–128.

Buznikov, G. A., Chudakova, I. V. and Zvezdina, N. D. (1964) The role of neurohumors in early embryogenesis. I. Serotonin content of developing embryos of sea urchin and loach. *J. Embryol. Exp. Morph.* 12: 563–573.

Buznikov, G. A., Gordeev, E. N., Markova, L. N. and Suvorov, N. N. (1981) Effect of tryptamine and serotonin on development of sea urchins. *Ontogenez*, 12: 414–417 (in Russian).

Buznikov, G. A., Kost, A. N., Kucherova, N. F., Mndzhoyan, A. L., Suvorov, N. N. and Berdysheva, L. V. (1970) The role of neurohumours in early embryogenesis. III. Pharmacological analysis of the role of neurohumours in cleavage divisions. *J. Embryol. Exp. Morph.*, 23: 549–569.

Buznikov, G. A., Malchenko, L. A., Rakić, L., Kovačević, N., Markova, L. N., Salimova, N. B. and Volina, E. V. (1984) Sensitivity of starfish oocytes and whole, half and enucleated embryos to cytotoxic neuropharmacological drugs. *Comp. Biochem. Physiol.*, 78C: 197–201.

Buznikov, G. A., Manukhin, B. N., Rakic, L., Aroyan, A. A., Kucherova, N. F. and Suvorov, N. N. (1975) On the mechanism of protective action of acetylcholine and serotonin against their cytotoxic analogs. *Zh. Evol. Biokhim. Fisiol.*, 11: 128–133 (in Russian).

Buznikov, G. A. and Shmukler, Y. B. (1981) Possible role of 'prenervous' neurotransmitters in cellular interactions of early embryogenesis. *Neurochem. Res.*, 6: 55–68.

Child, C. M. (1941) *Patterns and Problems of Development*, Univ. Chicago Press, Chicago.

Ciment, G. and Weston, J. (1985) Segregation of developmental abilities in neural crest-derived cells: identification of partially restricted intermediate cell types in the branchial arches of avian embryos. *Dev. Biol.*, 111: 73–83.

Crick, F. (1970) Diffusion in embryogenesis. *Nature*, 225: 420–422.

Darvas, Z., Swydan, R. and Csaba, G. (1985) Influence of benzodiazepine (diazepam) by single and repeated treatment on the growth of Tetrahymena. *Biomed. Biochim. Acta*, 11/12 (Suppl.): 1725–1728.

Deeb, S. S. (1972) Inhibition of cleavage and hatching of sea urchin embryos by serotonin. *J. Exp. Zool.*, 181: 79–87.

Driesch, H. (1908) *The Science and Philosophy of the Organism*, Black, London.

Eichele, G., Tickle, C. and Alberts, B. M. (1985) Studies on the mechanism of retinoid-induced pattern duplications in the early chick limb bud: Temporal and spatial aspects. *J. Cell Biol.* 101: 1913–1920.

Emanuelsson, H. (1974) Localization of serotonin in cleavage embryos of *Ophryotrocha labronica La Greca and Bacci. Roux' Arch. Entw.-mech.*, 175: 253–271.

Emanuelsson, H. (1976) Serotonin in chick embryo cells

during early embryogenesis. *J. Cell Biol.*, 70: 131a.

Emanuelsson, H. and Palen, K. (1975) Effects of L-tryptophan on morphogenesis and growth in the early chick blastoderm. *W. Roux's Arch.*, 177: 1–17.

Franquinet, R. (1979) Role de la serotonine et des catecholamines dans la regeneration de la planaire *Polycelis tenius*. *J. Embryol. Exp. Morph.*, 51: 85–95.

Franquinet, R. and Martelly, I. (1981) Effects of serotonin and catecholamines on RNA synthesis in planarians; in vitro and in vivo studies. *Cell Differentiation*, 10: 201–209.

Garbarino, M. and Greene, R. (1984) Identification of adenylate cyclase-coupled B-adrenergic receptors in the developing mammalian palate. *Biochem. Biophys. Res. Commun.*, 119: 193–202.

Gershon, M.D., Liu, K.P., Karpiak, S.E. and Tamir, H. (1983) Storage of serotonin in vivo as a complex with serotonin-binding protein in central and peripheral serotonergic neurons. *J. Neurosci.*, 3: 1901–1911.

Godin, I. (1986) Explanted and implanted notochord of amphibian anuran embryos. Histofluorescence study on the ability to synthesize catecholamines. *Anat. Embryol.*, 173: 393–399.

Godin, I. and Gipouloux, J.D. (1986) Notochordal catecholamines in exogastrulated *Xenopus* embryos. *Dev. Growth Diff.*, 28: 137–142.

Goldman, M.E., Gunderson, R.E., Erickson, C.K. and Thompson, G.A. (1981) High-performance liquid chromatographic analysis of catecholamines in growing and nongrowing *Tetrahymena pyriformis*. *Biochim. Biophys. Acta*, 676: 221–225.

Goulding, E.H. and Pratt, R.M. (1986) Isotretinoin teratogenicity in mouse whole embryo culture. *J. Craniofacial Genet. Dev. Biol.* 6: 99–112.

Grobstein, C. (1967) Mechanisms of organogenetic tissue interactions. *Natl. Cancer Inst. Monog.*, 26: 279–299.

Guram, M.S., Gill, T.S. and Geber, W.F. (1980) Teratogenicity of imipramine and amitriptyline in fetal hamsters. *Res. Commun. Psychol. Psychiat. Behav.*, 5: 275–282.

Guram, M.S., Gill, T.S. and Geber, W.F. (1982) Comparative teratogenicity of chlordiazepoxide, amitriptyline, and a combination of the two compounds in the fetal hamster. *Neurotoxicology*, 3: 83–90.

Gustafson, T. and Toneby, M. (1970) On the role of serotonin and acetylcholine in sea urchin morphogenesis. *Exp. Cell. Res.*, 62: 102–117.

Gustafson, T. and Toneby, M. (1971) How genes control morphogenesis. *Am. Sci.*, 59: 452–462.

Gustafson, T. and Wolpert, L. (1963) Cellular mechanisms in the morphogenesis of the sea urchin larva. *Exp. Cell Res.*, 27: 260–279.

Hall, J.C., Greenspan, R.J. and Kankel, D.R. (1979) Neural defects induced by genetic manipulation of acetylcholine metabolism in *Drosophila*. *Soc. Neurosci. Symp.*, 4: 1–42.

Handa, R.J., Hines, M., Schoonmaker, J.N., Shryne, J.E.

and Gorski, R.A. (1986) Evidence that serotonin is involved in the sexually dimorphic development of the preoptic area in the rat brain. *Dev. Brain Res.*, 30: 278–282.

Harris, W.A. (1981) Neural activity and development. *Annu. Rev. Physiol.*, 43: 689–710.

Herbst, C. (1901) *Formative Reize in der tierischen Ontogenese*, A. Georgi, Leipzig.

Holtfreter, J. (1968) On mesenchyme and epithelia in inductive and morphogenetic processes. In R. Fleischmajer and R.E. Billingham (Eds.) *Epithelial-Mesenchymal Interactions*, Williams and Wilkins, Baltimore, pp. 1–30.

Holtfreter, J. and Hamburger, V. (1955) Amphibians. In B.H. Willier, P.A. Weiss and V. Hamburger (Eds.), *Analysis of Development*, W.B. Saunders, Philadelphia and London, pp. 230–296.

Idänpään-Heikkilä, J. and Saxén, L. (1973) Possible teratogenicity of imipramine/chloropyramine. *Lancet*, ii: 282–284.

Ignarro, L.J. and Shideman, F.E. (1968a) Appearance and concentrations of catecholamines and their biosynthesis in embryonic and developing chick. *J. Pharmacol. Exp. Ther.*, 159: 38–48.

Ignarro, L.J. and Shideman, F.E. (1968b) Norepinephrine and epinephrine in the embryo and embryonic heart of the chick: uptake and subcellular distribution. *J. Pharmacol. Exp. Ther.*, 159: 49–58.

Iwata, H. and Kariya, K. (1973) Change in catecholamine content of *Tetrahymena pyriformis* during growth. *Jap. J. Pharmacol.*, 23: 751–755.

Johnston, M. (1974) Facial malformation in chick embryos resulting from removal of neural crest. *J. Dent. Res. (Suppl.)*, 43: 822.

Johnston, M.C. and Hazelton, R.D. (1972) Embryonic origins of facial structures related to oral sensory and motor functions. In J.F. Bosma (Ed.), *Third Symposium on Oral Sensation and Perception*, C.C. Thomas, Springfield, pp. 76–97.

Jonakait, G.M., Tamir, H., Gintzler, A.R. and Gershon, M.D. (1979) Release of [^{3}H]serotonin and its binding protein from enteric neurons. *Brain Res.*, 174: 55–69.

Jurand, A. (1980) Malformations of the central nervous system induced by neurotropic drugs in mouse embryos. *Dev. Growth Diff.*, 22: 61–78.

Kasschou, M.R. and Mansour, T.E. (1982) Serotonin-activated adenylate cyclase during early development of *Schistosoma mansoni*. *Nature*, 296: 66–68.

Kater, S.B. and Haydon, P.G. (1987) Multifunctional roles for neurotransmitters: the regulation of neurite outgrowth, growth cone motility and synaptogenesis. In A. Vernadakis, A. Privat, J.M. Lauder, P.S. Timiras and E. Giacobini (Eds.), *Model Systems of Development and Aging of the Nervous System*, Martinus Nijhoff, Boston, pp. 239–255.

Kirby, M.L. and Gilmore, S.A. (1972) A fluorescence study

on the ability of the notochord to synthesize and store catecholamines in early chick embryos. *Anat. Rec.*, 173: 469–478.

Kirschgessner, A.L., Liu, K.P., Gershon, M.D. and Tamir, H. (1987) Co-localization of serotonin with specific serotonin binding proteins in serotoninergic neurons of the rat brain and spinal cord. *Anat. Rec.*, 218: 73A.

Landauer, W. (1975) Cholinomimetic teratogens: studies with chicken embryos. *Teratology*, 12: 125–146.

Landauer, W. (1976) Cholinomimetic teratogens III. Interaction with amino acids known as neurotransmitters. *Teratology*, 13: 41–46.

Lankford, K., DeMello, F.G. and Klein, W.L. (1987) A transient embryonic dopamine receptor inhibits growth cone motility and neurite outgrowth in a subset of avian retina neurons. *Neurosci. Lett.*, 75: 169–174.

Lauder, J.M. (1987) Neurotransmitters as morphogenetic signals and trophic factors. In A. Vernadakis, A. Privat, J.M. Lauder, P.S. Timiras and E. Giacobini (Eds.), *Model Systems of Development and Aging of the Nervous System*, Martinus Nijhoff, Boston, pp. 219–237.

Lauder, J.M. and Krebs, H. (1978) Serotonin as a differentiation signal. *Dev. Neurosci.*, 1: 15–30.

Lauder, J.M. and Krebs, H. (1984) Humoral influences on brain development. *Adv. Cell. Neurobiol.*, 5: 3–51.

Lauder, J.M., Tamir, H. and Sadler, T.W. (1987) Sites of serotonin uptake and binding protein immunoreactivity in the cultured mouse embryo: roles in morphogenesis? *Soc. Neurosci. Abstr.*, 13: 254.

Lauder, J.M., Tamir, H. and Sadler, T.W. (1988) Serotonin and morphogenesis I. Sites of serotonin uptake and binding protein immunoreactivity in the midgestation mouse embryo. *Development*, in press

Lauder, J.M., Wallace, J.A., Krebs, H., Petrusz, P. and McCarthy, K. (1982) In vivo and in vitro development of serotonergic neurons. *Brain Res. Bull.*, 9: 605–625.

Lauder, J.M. and Zimmerman, E. (1988) Sites of serotonin uptake in the epithelium of the developing mouse palate, oral cavity and face: possible role in morphogenesis? *J. Craniofac. Genet. Dev. Biol.*, in press.

Lawrence, I.E., Jr. and Burden, H.W. (1973) Catecholamines and morphogenesis of the chick neural tube and notochord. *Am. J. Anat.*, 137: 199–208.

LeLièvre, C.S. and LeDouarin, N.M. (1975) Mesenchymal derivatives of the neural crest: analysis of chimeric quail and chick embryos. *J. Embryol. Exp. Morph.*, 34: 125–154.

Liu, K.P., Gershon, M.D. and Tamir, H. (1985) Identification, purification, and characterization of two forms of serotonin binding protein from rat brain. *J. Neurochem.*, 44: 1289–1301.

Liu, K.P., Hsiung, S.C., Kirschgessner, A.L., Gershon, M.D. and Tamir, H. (1987) Co-localization of serotonin with serotonin binding proteins in the rat CNS. *J. Neurochem. (Suppl.)*, 48: 63.

Mansour, T.E. (1983) Serotonin receptors in trematodes: characterization and function. In T.P. Singer, T.E. Mansour and R.N. Ondarza (Eds.), *Mechanism of Drug Action*, Academic Press, New York, pp. 197–205.

Manukhin B.N., Volina, E.V., Markova, L.N., Rakic, L. and Buznikov, G.A. (1981) Biogenic monoamines in early embryos of sea urchins. *Dev. Neurosci.*, 4: 322–328.

Marek, M. and Kubicek, M. (1981) Morphogen pattern formation and development in growth. *Bull. Math. Biol.*, 43: 259–270.

Markova, L.N., Buznikov, G.A., Kovačević, N., Rakić, L., Salimova, N.B. and Volina, E.V. (1985) Histochemical study of biogenic monoamines in early ('prenervous') and late embryos of sea urchins. *Int. J. Dev. Neurosci.*, 3: 493–499.

McMahon, D. (1974) Chemical messengers in development: a hypothesis. *Science*, 185: 1012–1021.

Meinhardt, H. (1978) Space-dependent cell determination under the control of a morphogen gradient. *J. Theor. Biol.*, 74: 307–321.

Morris, H.R., Taylor, G.W., Masento, M.S., Jermyn, K.A. and Kar, R.R. (1987) Chemical structure of the morphogen differentiation inducing factor from *Dictyostelium discoideum*. *Nature*, 328: 811–814.

Morse, D.E., Hooker, N., Duncan, H. and Jensen, L. (1979) γ-Amino-butyric acid, a neurotransmitter, induces planktonic abalonae larvae to settle and begin metamorphosis. *Science*, 204: 407–410.

Müller, W.A. (1984) Retinoids and pattern formation in a hydroid. *J. Embryol. Exp. Morph.*, 81: 253–271.

Müller, W.A., Mitze, A., Wickhorst, J.P. and Meier-Menge, H.M. (1977) Polar morphogenesis in early hydroid development: action of caesium, of neurotransmitters and of an intrinsic head activator on pattern formation. *W. Roux's Arch.*, 182: 311–328.

Newgreen, D.F., Allan, I.J., Young, H.M. and Southwell, B.R. (1981) Accumulation of exogenous catecholamines in the neural tube and non-neural tissues of the early fowl embryo. Correlation with morphogenetic movements. *W. Roux's Arch.*, 190: 320–330.

Nichols, D.H. (1986) Formation and distribution of neural crest mesenchyme to the first pharyngeal arch region of the mouse embryo. *Am. J. Anat.*, 176: 221–231.

Noden, D.M. (1983) The role of the neural crest in patterning of avian cranial skeletal, connective, and muscle tissues. *Dev. Biol.*, 96: 144–165.

Noden, D.M. (1984) Craniofacial development: new views on old problems. *Anat. Rec.*, 208: 1–13.

Palen, K., Thorneby, L. and Emanuelsson, H. (1979) Effects of serotonin and serotonin antagonists on chick embryogenesis. *W. Roux's Arch.*, 187: 89–103.

Parisi, E., De Prisco, P., Capasso, A. and del Prete, M. (1984) Serotonin and sperm motility. *Cell Biol. Int. Rep.*, 8: 95.

Patel, A.J., Barochovsky, O., Borges, S. and Lewis, P.D.

(1983) Effects of neurotropic drugs on brain cell replication in vivo and in vitro. *Monog. neural Sci.*, 9: 99–110.

Pienkowski, M.M. (1977) Involvement of biogenic amines in control of development of early mouse embryos. *Anat. Rec.*, 189: 550.

Pisano, M.M. and Greene, R.M. (1985) Hormone and growth factor involvement in craniofacial development. *IRCS Med. Sci.*, 14: 635–640.

Pisano, M., Schneiderman, M. and Greene, R. (1986) Catecholamine modulation of embryonic palate mesenchymal cell DNA synthesis. *J. Cell. Physiol.*, 126: 84–92.

Raïs, R., Girard, C. and Gipouloux, J.D. (1981) Mise en évidence de catécholamines dans la chorde dorsale des embryons d'amphibiens anoures. Relations possibles avec l'activité adénylate cyclasique de cet organe et la migration des cellules germinales primordinales. *Arch. Anat. Micr. Morphol. Exp.*, 70: 149–160.

Rakić, L.M., Buznikov, G.A., Manukhin, B.N. and Turpaev, T.M. (1978a) Binding of pharmacological drugs by sea urchin embryos. II. Influence of some substances on the binding of and the sensitivity to neuropharmaca. *Jugoslav. Physiol. Pharmac. Acta*, 14: 455–463.

Rakić, L.M., Manukhin, B.N., Buznikov, G.A. and Turpaev, T.M. (1978b) Binding of neuropharmacological drugs by sea urchin embryos. I. Early sea urchin embryos as experimental models in neuropharmaca binding studies. *Jugoslav. Physiol. Pharmac. Acta*, 14: 445–454.

Rand, J.B. and Russell, R.L. (1984) Choline acetyltransferase-dependent mutants of the nematode *Caenorhabditis elegans. Genetics*, 106: 227–248.

Renaud, F., Parisi, E., Capasso, A. and De Prisco, P. (1983) On the role of serotonin and 5-methoxytryptamine in the regulation of cell division in sea urchin eggs. *Dev. Biol.* 98: 37–46.

Rodriguez, N. and Renaud, F.L. (1980) On the possible role of serotonin in the regulation of regeneration of cilia. *J. Cell Biol.*, 85: 242–247.

Roth, J., Le Roith, D., Shiloach, J., Rosenzweig, J.L., Lesniak, M.A. and Havrankova, J. (1982) The evolutionary origins of hormones, neurotransmitters, biology. *N. Engl. J. Med.*, 306: 523–527.

Sadler, T.W. (1979) Culture of early somite mouse embryos during organogenesis. *J. Embryol. Exp. Morph.*, 49: 17–25.

Sako, H., Kojima, T. and Okado, N. (1986) Immunohistochemical study on the development of serotoninergic neurons in the chick: I. Distribution of cell bodies and fibers in the brain. *J. Comp. Neurol.*, 254: 61–78.

Santander, R.G. and Cuadrado, G.M. (1976) Ultrastructure of the neural canal closure in the chicken embryo. *Acta Anat.*, 95: 368–383.

Schaller, H.C. (1973) Isolation and characterization of a low molecular weight substance activating head and bud formation in hydra. *J. Embryol. Exp. Morph.*, 29: 27–38.

Schaller, H.C. (1975) A neurohormone from hydra is also present in the rat brain. *J. Neurochem.*, 25: 187–188.

Schaller, H.C., Schmidt, T. and Grimmelikhuijzen, C.J.P. (1979) Separation and specificity of action of four morphogens from Hydra. *W. Roux's Arch.*, 186: 139–149.

Schlumpf, M. and Lichtensteiger, W. (1979) Catecholamines in the yolk sac epithelium of the rat. *Anat. Embryol.*, 156: 177–187.

Schoots, A.F.M., Meijer, R.C. and Denuce, J.M. (1983) Dopaminergic regulation of hatching in fish embryos. *Dev. Biol.*, 100: 59–63.

Sherif, S. (1983) *Pharmacological control of ciliary activity in the young sea urchin larva. Cholinergic and monoaminergic effects and the role of calcium and cyclic nucleotides*, Wenner-Gren Inst., Stockholm.

Schreiner, C.M., Zimmerman, E.F., Wee, E.L. and Scott, W.J. (1986) Caffeine effects on cyclic AMP levels in the mouse embryonic limb and palate in vitro. *Teratology*, 34: 21–27.

Sims, T.J. (1977) The development of monoamine-containing neurons in the brain and spinal cord of the salamander, *Ambystoma mexicanum. J. Comp. Neurol.*, 173: 319–335.

Slack, J.M.W. (1987a) Morphogenetic gradients – past and present. *Trends Biochem. Sci.*, 12: 200–204.

Slack, J.M.W. (1987b) We have a morphogen! *Nature*, 327: 553–554.

Slack, J.M.W., Darlington, B.G., Heath, J.K. and Godsave, S.F. (1987) Mesoderm induction in early *Xenopus* embryos by heparin-binding growth factors. *Nature*, 326: 197–200.

Smith, J.C. (1987) A mesoderm-inducing factor is produced by a *Xenopus* cell line. *Development*, 99: 3–14.

Spemann, H. and Mangold, H. (1924) Uber Induktion von Embryonalanlagen durch Implantation artfremder Organisatoren. *Arch Mik. Anat. Entw-Mech.*, 100: 599–638.

Strudel, G., Meinel, P. and Gateau, G. (1977a) Recherches d'amines flurigènes dans les chordes d'embryons de poulet traites pas des cholinergiques. *C.R. Acad. Sci. Paris*, 284: 1097–1100.

Strudel, G., Recasens, M. and Mandel, P. (1977b) Identification de catécholamines et de serotonine dans les chordes d'embryons de poulet. *C.R. Acad. Sci. Paris*, 284: 967–969.

Sulik, K.K., Johnston, M.C., Ambrose, L.J.H. and Dorgan, D.R. (1979) Phenytoin (Dilantin)-induced cleft lip: a scanning and transmission electron microscopic study. *Anat. Rec.*, 195: 243–256.

Sulik, K.K., Johnston, M.C., Smiley, S.J., Speight, H.S. and Jarvis, B.E. (1987) Mandibulofacial dysostosis (Treacher Collins Syndrome): a new proposal for its pathogenesis. *Am. J. Med. Genet.*, 27: 357–372.

Sullivan, W.D. and Sullivan, C.F. (1964) The acetylcholine content and the effects of hexamethonium on this compound at various phases of division of *Tetrahymena pyriformis* Broteria. *Cienc. Natur.*, 33: 17–33.

Tamir, H. (1983) Serotonin-binding protein: function in synaptic vesicles. *Trans. N.Y. Acad. Sci.*, 41: 237–242.

386

Tamir, H., Brunner, W., Casper, D. and Rapport, M.M. (1980) Enhancement by gangliosides of the binding of serotonin to serotonin binding protein. *J. Neurochem.*, 34: 1719–1724.

Tamir, H. and Gershon, M.D. (1979) Storage of serotonin and serotonin binding protein in synaptic vesicles. *J. Neurochem.*, 33: 35–44.

Tamir, H. and Huang, Y.L. (1974) Binding of serotonin to soluble binding protein from synaptosomes. *Life Sci.*, 14: 83–93.

Tamir, H. and Liu, K.P. (1982) On the nature of the interaction between serotonin and serotonin binding protein: effect of nucleotides, ions, and sulfhydryl reagents. *J. Neurochem.*, 38: 135–141.

Tan, S.S. and Morriss-Kay, G. (1985) The development and distribution of the cranial neural crest in the rat embryo. *Cell Tissue Res.*, 240: 403–416.

Teitelman, G., Jaeger, C.B., Albert, V., Joh, T.H. and Reis, D.J. (1983) Expression of amino acid decarboxylase in proliferating cells of the neural tube and notochord of developing rat embryo. *J. Neurosci.*, 3: 1379–1388.

Thaller, C. and Eichele, G. (1987) Identification and spatial distribution of retinoids in the developing chick limb bud. *Nature*, 327: 625–628.

Tomkins, G. (1975) The metabolic code. *Science*, 189: 760–763.

Toneby, M. (1977a) *Functional aspects of 5-hydroxytryptamine and dopamine in early embryogenesis of Echinoidea and Asteroidea*, Wenner-Gren Institute, Stockholm.

Toneby, M. (1977b) Functional aspects of 5-hydroxytryptamine in early embryogenesis of the sea urchin *Paracentrotus lividus*. *W. Roux's Arch.*, 181: 247–259.

Turing, A.M. (1952) The chemical basis of morphogenesis. *Trans. R. Soc. Lond., Ser. B*, 237: 37–72.

Tyler, M.S. and Hall, B.K. (1977) Epithelial influences on skeletogenesis in the mandible of the embryonic chick. *Anat. Rec.*, 188: 229–240.

Van Cauteren, H., Vandenberghe, J. and Marsboom, R. (1986) Protective activity of ketanserin against serotonin-induced embryotoxicity and teratogenicity. *Drug Dev. Res.*, 8: 179–185.

Venkatasubramanian, K. and Zimmerman, E.F. (1983) Palate cell motility and substrate interaction. *J. Craniofacial Genet. Dev. Biol.*, 3: 143–157.

Vogt, W. (1929) Gestaltungsanalyse am Amphibienkeim mit örtlicher Vitalfärbung. *Roux' Arch. Entw.-Mech.*, 120: 384–706.

Volina, E.V., Markova, L.N., Rakić, L., Manukhin, B.N. and Buznikov, G.A. (1983) Serotonin and tryptamine binding by early embryos of sea urchin. *Zh. Evol. Biokhim. Fisiol.*, 19: 121–126.

Waddington, C.H. (1962) *New Patterns in Genetics and Development*, Columbia Univ. Press, New York.

Waddington, C.H. (1940) *Organizers and Genes*, Cambridge Univ. Press, Cambridge.

Wallace, J.A. (1979) *Biogenic Amines in the Development of the Early Chick Embryo*, Ph.D Thesis, Univ. California, Davis.

Wallace, J.A. (1982) Monoamines in the early chick embryo: demonstration of serotonin synthesis and the regional distribution of seotonin-concentrating cells during morphogenesis. *Am. J. Anat.*, 165: 261–276.

Wallace, J.A., Lilly, S. and Maez R.R. (1985) Characterization of serotonin uptake mechanisms in the region of the caudal neuropore of the early chick embryo. *Soc. Neurosci. Abstr.*, 11: 605.

Wallace, J.A., Petrusz, P. and Lauder, J.M. (1982) Serotonin immunocytochemistry in the adult and developing rat brain: methodological and pharmacological considerations. *Brain Res. Bull.*, 9: 117–129.

Waterman, R., Palmer, G., Palmer, J. and Palmer, S. (1976) Catecholamine-sensitive adenylate cyclase in the developing golden hamster palate. *Anat. Rec.*, 185: 125–138.

Webster, W.S., Johnston, M.C., Lammer, E.J. and Sulik, K.K. (1986) Isotretinoin embryopathy and the cranial neural crest: an in vivo and in vitro study. *J; Craniofacial Genet. Dev. Biol.*, 6: 211–222.

Wee, E.L., Babiarz, B.S., Zimmerman, S. and Zimmerman, E.F. (1979) Palate morphogenesis IV. Effects of serotonin and its antagonists on rotation in embryo culture. *J. Embryol. Exp. Morph.*, 53: 75–90.

Wee, E.L., Norman, E.J. and Zimmerman, E.F. (1986) Presence of γ-aminobutyric acid in embryonic palates of AJ and SWV mouse strains. *J. Craniofacial Genet. Dev. Biol.*, 6: 53–61.

Wee, E.L., Phillips, N.J., Babiarz, B.S. and Zimmerman, E.F. (1980) Palate morphogenesis V. Effects of cholinergic agonists and antagonists on rotation in embryo culture. *J. Embryol. Exp. Morph.*, 58: 177–193.

Wee, E.L. and Zimmerman, E.F. (1983) Involvement of GABA in palate morphogenesis and its relation to diazepam teratogenesis in two mouse strains. *Teratology*, 28: 15–22.

Wee, E.L. and Zimmerman, E.F. (1985) GABA uptake in embryonic palate mesenchymal cells of two mouse strains. *Neurochem. Res.*, 10: 1673–1688.

Williams, J.G., Ceccarelli, A., McRobbie, S., Mahbubani, H., Kay, R.R., Early, A., Berks, M. and Jermyn, K.A. (1987) Direct induction of *Dictyostelium* prestalk gene expression by DIF provides evidence that DIF is a morphogen. *Cell*, 49: 185–192.

Wolpert, L. (1969) Positional information and the spatial pattern of cellular differentiation. *J. Theor. Biol.*, 25: 1–47.

Wolpert, L. (1978) Pattern formation in biological development. *Sci. Am.*, 239: 154–164.

Wong, D.T., Horng, J.S., Bymaster, F.P., Hauser, K.L. and Molloy, B.B. (1974) A selective inhibitor of serotonin uptake: Lilly 11040, 3-(p-trifluoromethylphenoxyl)-N-methyl-3-phenylpropylamine. *Life Sci.*, 15: 471–479.

Zimmerman, E.F., Clark, R.L., Ganguli, S. and Venkatasubramanian, K. (1983) Serotonin regulation of palatal cell motility and metabolism. *J. Craniofacial Genet. Dev. Biol.* 3: 371–385.

Zimmerman, E. F. and Lauder, J. M. (1987) Sites of serotonin uptake in the epithelium of the developing mouse palate, oral cavity and face: possible role in morphogenesis? *Teratology*, 35: 39A.

Zimmerman, E. F. and Wee E. L. (1984) Role of neurotransmitters in palate development. In Zimmerman E. F. (Ed.), *Current Topics in Developmental Biology*: Vol. 19, *Palate Development*, Academic Press, New York, pp. 37–63.

Zimmerman, E. F., Wee, E. L., Phillips, N. and Roberts, N. (1981) Presence of serotonin in the palate just prior to shelf elevation. *J. Embryol. Exp. Morphol.*, 64: 233–250.

Discussion

A. Vaccari: You have just presented extremely interesting data showing a correlation between 5-HT (5-hydroxytryptamine or serotonin) uptake and serotonin binding protein (SBP) sites. Since we know of a transport process, a high-affinity binding process, and an association of 5-HT to the SBP, in order to rule out the possibility that at least a part of what you have measured was related to some kind of transport of 5-HT, have you checked the effects of specific 5-HT uptake inhibitors, such as citalopram?

J. M. Lauder: We have only worked with fluoxetine so far, but we intend to test a whole range of inhibitors for their ability to block 5-HT uptake into the sites in developmental embryonic tissues as well as for their effects on epithelia and mesenchyme grown in cell or tissue culture.

T. A. Slotkin: Since no 5-HT accumulates in the absence of a monoamine oxidase (MAO) inhibitor, how would you envision an action which would permit significant amounts to reach the SBP? Is there any evidence for existence of serotonergic receptors during this period?

J. M. Lauder: This is a very good question. However, one should keep in mind that 5-HT may be present in sites of uptake or even in the mesenchyme in amounts below the level of detection by immunocytochemistry, so that I would be reluctant to say that none accumulates in the absence of MAO inhibitor.

M. Mirmiran: In your presentation you indicated the trophic role of serotonin in early embryogenesis. However, later on you showed us the teratogenic effects of serotonin on the embryo. How do you reconcile this discrepancy?

J. M. Lauder: These are not discrepancies, since too much of a trophic substance can no doubt cause problems for developmental processes just as too little can. The teratogenic effects of serotonin in craniofacial development may relate to effects on the migration and proliferation of mesenchyme cells derived from the neural crest.

M. Mirmiran: Olson and Sieger (1972) as well as yourself have shown in rats the appearance of serotonin neurons of raphe nuclei in the brainstem on days 11–13 of gestation. Later biochemical studies have shown an active uptake system in the raphe not earlier than day 15 and in the cerebral cortex not earlier than early postnatally. How do you explain your very early uptake of serotonin, e.g. with fluoxetine?

J. M. Lauder: The sites of uptake we have shown in early embryos are clearly not in neuronal cells, although they seem to have some of the characteristics of high-affinity neuronal uptake sites. Since they are in non-neuronal cells, they need not develop with the same time course as those in neurons.

P. M. Rodier: You have shown SBP in the mesenchyme and serotonin uptake in epithelium. How do you think that serotonin will function in communication between the tissues?

J. M. Lauder: It is possible that serotonin is concentrated in these epithelia and then released onto the adjacent neural-crest-derived mesenchyme which possesses SBP, as we have shown in the head and facial mesenchyme. Alternatively, in regions such as the oral cavity and palate, where no SBP is present, the effects of serotonin might be receptor-mediated, as suggested by studies from Wee et al. (1979) and Zimmerman et al. (1983).

References

Olson, L. and Seiger, A. (1972) Early prenatal ontogeny of central monoamine neurons in the rat: fluorescence histochemical observations. *Z. Anat. Entwicklungsgesch.*, 137: 301–306.

Wee, E. L., Babiarz, B. S., Zimmerman, S. and Zimmerman, E. F. (1979) Palate morphogenesis IV. Effects of serotonin and its antagonists on rotation in embryo culture. *J. Embryol. Exp. Morphol.*, 53: 75–90.

Zimmerman, E. F., Clark, R. L., Ganguli, S. and Venkatasubramanian, K. (1983) Serotonin regulation of palatal cell motility and metabolism. *J. Craniofacial Genet. Dev. Biol.*, 3: 371–385.

G.J. Boer, M.G.P. Feenstra, M. Mirmiran, D.F. Swaab and F. Van Haaren
Progress in Brain Research, Vol. 73
© 1988 Elsevier Science Publishers B.V. (Biomedical Division)

CHAPTER 25

Brain cell acquisition and neurotropic drugs with special reference to functional teratogenesis

Ambrish J. Patel and Paul D. Lewis

MRC Developmental Neurobiology Unit, Institute of Neurology, 1 Wakefield Street, London, WC1N 1PJ, and Department of Histopathology, The Royal Postgraduate Medical School, Hammersmith Hospital, DuCane Road, London, W12 OHS, UK

Introduction

Much evidence indicates that substances which act as neurotransmitters in the developed brain may also function as neurohumoural agents, involved in the regulation both of the early phases of embryogenesis and of the subsequent stages of development in the nervous system (cf. Balazs et al., 1977; Patel and Lewis, 1982; Lauder and Krebs, 1984; Patel, 1987). These developmental effects may help to explain why certain neuroactive drugs specifically interfering with particular neurotransmitter systems produce persistent behavioural changes when given during the period of rapid brain growth (for reviews see Cuomo et al., 1983; Patel et al., 1983; Brown and Fishman, 1984; Boer and Swaab, 1985; Fujii and Adams, 1987). However, the basis for any functional changes produced by neuroactive drugs is likely to be complex, involving both neurobiological factors and environmental interactions. The latter would make it extremely difficult to evaluate specific effects of neuroactive drugs on mental development in man (see Nahas and Goujard, 1979; Balazs et al., 1986; Fujii and Adams, 1987). It is therefore not surprising that most investigations in this field of study have been carried out on rats or mice, where environmental interactions can be reasonably controlled. Though extrapolation of information from an animal model to the human

condition is not straightforward, it is made possible by the knowledge that in all mammalian species general aspects of brain development follow the same basic programme (see Jacobson, 1978). This begins with neurulation and continues through cell acquisition and differentiation to the formation of specific interneuronal connections. However, it must be borne in mind that the relationship of these developmental events to birth differs markedly with species (Dobbing and Sands, 1979; Kameyama, 1985), and drug-related neurobiological changes depend not only on the dose and pharmacological properties of the harmful agent but also on the stage of brain development at the time of exposure (see Vorhees, 1987). In this chapter we will confine ourselves to the effects of psychotropic drugs on cell acquisition in the rat brain, but it must be emphasized that, since normal brain development depends on the formation and differentiation of neural cells in an interrelated fashion, effects on cell differentiation may be of no less importance (Patel, 1987).

Assembly of cells in the normal brain

In recent years many reviews have been devoted to various aspects of cell proliferation in the mammalian nervous system, and these can be consulted for more detailed information and for references (Sidman and Rakic, 1973; Berry, 1974;

Balazs et al., 1977; Jacobson, 1978; Lewis, 1978; Patel and Balazs, 1980; Rodier, 1980; Patel and Lewis, 1982). Here we will deal only briefly with those aspects of cell acquisition for which there is some evidence of drug-induced perturbation.

The primordial nervous system is one of the first structures to appear in the embryo, its development beginning with the formation of a neural plate. This takes the form of a longitudinal mid-dorsal thickening which develops from the ectoderm and consists of a layer of neuroepithelial cells. As development continues, the induction of the neural ectoderm by chordamesoderm (notochord) elevates neural folds at the lateral edges of the plate, forming a neural groove near the midline. Later the edges of the neural folds fuse, forming a continuous neural tube. During the closure of the neural tube, some cells at the edges of the neural plate detach dorsally to form the neural crest. This seemingly homogeneous population of cells will give rise, depending on their routes of migration and final destination, to very diverse cell types (Le Douarin, 1980). The cranial portion of the neural tube expands to become the brain vesicles, while the caudal part develops into the spinal cord.

The walls of the brain vesicles are initially only one or two cells thick, but they increase in thickness with continuing cell division. A fraction of the daughter cells migrate into the periphery of the neural tube to form the mantle layer. The migration of the young neurons in the forebrain gives rise to five definitive laminae of cells (inward from the pial surface): the marginal layer, cortical plate, intermediate zone, subventricular zone and ventricular zone, the last zone constituting the primary germinal site. Neuroepithelium of the young fetus produces some glial precursor cells, including radial glia, but a large proportion of the cells originating from the primary germinal matrix are neurons.

In the rat, by about the 17th day of gestation the innermost cell layers of the developing forebrain differentiate into the ependyma which lines the ventricular system and a cellular periventricu-lar region called the subependymal layer. This secondary germinal layer persists around the forebrain lateral ventricles as a well-defined zone containing undifferentiated mitotic cells, found throughout in rodents and for some years, at least, in primates, and it is also prominent in the human neonatal brain. In the rat, it is much thinner by the end of the second postnatal week, but the primitive morphology of the constituent subependymal cells and some mitotic activity can be detected even in old age. This secondary germinal zone is a major source of neuroglia.

The production of long-axoned neurons is largely completed by the 19th day of gestation in the rat, following a rigid timetable (Fig. 1). Thereafter generation of nerve cells, mainly interneurons, continues at some of the secondary germinal sites up to about three postnatal weeks. The most important secondary site of neurogenesis, from the quantitative viewpoint, is the external granular layer of the cerebellum. This layer is derived from germinal cells produced by the neuroepithelium of the fourth ventricle, at about day 11 in the mouse fetus, before day 17 in the fetal rat and at 60 to 80 days gestation in man. These cells reach the surface of the cerebellum and replicate to form a layer several cells thick.

In man, the external granular layer is maximally developed by term, and the disappearance of this germinal zone parallels the five-fold increase in the concentration of cells in the internal granular layer of the cerebellum during the first two years after birth (Gadsdon and Emery, 1976). The external granular layer is a source of basket, stellate and granule cells and there is no evidence that this layer produces neuroglia. Cerebellar cortical neuroglia presumably originate from the periventricular matrix, and proliferate vigorously towards the end of the first postnatal week. With respect to other postnatally formed nerve cells, the granule cells in the fascia dentata and in the olfactory bulbs and also some neurons in the thalamus, in the inferior olive and in pontine nuclei (cochlear nuclei), are acquired from secondary germinal sites. In the fascia dentata

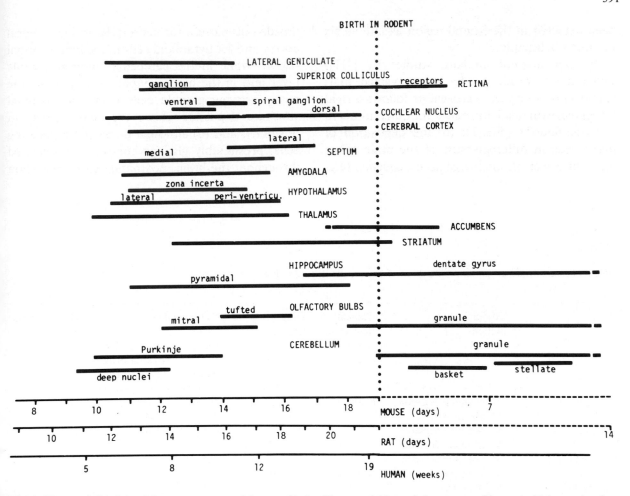

Fig. 1. Neuronal 'birthdays' in mouse, rat and human brain. The acquisition of the nerve cell type is high on the days corresponding with the middle of the horizontal bar and decreases gradually as one moves towards each end of the bar. The findings on the chronology of mouse neurogenesis are based on autoradiographic studies and are re-drawn from Rodier (1980), while the corresponding developmental periods in the rat and the approximate gestation periods in man are based on Dobbing and Sands (1979), Patel and Lewis (1982) and Kameyama (1985).

microneurons are generated into the third post-natal week in the rat and at least into the second postnatal month in man. In the rat olfactory bulbs the cell number increases about 4.5-fold between birth and the fifth postnatal week, but a slow rate of cell proliferation has been reported to continue for more than a year. A significant proportion of these postnatally formed cells in the olfactory bulbs are interneurons. A further secondary germinal zone, which appears to have been

adequately described only in the human brain, is the cerebral cortical subpial granular layer (Brun, 1965). This develops in the eighth week of gestation as a transitory layer of granule cells in the cell-free zone between the primitive cortical plate and the pia. It spreads laterally, anteriorly and posteriorly from the sylvian fissure, and increases up to the fifth month of intrauterine life. By the seventh month, it is already much involuted, although remnants are visible at term and have been detected in the frontal region as late as six months postnatally.

In experimental animals, studies by [³H]-thymidine autoradiography have revealed that: (a) the chronology of neurogenesis follows a rigid timetable, with fixed 'birthdays' for different nerve cell populations (Fig. 1); (b) the deposition of nerve cells in different parts of the brain takes place in a well-defined organized sequence (e.g. 'inside-out' pattern for nerve cells in the cerebral cortex and for pyramidal cells in the hippocampal region, while in the cerebellar internal granule layer and in the hippocampal dentate gyrus the newly arriving granule cells from the germinal sites are deposited above the cells already in position); and (c) although dispersed replicating cells, presumably glial precursors, are detected throughout the brain, postnatal cell proliferation

TABLE 1

Effects of neurotropic drugs on proliferation of brain cells in rat in vivo

Drug	Major known action	Clinical daily dose range (mg/kg)	Dose (mg/kg) and mode of injection	DNA labelling		Half-maximal effect (mg/kg)
				as a % of controls	during period (h) after drug administration	
Reserpine	Monoamine depletor	0.004–0.06	2.5, s.c.	30*	4–30	0.15
p-CPA	Monoamine depletor	–	300, × 2, i.p.	45*	1–96	–
α-M-p-T	Monoamine depletor	–	100, × 2, i.p.	65*	1–14	–
R04-1284	Monoamine depletor	0.3–2	10, s.c.	57*	1	–
Tetrabenazine	Monoamine depletor	1–3	10, s.c.	66*	1	–
Propranolol	β-Antagonist	0.3–10	10, s.c.	75*	5	–
Phenoxybenzamine	α-Antagonist	0.2–3	20, s.c.	71*	5	–
Chlorpromazine	DA-antagonist	2–30	50, s.c.	40*	14–30	10
Haloperidol	DA-antagonist	0.1–1.5	20, s.c.	50*	6–24	7
Thioridazine	DA-antagonist	0.5–12	15, s.c.	70*	3	15
LSD	5HT-antagonist	0.001–0.05	1, s.c.	54*	1–2	0.5
Nicotine	Nicotinic agonist	–	1, s.c.	96	0.5–24	–
Atropine	Muscarinic antagonist	0.004–0.06	50, s.c.	91	0.5	–
DBcAMP	'Second messenger'	–	2.5 µg, i.v.	116	0.16	–
DBcGMP	'Second messenger'	–	2.5 µg, i.v.	118	0.16	–

Eleven-day-old rats received either a single subcutaneous injection of drug or vehicle. The body temperature and nutritional status of the animals were maintained at normal levels. At the time indicated under 'period after drug administration', the rats received a subcutaneous injection of [³H]thymidine. Thirty minutes later they were killed and their forebrains removed and processed as described previously. The specific radioactivity of forebrain DNA (d.p.m./µg atom-P) was corrected on the basis of [³H]water-freed acid-soluble radioactivity (d.p.m./g) and the results in the drug-treated animals were expressed as a percentage of the control values. Significant differences ($P < 0.05$) between vehicle- and drug-treated groups are marked with an asterisk.

s.c., subcutaneous; i.p., intraperitoneal; i.v. intraventricular; p-CPA, DL-p-chlorophenylalanine; α-M-p-T, DL-α-methyl-p-tyrosine; R04-1284, (–)-threo-α-phenyl-α-piperid-2-yl methyl acetate hydrochloride; LSD, (+)-N,N-diethyl lysergamide; DBcAMP, dibutyryl adenosine 3',5'-cyclic monophosphate; DBcGMP, dibutyryl guanosine 3',5'-cyclic monophosphate; DA, dopamine; 5HT, 5-hydroxytryptamine.

The range of clinical daily doses are from Goodman and Gilman (1970) and Wade (1977). The other data are from Backhouse et al. (1982); Barochovsky et al. (1979); Lewis et al. (1977b, 1984); Patel et al. (1977, 1979, 1980, 1983).

largely occurs in circumscribed secondary germinal sites. Obviously the [³H]thymidine labelling procedure cannot be applied to man, but the findings of histological studies on postmortem material and on some in vitro studies of the incorporation of [³H]thymidine into human fetal brain tissue have indicated that the general pattern of brain cell proliferation is similar (Marin-Padilla, 1970; Sidman and Rakic, 1973; Berry, 1974; Gadsdon and Emery, 1976; Lewis, 1978; Dobbing and Sands, 1979).

In vivo studies with psychotropic drugs

In the experiments reviewed here, 11-day-old rats were used because at this age cell replication is occurring at a high level throughout the brain (Patel et al., 1973), and major secondary germinal zones are fully developed. Further, the cerebellar external granular layer mainly generates nerve cells, while the forebrain lateral ventricular subependymal layer largely produces neuroglial cells (see Patel and Lewis, 1982). The characterization of these germinal sites therefore permitted the differential analysis of proliferation kinetics of predominantly neuronal and glial precursors. Cell replication was assessed biochemically by measuring the rate of [³H]thymidine incorporation into DNA, and the findings were compared with morphologically derived estimates of cell proliferation.

Drugs affecting monoaminergic systems

Monoamine synthesis inhibitors. DL-*p*-Chlorophenylalanine methyl ester (p-CPA) and DL-α-methyl-*p*-tyrosine methyl ester (α-MPT) inhibit respectively tryptophan hydroxylase and tyrosine hydroxylase mediated enzymic reactions, and thus when given to developing rats produce a marked reduction in monoamine levels in the brain. Both compounds produced a severe reduction in the rate of [³H]thymidine incorporation into brain DNA (Table 1; Patel et al., 1983). After two doses of p-CPA (300 mg/kg, i.p.) or α-MPT

(100 mg/kg, i.p.) separated by 24 h, the rate of DNA labelling in the forebrain fell to 30–50% of controls for 96 and 14 h respectively.

Monoamine depletors. Reserpine, a well-known central nervous system depressant and antihypertensive agent, reversibly depletes brain monoamine stores. When reserpine was given to 11-day-old rats in a single dose (2.5 mg/kg, s.c.) it produced a severe reduction in the rate of [³H]thymidine incorporation into brain DNA (Patel et al., 1977; Lewis et al., 1977a). The depression in DNA labelling was already detectable 2 h after reserpine administration, and during the period 4–30 h after drug treatment the rate was about 30 and 60% of controls in the forebrain and cerebellum, respectively (Table 1). The effect of reserpine was dose-dependent and the half-maximal effect was produced with about 0.15 mg/kg in the forebrain and 0.5 mg/kg in the cerebellum (Patel et al., 1979). Parallel histological studies confirmed a depression of cell acquisition in both forebrain and cerebellar germinal sites (Table 2). In the forebrain subependymal layer, the labelling index was significantly depressed and cell cycle time, duration of DNA synthesis phase and the turnover time were clearly prolonged, indicating a reduction in the cell acquisition rate (Lewis et al., 1977a,b). In the cerebellar external granular layer, the major effect on the dividing cell population was a dramatic increase in cell death, paralleling a fall in the number of mitoses. A severe reduction in cell replication was not restricted to reserpine; the other monoamine depletors, including tetrabenazine and RO4–1284, also significantly inhibited brain DNA labelling (Table 1; Patel et al., 1983).

Adrenergic blockers. The results indicated that both the α- and the β-adrenergic systems may be involved in the control of brain cell replication. The administration of the α-antagonist phenoxybenzamine or the β-antagonist propranolol produced a marked reduction in [³H]thymidine incorporation into cerebral DNA (Table 1; Patel et al., 1983).

TABLE 2

Effects of psychotropic drugs on cell replication parameters and cell death in cerebellar external granular layer and forebrain subependymal layer

	Reserpine	Chlorpromazine	Haloperidol	LSD	Nicotine
1. External granular layer					
Mitotic index	79*	77*	95		
Labelling index	93	108	103	76*	
Cell cycle time	113	101	98		97
Duration of G_2-phase	107	176	181		150
Duration of S-phase	104	116	94		96
Turnover time	104	124	91		
Pyknotic index	268*	316*	135	100	
2. Subependymal layer					
Mitotic index	105	91	124		
Labelling index	71*	77*	100	83*	
Cell cycle time	149	117	106		100
Duration of G_2-phase	119	129	115		82
Duration of S-phase	114	109	118		110
Turnover time	160	143	118		
Pyknotic index	142	182*	118	101	

Eleven-day-old rats received a subcutaneous injection of [³H]thymidine at the specified time after administration of the neurotropic drug or vehicle, and they were killed at various times between 1 and 30 h later. Labelling indices were derived from counts of 1000 nuclei in rats killed 1 h after injection of [³H]thymidine, while mitotic and pyknotic indices were derived from counts of 2000 nuclei in each animal. Cell cycle parameters were derived from the computer-generated curves of percentage labelled mitoses at different times after injection of [³H]thymidine. Turnover time = 100 × computed S-phase duration/labelling index. The results are expressed as a percentage of control values. Significant differences ($P < 0.05$) between vehicle- and drug-treated groups are marked with an asterisk.
The data are from Lewis et al. (1977a,b, 1984); Barochovsky et al. (1979); Patel et al. (1980); Backhouse et al. (1982).

Dopamine antagonists. The neuroleptic drugs, chlorpromazine, thioridazine and haloperidol, are believed to act primarily on dopamine receptors. Of these one of the most widely used phenothiazines, chlorpromazine produced a severe reduction in the rate of [³H]thymidine incorporation into brain DNA (Tabel 1; Patel et al., 1980). The depression in DNA labelling was detectable by 6 h after chlorpromazine treatment (50 mg/kg, s.c.) and the rate of DNA synthesis was less than 30 and 60% of controls during the period 14–30 h in the forebrain and 6–30 h in the cerebellum, respectively. The effect was dose-dependent and a half-maximal effect was produced with approximately 10 mg/kg chlorpromazine (Table 1). The related phenothiazine drug, thioridazine, also produced a reduction in DNA labelling, the half-maximal effect in the forebrain occurring with a dose of about 15 mg/kg (Table 1). Parallel morphological analysis in chlorpromazine-treated rats revealed changes similar to those seen with reserpine (Table 2; Patel et al., 1980). The labelling index in subependymal cells was significantly depressed and the turnover time increased, indicating a decreased cell-acquisition rate. In the external granular layer there was a reduction in the mitotic index and a marked increase in cell degeneration (Table 2), thus reflecting the pattern of inhibition of DNA labelling (Table 1). More detailed analysis of autoradiographic results revealed that nuclear degeneration was a post-mitotic phenomenon. Feulgen cytophotometry confirmed that cell death occurred after division, although the relationship of this to the reduction in the number of mitoses was not clear.

Haloperidol, one of the butyrophenones, was also found to produce a severe reduction in DNA labelling (Backhouse et al., 1982). The significant depression was detectable by 4 h after haloperidol administration (20 mg/kg, s.c.), and over the period 10–24 h after drug treatment the rate in the forebrain was less than 50% of controls (Table 1). The effect was also dose-dependent, a half-maximal reduction in DNA labelling occurring with a dose of approximately 7 mg/kg haloperidol. In the cerebellum, the depression was similar but less pronounced than in the forebrain. Histological studies indicated that, though the changes were less severe, they were similar to those seen after reserpine and chlorpromazine treatments (Table 2; Backhouse et al., 1982).

Lysergic acid diethylamide (LSD). The effect on cell replication was not restricted to drugs influencing only dopaminergic transmitter systems in the brain. LSD, which is known to interfere mainly with the serotoninergic neurotransmitter system, also produced a severe dose–dependent, progressive reduction in the rate of [3H]thymidine incorporation into the brain DNA (Table 1; Barochovsky et al., 1979). The depression reached a nadir (40–50% of control value) throughout the brain at a dose of about 5 mg/kg. The half-maximum effect was obtained with 0.5 mg/kg in the forebrain and with 1 mg/kg in the cerebellum. Autoradiographic studies showed a dose–dependent decrease in the labelling index in both the forebrain subependymal and the cerebellar external granular layers, suggesting that entry of germinal cells into S-phase may have been affected in LSD-treated rats (Barochovsky et al., 1979).

Other drugs

In contrast to the drugs affecting mono-aminergic systems, the compounds influencing cholinergic systems, nicotine and atropine, had relatively little effect on brain cell replication in vivo (Tables 1 and 2; Patel et al., 1981; Lewis et al., 1984). Significant depression of DNA labelling was, however, seen at very high doses of nicotine. In rats given 2 mg/kg of nicotine [3H]thymidine incorporation into cerebellar DNA was reduced to 70% of the control values, while a reduction to 70% (of the control values) in forebrain and to 60% in cerebellum was observed after treatment with 4 mg/kg nicotine (Lewis et al., 1984). In a number of biological processes the effects of catecholaminergic agents are mediated through cyclic nucleotides, which have been implicated in the control of cell proliferation; our preliminary results indicated that intraventricular administration of relatively stable dibutyryl derivatives of cyclic nucleotides had very little effect on brain cell proliferation (Table 1; Patel et al., 1983).

In vitro studies with neurotropic drugs

In the in vivo studies a number of side-effects of drugs could be excluded as being responsible for the depressed rate of DNA labelling; the findings nevertheless provide only circumstantial evidence for the role of transmitters in the control of cell proliferation in the developing brain. In a further approach to this issue we have developed procedures which permit the study of cell replication in the brain in vitro (Barochovsky and Patel, 1982), without the complexity of the secondary reactions in in vivo studies. Brain slices from 11-day-old rats were incubated in Eagle's basal medium supplemented with 10% fetal calf serum at pH 7.4 in 95% oxygen and 5% carbon dioxide atmosphere. The incubation temperature was 37°C and slices were kept dispersed with the help of a shaking water bath. Under these conditions, the rate of in vitro [3H]thymidine incorporation into DNA was linear for periods much in excess of the S-phase duration: that is, more than 20 h in the forebrain and 14 h in the cerebellar slices (Barochovsky and Patel, 1982). During this period the in vitro rate of DNA labelling was about 3.36–times higher in the cerebellum than in the forebrain, a figure similar to the previously calculated ratio of in vivo cell acquisition rates (3.64) in these two brain regions (Patel et al., 1973; Barochovsky and Patel, 1982). Histological studies showed good morphological

TABLE 3

Effects of drugs interfering with particular neurotransmitter systems on replication of brain cells in vitro

Drug	Major known action	Forebrain		Cerebellum	
		% inhibition at 1 mM	half-maximum effect (mM)	% inhibition at 1 mM	half-maximum effect (mM)
Noradrenergic system					
(−)-Noradrenaline		77	0.11	91	0.55
(−)-Isoproterenol	β-Agonist	82	0.10	94	0.26
(−)-Alprenolol	β-Antagonist	39	–	96	0.32
Phenylephrine	α-Agonist	17	–	14	–
Clonidine	α-Agonist	2	–	15	–
Phenoxybenzamine	α-Antagonist	75	0.18	90	0.18
Dopaminergic system					
Dopamine		91	0.22		
A-6,7-DTN	Agonist	83	0.35		
Piribedil	Agonist	87	0.53		
Haloperidol	Antagonist	71	0.55		
Thioridazine	Antagonist	97	0.56		
Chlorpromazine	Antagonist	98	0.31		
Serotoninergic system					
5-Hydroxytryptamine		90	0.32	42	–
TFMTP	Agonist	95	0.41	78	0.60
Metergoline	Antagonist	91	0.31		
Cholinergic system					
Acetylcholine		4	–		
Carbamylcholine	Agonist	15	–	16	–
Atropine	Antagonist	5	–	18	–
Other drugs					
DBcAMP		17	–		
DBcGMP		4	–		

The slices of forebrain or cerebellum of 11-day-old rats were incubated in nutrient medium containing various concentrations of pharmacological agents. Four hours later the rate of [^{3}H]thymidine incorporation into DNA was measured and this was used as a measure of cell replication.
A-6,7-DTN, 6,7-dihydroxy-1,2,3,4-tetrahydronaphthalene; TFMTP, N-(α,α,α-trifluoro-m-tolyl)piperazine; DBcAMP, dibutyryl adenosine 3′,5′-cyclic monophosphate; DBcGMP, dibutyryl guanosine 3′,5′-cyclic monophosphate.
The data are from Barochovsky and Patel (1982).

preservation of the slices, while [3H]thymidine autoradiography demonstrated incorporation predominantly in cells of the germinal layer. Further, if the experiment was continued for a longer period, depending on the incubation time, labelled cells migrating from the germinal site were observed at different levels (Barochovsky and Patel, 1982). Thus, in our in vitro system, the operation of basic processes related to cell acquisition, including replication and migration, was more or less comparable to that in vivo.

The effects on cell replication of neurotransmitter compounds and psychotropic drugs were studied using this in vitro system (Barochovsky and Patel, 1982). The overall pattern of findings was consistent with the view that drugs affecting monoamine transmitter systems exert an influence on cell replication, as these compounds were found to produce a dose-dependent reduction in DNA labelling (Table 3). When various agonists and antagonists of the noradrenergic neurotransmitter systems were tested, it became apparent that only isoproterenol (β-agonist) and phenoxybenzamine (α-antagonist) resulted in dose-dependent reductions in DNA labelling, while phenylephrine and clonidine (α-agonists) showed relatively little effect both in the forebrain and in the cerebellar slices. Further, the action of isoproterenol was reversed by alprenolol (β-antagonist) and that of noradrenaline by a mixture of α- and β-antagonists. Moreover, in the forebrain slices the pharmacologically active isomers were several-fold more effective than the inactive isomers; however, the differences were smaller than usually encountered in this type of study. Like noradrenergic agents, pharmacological compounds affecting dopaminergic and serotoninergic neurotransmitter systems also resulted in a dose–dependent reduction in the rate of [3H]thymidine incorporation into DNA (Table 3; Barochovsky and Patel, 1982). There was no selectivity between agonists and antagonists, all showing more or less similar effects on DNA labelling. However, if brain slices were incubated in medium containing 1 mM of either dopamine

or serotonin antagonists, and then incubated for a further 2 h in a drug-free medium, the rate of DNA synthesis did not return to the control levels in these experiments. This contrasted with the effects of the other pharmacologically active compounds and may indicate that at a high concentration nonspecific effects may occur (Barochovsky and Patel, 1982).

In contrast to the marked effects of monoaminergic agents, but in agreement with in vivo findings (Table 1), the compounds influencing cholinergic systems have no appreciable effect on the rate of [3H]thymidine incorporation into DNA in either forebrain or cerebellar slices (Table 3; Barochovsky and Patel, 1982; Patel et al., 1981). Similar negative results were obtained with the relatively stable dibutyryl derivatives of cyclic nucleotides, and with cyclic nucleotides together with a phosphodiesterase inhibitor (Patel et al., 1983).

Comments

Possible limitations

A number of psychotropic drugs used in the present study are well-known for their side-effects, which may contribute to the observed reduction in the indices of brain cell replication. The possible secondary effects which may on their own interfere with cell proliferation include changes in body temperature, in circulating levels of corticosteroids and in entry of [3H]thymidine into the brain and its conversion to [3H]thymine nucleotides (Patel et al., 1979). Drug-induced food deprivation might also influence cell replication. Further, at high concentration, some of the effective drugs have been shown either to be toxic or to affect certain processes of cell proliferation not mediated through receptor stimulation (see Marx, 1976; Rebhun, 1977; Nahas et al., 1979; Patel et al., 1979; Dicker and Rozengurt, 1980). For example, some drugs can inhibit oxidative phosphorylation, which may restrict the energy supply for cell replication; they can interfere with microtubule assembly; or they can exert a local anaesthetic action on the cell membrane and disrupt both microtubules and microfilaments either directly or through an effect on the distribution of calcium ions in the cell; or associate tightly but nonspecifically with cell membrane and alter the operation of the normal cation pump activity of proliferating cells. It is also possible that the effect of some of these drugs may be related to their solubility in lipids and might be mediated, in part, through a common direct effect on the plasma membrane. However, some of these effects are irreversible, whereas most of the effects observed in our in vitro studies were not only reversible (when brain slices previously exposed to drugs were incubated in drug-free medium) but were also pharmacologically specific and obtained mainly with monoaminergic agents (Barochovsky and Patel, 1982). Further, in a few experiments, the radioactivity in thymidine and its nucleotide fraction was measured and the amount in the in vivo drug-treated brain or in the in vitro drug-treated brain slices was found not to differ significantly from the respective control value; thus, entry of the DNA precursor was not compromised (Patel et al., 1977, 1979, 1980, 1981; Barochovsky and Patel, 1982). Also, in in vivo studies certain side-effects of the drugs, such as restriction of food intake, induction of hypothermia, interference with the availability of energy supply and elevation of the level of blood corticosteroids, were excluded as being responsible for the depressed rate of cell proliferation (Patel et al., 1979, 1980).

In morphological studies it must be emphasized that the increased pyknotic index observed in the germinal zone in the drug-treated brain gives only a crude estimate of the lethally damaged newly formed cells. The number of cells with sublethal but functionally significant damage probably exceeds this value (Table 2; Lewis et al., 1977b; Patel et al., 1980). On the other hand, when comparing the results between experimental and control groups it should be borne in mind that substantial variation in the estimation of cell cycle length and the duration of its component phases is usually found in duplicate experiments on the same material carried out under stringently controlled conditions. Therefore, the changes of less than 20% must be interpreted with extreme caution. Further, turnover time should theoretically be of the same length as cell cycle time, but if all the cells in the renewing tissue are not involved in proliferation (as during early development) it will be greater and can vary considerably. The calculated values should be regarded as figures for comparison, rather than absolute (see Patel and Lewis, 1982).

Further remarks

Both the in vivo and the in vitro findings were consistent with an influence of monoamines and drugs affecting monoamine neurotransmitter systems on brain cell replication, although the precise mechanisms of their actions remain to be determined. Apart from effects on cell proliferation and cell death, our in vitro studies also suggest that monoamines may interfere with processes of cell migration in the developing brain (Barochovsky and Patel, 1982). In an experiment when serotoninergic neurons were transplanted into the fourth ventricle of the developing rat, some of these cells survived and grew their axons into the cerebellum (Yamamoto et al., 1980). In these hyperinnervated rats, clusters of ectopic granule cells were found in association with serotoninergic cell axons, suggesting that the presence of these fibers had altered the pattern of cerebellar granule cell migration. During the early phases of embryogenesis, monoamines have been detected in the neural plate and yolk material of the chick and in the yolk sac of rat, and drugs which interfere with monoamine metabolism are also found to disturb these neurulation processes (see Jurand, 1980; Schlumpf and Lichtensteiger, 1979; Wallace, 1982). It is also possible that neurotransmitter compounds may play a dual regulatory role in brain maturation, depending on the stage of development at the time of action (see also Vorhees, 1987). For example, during the early embryonic stage serotonin is found to inhibit the outgrowth of neurites to target areas and to promote short neuronal processes (autoregulation), while at mid-gestation pharmacological depletion of serotonin appeared to cause retardation in the genesis of those cells which eventually receive serotoninergic innervation (maturational signal for target regions) (see Lauder and Krebs, 1984; Whitaker-Azmitia et al., 1987).

Furthermore, several lines of evidence suggest that, apart from monoamines, other neuroactive substances including neuropeptides and opioid compounds may also modulate cell proliferation in the brain (Boer and Swaab, 1985; Zagon and McLaughlin, 1987). The presence of putative neuropeptide transmitters and opioid systems can be demonstrated immunocytochemically early in development, and treatment with these substances has been found to cause significant alterations in the overall growth of the brain and in the

replication of neural cells (Boer and Patel, 1983; Boer and Swaab, 1985; Johannesson and Steele, 1975; Vertes et al., 1982; Zagon and McLaughlin, 1987).

Some functional implications

In the context of functional neuroteratology, it should be noted that the chronology of neurogenesis in the developing brain follows a rigid timetable: the 'birthdays' of different nerve cell populations are fixed (Fig. 1; for references see Rodier, 1980; Patel and Lewis, 1982). So inflexible is this chronological programme for neurogenesis that perturbation of cell generation during the limited period in which any nerve cell type is normally produced will inevitably lead to numerical alterations and changes in the formation of neural networks. In support of this

TABLE 4

Effect of treatment with chlorpromazine during gestation and postnatal periods on the acquisition of Purkinje and granule cells in the rat cerebellum

Period of chlorpromazine treatment	Parameter	Control	Chlorpromazine	Significance (P)
I. 12–15 days of gestation:				
	Purkinje cells (No. per mm)	16.44 ± 0.35	14.89 ± 0.25	< 0.001
	Granule cells (No. per section)	9616 ± 290	9853 ± 267	ns
II. 10–13 days after birth:				
	Purkinje cells (No. per mm)	15.90 ± 0.44	15.41 ± 0.38	ns
	Granule cells (No. per section)	9320 ± 358	7731 ± 180	< 0.001

In Group I pregnant female rats received daily subcutaneous injections of chlorpromazine (50 mg/kg) during the period 12–15 days of gestation, while in Group II young rats received daily subcutaneous injections of chlorpromazine (25 mg/kg) during the period 10–13 days after birth. Controls received vehicle only. About 12 rats in each group were killed by aortic perfusion when they were 65 days old. Mid-sagittal 10-μm sections of the cerebellum were prepared and stained with haematoxylin and eosin. The number of Purkinje cells and granule cells was measured in three cerebellar lobules. Each of the values is mean $\pm$ S.E.M. of 36 observations; ns, no significant difference ($P > 0.05$).

hypothesis we have examined the effects on neurogenesis of chlorpromazine exposure at different stages of development (Table 4). Daily administration of chlorpromazine during the period of 12–15 days of gestation resulted in cerebellar cortex in a selective reduction in Purkinje cell numbers, but no effect on the granule cell numbers. In contrast, daily treatment with chlorpromazine during the period 10–13 days after birth decreased granule cell numbers in the different lobules of the cerebellum but it had no significant effect on Purkinje cell numbers. As Purkinje cells are formed before birth and granule cells are mainly acquired postnatally (Fig. 1), these findings provide direct evidence for chronologically determined interference with neurogenesis by chlorpromazine.

Our results show effects of various centrally active neuropharmacological agents on cell proliferation in the developing brain, and provide a basis, partial at least, for the understanding of behavioural teratogenesis. These experimental findings need, however, to be correlated with behavioural measures. Buelke-Sam (1987) has outlined strategies for the investigation of behavioural and physiological effects following prenatal drug exposure, and discussed the interpretation of animal findings in relationship to man. There is need for as much caution in making inferences from data such as those described here as there is in the laboratory evaluation of pharmacological substances designed for human use, particularly for pregnant and breast-feeding mothers and developing children.

Summary

Persistent changes in higher nervous function are often seen in experimental animals after exposure to neurotropic drugs during the period of rapid brain development. We have examined the possibility that such abnormalities have a structural basis and may be due to drug-induced perturbations of cell acquisition in the brain.

Cell proliferation in the mammalian brain occurs over a relatively restricted period, up to about 3 weeks postnatally in the rat, and probably up to 2 years in man. The 'birthdays' of many different nerve cell populations are fixed, indicating that the chronology of neurogenesis follows a rigid timetable. Although dispersed replicating cells, presumably glial precursors, are detected throughout the brain, postnatal cell proliferation occurs largely in circumscribed secondary germinal sites. Cell proliferation was assessed biochemically (by measuring the rate of incorporation of labelled thymidine into DNA in the forebrain and in the cerebellum in vivo and in morphologically well-preserved brain slices in vitro) and histologically (by measuring the estimates of cell replication) with emphasis on the cerebellar external granular layer, a source of nerve cells, and on the forebrain lateral ventricular subependymal layer, a source of neuroglia. In the brain, cell proliferation was significantly reduced by a number of psychoactive drugs. These were the monoamine depletors, reserpine, tetrabenazine and RO4–1284; inhibitors of monoamine synthesis, DL-p-chlorophenylalanine and DL-α-methyl-p-tyrosine; dopamine antagonists, chlorpromazine, thioridazine and haloperidol; and the antiserotonin drug, lysergic acid diethylamide. Morphological analysis confirmed a depression of cell acquisition in both forebrain and cerebellar germinal sites. In the subependymal layer, the rate of cell acquisition was markedly reduced and cell cycle time and the duration of the DNA synthesis phase were prolonged. In the cerebellar external granular layer, the major effect was a decrease in the mitotic index and an increase in the degeneration of postmitotic cells. In vitro studies showed that the drugs affecting monoamine neurotransmitter systems reduced the rate of DNA labelling in a dose-dependent manner. The drugs affecting cholinergic systems and cyclic nucleotides were apparently ineffective. Further, direct evidence for chronologically determined interference with neurogenesis was provided by the observation that temporary exposure to chlorpromazine during gestation or in the neonatal period results in a selective reduction of the prenatally generated Purkinje cells or of the postnatally formed granule cells. These results support the view that the changes in neuronal composition (and circuitry in 'functionally sensitive' brain regions) may be involved in behavioural deficits seen after exposure to neurotropic drugs in early life.

Acknowledgements

We would like to acknowledge the collaboration of Mrs. O. Barochovsky, Dr. G. Bendek, Dr. S. Borges and Dr. Z. Vertes, and we are grateful to Mr. B. Backhouse, Mrs. P. Bailey, Miss M. Lai and Mrs. C. Malik for expert help in part of these studies. Gratitude is expressed to Dr. R. Balázs for his advice and encouragement.

References

Backhouse, B., Barochovsky, O., Malik, C., Patel, A.J. and Lewis, P.D. (1982) Effect of haloperidol on cell proliferation in the early postnatal rat brain. *Neuropath. Appl. Neurobiol.*, 8: 109–116.

Balázs, R., Patel, A.J. and Lewis, P.D. (1977) Metabolic influences on cell proliferation in the brain. In A.N. Davison (Ed.), *Biochemical Correlates of Brain Structure and Function*, Academic Press, New York, pp. 43–83.

Balázs, R., Jordan, T., Lewis, P.D. and Patel, A.J. (1986) Undernutrition and brain development. In F. Frank, and J.M. Tanner (Eds.), *Human Growth, Vol. 3*, 2nd Edn., Plenum Press, New York, pp. 415–473.

Barochovsky, O. and Patel, A.J. (1982) Effect of central nervous system acting drugs on brain cell replication in vitro. *Neurochem. Res.*, 7: 1059–1074.

Barochovsky, O., Patel, A.J. and Balázs, R. (1979) Neurohumors and cell proliferation in the developing brain: effect of lysergic acid diethylamide (LSD). In *Proc. 7th Meet. Int. Soc. Neurochem.*, Jerusalem, p. 212.

Berry, M. (1974) Development of the cerebral neocortex of the rat. In G. Gottlieb (Ed.), *Aspects of Neurogenesis. Studies on the Development of Behaviour and the Nervous System, Vol. 2*, Academic Press, London, pp. 7–67.

Boer, G.J. and Patel, A.J. (1983) Disorders of cell acquisition in the brain of rats deficient in vasopressin (Brattleboro mutant). *Neurochem. Int.*, 5: 463–469.

Boer, G.J. and Swaab, D.F. (1985) Neuropeptide effects on

brain development to be expected from behavioral teratology. *Peptides (Suppl. 2)*, 6: 21–28.

Brown, R.M. and Fishman, R.H.B. (1984) An overview and summary of the behavioural and neural consequences of perinatal exposure to psychotropic drugs. In J. Yanai (Ed.), *Neurobehavioral Teratology*, Elsevier, Amsterdam, pp. 3–54.

Brun, A. (1965) The subpial granular layer of the foetal cerebral cortex in man. *Acta Path. Microbiol. Scand. (Suppl.)*, 179: 1–98.

Buelke-Sam, J. (1987) Behavioral and physiological effects following prenatal exposures: relationships among human and animal findings. In T. Fujii and P.M. Adams (Eds.), *Functional Teratogenesis. Functional Effects on the Offspring After Parental Drug Exposure*, Teikyo University Press, Tokyo, pp. 217–233.

Cuomo, V., Cagiano, R., Mocchetti, I., Coen, E., Cattabeni, F. and Racagni, G. (1983) Biochemical and behavioral effects after early postnatal administration of neuroleptics in rats. In G. Zbinden, V. Cuomo, G. Racagni and B. Weiss (Eds.), *Application of Behavioral Pharmacology in Toxicology*, Raven Press, New York, pp. 173–185.

Dicker, P. and Rozengurt, E. (1980) Phorbol esters and vasopressin stimulate DNA synthesis by a common mechanism. *Nature*, 287: 607–612.

Dobbing, J. and Sands, J. (1979) Comparative aspects of the brain growth spurt. *Early Human Dev.*, 3: 79–83.

Fujii, T. and Adams, P.M. (Eds.) (1987) *Functional Teratogenesis. Functional Effects on the Offspring after Parental Drug Exposure*, Teikyo University Press, Tokyo.

Gadsdon, D.R. and Emery, J.L. (1976) Some quantitative morphological aspects of postnatal human cerebellar growth. *J. Neurol. Sci.*, 29: 137–148.

Goodman, L.S. and Gilman, A. (Eds.) (1970) *The Phamacological Basis of Therapeutics*, Macmillan, London.

Jacobson, M. (1978) *Devolopmental Neurobiology*, Plenum Press, New York.

Johannesson, T. and Steele, W.J. (1975) Effects of prenatally-administered morphine on brain development and resultant tolerance to the analgesic effect of morphine treated rats. *Acta Pharmacol. Toxicol.*, 36: 243–256.

Jurand, A. (1980) Malformations of the central nervous system induced by neurotropic drugs in mouse embryos. *Dev. Growth Diff.*, 22: 61–70.

Kameyama, Y. (1985) Comparative developmental pathology of malformations of the central nervous system. *Prog. Clin. Biol. Res.*, 163A: 143–156.

Lauder, J.M. and Krebs, H. (1984) Humoral influences on brain development. *Adv. Cell. Neurobiol.*, 5: 3–50.

Le Douarin, N.M. (1980) The ontogeny of the neural crest in avian embryo chimaeras. *Nature*, 286: 663–669.

Lewis, P.D. (1978) The application of cell turnover studies to neuropathology. In W.T. Smith and J.B. Cavanagh (Eds.),

Recent Advances in Neuropathology, Churchill Livingstone, London, pp. 41–65.

Lewis, P.D., Patel, A.J., Bendek, G. and Balázs, R. (1977a) Do drugs acting on the nervous system affect cell proliferation in the developing brain? *Lancet*, i: 399–401.

Lewis, P.D., Patel, A.J., Bendek, G. and Balázs, R. (1977b) Effect of reserpine on cell proliferation in the developing rat brain: a quantitative histological study. *Brain Res.*, 129: 299–308.

Lewis, P.D., Backhouse, B. and Patel, A.J. (1984) A study of nicotine effects on cell proliferation in developing brain. In F. Caciagli, E. Giacobini and R. Paoletti (Eds.), *Developmental Neuroscience: Physiological, Pharmacological and Clinical Aspects*, Elsevier, Amsterdam, pp. 123–126.

Marin-Padilla, M. (1970) Prenatal and early postnatal ontogenesis of the human motor cortex: a Golgi study. *Brain Res.*, 23: 167–191.

Marx, J.L. (1976) Cell biology: cell surface and the regulation of mitosis. *Science*, 192: 455–457.

Nahas, G. and Goujard, J. (1979) Phenothiazines, benzodiazepines, and the fetus. In E.M. Scarpelli and E.V. Cosmi (Eds.), *Reviews in Perinatal Medicine, Vol. 3*, Raven Press, New York, pp. 243–280.

Nahas, G., Desoize, B. and Leger, C. (1979) Effects of psychotropic drugs on DNA synthesis in cultured lymphocytes. *Proc. Soc. Exp. Biol. Med.*, 160: 344–348.

Patel, A.J. (1987) Neurobiological aspects of functional teratogenesis: cell proliferation and development of certain neurotransmitter systems. In T. Fujii and P.M. Adams (Eds.), *Functional Teratogenesis. Functional Effects on the Offspring after Parental Drug Exposure*, Teikyo University Press, Tokyo, pp. 3–15.

Patel, A.J. and Balázs, R. (1980) Hormones and cell proliferation in the rat brain. In F. Brambilla, G. Racagni and D. de Wied (Eds.), *Progress in Psychoneuroendocrinology*, Elsevier, Amsterdam, pp. 621–632.

Patel, A.J. and Lewis, P.D. (1982) Effects on cell proliferation of pharmacological agents acting on the central nervous system. In K.N. Prasad and A. Vernadakis (Eds.), *Mechanisms of Actions of Neurotoxic Substances*, Raven Press, New York, pp. 181–218.

Patel, A.J., Balázs, R. and Johnson, A.L. (1973) Effect of undernutrition on cell formation in the rat brain. *J. Neurochem.*, 20: 1151–1165.

Patel, A.J., Bendek, G., Balázs, R. and Lewis, P.D. (1977) Effect of reserpine on cell proliferation in the developing rat brain: a biochemical study. *Brain Res.*, 129: 283–297.

Patel, A.J., Bailey, P. and Balázs, R. (1979) Effect of reserpine on cell proliferation and energy stores in the developing rat brain. *Neuroscience*, 4: 139–143.

Patel, A.J., Vertes, Z., Lewis, P.D. and Lai, M. (1980) Effect of chlorpromazine on cell proliferation in the developing rat brain. A combined biochemical and morphological study. *Brain Res.*, 202: 415–428.

Patel, A.J. Barochovsky, O. and Lewis, P.D. (1981) Psychotropic drugs and brain development: effects on cell replication in vivo and in vitro. *Neuropharmacology*, 20: 1243–1249.

Patel, A.J., Barochovsky, O., Borges, S. and Lewis P.D. (1983) Effects of neurotropic drugs on brain cell replication in vivo and in vitro. *Monogr. Neural Sci.*, 9: 99–110.

Rebhun, L.I. (1977) Cyclic nucleotides, calcium and cell division. *Int. Rev. Cytol.*, 49: 1–54.

Rodier, P.M. (1980) Chronology of neuron development: animal studies and their clinical implications. *Dev. Med. Child Neurol.*, 22: 525–545.

Schlumpf, M. and Lichtensteiger, W. (1979) Catecholamines in the yolk sac epithelium of the rat. *Anat. Embryol.*, 156: 177–187.

Sidman, R.L. and Rakic, P. (1973) Neuronal migration, with special reference to developing human brain: a review. *Brain Res.*, 62: 1–35.

Vertes, Z., Melegh, H., Vertes, M. and Kovacs, S. (1982) Effect of naloxane and D-met²-pro⁵-enkephalinamide treatment on the DNA synthesis on the developing rat brain. *Life Sci.*, 31: 119–126.

Vorhees, C.V. (1987) Dependence on the stage of gestation: prenatal drugs and offspring behavior as influenced by different periods of exposure in rats. In T. Fujii and P.M. Adams (Eds.), *Functional Teratogenesis. Functional Effects in the Offsprings After Parental Drug Exposure*, Teikyo University Press, Tokyo, pp. 39–51.

Wade, A. (1977) *Martindale: The Extra Phamacopocia*, 27th Edn., The Pharmaceutical Press, London.

Wallace, J.A. (1982) Monoamines in the early chick embryo: demonstration of serotonin synthesis and the regional distribution of serotonin-concentrating cells during morphogenesis. *Am. J. Anat.*, 165: 261–276.

Whitaker-Azmitia, P.M., Lauder, J.M., Shemmer, A. and Azmitia, E.C. (1987) Postnatal changes in serotonin-1 receptors following prenatal alterations in serotonin level: further evidence for functional fetal serotonin-1 receptors. *Dev. Brain Res.*, 33: 285–289.

Yamamoto, M., Chan-Palay, V., Steinbusch, H.W.M. and Palay, S.L. (1980) Hyperinnervation of arrested granule cells produced by transplantation of monoamine-containing neurons into the fourth ventricle of rat. *Anat. Embryol.*, 159: 1–15.

Zagon, I.S. and McLaughlin, P.J. (1987) Endogenous opioid systems regulate cell proliferation in the developing rat brain. *Brain Res.*, 412: 68–72.

Discussion

A. Vaccari: I have been impressed by the potency of reserpine in inhibiting DNA labelling. I would have expected a similar inhibition by tetrabenazine, which, however, resulted in a lot weaker inhibition. It has been shown that in the CNS both reserpine and tetrabenazine have specific high-affinity binding sites, which, however, are different from each other, and which are related to the transmitter systems of dopamine. So, I am wondering whether the different activities of the two depletors are somehow related to reserpine or tetrabenazine binding sites.

A.J. Patel: It is possible that differences in the reserpine and tetrabenazine binding sites may produce differential effects on brain DNA labelling by these monoamine depletors. However, I would like to remind you that the results summarized on the effects of reserpine are based on very comprehensive studies, while those on tetrabenazine are rather preliminary in nature and carried out at one time-point with a single dose of drug administration. A more detailed study of the effect of tetrabenazine on brain cell proliferation is required before one starts thinking along the lines you indicated.

J.A. Slotkin: Could the transmitter be acting in a dual fashion, with low levels stimulating DNA synthesis, particularly during early development, and at high levels shutting off cell replication during later developmental stages?

A.J. Patel: There are a number of findings in the literature showing a biphasic effect of neurotransmitter compounds on various biological systems. However, I would prefer to think that the effects of neurotransmitter compounds during embryogenesis and during the perinatal period are not contradictory but that they are aimed towards achieving the same objectives. During embryogenesis, there is a requirement for a large increase in cell number; thus, the transmitter compounds are involved in controlling this massive increase in the population of cells. On the other hand, at later stages of development cells are normally generated in excess of their final requirement. Thus, at these stages of development, monoamines appear to control the processes related to the reduction in cell number.

M. Weinstock: Why do you need concentrations of this magnitude to influence cell proliferation when in in vitro cell systems one requires much less (2 to 3 orders of magnitude) to stimulate/inhibit receptors and induce formations of second messengers or open channels for ions?

A.J. Patel: Yes, you are right that in our in vitro studies, although the influence on cell proliferation in dose-dependent, half-maximal effects are obtained at higher concentrations than those necessary in in vivo cell replication studies and in the therapeutic dose-range in man. This also worries us considerably. However, I would like to emphasize that the requirement of high concentrations of neurotropic drugs is by no means a rare occurrence in our in vitro experiments. For example: (a) a significant release of [^{14}C]-dopamine in rat striatal synaptosomes cannot be effected by 5-hydroxytryptamine at concentrations of less than 10^{-4} M; (b) similarly, dopamine receptor-mediated half-maximal inhibition of [^{14}C]dopamine synthesis from [^{14}C]tyrosine is obtained at about 1.3×10^{-6} M haloperidol, 3.3×10^{-5} chlorpromazine or 4.0×10^{-4} M thioridazine; (c) about 10^{-4} M norepinephrine or 10^{-2} M carbamylcholine is needed to enhance the incorporation of inorganic [^{32}P]phosphate into phosphatidic acid and phosphatidylinositol through the stimulation of α_1-adrenergic and muscarinic receptors in in vitro preparations of the cerebral cortex; (d) in non-neural systems, comparatively high concentrations of haloperidol (IC$_{50}$, 10^{-5} M) and chlorpromazine (IC$_{50}$, 1.30×10^{-5} M) are needed to inhibit [^{3}H]thymidine incorporation into cultured human phytohaemagglutinin–stimulated T-lymphocytes (for references, see Barochovsky and Patel, 1982).

J. Lauder: I have one comment and one question. The comment is that perhaps you should also consider the possibility that differences in the amount of binding proteins or of transmitter compounds in serum could be responsible, in part, for the differential effects of drugs and doses required in vivo and in vitro. Now the question is: I would like to know your thoughts on the role of neurotransmitters in the control of cell proliferation, i.e. whether this is related to innervation or to those substances coming from the circulation and acting as diffuse modulators, or both these processes?

A.J. Patel: The short answer is that both the innervation and the diffuse modulation appear to be involved in the regulation of brain cell proliferation. However, the modulating compounds do not need to come from the blood circulation. Much evidence in recent years indicates that a number of compounds released at nerve endings also act as diffuse modulators in the brain. Furthermore, our results are consistent with an influence of monoamines and drugs affecting monoamine neurotransmitter systems on brain cell replication, although, as I am sure you will be the first to agree, the precise mechanisms of their actions remain to be determined. It is also possible that the 'classical pharmacological (i.e. high-affinity–low-capacity)' receptors may not be involved in cell proliferation. At present this issue is in flux, and much work is needed to clarify these important points.

Reference
Barochovsky, O. and Patel, A.J. (1982) Effect of central nervous system acting drugs on brain replication in vitro. *Neurochem. Res.*, 7: 1059–1074.

G.J. Boer, M.G.P. Feenstra, M. Mirmiran, D.F. Swaab and F. Van Haaren
Progress in Brain Research, Vol. 73
© 1988 Elsevier Science Publishers B.V. (Biomedical Division)

CHAPTER 26

Reorganization of noradrenergic neuronal systems following neonatal chemical and surgical injury

Richard M. Kostrzewa

Department of Pharmacology, Quillen-Dishner College of Medicine, East Tennessee State University, Johnson City, TN 37614, USA

Introduction

The topic neuroteratology of monoaminergic neurons represents an ever-expanding area of research. In recent decades many studies have focused on the noradrenergic system.

The purpose of the present review is (a) to relate the actions of the major toxins used to study development of monoaminergic neurons, (b) to compare the principal agents, and discuss the major advantages and disadvantages of each, in order that a reader may understand the rationale for selecting one agent over another in any particular study, (c) to summarize results of studies which have been conducted with the variety of chemical agents and by surgical means, and (d) to reconstruct some of the principles of development of monoaminergic neurons that have been garnered with the variety of chemical tools. The principal neuroteratogens will be discussed separately in the approximate order of their discovery, and related agents will be compared when appropriate.

Synthetic catecholamine-neuroteratogens

A major breakthrough in the neuroteratology of aminergic neuronal systems came when Tranzer and Thoenen (1967) were searching for tri-hydroxyphenethylamines which would be visible in sympathetic neurons at the ultrastructural level.

They discovered that the norepinephrine (NE) isomer, 6-hydroxydopamine (6-OHDA), produced an actual destruction of peripheral sympathetic neurons. Analogues of these agents have been discovered, including the substance 6-hydroxydopa (6-OHDOPA), which crosses the blood-brain barrier and is metabolically converted to 6-OHDA. Several other substances, unrelated chemically to 6-OHDA, most notably guanethidine and N-(2-chloroethyl)-N-ethyl-bromobenzylamine (DSP-4), produce a similar destructive action on noradrenergic neurons.

6-Hydroxydopamine

The in vivo administration of 6-OHDA produces reversible loss of a large portion of the post-ganglionic sympathetic (noradrenergic) nerve terminals, a procedure that has been termed a 'chemical sympathectomy' (Thoenen and Tranzer, 1968). Because of its polar nature, entry of 6-OHDA into the adult CNS is prevented by the blood-brain barrier. However, by administering 6-OHDA directly into one of the ventricles (intracerebroventricular route, i.c.v.) (Bloom et al., 1969; Uretsky and Iversen, 1969) or one of the cisternae (intracisternal route, i.c.) (Breese and Traylor, 1970), or into the parenchyma per se (Ungerstedt, 1968), destruction of central noradrenergic and dopaminergic neurons is attained. In contrast to the regeneration of sympathetic noradrenergic fibers which is seen in the peripheral nervous system, little regeneration of catecholamine (CA)-containing fibers is found in the CNS after 6-OHDA treatment of adult animals.

Actions of 6-OHDA in the peripheral nervous system. When injected s.c. or i.p. in neonatal mice or rats, the action of 6-OHDA extends to sympathetic para- and prevertebral ganglion cells, resulting in their extensive destruction and marked reduction in size of the ganglion. As a consequence, sympathetic innervation of peripheral tissues is permanently reduced and adrenal hypertrophy occurs (Angeletti and Levi-Montalcini, 1970; Angeletti, 1971). Electron microscopic observation of ganglia demonstrates that surviving ganglion cells have a normal appearance (Jaim-Etcheverry and Zieher, 1971). Peripheral tissues display different degrees of sympathetic input in adulthood after the neonatal 6-OHDA treatment. The vas deferens has a normal complement of sympathetic fibers, while the heart has about half of the normal sympathetic innervation, with the spleen having only 10% of the control number of sympathetic fibers (Jaim-Etcheverry and Zieher, 1971; Lew and Quay, 1971; Clark et al., 1972; Sachs and Jonsson, 1972b; Jacobowitz, 1975).

Ganglionic cell death is thought to occur in the following way. The sympathetically innervated organs are believed to synthesize NGF, which is then taken up by sympathetic nerve terminals and transported to the sympathetic ganglion cell body. In the nucleus NGF exerts a trophic action. When 6-OHDA destroys the sympathetic nerve endings and/or axonal segments, NGF cannot be transported to the cell body, which requires this protein for survival. Lacking the protein, the cell dies. Convincingly, exogenous administration of NGF to 6-OHDA-treated neonatal rats increases survival of sympathetic ganglion cells (Aloe et al., 1975; Levi-Montalcini et al., 1975). The same protection from death after neonatal surgical axotomy is afforded to sympathetic ganglion cells by the NGF (Hendry, 1975).

Actions of 6-OHDA in the CNS. Breese and Traylor (1972) published the first study on neuroteratological actions of 6-OHDA on central CA-containing neurons. Following 6-OHDA (100 µg), administered i.c. to rat pups 7 days after birth, whole brain NE and dopamine (DA), as well as tyrosine hydroxylase (T-OH) activity were reduced within 3 h. At 3–4 months of age, rat brain NE, DA and T-OH were still reduced by 80%, 90% and 98%, respectively. Animals treated with 150 µg of 6-OHDA at 14 days after birth had similar alterations. These findings demonstrated that the development of both noradrenergic and dopaminergic neurons in the brain would be impaired when 6-OHDA was administered during ontogeny.

Other reports at about the same time showed that central noradrenergic neurons are far more sensitive to 6-OHDA action than dopaminergic neurons (Lytle et al., 1972; Sachs and Jonsson, 1972b). A 50 µg i.c. dose of 6-OHDA reduces whole brain NE content by about 90%, but alters DA by only 40%. This resistance to 6-OHDA damage is exhibited by both nigrostriatal (Sachs and Jonsson, 1972b) and mesolimbic (Schmidt and Bhatnagar, 1979a) dopaminergic systems. It has also been demonstrated that CA-containing neurons are most sensitive to 6-OHDA action at earlier stages of ontogeny (ie. treatment at birth vs. 12 d vs. 24 d after birth) (Lytle et al., 1972).

By administering divided low doses of 6-OHDA (15 and 25 µg i.c., respectively, at 5 and 7 d after birth), whole brain NE could be more selectively reduced than DA (54% for NE vs. 28% for DA). Also by pretreatment with desmethylimipramine (20 mg/kg i.p., 1 h), whole brain DA could be selectively depleted by 90%, while NE content was unaltered. When brain regions were analysed separately, NE levels were still consistently reduced, although the brain stem appeared to be the least sensitive region to 6-OHDA (Smith et al., 1973).

Shortly before the appearance of these reports on the CNS effects of 6-OHDA, the noradrenergic neuronal systems in the brain had been exten-

PROJECTIONS OF THE NUCLEUS LOCUS COERULEUS

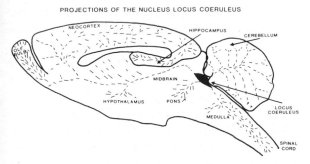

Fig. 1 Schematic illustration of the noradrenergic fiber distribution from the nucleus locus coeruleus. Virtually all of the dorsal aspect of the brain is supplied by fibers from the locus coeruleus. The neocortex, hippocampus olfactory bulbs, brain stem, cerebellum and spinal cord all receive inputs from the locus coeruleus. A small portion of noradrenergic innervation of the hypothalamus is derived from the coeruleus.

sively mapped (Ungerstedt, 1971b). Illustrated in Fig. 1 is a schematic representation of the fiber distribution from the nucleus locus coeruleus – the central noradrenergic system that is most sensitive to the actions of neurotoxins.

It is now known that neonatal i.c. or i.c.v. 6-OHDA in low doses (10–50 μg) typically produces a permanent destruction of the majority of noradrenergic fibers innervating the neocortex and hippocampus. At this dosage level, 6-OHDA also initially destroys noradrenergic fibers in the hindbrain, but a proliferative growth of noradrenergic fibers ensues in this brain region, resulting in a permanent hyperinnervation of the brain stem and cerebellum (Jaim-Etcheverry and Zieher, 1975; Zieher and Jaim-Etcheverry, 1979; Schmidt and Bhatnagar, 1980; Schmidt et al., 1980; Pappas et al., 1976). At higher doses of i.c. or i.c.v. 6-OHDA, a marked proliferation of noradrenergic fibers in the hindbrain does not occur. Noradrenergic innervation of brain stem of adult rats is little changed from control, while that of the cerebellum is reduced. While noradrenergic neurons seem to be most sensitive to 6-OHDA in younger animals, it is also notable that the noradrenergic fiber proliferation in hindbrain is greater in younger animals (Schmidt et al., 1980).

When neonatal dopaminergic fibers are de-

stroyed by high i.c. or i.c.v. doses of 6-OHDA, ingestive behavior is not impaired (Stachowiak et al., 1984) as is found in adult lesioned rats (Ungerstedt, 1971a). However, as adults, these animals are particularly sensitive to dopaminergic agonists which produce a variety of stereotyped activities, including self-biting and self-mutilation behaviors (Breese et al., 1984). While development of striatal dopaminergic fiber innervation is permanently impaired by neonatal 6-OHDA, elevated levels of serotonin (5-hydoxytryptamine, 5-HT) are found in the rostral striatum (Breese et al., 1984; Stachowiak et al., 1984), which represents a serotoninergic hyperinnervation of this region (Berger et al., 1985; Snyder et al., 1986). Therefore, it can be seen that neonatal intracerebral 6-OHDA produces an altered developmental pattern for the three major monoaminergic neuronal systems in the brain.

In mature animals, peripherally administered 6-OHDA is unable to gain entry to the CNS because of the presence of a blood-brain barrier (Stone et al., 1963; Laverty et al., 1965). In perinatal rodents, however, this barrier is incompletely developed, and central monoaminergic neurons are affected by peripheral doses of 6-OHDA. Neonatal treatment of mice or rats with 6-OHDA by an i.p. or s.c. route produces actions on central catecholaminergic neurons which are quite similar to those produced after i.c. or i.c.v. administration of 6-OHDA (Uretsky and Iversen, 1969; Bloom et al., 1969; Breese and Traylor, 1970). Acutely, after peripheral 6-OHDA, nerve fibers in any portion of the brain will be destroyed if sufficiently high amounts of the neurotoxin are accumulated (Brus, 1973). Noradrenergic nerve terminals are far more susceptible to 6-OHDA destruction than are the axonal segments of the neuron. Cell bodies are most resistant to damage.

The earliest reports on peripheral neonatal 6-OHDA treatment contain a cautionary note. Should whole brain be assessed for noradrenergic neuronal alteration by assaying for NE, rather than on a regional basis, then reduced NE in the forebrain may be masked by elevated NE in the hindbrain. Total NE content may be little altered (Jaim-Etcheverry and Zieher, 1971; Clark et al., 1972; Jacks et al., 1972) and one may be tempted to conclude that central noradrenergic neurons are unaltered by neonatal 6-OHDA.

When the brain is assayed regionally, it is evident that noradrenergic input to the forebrain is markedly impaired when 6-OHDA neonatally treated rats are studied after attainment of maturity. In the forebrain NE content is reduced in a dose-dependent manner (Clark et al., 1972; Jacks et al., 1972; Pappas and Sobrian, 1972; Sachs and Jonsson, 1972b; Singh and De-Champlain, 1972; Taylor et al., 1972) and the reduction of NE content is associated with a decrease in [^{3}H]NE uptake by homogenates of cortex (Sachs and Jonsson, 1972b; Jonsson et al., 1974), and an observed reduction in the numbers of NE-containing fibers in the forebrain structures (Jonsson et al., 1974). Impaired development of noradrenergic innervation to the spinal cord apparently reflects those same alterations, as in the forebrain after 6-OHDA (Clark et al., 1972; Sachs and Jonsson, 1972b; Taylor et al., 1972).

In contrast to the alterations observed in the above distal targets, enhanced development and hyperinnervation of the brain stem ensues after neonatal 6-OHDA. Brain stem concentration of NE is typically elevated (Clark et al., 1972; Jacks et al., 1972; Pappas and Sobrian, 1972; Sachs and Jonsson, 1972b; Singh and DeChamplain, 1972; Taylor et al., 1972). Initially, it was thought that elevated brain stem NE levels reflected retrograde accumulation within the noradrenergic axons coursing through this brain region, as occurred in adult brain after 6-OHDA (Ungerstedt, 1971b). However, Jonsson et al. (1974) demonstrated that elevated brain stem NE levels are due in part to an accumulation of NE in collateral nerve fibers, but are also correlated with an increase in the V_{max} for in vitro [^{3}H]NE uptake by homogenates of the pons-medulla portion of the brain stem. This indicated an actual increase in the number of uptake sites for NE, and is suggestive of an increase in the numbers of nor-

adrenergic fibers innervating this brain region. Visualizaton of NE-containing fibers, by histofluorescence microscopy, demonstrated the noradrenergic hyperinnervation of brain stem. More recent studies have extended these early findings (Schmidt and Bhatnagar, 1979d).

Alterations of noradrenergic input to the cerebellum, following neonatal 6-OHDA, initially reflected an impairment of development, as evidenced by reduced NE content of this region when treated animals were studied as adults (Clark et al., 1972; Taylor et al., 1972), and a reduced uptake of [^{3}H]NE by homogenates of cerebellum (Jonsson et al., 1974).

Selectivity of neonatal peripheral 6-OHDA-treatment for noradrenergic neurons was indicated by the lack of this treatment on development of DA (Brus, 1973; Sachs and Jonsson, 1972b), acetylcholine, GABA, and a host of amino acids (Jacks et al., 1972), 5-HT content or [^{3}H]5-HT uptake by homogenates of brain regions (Sachs and Jonsson, 1972b).

These earliest reports on the actions of 6-OHDA on ontogeny of noradrenergic neurons established that this treatment would result in a permanent noradrenergic hypoinnervation of forebrain regions and a hyperinnervation of the brain stem. Other neuronal types were little affected by the 6-OHDA.

6-Hydroxydopa

One of the disadvantages of 6-OHDA as an experimental neurotoxin is that it is unable to efficiently cross the blood-brain barrier. This barrier appears to develop in rats at about 9 days after birth (Sachs, 1973), but is 'leaky' with high doses of 6-OHDA (Sachs and Jonsson, 1973). Therefore, in order to study the ontogenic effects of 6-OHDA at different times in development, one must consider changes in the neuronal responsiveness to 6-OHDA, as well as changes in the blood-barrier to 6-OHDA. A neurotoxin which overcomes this limitation is 6-hydroxydopa (6-OHDOPA).

6-OHDOPA effectively crosses the blood-brain barrier and is metabolically converted to 6-OHDA by a decarboxylase enzyme (Ong et al., 1969; Berkowitz et al., 1970; Corrodi et al., 1971; Jacobowitz and Kostrzewa, 1971). In adults this substance produces a destruction of noradrenergic neurons in the peripheral and central nervous system, while leaving central dopaminergic neurons relatively intact. In time, peripheral noradrenergic neurons regenerate, so that only central noradrenergic neurons are permanently altered (Jacobowitz and Kostrzewa, 1971; Kostrzewa and Jacobowitz, 1972, 1973; Sachs and Jonsson, 1972a,c).

In developmental studies it has been shown that prenatal development of noradrenergic neurons can be altered by administering 6-OHDOPA to pregnant rats (Jaim-Etcheverry and Zieher, 1975; Zieher and Jaim-Etcheverry, 1975 a,b) and mice (Kostrzewa et al., 1978), since this agent is able to cross the placenta. Development of noradrenergic neurons into the telencephalon is altered by treatment with 6-OHDOPA at 16 or 17 days from conception (C16, C17), in the brain stem by 6-OHDOPA at C14 to C17, and in the cerebellum by 6-OHDOPA at C13 to C16. The perinatal actions of 6-OHDOPA are analogous to those of 6-OHDA: telencephalic noradrenergic innervation is reduced, while brain stem noradrenergic input is elevated (Sachs and Jonsson, 1972a; Zieher and Jaim-Etcheverry, 1973, 1975a,b; Kostrzewa and Harper, 1974; Kostrzewa, 1975; Kostrzewa and Garey, 1976).

A disadvantage of 6-OHDOPA is that only a moderate degree of neuronal destruction is produced, and higher doses of 6-OHDOPA cannot be used because of increased lethality (Corrodi et al., 1971). The central destructive action of 6-OHDOPA can be enhanced with a peripherally acting dopa decarboxylase inhibitor, thereby allowing a greater number of intact molecules to enter the brain (Kostrzewa and Jacobowitz, 1973). However, the enhancement of potency is not dramatic.

Despite these limitations, 6-OHDOPA is of immense value in studying the ontogeny of central noradrenergic neurons. The ability to penetrate the blood-brain barrier makes 6-OHDOPA a valuable chemical tool for examining nerve regeneration and sprouting at any stage of pre- or postnatal development.

DSP-4

DSP-4 (N-(2-chloroethyl)-N-ethyl-2-bromobenzylamine), a strong alkylating agent similar in structure to bretylium, is a relatively selective noradrenergic neuronal neurotoxin which is able to cross the blood-brain barrier. Therefore, both central and peripheral noradrenergic neurons are damaged by this agent, as evidenced by reduced NE content, reduced [^{3}H]NE uptake and reduced dopamine-β-hydroxylase (DBH) activity in the different tissues studied (Ross et al., 1973; Ross, 1976; Ross and Renyi, 1976).

When administered to developing rats, DSP-4 produces effects on central noradrenergic neurons that are similar to those produced by 6-OHDOPA. Noradrenergic fibers in the peripheral nervous system recover from damage, while, in the CNS, telencephalic and spinal cord regions remain hypoinnervated, and brain stem regions become hyperinnervated by noradrenergic fibers (Jaim-Etcheverry and Zieher, 1980; Jonsson et al., 1982). Selectivity of DSP-4 for noradrenergic neurons is indicated by its lack of effect on brain levels of DA, epinephrine, acetylcholine, GABA, glycine, glutamic acid and aspartic acid (Ross, 1976; Dudley et al., 1981; Jonsson et al., 1982; Dooley et al., 1983). Levels of 5-HT are altered only slightly (Ross, 1976; Jonsson et al., 1982).

Guanethidine

At about the same time that the actions of 6-OHDA on neonatal animals were described, it was found that guanethidine, a sympathetic neuronal blocking agent, also produced a destructive lesion in immature sympathetic ganglion cells (Burnstock et al., 1971; Eränkö and Eränkö, 1971; Angeletti and Levi-Montalcini, 1972). The actions of this agent have been well characterized and have been shown to be limited to noradrenergic fibers outside the CNS (Johnson and Hunter, 1979). The mechanism of destruction is known to involve lymphocytic infiltration of the ganglion, associated with immune processes (Manning et al., 1982, 1983). Thus, the mechanism of action is distinct from that of 6-OHDA.

Hypo- or hyperinnervation of cerebellum as a result of noradrenergic neuroteratology

It was initially concluded that neonatal 6-OHDA would produce a permanent noradrenergic hypoinnervation of the cerebellum (Clark et al., 1972; Taylor et al., 1972; Jonsson et al., 1974). However, it was later found that when newborn rats were treated with a single dose of 6-OHDA or 6-OHDOPA, noradrenergic hyperinnervation developed (Jaim-Etcheverry and Zieher, 1975; Kostrzewa, 1975; Kostrzewa and Harper, 1975; Zieher and Jaim-Etcheverry, 1975a; Kostrzewa and Garey, 1976, 1977). When animals received a single dose of 6-OHDA or 6-OHDOPA at 3 days of age or later, then either no change in innervation or a permanent noradrenergic hypoinnervation of the cerebellum ensued (Fig. 2), and the reduced NE content was associated with a reduction in the number of uptake sites for NE. When multiple injections of neurotoxin were given over several days from birth, then the hyperinnervation of the cerebellum became progressively diminished (Kostrzewa, 1975; Kostrzewa and Garey, 1976). This effect accounted for the early reports that 6-OHDA produced hypoinnervation of the cerebellum by noradrenergic neurons.

It is now known that the s.c. and i.p. treatment of neonates with 6-OHDA or 6-OHDOPA in the first 2 days after birth results in noradrenergic hypoinnervation of forebrain regions and hyperinnervation of both brain stem and cerebellum. Treatment with 6-OHDOPA or 6-OHDA from 3 to 9 days after birth results in noradrenergic hyperinnervation of brain stem and hypoinnervation of cerebellum. Treatment at a later time results in

hypoinnervation of both regions (Kostrzewa and Harper, 1974; Jaim-Etcheverry and Zieher, 1975; Kostrzewa and Garey, 1977; Schmidt and Bhatnagar, 1979b). Following i.c. 6-OHDA, development of cerebellar noradrenergic hyperinnervation occurs with treatment up to 5 or 7 days after birth (Schmidt et al., 1980; Schmidt and Bhatnagar, 1980). Similar kinds of age-related responses have also been shown now for DSP-4 (Jonsson et al., 1982).

It is noteworthy that the collateral fiber sprouting is greater in the brain stem than cerebellum after 6-OHDA or 6-OHDOPA. However, following neonatal DSP-4 treatment the collateral sprouting is greater in the cerebellum than brain stem (Jaim-Etcheverry and Zieher, 1980). The reason for this difference is unknown.

It has been suggested that the proliferative sprouting into cerebellum can occur only if noradrenergic fibers are injured prior to a time of critical developmental growth into the cerebellum (Schmidt et al., 1980). However, since noradrenergic fibers are able to sprout into and hyperinnervate the cerebellum after surgical lesion of the

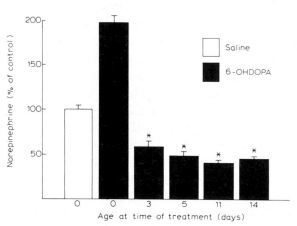

Fig. 2 Percentage alterations in cerebellar norepinephrine (NE) concentrations by neonatal 6-OHDOPA treatment (60 μg/g i.p.) of the rat at different postnatal ages. Day of birth is indicated by age '0'. All animals were killed at 5 weeks of age. Each bar is the mean $\pm$ S.E.M. of 4–7 rats. Control level of NE was 0.19 $\pm$ 0.01 μg/g. * Significance of difference in NE level between control and 6-OHDOPA-treated group, $P < 0.005$. (From Kostrzewa and Garey, 1977).

dorsal bundle at one week after birth (Jonsson and Sachs, 1982), it appears that the capacity of proliferative noradrenergic fiber growth in the cerebellum is retained for a long time. Therefore, the expression of that capacity is a determinant that is governed within the noradrenergic cell per se and/or the cerebellum or other target tissues.

Responsiveness of noradrenergic neurons to injury

In the peripheral nervous system axonal segments of noradrenergic neurons typically regenerate after injury, and reinnervate peripheral organs and tissues. This response occurs whether injury is produced in adult or in developing animals (see previous discussion).

In the central nervous system noradrenergic neurons derived from the locus coeruleus seem to be particularly susceptible to neurotoxins, while those noradrenergic neurons with axons coursing through the ventral bundle seem to be resistant to injury (Levitt and Moore, 1980; Versteeg et al., 1980). Uptake and storage processes in each group of neurons are similar, and so, apparently, are intraneuronal synthetic and degradative enzymes for catecholamines. Since neurotoxin injury is related to attainment of critical intraneuronal concentrations of the substance, it would appear that fibers of the ventral bundle accumulate less neurotoxin. It is also hypothesized that distribution of the neurotoxin in the brain by the circulation could account for part of this difference, with less neurotoxin being transported to the more ventral portions of the brain. Another possible factor is that the denser noradrenergic terminal plexus in the ventral aspects of the brain may serve as a protective mechanism. Each of the many nerve terminals in this portion of the brain may compete for the limited amount of neurotoxin, with the various terminals accumulating amounts that are sub-threshold for producing destruction. Higher intraneuronal NE concentrations would also protect against 6-OHDA damage (Sachs et al., 1975), as would a greater level of monoamine oxidase (MAO).

Injury to locus coeruleus noradrenergic neurons early in development seems to have a 'priming' influence. The response to injury is a collateral sprouting and hyperinnervation of hindbrain regions. This effect is not normally produced when injury is severe, as evidenced by lack of the response following i.c. or i.c.v. injection of high doses of 6-OHDA (Schmidt et al., 1980). However, even in this instance there appears to be a priming effect, since additional injury with 6-OHDOPA, several days after 6-OHDA, restores the sprouting response in the brain stem (Zieher and Jaim-Etcheverry, 1979). Thus, additional injury may unmask the priming effect on developing noradrenergic neurons, and stimulate a regenerative process. The mechanisms associated with this effect still need to be explored.

Functional nature of reorganized catecholamine neurons

The status of noradrenergic neurons in brain regions that are either hypo- or hyperinnervated after neonatal neurotoxin treatment was in question for a long time. Regenerated or sprouted neurons might not have established normal synaptic contact and could have represented nonfunctional neurons. Jonsson et al. (1974, 1979), by administering a T-OH inhibitor to adult rats prior to death, found that the turnover rate of NE was the same in neonatally 6-OHDA-treated and control groups, irrespective of whether a brain region was hypo- or hyperinnervated. At the same time β-adrenoceptor number was increased by 40–75% (Harden et al., 1977, 1979; Jonsson and Hallman, 1978; Sporn et al., 1976), and isoproterenol-stimulated cyclic AMP accumulation was enhanced by 40–65% in the hypoinnervated neocortex (Harden et al., 1977), while the converse alteration was found in the hyperinnervated cerebellum (Jonsson and Hallman, 1978; Harden et al., 1979). It has been further demonstrated by chronic (9 d) i.c.v. infusion of NE to the adult 6-OHDA-group that when endogenous neocortical NE content becomes elevated toward control

412

levels, β-adrenoceptor binding of this brain region decreases to control levels (Biswas and Jonsson, 1981).

This series of studies indicates that the noradrenergic neurons in both hypo- and hyperinnervated regions exhibit normal neurochemical synthetic/release patterns, and an interplay with the receptor field.

Collateral sprouting of noradrenergic fibers into hindbrain regions occurs whether the denervation of forebrain regions is produced in neonates by neurotoxin (Jonsson et al., 1974) or surgical means (Jonsson and Sachs, 1982). Elevated levels of NE, T-OH and DBH in brain stem and cerebellum after neonatal 6-OHDOPA/6-OHDA reflect two events: an intraneuronal increase in the amount of these substances and an actual increase in the number of noradrenergic nerve terminals (Jonsson et al., 1974; Kostrzewa and Garey, 1977; Schmidt and Bhatnagar, 1979c).

Jonsson et al. (1974) have hypothesized that noradrenergic neurons have a strict developmental program to express a defined number of nerve terminals, so that pruning of one axonal branch promotes the formation of collateral branches. This proposal is known as the 'pruning hypothesis'. In support of this hypothesis is the work with the antimitotic agent methylazoxymethanol, which markedly impairs development and size of the neocortex when given to fetal rats. However, the number of noradrenergic terminals which grow into and supply the neocortex is the same as in intact controls (Johnston and Coyle, 1979; Jonsson and Hallman, 1981). A similar situation prevails in mouse genetic mutants which are characterized by impaired development of brain regions, yet still have the same number of noradrenergic fibers as in the normally developing heterozygote control (Landis et al., 1975, 1978; Kostrzewa et al., 1982; Roffler-Tarlov et al., 1984; Kostrzewa and Harston, 1986; Felton et al., 1986). These observations suggest that neurons are 'programmed' to express a specific number of terminals, independent of the developmen-

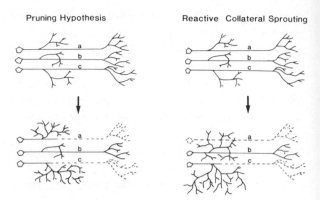

Pruning Hypothesis   Reactive Collateral Sprouting

Fig. 3 Contrast of the pruning hypothesis with reactive collateral fiber sprouting. According to the pruning hypothesis, damage of one of the fiber tracts (eg. dorsal noradrenergic bundle) in developing animals (stippled lines, lower left) results in hypoinnervation of regions normally supplied by fibers of this tract. As fiber growth is impeded in this tract, collateral sprouting of fibers nearer the cell body occurs, resulting in hyperinnervation of regions supplied by these fibers (lower left). Presumably, nerve cells are 'programmed' to grow a predetermined number of nerve terminals. The final state would represent one in which the injured neuron would have the same number of nerve terminals as for an intact neuron, except that the fibers and terminals would have different regional distributions (neurons a and c, left). It should be noted that intact neurons situated among injured neurons would not demonstrate collateral sprouting or an alteration in fiber distribution (neuron b, left). For reactive collateral sprouting it is postulated that injury to one of the fiber tracts in developing animals results in collateral sprouting of fibers near the cell body. It is proposed that both injured and uninjured neurons may sprout fibers, and that the final state may represent one in which the injured neuron has fewer, the same, or a greater number of fibers than for intact neurons. The figure on the right shows the complete degeneration of neuron a, and the loss of one of the tracts of neuron c. Illustrated is fiber sprouting of both the uninjured neuron b and the injured neuron c. The ultimate number of nerve fibers and terminals may be greater or less than that in the uninjured state.

tal characteristics of the target tissue. An illustration of the pruning hypothesis is given in Fig. 3.

While collateral fiber sprouting is an accepted neuronal response to neonatal damage of the dorsal bundle, not all findings support the contention that noradrenergic neurons are programmed to express a specific number of terminals. Prenatal treatment of rodents with 6-

OHDOPA on critical days has resulted in the apparent sprouting of noradrenergic fibers into brain stem or cerebellum in the absence of telencephalic alterations (Jaim-Etcheverry and Zieher, 1975; Zieher and Jaim-Etcheverry, 1975b; Kostrzewa et al., 1978). Also, following a high dose of 6-OHDA at birth, which permanently reduces telencephalic NE but suppresses the elevation of brain stem NE in the adult, 6-OHDOPA at 3 days after birth does not further alter telencephalic NE but induces an elevation of brain stem NE in the adult (Zieher and Jaim-Etcheverry, 1979). After neonatal 5,7-DHT there is not a good correlation between forebrain hypoinnervation and hindbrain hyperinnervation by noradrenergic fibers (Sachs and Jonsson, 1975). And finally, recovery of telencephalic NE from a dorsal bundle lesion did not modify the noradrenergic hyperinnervation of cerebellum (Klisans-Fuenmayor et al., 1986). Similar marked degrees of sprouting of the hindbrain noradrenergic fibers occur despite different telencephalic NE alterations induced by various doses of 6-OHDA or 6-OHDOPA (Kostrzewa and Harper, 1975).

The collateral sprouting in hindbrain is critically dependent on the stage of development of the noradrenergic system at the time of injury (Kostrzewa and Harper, 1975; Schmidt and Bhatnagar, 1979b; Schmidt et al., 1980; Jaim-Etcheverry and Zieher, 1975). Treatment with a neurotoxin even several days after birth does not result in collateral sprouting. Moreover, if injury is too great after neurotoxin treatment, collateral sprouting does not occur (Schmidt and Bhatnagar, 1980; Jaim-Etcheverry and Zieher, 1975a). Each of these conditions limits the applicability of the pruning hypothesis and promotes a reactive collateral sprouting hypothesis (see Fig. 3).

Additionally, based on histofluorescent observations, it has been assumed that numbers of locus coeruleus cells are unaltered after neonatal 6-OHDA treatment. However, studies with neonatal 6-OHDOPA indicate that lower doses do not destroy coeruleus cells (Kostrzewa, unpublished data), while higher doses do destroy coeruleus cells (Clark et al., 1979). In each of these three experimental paradigms the noradrenergic fiber sprouting in the brain stem and cerebellum is similar. Therefore, it would appear that when fewer cells are present, the numbers of fibers/terminals per cell increase.

The pruning hypothesis has been a valuable one, because of the foundation and direction it has provided for research on nerve regeneration and sprouting in general, and more specifically in regard to those same processes in noradrenergic neurons. It is acknowledged that this hypothesis may be valid for undamaged neurons. However, once perturbations of those neurons are introduced, then a variety of regeneration and sprouting phenomena may come into play, which are not specifically applicable to the pruning hypothesis. For reasons stated above, the following, more general hypothesis is suggested – that of reactive collateral sprouting. This hypothesis has been considered in the literature for a number of years. Implicit in this hypothesis is that a 'pruning' effect may occur, so that lesion of a long axon may result in collateral fiber sprouting. This is shown in Fig. 3 by the response of neuron c. No assumption is made about survival of cells in the nucleus, except that a response cannot be produced if a neuron is not present (neuron a). The possibility of a sprouting response by uninjured neurons remains, and this is shown by neuron b. According to this latter proposal target tissue may be stimulated, after injury to axonal segments of other neurons, to produce a nerve growth-promoting factor. The promotion of central noradrenergic fiber growth into implants or from implanted noradrenergic cells into CNS regions is a process that apparently is governed by the liberation of a nerve growth-promoting factor (Björklund et al., 1976; Björklund and Stenevi, 1971; Olson et al., 1980). The accelerated collateral fiber growth of injured neurons could be a signal for the onset of such a process. McBride et al. (1985) have concluded from their neonatal 6-OHDA studies that axon damage is not essential for collateral fiber growth. Study of the con-

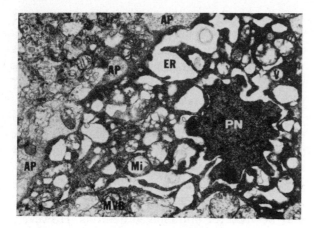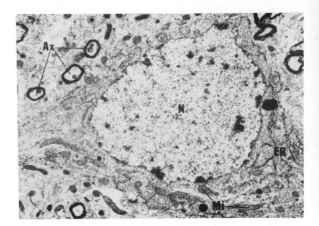

Fig. 4 (left) Electron micrograph illustrating a typical neuronal profile seen in the locus coeruleus 14 days after 6-OHDOPA (60 μg/g i.p. × 3, 48 h intervals from birth). Degenerative changes in this cell are typified by an extreme electron-opacity of the cellular matrix and a shrunken, pyknotic nucleus (PN). Extensive dilation of the endoplasmic reticulum cisternae (ER) is apparent, and swollen, fragmented mitochondria (Mi) are present. Multivesicular bodies (MVB), large vacuoles (V) and dissociated polyribosomes can be seen in the cytoplasm of the cell. Abnormally large astrocytic processes (AP) frequent the neuropil surrounding the cell. (right) Electron micrograph of a neuron in the nucleus tegmenti dorsalis taken from the same section as the tissue specimen in the left-hand micrograph. No abnormal ultrastructural changes are observed in this cell or in the adjacent neuropil. N, nucleus; Mi, mitochrondrion; ER, endoplasmic reticulum; Ax, myelinated axons. × 7130. (From Kostrzewa and Harper, 1974.)

ditions of collateral fiber growth could provide valuable clues to the factors that are associated with nerve regeneration in the CNS.

Destruction of locus coeruleus noradrenergic perikarya

Descarries and Saucier (1972), by means of the fluorescence technique and conventional histology, demonstrated that i.c.v. 6-OHDA (300 μg) destroyed approximately 85% of locus coeruleus cells in adult rats. This finding was confirmed by Lewis and Schon (1975), who used a lower dose of 6-OHDA (150 μg, i.c.v.) and followed the disappearance of acetylcholinesterase-containing cells in the nucleus. In developing animals the locus coeruleus perikarya appear to be unaffected by 6-OHDA (s.c.), as evidenced by lack of a change in histofluorescence morphology of the cell bodies (Jonsson et al., 1974; Sachs et al., 1974).

Kostrzewa and Harper (1974, 1975) found that neonatal 6-OHDOPA (i.p.) produced overt destruction of locus coeruleus cells at the ultrastructural level (Fig. 4). Nuclei became pyknotic, and axons emerging from the coeruleus underwent degenerative changes, as indicated by a Fink-Heimer stain. It was subsequently found that 6-OHDOPA (60 μg/g i.p. × 3, 48 h intervals from birth) produced degeneration of about 33% of the cells in the locus coeruleus. A regional cell loss was found, with virtually all cells in the rostral 40% of the nucleus remaining intact, and 50% of the cells in the remainder of the nucleus being destroyed (Clark et al., 1979).

A discrepancy between the 6-OHDA and 6-OHDOPA data still remains. Direct injection of 6-OHDA into the newborn rat locus coeruleus destroys almost 90% of histofluorescent cell bodies (Lanfumey et al., 1981), as might be expected from similar treatment effects in adults (Koda et al., 1978). With i.c. administration of high doses of 6-OHDA (80 or 100 μg) to neonatal rats, destruction of cells in the locus coeruleus has been reported (Sievers et al., 1980; Schmidt et al., 1980), with the major portion of cell loss occurring in the mid- and caudal regions of the nucleus (Sievers et al., 1980) – as was found after i.p. 6-OHDOPA. However, when observed only by histofluorescence microscopy, locus coeruleus cells have also been reported to have a normal appearance, and not show evidence of destruction after 6-OHDA ($\leq 100\ \mu$g i.c.) (Konkol et al., 1978). Given peripherally, 200 μg/g of 6-OHDA (100 μg/g s.c. $\times$ 2, 24 h intervals from birth) did not alter locus coeruleus cell number, and 400 μg/g (i.e., 200 μg/g $\times$ 2, 24 h) destroyed only 18% of cells in the nucleus, primarily those cells in the anterior pole (McBride et al., 1985).

These findings suggest that 6-OHDA and 6-OHDOPA have quite different neurotoxic potentials. Noradrenergic nerve terminal destruction is far greater after 6-OHDA than after an equimolar amount of 6-OHDOPA. However, noradrenergic cell bodies are seemingly more susceptible to 6-OHDOPA than to 6-OHDA destruction. The differences in destructive actions between 6-OHDOPA and 6-OHDA are not known, but are not considered to involve the decarboxylation step for conversion of 6-OHDOPA to 6-OHDA.

Similarity of neonatal 6-OHDOPA/6-OHDA effects to an ascending-tract surgical lesion

While surgical transection of the medial forebrain bundle did not produce any apparent sprouting of brain stem or cerebellar noradrenergic fibers (Iacovitti et al., 1981), knife cut of the dorsal bundle did produce collateral noradrenergic fiber sprouting in those hindbrain regions (Jonsson and Sachs, 1982; Klisans-Fuenmayor et al., 1986). Little regeneration of the transected ascending noradrenergic tract is seen (Fig. 5; Kostrzewa et al., 1988), so that the forebrain and hippocampus remain hypoinnervated by noradrenergic fibers following the neonatal lesion.

The reorganization of noradrenergic fiber distribution to the brain after neonatal transection of the dorsal bundle is analogous to that found after treatment of newborn rats or mice with CA neurotoxins. However, it is noted that changes in locus coeruleus cell survival are quite different. Iacovitti et al. (1981) reported that retrograde changes in locus coeruleus cells were unaltered after section of the medial forebrain bundle, a finding similar to that after 6-OHDA treatment (Jonsson et al., 1974; McBride et al., 1975). However, Kostrzewa et al. (1988) found that 17% of locus coeruleus cells were destroyed after midbrain lesions of the dorsal bundle. The cell loss is qualitatively similar to that reported after neonatal 6-OHDOPA, except that the axonal lesion preferentially destroys those cells in the midportion of the locus coeruleus (20–25% cell loss; Fig. 6), while 6-OHDOPA destroys cells in the caudal locus coeruleus (Clark et al., 1979).

One distinction between neonatal surgical and neurotoxin lesions is that the former procedure is associated with a greater proliferative growth of noradrenergic fibers into the cerebellum, while with 6-OHDOPA/6-OHDA a greater degree of noradrenergic hyperinnervation occurs in the brain stem. Another distinction between surgical and neurotoxin lesions is that 6-OHDA at 3 days or later, from birth, is not consistently associated with the development of noradrenergic hyperinnervation of the cerebellum (Jaim-Etcheverry and Zieher, 1975; Kostrzewa and Harper, 1975; Kostrzewa and Garey, 1977; Schmidt and Bhatnagar, 1979b; Schmidt et al., 1980), while surgical axonal lesions at 7 days are still associated with the latter event (Jonsson and Sachs, 1982). For unknown reasons, neurotoxins appear to eliminate the sprouting capacity.

Cerebellectomy in rat pups up to 9 days after birth, with consequent removal of noradrenergic tracts to this region, results in the development of noradrenergic hyperinnervation of the brain stem, with no changes occurring in the forebrain (Iacovitti et al., 1981). Cerebellectomy at 18 days after birth does not produce alterations in T-OH activity of the pons-medulla 30 days later. Thus, section of a relatively short noradrenergic tract

416

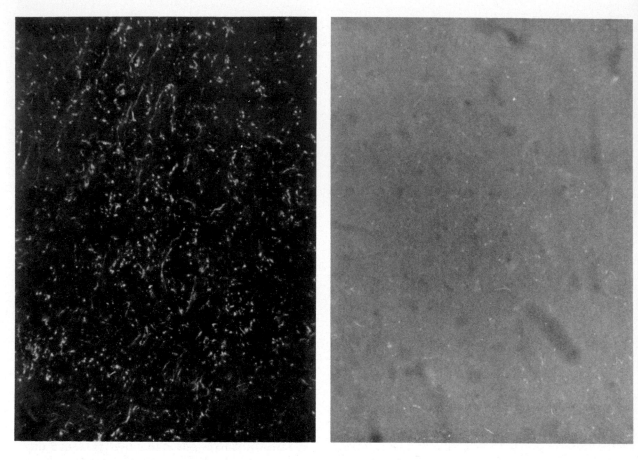

Fig. 5 Loss of axons in the dorsal bundle of adult rat following a neonatal midbrain lesion. An immunocytochemical procedure for dopamine-β-hydroxylase was employed on brain sections in both control (left) and lesioned rats. × 223. (From Kostrzewa et al., 1988.)

will still produce noradrenergic collateral fiber sprouting. While noradrenergic tracts to the spinal cord have not been removed surgically in neonatal rats, Jonsson and Sachs (1982) have shown that 6-OHDA removal of this tract in newborn rats results in elevations in NE content of the pons-medulla 8 days afterwards. This finding suggests that neonatal removal of descending long noradrenergic fiber tract will also result in collateral sprouting of noradrenergic fibers.

The above studies, primarily on surgical lesions, indicate that damage to one of several noradrenergic axonal tracts will promote collateral fiber sprouting. The major distinction between chemical and surgical lesioning is that the latter

procedure does not directly alter other segments of the noradrenergic system, and does not reduce the regenerative potential of noradrenergic neurons, at least not to the degree found with the neurotoxin. Surgical lesioning of the developing noradrenergic system in the brain represents an alternative approach to the study of the recovery of the noradrenergic system from damage.

Modulation of the actions of 6-OHDOPA/6-OHDA

The possible influence of other neuronal systems in modulating neuroteratological actions of 6-OHDOPA/6-OHDA was considered in a series

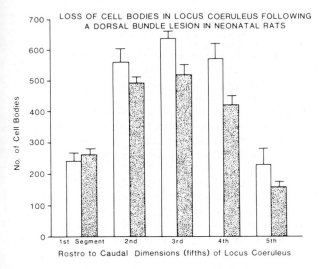

Fig. 6 Loss of locus coeruleus (LC) cells along the rostro-caudal axis following bilateral transection of the dorsal bundle in neonatal rats. A midbrain lesion was made in rat pups 3 days after birth, and animals were killed at 8–10 weeks. After counting the total number of locus coeruleus cells for each animal, and recording the numbers of cells along the rostro-caudal axis, the nucleus was divided into five segments, and the number of coeruleus cells in each segment was determined. Each bar represents the mean number of cells ± S.E.M. for each segment of both control (N = 4, open column and lesioned (N = 6, stippled column) animals. Cell counts in the 2nd to 4th segments were significantly different between control and lesioned groups (Student's 't' test, P < 0.05) (From Kostrzewa et al., 1987.)

of studies that were begun about 10 years ago. When morphine was co-administered with 6-OHDOPA to rat pups at birth, the ensuing developmental response of noradrenergic hyperinnervation of brain stem and cerebellum was enhanced (Harston et al., 1980, 1982). This effect of morphine was mimicked by met- and leu-enkephalin, β-endorphin and D-ala²-met-enkephalinamide (Harston et al., 1981). Although the action of morphine was not antagonized by naloxone in newborn rats, it was later found that the opioid action was receptor-mediated in rats 3 days after birth (Kostrzewa and Klisans-Fuenmayor, 1984). It has now been found that morphine enhances the neurotoxicity of 6-OHDOPA, by promoting a

destructive loss of locus coeruleus cells (Kostrzewa, unpublished data). Thus, a developmental change in the opioid system has an interactive role on the neuroteratological actions of neurotoxins.

Locus coeruleus perikarya are known to be innervated by enkephalin-containing fibers (Sar et al., 1978) and substance P-containing fibers (Ljungdahl et al., 1978). Opioids are associated with analgesic actions, while substance P systems are associated with algesic effects. Opioids exert an inhibitory action on locus coeruleus cell firing (see North, 1979), while substance P exerts an excitatory action (Guyenet and Aghajanian, 1977). Jonsson and Hallman (1982a,b,c) have demonstrated that the modulatory actions of substance P are distinctly opposite to those of opioids. Substance P appears to have a neuroprotective action, since noradrenergic denervation of forebrain regions after 6-OHDA is not as severe after substance P co-treatment. At the same time, the degree of collateral sprouting of noradrenergic fibers and hyperinnervation of hindbrain is reduced.

The mechanisms associated with the neuromodulatory actions of opioids and substance P have not been resolved. Modification of the neurodegenerative effects of 6-OHDA by these substances is not necessarily a critical component, since these agents are effective when given several hours after 6-OHDA. The degenerative effects of 6-OHDA are complete within minutes to less than 2 h, and neither of the agents necessarily alters the initial neurodegenerative effects in neonates (Jonsson and Hallman, 1982b). Nevertheless, morphine does promote locus coeruleus cell death when given concurrently with 6-OHDOPA (Kostrzewa, unpublished data). Based on the finding that substance P enhances noradrenergic fiber sprouting in hindbrain after surgical transection of the dorsal bundle, it has been hypothesized that substance P has a growth-stimulatory effect on damaged noradrenergic fibers, at least in brain regions which are proximal to the locus coeruleus (Jonsson and Hallman, 1983). This effect could be related to the excitatory action of substance P on locus coeruleus cells, since nicotine also produces excitation and a neuroteratological action similar to that of substance P (Jonsson and Hallman, 1980).

More studies with these and other neurochemical agents are required to obtain a clearer understanding of the regulation of degenerative and regenerative processes of developing neurons.

Summary

A variety of chemical agents and surgical procedures have dramatic influences on the ontogenetic development of noradrenergic neurons. Because of space limitations, in-depth descriptions of each of the neurotoxins could not be given, and the reader is referred to review articles which present a different perspective on uses of the agents (Breese, 1975; Jonsson, 1980; Kostrzewa, 1988; Kostrzewa and Jacobowitz, 1974; Thoenen and Tranzer, 1973).

The studies involving an intervention in monoaminergic neuronal development have provided the field of neuroscience with an abundance of information on neuronal cell/fiber susceptibility to destruction, neuronal fiber regeneration, collateral fiber sprouting, neuroteratological responses to injury, regional differences in blood-brain barrier formation, pre- and post-synaptic interactive events, and a host of other aspects. These data have served to generate new hypotheses on neuronal function, neuronal modulation and neuronal regeneration/sprouting. This chapter is an attempt to put the different studies and findings into perspective, in order to aid the development of novel experiments that will further probe neuronal mechanisms and lead to new vistas in our understanding of neuronal function.

Acknowledgement

The author wishes to thank Ms. Betty Hughes for typing the manuscript.

References

Aloe, L., Mugnaini, E. and Levi-Montalcini, R. (1975) Light and electron microscope studies on the excessive growth of sympathetic ganglia in rats injected with 6-OHDA and NGF. *Arch. Ital. Biol.*, 113: 326–353.

Angeletti, P. U. (1971) Chemical sympathectomy in newborn animals. *Neuropharmacology*, 10: 55–59.

Angeletti, P. U. and Levi-Montalcini, R. (1970) Sympathetic nerve cell destruction in newborn mammals by 6-hydroxydopamine. *Proc. Natl. Acad. Sci. USA*, 65: 114–121.

Angeletti, P. U. and Levi-Montalcini, R. (1972) Growth inhibition of sympathetic cells by some adrenergic blocking drugs. *Proc. Natl. Acad. Sci. USA*, 69: 86–88.

Berger, T. W., Kaul, S., Stricker, E. M. and Zigmond, M. J. (1985) Hyperinnervation of the striatum by dorsal raphe afferents after dopamine-depleting brain lesions in neonatal rats. *Brain Res.*, 336: 354–358.

Berkowitz, B. A., Spector, S., Brossi, A., Focella, A. and Teitel, S. (1970) Preparation and biological properties of (−) and (+)-6-hydroxydopa. *Experientia (Basel)*, 26: 982–983.

Biswas, B. and Jonsson, G. (1981) Reversal of noradrenaline denervation-induced increase of β-adrenoreceptor binding in rat neocortex by noradrenaline infusion. *Eur. J. Pharmacol.*, 69: 341–346.

Björklund, A. and Stenevi, A. (1971) Growth of central catecholamine neurons into smooth muscle grafts in the rat mesencephalon. *Brain Res.*, 31: 1–20.

Björklund, A., Stenevi, U. and Svendgaard, N.-A. (1976) Growth of transplanted monoaminergic neurons into the adult hippocampus along the perforant path. *Nature*, 262: 787–790.

Bloom, F. E., Algeri, S., Gropetti, A., Revuelta, A. and Costa, E. (1969) Lesions of central norepinephrine terminals with 6-OH-dopamine: Biochemistry and fine structure. *Science*, 166: 1284–1286.

Breese, G. R. (1975) Chemical and immunochemical lesions by specific neurotoxic substances and antisera. In L. L. Iversen, S. D. Iversen and S. H. Snyder (Eds.), *Handbook of Psychopharmacology*, Vol. 1, Plenum, New York, pp. 137–189.

Breese, G. R. and Traylor, T. D. (1970) Effect of 6-hydroxydopamine on brain norepinephrine and dopamine: evidence for selective destruction of catecholamine neurons. *J. Pharmacol. Exp. Ther.*, 174: 413–420.

Breese, G. R. and Traylor, T. D. (1972) Developmental characteristics of brain catecholamines and tyrosine hydroxylase in the rat: effects of 6-hydroxydopamine. *Br. J. Pharmacol.*, 44: 210–222.

Breese, G. R., Baumeister, A. A., McCown, T. J., Emerick, S. G., Frye, G. D., Crotty, K. and Mueller, R. A. (1984)

Behavioral differences between neonatal and adult 6-hydroxydopamine-treated rats to dopamine agonists: relevance to neurological symptoms in clinical syndromes with reduced brain dopamine. *J. Pharmacol. Exp. Ther.*, 231: 343–354.

Brus, R. (1973) Effect of 6-hydroxydopamine on the level of the catecholamines in the brain of developing rats. *Arch. Int. Pharmacodyn. Ther.*, 201: 71–76.

Burnstock, G., Doyle, A.E., Gannon, B.J., Gerkens, J.F., Iwayama, T. and Mashford, M.L. (1971) Prolonged hypotension and ultrastructural changes in sympathetic neurons following guanacline treatment. *Eur. J. Pharmacol.*, 13: 175–187.

Clark, D.W.J., Laverty, R. and Phelan, E.L. (1972) Long-lasting peripheral and central effects of 6-hydroxydopamine in rats. *Br. J. Pharmacol.*, 44: 233–243.

Clark, M.B., King, J.C. and Kostrzewa, R.M. (1979) Loss of nerve cell bodies in caudal locus coeruleus following treatment of neonates with 6-hydroxydopa. *Neurosci. Lett.*, 13: 331–336.

Corrodi, H., Clark, W.G. and Masuoka, D.I. (1971) The synthesis and effects of DL-6-hydroxydopa. In T. Malmfors and H. Thoenen (Eds.), *6-Hydroxydopamine and Catecholamine Neurons*, North-Holland, Amsterdam, pp. 187–192.

Descarries, L. and Saucier, G. (1972) Disappearance of the locus coeruleus in the rat after intraventricular 6-hydroxydopamine. *Brain Res.*, 37: 310–316.

Dooley, D.J., Bittiger, H., Hauser, K.L., Bischoff, S.F. and Waldmeier, P.C. (1983) Alteration of central alpha 2 and beta-adrenergic receptors in the rat after DSP-4, a selective noradrenergic neurotoxin. *Neuroscience*, 9: 889–898.

Dudley, M.W., Butcher, L.L., Kammerer, R.C. and Cho, A.K. (1981) The actions of xylamine on central noradrenergic neurons. *J. Pharmacol. Exp. Ther.*, 217: 834–840.

Eränkö, L. and Eränkö, O. (1971) Effect of guanethidine on nerve cells and small intensely fluorescent cells in sympathetic ganglia of newborn and adult rats. *Acta Pharmacol. Toxicol.*, 30: 403–416.

Felten, D.L., Felten, S.Y., Perry, K.W., Fuller, R.W., Nurnberger, J.I. and Ghetti, B. (1986) Noradrenergic innervation of the cerebellar cortex in normal and in Purkinje cell degeneration mutant mice: evidence for long term survival following loss of the two major cerebellar cortical neuronal populations. *Neuroscience*, 18: 783–793.

Guyenet, P.G. and Aghajanian, G.K. (1977) Excitation of neurons in the locus coeruleus by substance P and related peptides. *Brain Res.*, 136: 178–184.

Harden, T.K., Wolfe, B.B., Sporn, J.R., Poulos, B.K. and Molinoff, P.B. (1977) Effects of 6-hydroxydopamine on the development of the β-adrenergic receptor adenylate cyclase system in rat cerebral cortex. *J. Pharmacol. Exp. Ther.*, 203: 132–143.

Harden, T.K., Mailman, R.B., Mueller, R.A. and Breese, G.R. (1979) Noradrenergic hyperinnervation reduces the density of β-adrenergic receptors in rat cerebellum. *Brain Res.*, 166: 194–198.

Harston, C.T.,Morrow, A. and Kostrzewa, R.M. (1980) Enhancement of sprouting and putative regeneration of central noradrenergic fibers by morphine. *Brain Res. Bull.*, 5: 421–424.

Harston, C.T., Clark, M.B., Hardin, J.C. and Kostrzewa, R.M. (1981) Opiate-enhanced toxicity and noradrenergic sprouting in rats treated with 6-hydroxydopa. *Eur. J. Pharmacol.*, 71: 365–373.

Harston, C.T., Clark, M.B., Hardin, J.C. and Kostrzewa, R.M. (1982) Developmental localization of noradrenergic innervation to the rat cerebellum following neonatal 6-hydroxydopa and morphine treatment. *Dev. Neurosci.*, 5: 252–262.

Hendry, I.A. (1975) The response of adrenergic neurons to axotomy and nerve growth factor. *Brain Res.*, 94: 87–97.

Iacovitti, L., Reis, D.J. and Joh, T.H. (1981) Reactive proliferation of brain stem noradrenergic nerves following neonatal cerebellectomy in rats: role of target maturation on neuronal response to injury during development. *Dev. Brain Res.*, 1: 3–24.

Jacks, B.R., DeChamplain, J. and Cordeau, J.P. (1972) Effects of 6-hydroxydopamine on putative transmitter substances in the central nervous system. *Eur. J. Pharmacol.*, 18: 353–360.

Jacobowitz, D.M. (1975) Long-term effects on peripheral adrenergic nerves of 6-hydroxydopamine injected into newborn rats. In G. Jonsson, T. Malmfors and C. Sachs (Eds), *Chemical Tools in Catecholamine Research, Vol. 1*, North-Holland, Amsterdam, pp. 153–162.

Jacobowitz, D. and Kostrzewa, R. (1971) Selective action of 6-hydroxydopa on noradrenergic terminals: mapping of preterminal axons of the brain. *Life Sci.*, 10: 1329–1341.

Jaim-Etcheverry, G. and Zieher, L.M. (1971) Permanent depletion of peripheral norepinephrine in rats treated at birth with 6-hydroxydopamine. *Eur. J. Pharmacol.*, 13: 272–276.

Jaim-Etcheverry, G. and Zieher, L.M. (1975) Alterations of the development of central adrenergic neurons produced by 6-hydroxydopa. In G. Jonsson, T. Malmfors and C. Sachs (Eds), *Chemical Tools in Catecholamine Research, Vol. 1*, North-Holland, Amsterdam, pp.173–180.

Jaim-Etcheverry, G. and Zieher, L.M. (1980) DSP-4: A novel compound with neurotoxic effects on noradrenergic neurons of adult and developing rats. *Brain Res.*, 188: 513–523.

Johnson, E.M. and Hunter, F.E. (1979) Chemical sympathectomy by guanidinium adrenergic blocking agents. *Biochem. Pharmacol.*, 28: 1525–1531.

Johnston, M.V. and Coyle, J.T. (1979) Histological and neurochemical effects of fetal treatment with methylazoxymethanol on rat neocortex in adulthood. *Brain Res.*, 170: 135–155.

Jonsson, G. (1980) Chemical neurotoxins as denervating tools in neurobiology. *Annu. Rev. Neurosci.*, 3: 169–187.

420

Jonsson, G. and Hallman, H. (1978) Changes in β-receptor binding sites in rat brain after neonatal 6-hydroxydopamine treatment. *Neurosci. Lett.*, 9: 27–32.

Jonsson, G. and Hallman, H. (1980) Effect of neonatal nicotine administration on the postnatal development of central noradrenaline neurons. *Acta Physiol. Scand. Suppl.*, 479: 25–26.

Jonsson, G. and Hallman, H. (1981) Effects of prenatal methylazoxymethanol treatment on the development of central monoamine neurons. *Dev. Brain Res.*, 2: 513–530.

Jonsson, G. and Hallman, H. (1982a) Modulation of 6-hydroxydopamine induced alteration of the postnatal development of central noradrenaline neurons. *Brain Res. Bull.*, 9: 635–640.

Jonsson, G. and Hallman, H. (1982b) Substance P counteracts neurotoxin damage on norepinephrine neurons in rat brain during ontogeny. *Science*, 215: 75–77.

Jonsson, G. and Hallman, H. (1982c) Substance P modifies the 6-hydroxydopamine induced alteration of postnatal development of central noradrenaline neurons. *Neuroscience*, 7: 2909–2918.

Jonsson, G. and Hallman, H. (1983) Effect of substance P on neonatally axotomized noradrenaline neurons in rat brain. *Med. Biol.*, 61: 179–185.

Jonsson, G. and Sachs, C. (1982) Changes in the development of central noradrenaline neurons after neonatal axon lesions. *Brain Res. Bull.*, 9: 641–650.

Jonsson, G., Pycock, C., Fuxe, K. and Sachs, C. (1974) Changes in the development of central noradrenaline neurons following neonatal administration of 6-hydroxydopamine. *J. Neurochem.*, 22: 419–426.

Jonsson, G., Wiesel, F.-A. and Hallman, H. (1979) Developmental plasticity of central noradrenaline neurons after damage – changes in transmitter functions. *J. Neurobiol.*, 10: 337–353.

Jonsson, G., Hallman, H. and Sundström, E. (1982) Effects of the noradrenaline neurotoxin DSP-4 on the postnatal development of central noradrenaline neurons in the rat. *Neuroscience*, 7: 2895–2907.

Klisans-Fuenmayor, D., Harston, C.T. and Kostrzewa, R.M. (1986) Alterations in noradrenergic innervation of the brain following dorsal bundle lesions in neonatal rats. *Brain Res. Bull.*, 16: 47–54.

Koda, L.Y., Schulman, J.A. and Bloom, F.E. (1978) Ultrastructural identification of noradrenergic terminals in rat hippocampus: unilateral destruction of the locus coeruleus with 6-hydroxydopamine. *Brain Res.*, 145: 190–195.

Konkol, R.J., Bendeich, E.G. and Breese, G.R. (1978) A biochemical and morphological study of altered growth pattern of central catecholamine neurons following 6-hydroxydopamine. *Brain Res.*, 140: 125–135.

Kostrzewa, R.M. (1975) Effects of neonatal 6-hydroxydopa on monamine content of rat brain and peripheral tissues. *Res. Commun. Chem. Pathol. Pharmacol.*, 11: 567–579.

Kostrzewa, R.M. (1988) Neurotoxins that effect central and peripheral catecholamine neurons. In A.A. Boulton, G.B. Baker and J.M. Baker (Eds.), *Neuromethods, Vol. 12*, Humana Press, Clifton, NJ, in press.

Kostrzewa, R.M. and Garey, R.E. (1976) Effects of 6-hydroxydopa on noradrenergic neurons in developing rat brain. *J. Pharmacol. Exp. Ther.*, 197: 105–118.

Kostrzewa, R.M. and Garey, R.E. (1977) Sprouting of noradrenergic terminals in rat cerebellum following neonatal treatment with 6-hydroxydopa. *Brain Res.*, 124: 385–391.

Kostrzewa, R.M. and Harper, J.W. (1974) Effect of 6-hydroxydopa on catecholamine-containing neurons in brains of newborn rats. *Brain Res.*, 69: 174–181.

Kostrzewa, R.M. and Harper, J.W. (1975) Comparison of the neonatal effects of 6-hydroxydopa and 6-hydroxydopamine on growth and development of noradrenergic neurons in the central nervous system. In T. Malmfors, G. Jonsson and C. Sachs (Eds.), *Chemical Tools in Catecholamine Research, Vol. 1*, North-Holland, Amsterdam, pp. 181–189.

Kostrzewa, R.M. and Harston, C.T. (1986) Altered histofluorescent pattern of noradrenergic innervation of the cerebellum of the mutant mouse 'Purkinje cell degeneration.' *Neuroscience*, 8: 809–815.

Kostrzewa, R. and Jacobowitz, D. (1972) The effect of 6-hydroxydopa on peripheral adrenergic neurons. *J. Pharmacol. Exp. Ther.*, 183: 284–297.

Kostrzewa, R. and Jacobowitz, D. (1973) Acute effects of 6-hydroxydopa on central monoaminergic neurons. *Eur. J. Pharmacol.*, 21: 70–80.

Kostrzewa, R.M. and Jacobowitz, D.M. (1974) Pharmacological actions of 6-hydroxydopamine. *Pharmacol. Rev.*, 26: 199–288.

Kostrzewa, R.M. and Klisans-Fuenmayor, D. (1984) Development of an opioid-specific action of morphine in modifying recovery of neonatally-damaged noradrenergic fibers in rat brain. *Res. Commun. Chem. Pathol. Pharmacol.*, 46: 3–11.

Kostrzewa, R.M., Klara, J.W., Robertson, J. and Walker, L.C. (1978) Studies on the mechanism of sprouting of noradrenergic terminals in rat and mouse cerebellum after neonatal 6-hydroxydopa. *Brain Res. Bull.*, 3: 525–531.

Kostrzewa, R.M., Harston, C.T., Fukushima, H. and Brus, R. (1982) Noradrenergic fiber sprouting in the cerebellum. *Brain Res. Bull.*, 9: 509–517.

Kostrzewa, R.M., Hardin, J.C. and Jacobowitz, D.M. (1988) Destruction of cells in the midportion of the locus coeruleus by a dorsal bundle lesion in neonatal rats. *Brain Res.*, 442: 321–328.

Landis, S.C. and Mullen, R.J. (1978) The development and degeneration of Purkinje cells in pcd mutant mice. *J. Comp. Neurol.*, 177: 125–143.

Landis, S.C., Shoemaker, W.J., Schlumpf, M. and Bloom, F.E. (1975) Catecholamines in mutant mouse cerebellum:

fluorescence microscopic and chemical studies. *Brain Res.*, 93: 253–266.

Lanfumey, L., Arluison, M. and Adrien, J. (1981) Destruction of noradrenergic cell bodies by intracerebral 6-hydroxydopamine in the newborn rat. *Brain Res.*, 214: 445–450.

Laverty, R., Sharman, D. E. and Vogt, M. (1965) Action of 2,4,5-trihydroxyphenylethylamine on the storage and release of noradrenaline. *Br. J. Pharmacol.*, 24: 549–560.

Levi-Montalcini, R., Aloe, L., Mugnaini, E., Oesch, F. and Thoenen, H. (1975) Nerve growth factor induces volume increase and enhances tyrosine hydroxylase in sympathetic ganglia of newborn rats. *Proc. Natl. Acad. Sci. USA*, 72: 595–599.

Levitt, P. and Moore, R. Y. (1980) Organization of brain stem noradrenaline hyperinnervation following neonatal 6-hydroxydopamine treatment in rat. *Anat. Embryol.*, 158: 133–150.

Lew, G. M. and Quay, W. B. (1971) Noradrenaline contents of hypothalamus and adrenal gland increased by postnatal administration of 6-hydroxydopamine. *Res. Commun. Chem. Pathol. Pharmacol.*, 2: 807–812.

Lewis, P. R. and Schon, F. E. G. (1975) The localization of acetylcholinesterase in the locus coeruleus of the normal rat and after 6-hydroxydopamine treatment. *J. Anat.*, 120: 373–385.

Ljungdahl, A., Hokfelt, T. and Nilsson, G. (1979) Distribution of substance P-like immunoreactivity in the central nervous system of the rat. *Neuroscience*, 3: 861–943.

Lytle, L. D., Shoemaker, W. J., Cottman, K. and Wurtman, R. J. (1972) Long-term effects of postnatal 6-hydroxydopamine treatment on tissue catecholamine levels. *J. Pharmacol. Exp. Ther.*, 183: 56–64.

Manning, P. T., Russell, J. H. and Johnson, E. M. (1982) Immunosuppressive agents prevent guanethidine-induced destruction of rat sympathetic neurons. *Brain Res.*, 241: 131–143.

Manning, P. T., Powers, C. W., Schmidt, R. E. and Johnson, E. M. (1983) Guanethidine-induced destruction of peripheral sympathetic neurons occurs by an immune-mediated mechanism. *J. Neurosci.*, 3: 714–724.

McBride, R. L., Ozment, R. V. and Sutin, J. (1985) Neonatal 6-hydroxydopamine destroys spinal cord noradrenergic axons from the locus coeruleus, but not those from lateral tegmental cell groups. *J. Comp. Neurol.*, 235: 375–383.

North, R. A. (1979) Mini review: opiates, opioid peptides and single neurons. *Life Sci.*, 24: 1527–1546.

Olson, L., Seiger, Å., Taylor, D., Freedman, R. and Hoffer, B. J. (1980) Conditions for adrenergic hyperinnervation in hippocampus. I. Histochemical evidence from intraocular double grafts. *Exp. Brain Res.*, 39: 277–288.

Ong, H. H., Creveling, C. R. and Daly, J. W. (1969) The synthesis of 2,4,5-trihydroxyphenylalanine (6-hydroxydopa). A centrally active norepinephrine-depleting agent. *J. Med. Chem.*, 12: 458–469.

Pappas, B. A. and Sobrian, S. K. (1972) Neonatal sympathectomy by 6-hydroxydopamine in the rat: No effects on behavior but changes in endogenous brain norepinephrine. *Life Sci.*, 11: 653–659.

Pappas, B. A., Saari, M. and Peters, D. A. V. (1976) Regional brain catecholamine levels after intraventricular 6-hydroxydopamine in the neonatal rat. *Res. Commun. Chem. Pathol. Pharmacol.*, 14: 751–754.

Roffler-Tarlov, S., Landis, S. C. and Zigmond, M. J. (1984) Effects of Purkinje cell degeneration on the noradrenergic projection to mouse cerebellar cortex. *Brain Res.*, 298: 303–311.

Ross, S. B. (1976) Long-term effects of N-2-chloroethyl-N-ethyl-2-bromobenzylamine hydrochloride on noradrenergic neurons in the rat brain and heart. *Br. J. Pharmacol.*, 58: 521–527.

Ross, S. B. and Renyi, A. L. (1976) On the long-lasting inhibitory effect of N-(2-chloroethyl)-N-ethyl-2-bromobenzylamine (DSP-4) on the active uptake of noradrenaline. *J. Pharm. Pharmacol.*, 28: 458–459.

Ross, S. B., Johansson, J. B., Lindborg, B. and Dahlbom, R. (1973) Cyclizing compounds. I. Tertiary N-(2-bromobenzyl)-N-haloalkylamines with adrenergic blocking actions. *Acta Pharm. Suec.*, 10: 29–42.

Sachs, C. (1973) Development of the blood-brain barrier for 6-hydroxydopamine. *J. Neurochem.*, 20: 1753–1760.

Sachs, C. and Jonsson, G. (1972a) Degeneration of central and peripheral noradrenergic neurons produced by 6-hydroxydopa. *J. Neurochem.*, 19: 1561–1575.

Sachs, C. and Jonsson, G. (1972b) Degeneration of central noradrenaline neurons after 6-hydroxydopamine in newborn animals. *Res. Commun. Chem. Pathol. Pharmacol.*, 4: 203–220.

Sachs, C. and Jonsson, G. (1972c) Selective 6-hydroxy-DOPA induced degeneration of central and peripheral noradrenaline neurons. *Brain Res.*, 40: 563–568.

Sachs, C. and Jonsson, G. (1973) Changes in central noradrenaline neurons after systemic 6-hydroxydopamine administration. *J. Neurochem.*, 21: 1517–1524.

Sachs, C. and Jonsson, G. (1975) 5,7-Dihydroxytryptamine induced changes in the postnatal development of central 5-hydroxytryptamine neurons. *Med. Biol.*, 53: 156–164.

Sachs, C., Pycock, C. and Jonsson, G. (1974) Ontogenesis of central noradrenaline neurons after 6-hydroxydopamine treatment at birth. In K. Fuxe, L. Olson and G. Zotterman (Eds.), *Dynamics of Degeneration and Growth in Neurons*, Pergamon, Oxford, pp. 479–484.

Sachs, C., Jonsson, G., Heikkila, R. and Cohen, G. (1975) Control of the neurotoxicity of 6-hydroxydopamine by intraneuronal noradrenaline in rat iris. *Acta. Physiol. Scand.*, 93: 345–351.

Sar, M., Stumpf, W. E., Miller, R. J., Chang, K. and Cuatrecasas, P. (1978) Immunohistochemical localization of enkephalin in rat brain and spinal cord. *J. Comp. Neurol.*, 182: 17–38.

Schmidt, R.H. and Bhatnagar, R.K. (1979a) Assessment of the effects of neonatal subcutaneous 6-hydroxydopamine on noradrenergic and dopaminergic innervation of the cerebral cortex. *Brain Res.*, 166: 309–319.

Schmidt, R.H. and Bhatnagar, R.K. (1979b) Critical periods for noradrenergic regeneration in rat brain regions following neonatal subcutaneous 6-hydroxydopamine. *Life Sci.*, 25: 1641–1650.

Schmidt, R.H. and Bhatnagar, R.K. (1979c) Distribution of hypertrophied locus coeruleus projection to adult cerebellum after neonatal 6-hydroxydopamine. *Brain Res.*, 172: 23–33.

Schmidt, R.H. and Bhatnagar, R.K. (1979d) Regional development of norepinephrine, dopamine-β-hydroxylase and tyrosine hydroxylase in the rat brain subsequent to neonatal treatment with subcutaneous 6-hydroxydopamine. *Brain Res.*, 166: 293–308.

Schmidt, R.H. and Bhatnagar, R.K. (1980) Intracisternal dose-response analysis of 6-hydroxydopamine-induced noradrenergic sprouting in the neonatal rat cerebellum. *J. Pharmacol. Exp. Ther.*, 212: 456–461.

Schmidt, R.H., Kasik, S.A. and Bhatnagar, R.K. (1980) Regenerative critical periods for locus coeruleus in postnatal rat pups following intracisternal 6-hydroxydopamine: a model of noradrenergic development. *Brain Res.*, 191: 173–190.

Sievers, J., Klemm, H.P., Jenner, S., Baumgarten, H.G. and Berry, M. (1980) Neuronal and extraneuronal effects of intracisternally administered 6-hydroxydopamine on the developing rat brain. *J. Neurochem.*, 34: 765–771.

Singh, B. and DeChamplain, J. (1972) Altered ontogenesis of central noradrenergic neurons following neonatal treatment with 6-hydroxydopamine. *Brain Res.*, 48: 432–437.

Smith, R.D., Cooper, B.R. and Breese, G.R. (1973) Growth and behavioral changes in developing rats treated intracisternally with 6-hydroxydopamine: evidence for involvement of brain dopamine. *J. Pharmacol. Exp. Ther.*, 185: 609–619.

Snyder, A.M., Zigmond, M.J. and Lund, R.D. (1986) Sprouting of serotoninergic afferents into striatum after dopamine-depleting lesions in infant rats: a retrograde transport and immunocytochemical study. *J. Comp. Neurol.*, 245: 274–281.

Sporn, J.R., Harden, T.K., Wolfe, B.B. and Molinoff, P.B. (1976) Beta-adrenergic receptor involvement of 6-hydroxydopamine induced supersensitivity in rat cerebral cortex. *Science*, 194: 624–626.

Stachowiak, M.K., Bruno, J.P., Snyder, A.M., Stricker, E.M. and Zigmond, M.J. (1984) Apparent sprouting of striatal serotonergic terminals after dopamine-depleting brain lesions in neonatal rats. *Brain Res.*, 291: 164–167.

Stone, C.A., Stavorski, J.M., Ludden, C.T., Wengler, H.C., Ross, C.A., Totaro, J.A. and Porter, C.C. (1963) Comparison of some pharmacological effects of certain 6-substituted dopamine derivatives with reserpine, guanethidine and metaraminol. *J. Pharmacol. Exp. Ther.*, 142: 147–156.

Taylor, K.M., Clark, D.W.J., Laverty, R. and Phelan, E.L. (1972) Specific noradrenergic neurons destroyed by 6-hydroxydopamine injection into newborn rats. *Nature, (New Biol)*, 239: 247–248.

Thoenen, H. and Tranzer, J.P. (1968) Chemical sympathectomy by selective destruction of adrenergic nerve endings with 6-hydroxydopamine. *Naunyn-Schmiedebergs Arch. Pharmakol. Exp. Pathol.*, 261: 271–288.

Thoenen, H. and Tranzer, J.P. (1973) The pharmacology of 6-hydroxydopamine. *Annu. Rev. Pharmacol.*, 13: 169–180.

Tranzer, J.P. and Thoenen, H. (1967) Ultra-morphologische Veranderungen der sympatischen Nervendigunden der Katz nach Vorbehandlung mit 5- und 6-hydroxydopamine. *Naunyn-Schmiedebergs Arch. Pharmakol. Exp. Pathol.*, 257: 343–344.

Ungerstedt, U. (1968) 6-Hydroxydopamine induced degeneration of central monoamine neurons. *Eur. J. Pharmacol.*, 5: 107–110.

Ungerstedt, U. (1971a) Adipsia and aphagia after 6-hydroxydopamine-induced degeneration of the nigro-striatal dopamine system. *Acta Physiol. Scand. Suppl.*, 367: 95–122.

Ungerstedt, U. (1971b) Stereotaxic mapping of the monoamine pathways in the rat brain. *Acta Physiol. Scand. Suppl.*, 367: 1–48.

Uretsky, N.J. and Iversen, L.L. (1969) Effects of 6-hydroxydopamine on noradrenaline-containing neurons in the rat brain. *Nature*, 221: 557–559.

Versteeg, D.H.G., Wijnen, H.J.L.M., DeKloet, E.R. and DeJong, W. (1980) Differential effects of neonatal 6-hydroxydopamine treatment on the catecholamine content of hypothalamic nuclei and brain stem regions. *Neurosci. Lett.*, 7: 341–346.

Zieher, L.M. and Jaim-Etcheverry, G. (1973) Regional differences in the long-term effect of neonatal 6-hydroxydopa treatment on rat brain noradrenaline. *Brain Res.*, 60: 199–207.

Zieher, L.M. and Jaim-Etcheverry, G. (1975a) Different alterations in the development of the noradrenergic innervation of the cerebellum and the brain stem produced by neonatal 6-hydroxydopa. *Life Sci.*, 17: 987–992.

Zieher, L.M. and Jaim-Etcheverry, G. (1975b) 6-Hydroxydopa during development of central adrenergic neurons produces different long-term changes in rat brain noradrenaline. *Brain Res.*, 86: 271–281.

Zieher, L.M. and Jaim-Etcheverry, G. (1979) 6-Hydroxydopamine during development: relation between opposite regional changes in brain noradrenaline. *Eur. J. Pharmacol.*, 58: 217–223.

Discussion

I. Reisert: Do neonatally 6-hydroxy-dopa(6-OHDOPA)-treated animals behave differently in comparison to controls?

R.M. Kostrzewa: A number of investigators have studied the adult behavior of rats treated as neonates with either 6-hydroxydopamine (6-OHDA) or 6-OHDOPA. By gross observations, treated and control animals are similar. In behavioral tests it has been found that 6-OHDA-treated neonatal rats, tested as adults, showed decrements in eating and drinking – including intake of a sucrose solution. These animals also displayed impaired performance in acquisition of a shuttle-box avoidance response, and reduced performance in reward tasks (Smith et al., 1973). In rats treated with 6-OHDOPA by an i.p. route, it has been found that exploratory behavior is increased in the open field, and that these animals are less aggressive (McLean et al., 1976).

G.J. Boer: Since the blood brain barrier (BBB) develops regionally in different ways in the brain (e.g. in the cerebellum later than the cerebral cortex; Johanson, 1980), could you not explain the regional differences in chemical lesions in the noradrenalin (NA) system for cerebellum and cortex on the basis of differences in BBB at the moment of administration of the compound?

R.M. Kostrzewa: In undertaking these studies we were well aware of regional differences in the brain for development of BBB. In studying the effects of neonatal administration of 6-OHDA, Sachs (1973) found that the BBB formed in the telencephalon by 9 days after birth. Our own data on 6-OHDA indicate formation of the BBB in rat neocortex by 3 days, in the cerebellum after 14 days and at different times in other brain regions (Kostrzewa and Harper, 1975). Other data on the accumulation of [³H]metaraminol by different brain regions, following acute administration at different times after birth, support the 6-OHDA results. In order to circumvent possible confounding results, arising from the above differences in BBB formation, we have purposely selected 6-OHDOPA as a neurotoxin in these studies. The 6-OHDOPA is able to cross the BBB, and therefore this neurotoxin gains access to all brain regions when given at any time during development.

J. Sweeney: Could you speak about the differential sensitivity of the locus coeruleus cells to the effects of 6-OHDA, with caudal cells being more sensitive than rostral?

R.M. Kostrzewa: It is well known that neonatal 6-OHDA and 6-OHDOPA treatments produce a relatively selective effect on the neurons of the locus coeruleus. Other cell groups, particularly those that provide noradrenergic innervation of the hypothalamus, are relatively resistant to neurotoxin destruction. This could be related to differences in blood transport of the neurotoxin to the various brain regions. Alternatively, in areas with a dense input of noradrenergic fibers, critical intraneuronal concentrations of 6-OHDA may not be attained. That is, each of the many fibers may accumulate a relatively small amount of neurotoxin which is not capable of overwhelming the cells' protective mechanism, and therefore damage might not result.

References

Johanson, C.E. (1980) Permeability and vascularity of the developing brain: cerebellum vs cerebral cortex. *Brain Res.*, 190: 3–16.

Kostrzewa, R.M. and Harper, J.W. (1975) Comparison of the neonatal effects of 6-hydroxydopa and 6-hydroxydopamine on growth and development of noradrenergic neurons in the central nervous system. In T. Malmfors, G. Jonsson and C. Sachs (Eds.), *Chemical Tools in Catecholamine Research, Vol. 1*, North-Holland, Amsterdam, pp. 181–189.

McLean, J.H., Kostrzewa, R.M. and May, J.G. (1976) Behavioral and biochemical effects of neonatal treatment of rats with 6-hydroxydopa. *Pharmacol. Biochem. Behav.*, 4: 601–607.

Sachs, C. (1973) Development of the blood-brain barrier for 6-hydroxydopamine. *J. Neurochem.*, 20: 1753–1760.

Smith, R.D., Cooper, B.R. and Breese, G.R. (1973) Growth and behavioral changes in developing rats treated intracisternally with 6-hydroxydopamine: evidence for involvement of brain dopamine. *J. Pharmacol. Exp. Ther.*, 185: 609–619.

G.J. Boer, M.G.P. Feenstra, M. Mirmiran, D.F. Swaab and F. Van Haaren
Progress in Brain Research, Vol. 73
© 1988 Elsevier Science Publishers B.V. (Biomedical Division)

CHAPTER 27

Use of toxins to disrupt neurotransmitter circuitry in the developing brain

Michael V. Johnston[1-4], John Barks[1], Timothy Greenamyre[2,3] and Faye Silverstein[1,2]

Departments of [1]Pediatrics, [2]Neurology, [3]Medical School, The Neuroscience Graduate Program and [4]The Center for Human Growth and Development, The University of Michigan, Ann Arbor, MI 48104, USA

Introduction

Many teratogens and drugs disrupt developing neuronal circuitry. The mechanisms for these effects and their relationship to neurobehavioral abnormalities are poorly understood. Studies of animal models prepared by exposing the fetal brain to specific neurotoxins are useful for studying behavioral outcome from a toxic exposure. They may also be useful for examining the basic rules which determine assembly of neuronal circuitry. This review describes use of two major groups of developmental neurotoxins. The first, mitotic disrupters (e.g., methylazoxymethanol acetate (MAM)) delete populations of rapidly dividing neuroepithelial cells. Their effects are limited to phases of rapid embryonic neurogenesis. Due to the restricted birthdays of certain groups of neurons, mitotic disruptors administered at appropriate times lead to atrophic brain regions and major imbalances in remaining neurotransmitter-specific neuronal circuitry. Several mitotic disruptors are rapidly eliminated from the brain and have negligible effects on the differentiation of postmitotic neurons or other brain structures.

In contrast, synaptic disruptors destroy neurons and possibly other structures bearing specific neurotransmitter receptors. The proliferative neuroepithelium may be less vulnerable to toxins of this group, which act primarily on maturing synapses associated with postmitotic neurons. Examples of this group are analogues of the excitatory amino acid neurotransmitter glutamate. These chemicals are neurotoxic in the immature brain and studies of animals and human fetuses indicate that receptors for glutamate appear early in brain development. In certain immature regions, such as the hippocampus and globus pallidus, glutamate recognition sites are expressed in higher numbers than are seen in the adult brain. The appearance of these receptors may form a neurochemical substrate for selective vulnerability of those neurons during critical periods.

The two groups of neurotoxins act by distinct mechanisms, at discrete times in brain development, and produce different patterns of morphologic injury. They also produce a diverse spectrum of changes in biochemical markers for neurotransmitter circuitry as well as behavioral changes.

Correspondence: Michael V. Johnston, M.D., 1120 Neuroscience Laboratory Building, 1103 E. Huron, The University of Michigan, Ann Arbor, MI 48104, U.S.A.

Mitotic disruptors

Chemicals which kill mitotically active neurons selectively may be used to make lesions in the brain if given at critical times during neurogenesis. Neuronal groups which are intimately associated in the adult nervous system can be dissociated using these compounds. For example, rat fetuses exposed to chemicals such as methylazoxymethanol acetate (MAM) or 5-azacytidine on day 15 of gestation grow to adulthood lacking superficial neocortical layers II–IV. In contrast, layers V and VI, thalamocortical afferents and other cortical inputs remain relatively intact (Jones et al., 1982). The subcortical afferents and deep cortical layers originate predominantly in the first two fetal weeks but cells destined for outer cortical layers divide in the third week. Similarly, rodents treated postnatally with mitotic disruptors develop atrophic cerebella which lack late-dividing granule cells and other interneurons but retain normal numbers of Purkinje cells.

Neurogenetic patterns and action of mitotic disrupters

Several factors determine the lesion produced by mitotic disrupting drugs (Table 1). Since these toxins kill rapidly dividing cells preferentially, the most important factor is the timing of treatment in relationship to the brain's neurogenetic time-

TABLE 1

Factors influencing patterns of brain injury from mitotic disruptors

1. Timing of treatment in relationship to regional cell replication timetables
2. Timing of toxin's action in cell cycle
3. Variations in brain cell cycle kinetics
4. Cell killing potency (vs. ability to damage without killing)
5. Dose of toxin
6. Pattern of activation to proximate toxin
7. Duration of brain exposure to proximate toxin

tables. [^{3}H]Thymidine autoradiographic studies have been used to determine neurogenetic sequences (Fig. 1: Schultze et al., 1974). Genetically similar animals have virtually identical start and stop times for generation of distinct neuronal groups. In general, neurogenesis proceeds in a caudal to rostral time gradient with cortical neurogenesis in the germinal matrix generating deeper cortical neurons before superficial ones (Fig. 2; Angevine and Sidman, 1961; Hicks and D'Amato, 1968). Cerebellar neurogenesis occurs in two distinct phases: the first phase of Purkinje cell production occurs relatively early in concert with the brainstem, but granule cells and other interneurons lag behind until the neocortex has divided (Altman, 1969). Most neocortical cell division in rodents is completed in the last week of a 3 week gestation, and cerebellar replication continues for the next three postnatal weeks. Areas such as olfactory bulb and hippocampus contain some neuronal populations which are among the last to divide.

Although the order of neurogenesis is similar across species, timing in relationship to birth is quite variable. Neurogenesis in the guinea pig occurs much earlier than it does in mice and rats. The latter two species have parallel timetables within 48 h of each other. It is noteworthy that the same neurogenetic sequences, such as the inside-out sequence in neocortex, are less rigid in rodents than in primates. The distribution of neuronal deficits resulting from a single dose of an antiproliferative chemical generally correlates well with autoradiographic dating of cells undergoing peak mitosis at the same time.

The toxin's molecular action on the cell cycle and variations in cycle kinetics are also major determinants of the severity of the neuronal deficit. The cell's replicative cycle is divided into distinct stages in which the cell moves from a non-proliferative phase (G_0) through DNA synthetic (S) and mitotic (M) phases (Fig. 3). Data from rapidly proliferating neoplastic cell systems indicate that antiproliferative toxins vary in their spectrum of action on different phases. Some, like

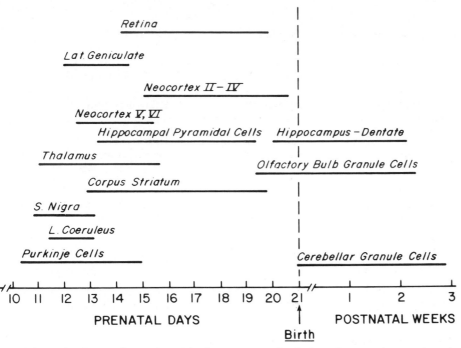

Fig. 1 Schematic of approximate timetables for neurogenesis of selected neuronal groups in rodents. Based on [³H]thymidine autoradiographic studies of Altman (1966, 1969), Angevine and Sidman (1961), Hicks and D'Amato (1968) and others (Rodier and Reynolds, 1977 and Rodier, 1977, 1980).

cytosine arabinoside, are selective for the S phase while others, such as MAM, are active in all phases except G_0 (Table 2; Calabresi and Parks, 1980). Toxins which are relatively nonselective for

stages in the cell cycle have the opportunity to damage more cells than toxins which are cycle phase specific. This factor is minimally important for a very rapidly dividing cell population, but

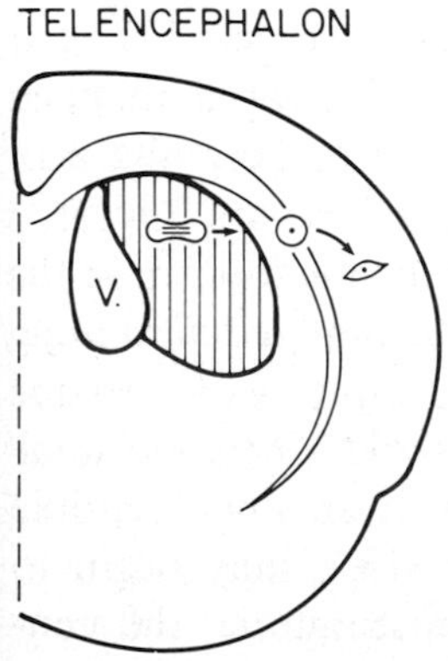

TELENCEPHALON

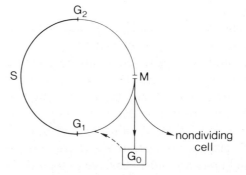

Fig. 2 Schematic diagram of one half of a fetal telencephalon in the rat showing neurogenesis in the germinal matrix (vertical lines) with postmitotic neurons migrating to cerebral cortex (From Johnston and Coyle, 1982).

Fig. 3 Schematic of stages of the neurogenetic cycle in germinal matrix. G_1 and G_2 are nonproliferative stages, and S is the DNA synthetic phase. M is the mitotic stage, from which neuroblasts may become either permanently postmitotic, proceed through another cycle or enter the G_0 pool of neuroblasts destined to re-enter the neurogenetic cycle at a later time.

TABLE 2

Antiproliferative chemicals used as neurotoxins in the developing brain

Agent	Action	Cell cycle phase	In vivo activation steps
Methylazoxymethanol (MAM)	Methylation of DNA and RNA	All except G_0; late G_1 and S	Rapid hydrolysis to carbonium ion
Cyclophosphamide	Alkylation of DNA and RNA	All except G_0; late G_1 and S	Hydroxylated in liver by P450 system; oxidized at active site to phosphoramide mustard + acrolein
Ethylnitrosourea (ENU)	Alkylation of nucleic acids; carbamolyation of proteins	All except G_0; late G_1 and S	Nonenzymatic degradation to carbonium ions
Cytosine arabinoside (Ara-C)	Competitive inhibition of DNA polymerase	S	Enzymatic, three step activation to Ara-C triphosphate
5-Azacytidine	Inhibits sequential RNA processing, DNA synthesis	S, probably others	Enzymatic activation to 5-azacytidine triphosphate
Fluorodeoxyuridine (FUdR)	Inhibits thymidylate synthetase, rate limiting for DNA synthesis	S, probably others	Converted to 5-fluoro-2'-deoxyuridine-5'-phosphate (F-dUMP) by intracellular kinase
Hydroxyurea	Inhibits ribonucleoside diphosphate reductase, rate limiting step in DNA synthesis	S, probably others	None

assumes greater relevance if fewer and/or longer cycles generate the target population.

Kinetic studies in the rodent brain indicate that cycle times approximate 12 h before 16 days gestation but at later times the cycles lengthen with variation from population to population (Schultze et al., 1974). If other factors are the same, cell groups with relatively short, intense replicative bursts are most sensitive to total decimation by a single dose of mitotic disruptors. Cell groups generated over an extended period (e.g., neuroglia) are less likely to be ablated by single doses of mitotic disruptors. Furthermore, work with antineoplastic agents indicates that they kill by first-order kinetics, i.e., a constant percentage

of vulnerable cells die (Chabner et al., 1977). It follows that a distinct neuronal group is reduced most by toxin exposure at the earliest phase of replication when absolute numbers are lowest.

The chemical's dose and its metabolism in the animal are also critically important in determining the final brain lesion. Dose responses for toxins such as MAM exhibit a threshold. There is a small difference between doses with an imperceptible effect and higher amounts which may begin to disrupt non-dividing or post-mitotic differentiating cells as well as the target group. Dose requirements may be influenced by in vivo activation and/or degradative steps (Table 2). Toxins such as cyclophosphamide must be metabolized by the liver and target cell enzymes to active 'proximate' toxins. The kinetics of other drugs (e.g., Ara-C) are influenced in a major way by activities of degradative enzymes. In addition, dose, metabolic disposition and excretion patterns determine the duration of brain exposure to the proximate toxin. Metabolic disposition in the animal is altered by species or strain differences. Prolonged retention of the proximate toxin makes the treatment less selective for specific groups of neurons and increases the chances for the toxin to exert generalized effects on the rest of the body.

Alkylating agents used for neuroteratology

Three alkylating agents (MAM, cyclophosphamide and cthylnitrosourea) have been used as neurotoxins in the developing CNS (Table 2). Their cytotoxic effects are thought to be related directly to covalent alkylation of components of DNA, especially the 7-nitrogen atom of guanine. Other purine and pyrimidine bases, nuclear proteins and RNA constituents are also alkylated. These reactions probably are cytotoxic because of genetic miscoding, excision of guanine residues and cross-linking of DNA chains (Shapiro, 1968). Besides the three toxins discussed here, others might produce similar lesions but have not been studied in detail in developing brain.

Methylazoxymethanol acetate (MAM)

MAM is an ester synthetized from the naturally occurring substance, methylazoxymethanol β-glucoside or cycasin. When injected intraperitoneally into pregnant animals it readily crosses into the brain, decomposing to carbonium ions which methylate DNA (Fig. 4). Kinetic studies with [^{3}H]MAM indicate that its intense cytotoxic action is relatively brief since it is cleared from the body in 12–24 h (Nagata and Matsumoto, 1969).

For fetal rat brain lesions, MAM (liquid from Aldrich Chemical Company, St. Louis, MO) is mixed with 0.9% NaCl (10 mg/ml) immediately before administration to the pregnant dam.

Appropriate precautions should be used (ventilated hood, disposable gloves and syringes) to avoid contamination of personnel since the compound is a potent carcinogen. Timed pregnant rats are injected intraperitoneally on the chosen day of gestation (DG), counting the morning on which the vaginal plug is found as day 1. For comparisons of effects at different days it is worthwhile to make all injections at the same time each day. Pups are born on days 21 or 22 of gestation and are reduced to fewer than ten per litter.

Effects of MAM on telencephalon

A number of studies have examined effects of MAM at 15 DG days gestation in the rat (Haddad et al., 1969; 1979; Johnston et al., 1979; Johnston and Coyle, 1979; Matsutani et al., 1980; Jonsson and Hallman, 1982). A dose of 20 mg/kg produces a 50% reduction in telencephalic mass but no change in the mass or histology of the cerebellum or brainstem. Doses of less than 20 mg produce less reproducible effects and higher doses may produce pervasive effects on development. The DNA content of the telencephalon is reduced commensurate with the reduction in mass indicating that the microcephaly is primarily related to a change in cell number

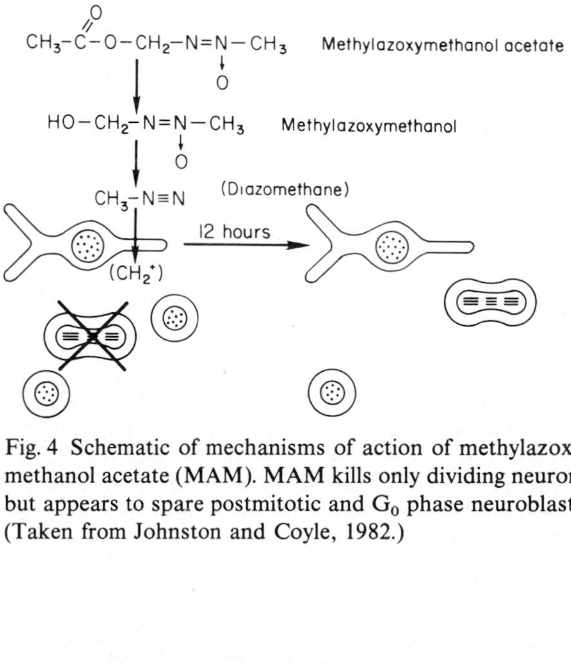

Fig. 4 Schematic of mechanisms of action of methylazoxymethanol acetate (MAM). MAM kills only dividing neurons but appears to spare postmitotic and G_0 phase neuroblasts. (Taken from Johnston and Coyle, 1982.)

(Matsumoto et al., 1972). This is consistent with histologic studies showing that early damage is confined to the periventricular germinal matrix so that many neurons are prevented from migrating to the cortex and other forebrain areas (Spatz and Laqueur, 1968; Johnston and Coyle, 1980; Fig. 5). Since neurons destined to occupy deep regions of cerebral cortex have already been generated by day 15, the outer layers are much more heavily damaged. Other regions such as the corpus striatum are also markedly reduced in size (Beaulieu and Coyle, 1981; Balduini, et al., 1984).

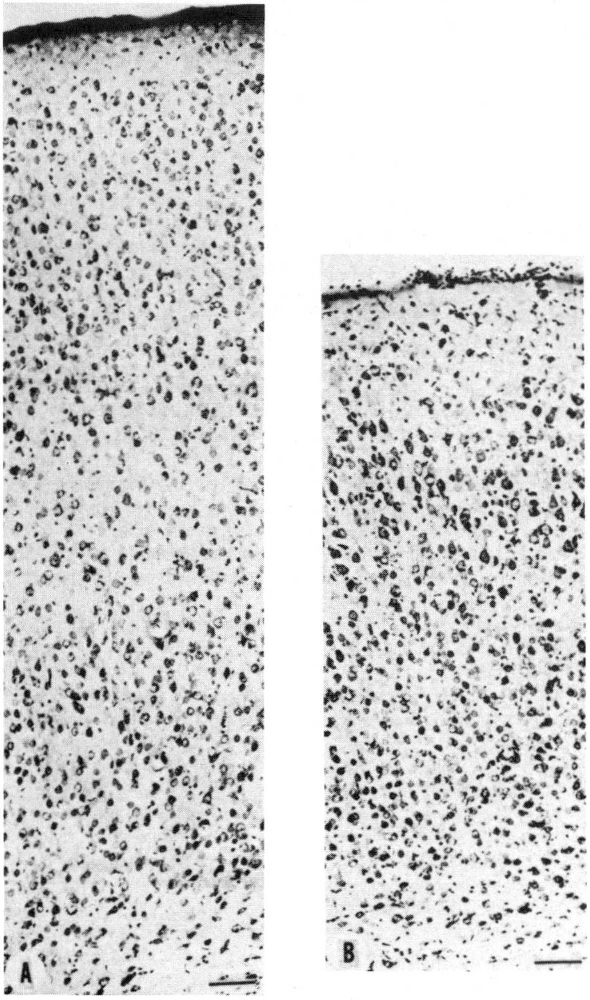

MAM injected at 15 DG has been shown to be remarkably uniform and selective in its effects. We found that the bodily growth and development of the microcephalic pups from the Sprague-Dawley strain is normal (Johnston and Coyle, 1980). However, several authors reported that the toxin produced generalized growth retardation (Fischer et al., 1972; Vorhees et al., 1984; Balduini et al., 1986). In adult animals, neurons with perikarya remaining in the cortex have the normal histological appearance of layers V and VI of untreated animals (Johnston and Coyle, 1979; Jones et al., 1982; Fig. 5). Similarly, neurons in other regions with 'birthdays' before or after 15 DG (thalamus, brainstem, cerebellum) appear normal. The lack of effect on cerebellar granule cells is noteworthy since their precursors are in Go phase when the toxin is administered at 15 DG. In Golgi-stained material, most remaining cortical pyramidal cells are normal, though some are inverted and other superficial ones have unusual apical dendrites (Jones et al., 1982). In spite of the loss of many target neurons, thalamocortical afferents retain their normal bilaminar distribution in the dystrophic cortex. Many animals have a few abnormal islands of cells in the subcortical white matter and hippocampus, apparently due to migrational arrest (Singh, 1977). MAM-treated rats have also been reported to have aberrant mossy fibers in hippocampus (Chema and Lauder, 1983). Nevertheless, the predominant impression from histological analysis is that MAM's effect is short lived and localized (Jones et al., 1982).

Fig. 5 Nissl-stained coronal section of control (A) and MAM-treated lateral neocortex (B) at the level of the anterior commissure. The rats were 7 weeks old and were born to dams treated with saline or MAM (20 mg/kg^{-1}) on day 15 of gestation. Architectonic layers II–IV are depleted in the thinner MAM treated cortex. Bar = 100 um (From Johnston and Coyle, 1979.)

Neurochemical abnormalities induced by MAM

MAM eliminates a large group of intrinsic cortical interneurons destined to form outer layers of cerebral cortex. Many GABAergic interneurons are among those lesioned. Analysis of biochemical markers for GABAergic inter-

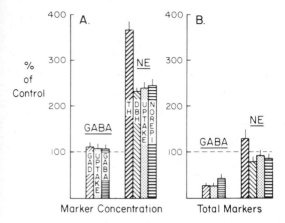

Fig. 6 Neurochemical data from lateral cortex of adult rats treated on gestational day 15 with MAM represented as percent of activity or concentration in cortex from saline-treated rats. Panel A shows the concentration of markers for GABAergic and noradrenergic neurons per mg of wet weight. GABAergic markers are (from left to right): L-glutamate decarboxylase (GAD), [³H]GABA synaptosomal uptake and endogenous GABA. Noradrenergic markers are: tyrosine hydroxylase (TH), dopamine β-hydroxylase (DBH), [³H]norepinephrine synaptosomal uptake and endogenous norepinephrine (NE). Panel B shows the results of calculating total amounts of the same markers in cortical slabs carefully dissected to include analogous areas from the control and microcephalic rats. The wet weight of these cortical slabs was reduced by 67% compared with the control rats. (From Johnston and Coyle, 1982.)

neurons in the cortex of adult animals treated on day 15 of fetal life with MAM showed that their concentration was identical to control cortex (Fig. 6). In contrast, markers for noradrenergic axons in the atrophic cerebral cortex were markedly elevated (Johnston and Coyle, 1982). This suggested that the GABAergic neurons are eliminated in proportion to the loss of other non-GABA neurons in the cortex but noradrenergic axons were relatively unaffected by the lesion. Biochemical markers for cholinergic and serotonin axons are also relatively enriched in the MAM-lesioned cortex.

Ontogenetic studies of cortex in MAM-treated rats showed that the pattern for biochemical GABA markers is similar to control (Fig. 7). When calculated in terms of total noradrenergic markers per cortex, analysis suggests that the total noradrenergic arbor develops normally despite the loss of surrounding cortical neurons. Total [³H]norepinephrine uptake into synaptosomes is virtually unchanged throughout postnatal development (Fig. 8). We interpret this to mean that noradrenergic perikarya which are 'born' on gestational day 13 continue to project an axonal arbor to the shrunken cortex which is quantitatively nearly identical to untreated animals (Johnston and Coyle, 1980; Fig. 9). Neurons born during chemical exposure are reduced, but later dividing groups survive. Loss of potential target neurons appears to have little effect on the development of the full noradrenergic axonal arbor. MAM has similar effects on the developing corpus striatum (Beaulieu and Coyle, 1981; Balduini et al., 1984).

In contrast to the effects on the total axonal arbor, fetal treatment does disrupt the organization of axons in the atrophic cortex. Using an antibody directed at dopamine-β-hydroxylase, we showed that the normal laminar pattern of noradrenergic fibers was compressed and disorganized (Johnston et al., 1979). These results were consistent with the neurochemical data suggesting noradrenergic hyperinnervation in MAM-treated cortex. They indicate that target neurons in the cortex influence the distribution of developing noradrenergic axons. The noradrenergic hyperinnervation is associated with a 2-fold increase in the concentration of the norepinephrine metabolite, 3-methoxyl-4-hydroxy-phenylglycol (MHPG) sulfate, and a 26% decrease in the B_{max} of β-adrenergic receptors labelled by [³H]-dihydroalprenolol. This suggests that the denser noradrenergic innervation is functionally active (Beaulieu and Coyle, 1982).

MAM given on gestational days other than day 15 produces reciprocal changes in cortical mass and concentration of axons of aminergic brainstem projections. MAM, given in a dose of 20 mg/kg to the pregnant rat on 14 DG, produces greater reductions in cortical neurons than on 15 DG. Injection on 13 or 17 DG produces

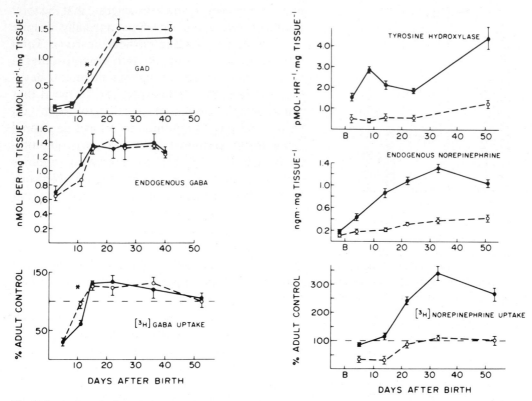

Fig. 7 Ontogeny of neurochemical markers for GABAergic neurons (left panel) and noradrenergic (right panel) axons in lateral neocortex of rats exposed to MAM as fetuses on gestational day 15. Prenatal MAM treatment produced little change in any of the three neurochemical markers for GABA neurons in the atrophic MAM exposed cortex. In contrast, the neurochemical markers for noradrenergic axons, tyrosine hydroxylase and [³H]norepinephrine uptake, were already higher in the MAM treated cortex on postnatal day 5. Although the markers for noradrenergic axons were elevated, the treatment had little detectable effects on the ontogenetic pattern in either group. * $P < 0.05$ (Data from Johnston and Coyle, 1980.)

definite but less marked reduction in cortical mass than injection at intermediate times (Johnston et al., 1981). The elevations in neurotransmitter markers for serotonergic and noradrenergic neurons vary inversely to the change in cortical mass from treatments on various days (Fig. 10). This supports the contention that these markers are elevated because they persist within a neuron-depleted cortex. Injections earlier than 12 DG cause major anomalies and fetal wastage.

Myelin in forebrain structures such as the corpus callosum is reduced in the MAM-treated animals, probably related to reduced commissural connections. Myelin in the brainstem is not altered by MAM, and CNPase activity (2,3-cyclic

nucleotide 3-phosphohydrolase) a marker for cerebral myelin indicates that oligodendroglia are relatively spared (Matsutani et al., 1980).

Microcephaly from fetal MAM treatment has also been produced in hamsters, gerbils and ferrets (Haddad et al., 1972). At a dose of 20 mg/kg, MAM is lethal for a high percentage of ferrets but 15 mg/kg on 33 DG produces live microcephalic pups. This treatment reduces brain weight by 28% and markedly impairs the normal development of the gyral patterns (Johnston et al., 1982). There is considerable regional variation within the cortex with the temporal-occipital region the most heavily affected. In general the neurochemical changes resemble those found in the rat.

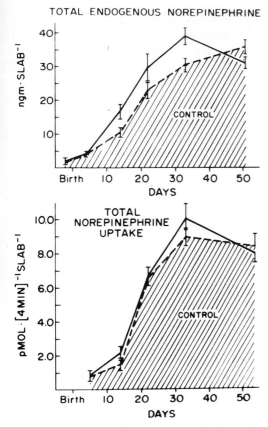

TOTAL ENDOGENOUS NOREPINEPHRINE

TOTAL
NOREPINEPHRINE
UPTAKE

Fig. 8 Ontogeny of total neurochemical markers for nor-adrenergic axons. Norepinephrine content (NE) and [³H]NE uptake per cortex slab in animals exposed to MAM (20 mg kg⁻¹) on day 15 of gestation. Despite the effect of MAM to deplete cortical neurons, the treatment had a negligible effect on the development of the total markers for these axons. The data suggest that the total extent of the NE axonal arbor projected into cortex develops fully despite the early injury to intrisic cortical neurons. (Data from Johnston and Coyle, 1980.)

Behavioral deficits in offspring of MAM-treated rats

Prenatally, MAM-treated microencephalic rats are useful for understanding prenatal effects on behavior and for testing effects of drugs on cognitive disorders (Balduini et al., 1986; Sanberg et al., 1987). Haddad et al. (1969) found that rats treated on day 15 of gestation performed poorly on a Hebb-Williams maze test though they appeared normal on casual observation. However, MAM rats appeared to be able to acquire

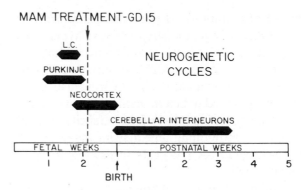

Fig. 9 Schematic of periods of neurogenesis for selected neuronal groups in the rat in relation to the treatment of MAM on gestational day 15 (GD15). See also fig. 1. L.C. = locus coeruleus. (From Johnston and Coyle, 1982.)

simple behaviors including left-right discrimination and a single T-maze (Rabe and Haddad, 1972). Cannon-Spoor and Freed (1984) showed that MAM rats are deficient in their ability to inhibit responses and may perseverate. MAM-treated rats had less ability to suppress intake of flavored water on first reexposure and also showed deficits and reversal of passive avoidance.

Vorhees et al. (1984) studied the behavior of rats exposed to MAM as fetuses (30 mg/kg on

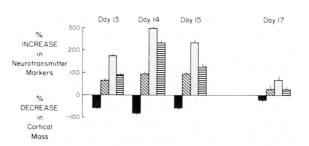

Fig. 10 Relationship between the reduction in cortical mass (black bars) and elevation in cortical neurotransmitter markers in adult rats exposed to MAM (20 mg kg⁻¹) on gestational days 13, 14, 15 or 17. Diagonally lined bars represent choline acetyltransferase activity, a marker for cholinergic axons; stippled bars represent endogenous serotonin; horizontally lined bars are endogenous norepinephrine. (From Johnston and Coyle, 1982.)

day 14 of gestation). They reported that, from 49 to 192 days of age, the offspring were hyperactive and females exhibited impaired activity habituation patterns. Males exhibited impaired passive avoidance performance. The offspring also showed a pronounced deficit in learning a water maze. Mohammed et al. (1986) found deficits in taste aversion conditioning and a swim maze task in MAM-treated (14 DG) rats suggesting attention deficits.

Sanberg et al. (1987) studied MAM rats on a passive avoidance test. They measured acquisition as well as retention and shock sensitivity. They studied rats which had been injected on day 15 of gestation with 20 mg/kg of MAM. At 90 days of age, the rats were tested on a platform shelf and their attempts to step down were recorded. Upon stepping off the platform, the rat received a foot shock until returning to the platform. The investigators found no differences in the initial step down latencies when rats were first placed on the platform. However, acquisition was impaired in terms of the number of descents and time spent being shocked. Cannon-Spoor and Fried (1984) also found a deficit in acquisition of passive-avoidance responses. These behavioral deficits may be related more to the inability of the MAM animals to inhibit behavior than to a cognitive deficit. Therefore, behavior in MAM-exposed microencephalic rats points to deficits in reference and working memory with equally or more prominent abnormalities in response inhibition.

MAM rats have also been reported to have abnormalities in activity. Studies summarized by Sanberg et al. (1987) suggested a profound hyperkinesis during times of arousal. Activity measured during the daytime was generally normal unless rats were awake and actively exploring their environment. When MAM animals are tested for activity in an open field over a 24-h period, significant increases in activity appeared only during night-time (Sanberg et al., 1987). Adult MAM rats tended to travel further than control rats and had a marked increase in rearing

or vertical activity. The contribution of these abnormal activity patterns to deficits in tests of learning and memory remains unclear.

Significant abnormalities have also been reported in prenatally treated MAM rats in behavioral development and response to drugs. Moran et al. (1986) found significant delays in development of organized behavior in response to electrical stimulation paradigms. Sanberg et al. (1987) found that the MAM-treated animals respond to drugs affecting the dopamine receptors as if the receptors had been desensitized by dopamine hyper-innervation. Alternatively, loss of receptors due to the toxin may have eliminated portions of pathways which normally respond to these drugs. Giurgea et al. (1982) treated MAM rats with the nootropic drug, piracetam, and reported improved cognitive function.

The obvious cortical hypoplasia produced by MAM and their behavioral abnormalities suggest that the animals may be suitable models for effects of toxins on learning memory activity. Although the deficits induced by MAM are relatively selective dependent on the timing of injection, the morphologic deficits are widespread. Furthermore, as shown by neurochemical studies, the remaining brain is characterized not only by a reduced size but by major imbalances in residual neurotransmitter circuits. More work is needed to attempt to segregate effects of regional and generalized neuronal loss from those directed by reorganized neurotransmitter circuitry. Careful behavioral characterization of these models might provide useful models for testing cognition enhancing drugs. Prenatal MAM treatment has also been suggested as a positive control for screening other developmental neurotoxins. The malformed brain produced by a prenatal exposure to MAM is thus of considerable theoretical and practical importance in neurotoxicology.

Cerebellar lesions induced by MAM

Mitotic cell disruptors administered to postnatal animals have provided information about cerebellar circuitry, complementing data from genetic models (DeBarry et al., 1987). Postnatal injection of MAM produces cerebellar hypoplasia in a variety of species (Haddad et al., 1972). In rats, mice and hamsters, treatment shortly after birth kills interneuronal populations (granule, basket and stellate neurons) but spares early dividing Golgi II and Purkinje neurons (Shimada and Langman, 1970; Sanger et al., 1972; Grondin et al., 1975; Lovell et al., 1980). The loss of basket and stellate cells, which mature slightly in advance of granule cells, is less severe than that of granule cells after neonatal injection. The Purkinje neurons are usually clumped in disarray and their dentritic arbors are hypoplastic because of reduced granule cell input.

Cerebellar interneurons are generated in the external granular layer over the first three postnatal weeks in rodents, and considerable regeneration may take place after MAM or radiation are administered during this period. Regeneration appears more vigorous in rats than mice. Several daily injections in rats are required to achieve the same neuronal depletion produced by a single injection in neonatal mice. Necrosis is apparent in the mouse external granule layer shortly after MAM injection, and necrotic debris is removed within 4 days. Some islands of the external granule cell layer reappear by 5 days (Jones and Gardner, 1976; Lovell et al., 1980). Regeneration after MAM treatment may be enhanced by a transient increase in the proliferative rate of remaining cells, which has been noted following radiation-induced lesions.

A variety of dosage schedules can be used to produce MAM cerebellar lesions. Slevin et al. (1982) found a 47% reduction in adult cerebellar weight in Blu-Ha mice injected subcutaneously with a single dose of 30 mg/kg given within 24 h after birth. Grondin et al. (1975), Lovell et al. (1980) and Shimada and Langman (1970) reported slightly different effects of particular protocols. It is prudent to use the lowest dose that produces a suitable lesion since MAM may interfere with postnatal weight gain at higher doses.

MAM lesions have been used to explore the organization of neurotransmitter circuitry in the cerebellum. Slevin et al. (1982) found an increase in receptor binding of [^{3}H]glutamate corresponding to an increased concentration of GABAergic markers localized predominantly in Purkinje and other cerebellar interneurons (Golgi II and basket cells). Markers for glutamate nerve endings ([^{3}H]glutamate uptake, endogenous glutamate) are reduced, as previously reported in other granuloprival models. Olson et al. (1987) used in vitro receptor autoradiography for [^{3}H]glutamate receptors to examine the distribution of receptor subtypes in cerebellum. In the molecular layer of MAM granuloprival mice, the number of quisqualate-preferring binding sites increased to 214% of control while N-methyl-D-aspartate (NMDA) preferring sites decreased by 38%. In contrast, in a genetic mutant lacking Purkinje cells, quisqualate-sensitive sites were reduced by 71% and NMDA sites were unchanged. The MAM experiments suggest that the quisqualate sites are localized predominantly on dendrites of Purkinje cells while NMDA sites are localized on granule cells and other interneurons.

MAM has been used to produce cerebellar lesions in a variety of other species (Haddad et al., 1972). In ferrets, 5 mg/kg at birth produces no lesion, 10 mg/kg produces cerebellar malformations and 20 mg/kg kills the animal. Kittens develop lesions with 10 mg/kg and beagle pups develop lesions after 20 mg/kg. Neonatal rabbits and piglets develop cerebellar dysgenesis after doses of 20 mg/kg. MAM has also been used to inhibit replication of granule cells in newborn rat cerebellar explant cultures (Calvet et al., 1974). In these granuloprival cultures, electron microscopy and electrophysiological monitoring suggest that abnormal synaptic connections are established on Purkinje cells by axon recurrent collateral endings.

Effects of alkylating agents other than MAM

Other alkylating agents appear to be less selective for dividing cells and therefore less useful for experimental teratology than MAM. Nathanson et al. (1969) reported the effects of cyclophosphamide on cerebellar development in suckling rats. The drug generally produces more subtle lesions than produced by MAM. The major effect was to produce prominent clumps of heterotopic granule cells in the molecular layer of the cerebellum. Doses of 25–200 mg/kg produced heterotopias when injected at 2–3 or 7–8 days but not at later times. Ethylnitrosourea (ENU), another alkylating agent produces microcephaly when administered on days 14–20 of gestation at a dose of 60 mg/kg (Das and Pfaffenroth, 1972). ENU produces prominent heterotopias (Hallas and Das, 1979) and brain tumors (Druckrey et al., 1966) and may be cytotoxic for certain differentiating as well as dividing cells.

Antimetabolites

Cytosine arabinoside (Ara-C)

This pyrimidine analog is a potent antineoplastic and antiviral agent which acts primarily to inhibit DNA polymerase. It is thought to act primarily on the S phase of the cell cycle. It must be phosphorylated intracellularly to 5-monophosphate nucleotide and subsequently to triphosphate nucleotides to have an antiproliferative effect. The kinetics of Ara-C in the body depend heavily on the catabolic enzyme, cytidine deaminase.

Ara-C produces telencephalic and cerebellar lesions that generally resemble those produced by alkylating agents given at the same time in development. Fishaut et al. (1974) produced cerebellar hypoplasia with four daily injections of Ara-C into Sprague-Dawley rats starting on the second day of life. Damage was dose related: a daily dose of 15 mg/kg almost completely inhibited cerebellar granule cell proliferation while a dose of 3 mg/kg/day produced temporary damage with later repair. Doses of 5 and 10 mg/kg/day inhibited cerebellar growth to an intermediate degree. Behavior abnormalities such as ataxia also correlated with the histopathologic changes.

Adlard et al. (1975) produced cerebellar hypoplasia in postnatal rats using single doses of 50 or 250 mg/kg of Ara-C on the 5th day of life. At 25 days, the lower dose reduced cerebellar weight by 8% and the higher dose lowered it by 22%. The weight of the rest of the brain was unaffected. Granuloprival cerebellar explants from neonatal mice have also been produced using Ara-C (Seil et al., 1980). Cultures were exposed to concentrations from 2.5 to 10 µg/ml for 4–9 days post explant. Like the in vivo Ara-C treated cerebella, granule cells were absent in older cultures but Golgi cells and Purkinje cells survived. These culture preparations resembled those treated with MAM in that excess axon collaterals formed on Purkinje cells. However, unlike the MAM-treated cultures, Ara-C-treated cerebella did not myelinate normally.

Ara-C treatment of pregnant animals results in reduction in cell number in the forebrain. A dose of 50 mg/kg on day 14 in rats reduced brain weight at birth by 17% and total DNA by 29% (Adlard et al., 1975). A dose of 30 mg/kg in mice on gestational day 13 produced necrotic germinal matrix cells within several hours lasting up to 16 h. Two injections, one on day 13 and another on day 14, produced more severe destruction of the germinal matrix, but these animals failed to thrive and died prematurely. These mice also developed hydrocephalus (Kasubuchi et al., 1977). Assay of neurotransmitter concentrations in Ara-C-induced microcephaly indicates that the cortex resembles the MAM preparation in being markedly enriched in markers for catecholamine and serotonin axons (Matsutani et al., 1980).

5-Azacytidine

This antimetabolite is a cytotoxic analog of cytidine and inhibits the cytosine pathway in RNA and DNA synthesis. Activation occurs through an initial phosphorylation by uridine-cytidine kinase. Its site of action is thought to be primarily inhibition of RNA processing. In vivo disposition is influenced by spontaneous decomposition and cytidine deaminase activity (Chabner et al., 1977).

Langman and Shimada (1971) studied the effects of 5-azacytidine on fetal mice at DG 15 using a single dose of 4 mg/kg. Within 3–4 h of injection the fetal germinal matrix contained abnormal mitotic figures. Many abnormal chromosomal figures were seen over the next 10 h when some recovery began. Mice given 2 mg/kg dose on days 13, 14 and 15 were also studied. In both preparations, neuronal deficits were found in hippocampal and cortical regions though it was difficult to pinpoint the precise nature of the neuronal losses. Rodier and Reynolds (1977) and Rodier (1977) performed detailed behavioral studies of mice exposed as fetuses to the drug in two doses (4 mg/kg) 6 h apart. When the animals were treated on 15 DG, 19 DG or postnatal day 3, cell loss followed predicted patterns based on [^{3}H]thymidine autoradiography data. The morphological changes were difficult to appreciate without direct comparison to a number of normal specimens, and statistical comparisons of regional measurements were used to quantitate changes. These measurements documented shifting patterns of cell loss depending on the time of injection. For example, injection on day 16 led to significant reduction in cortex thickness, and depletion in the pyramidal cell layer of the hippocampus, while injection on DG 18 produced reduction in the hippocampal dentate gyrus. Jones et al. (1982) also studied effects of fetal 5-azacytidine injection (1–1.5 mg per pregnant rat) and found the morphological effects on cortex to be similar to those of MAM.

Fluorodeoxyuridine (FUdR)

This fluorinated pyrimidine antimetabolite is converted by intracellular thymidine kinase into a potent inhibitor of thymidylate kinase. Langman and Cardell (1977) found that necrotic cells appeared in the neuroepithelial layer within 2 h of a dose of 45 mg/kg on day 12 of gestation in mice. The drug ceased to act within about 12 h after injection as mitotic figures returned. Within 48 h a morphologically normal neuroepithelium was rebuilt.

FUdR's effect on the cerebellum has also been studied (Langman et al., 1972). In 2-day-old mice treated with three injections of 5-FUdR (50 mg/kg), granule cell damage similar to that produced by radiation and other toxins was produced.

Hydroxyurea

This simple compound is chemically unrelated to the others and inhibits ribonucleoside diphosphate reductase which is important for DNA synthesis. Adlard and Dobbing (1975) studied the brains of rats whose mothers received hydroxyurea (1 or 2 g/kg) at 14 days of gestation. At birth, rats exposed to 1 g/kg suffered a 27% reduction in body weight and 34% reduction in brain DNA, with the forebrain predominantly affected. Two g/kg produced somewhat more effect on body weight but no more reduction in brain weight. Behavior on maze tasks was impaired. The precise neuronal deficits produced by hydroxyurea treatment of developing rats have not been reported.

Synaptic disruptors

Chemical synaptic disruptors ablate neurons which have expressed specific synaptic markers. Toxins in this group may be expected to spare neurons which have not yet extended neuronal processes and differentiated along a specific neurotransmitter phenotype. Many toxins might act through synaptic mechanisms in the developing brain. However, relatively few have been examined in detail (Jonsson, 1980).

The neurotoxic effects of glutamate and several excitatory amino acid analogues have been explored in the neonatal period (Olney, 1971). Their destructive actions appear to differ at this age from effects in mature animals. The neurotoxicity of glutamate itself in newborn animals is very restricted, in part because a very active reuptake system limits the duration of high concentrations of transmitter in the synapse. A hypothalamic toxicity syndrome has been described after neo-

438

natal glutamate administration (Olney, 1969). In the mature brain, the toxicity of glutamate and its analogs has been linked to their actions on specific subtypes of excitatory amino acid neurotransmitter receptors. Autoradiographic examination of the ontogeny of these receptors in the human fetus and newborn as well as in rats shows that they are transiently expressed in several regions and then lost during postnatal development. This pattern of transient expression and reorganization during the differentiation of amino acid pathways could provide a substrate for shifting patterns of synaptic disruption and selective cell death in the developing brain. Although this group of toxins has not yet been exploited extensively for teratology studies in the fetal brain, they may prove to be useful tools for producing selective lesions.

Differential sensitivity to glutamate analogs during development

Neurotoxic analogs of glutamate may cause neuronal death by interacting with one of three types of recognition sites preferring kainic acid, quisqualic acid or N-methyl-D-aspartate (NMDA) (Zaczek and Coyle, 1982; Watkins and Olverman, 1987). Kainic acid requires the presence of glutamate released from presynaptic nerve terminals as well as specific receptors to exert its neurotoxic action. Kainate is relatively inactive as a neurotoxin in the striatum of newborn rats. Presynaptic glutamate terminals are relatively immature at that age. At high concentrations toxicity has been reported in the neonatal hippocampus (Cook and Crutcher, 1986). Development of toxicity with age in striatum correlates with the ontogenetic rise in synaptosomal uptake of [³H]glutamate into nerve terminals and addition of specific receptors for [³H]kainate (Campochiaro and Coyle, 1978). In contrast, NMDA and quisqualic acid both produce neurotoxic lesions in immature rat brain. Silverstein et al. (1986b) showed that 100 nmol of quisqualic acid injected into the striatum cause neuronal loss in the stria-

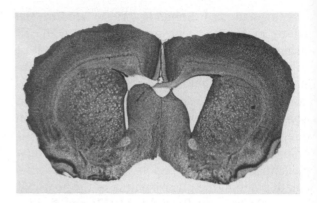

Fig. 11 Effect of injection of the glutamate analogue, quisqualic acid (0.1 μmol in 1 μl 0.01 M Tris, pH 7.4) at 7 days of age. At 12 days, the sections showed reduction in the size of the striatum and neuronal loss with asymmetric dilatation of the ventricle. (From Silverstein et al., 1986b).

tum and adjacent hippocampus (Figs. 11 and 12). The hippocampal lesion produced by quisqualate is distinctive in that damage is limited to the CA3 and 4 regions of the hippocampus with some injury to dentate gyrus. Quisqualic acid appears to produce less injury in adult animals (Zaczek and Coyle, 1982). Because no specific inhibitor of quisqualic acid is available, direct proof that it acts through the quisqualate receptors is lacking. Ibotenic acid, a preferential but nonspecific NMDA agonist produces lesions in the immature brain (Steiner et al., 1984). NMDA injection into the immature striatum (10–100 nmol) produces extensive necrosis of the hemisphere, including cortex, hippocampus and striatum. NMDA effects are blocked by the non-competitive antagonist MK-801 (McDonald and Johnston, unpublished).

The possible sites of action for these toxins, glutamate neurotransmitter recognition sites, undergo considerable reorganization in the fetal and neonatal brain. The human fetal and neonatal brain and the developing rat brain contain high densities of glutamate recognition sites in several regions where few glutamate sites are found in the mature brain (Greenamyre et al., 1987; Barks et al., 1986). Fig. 13 shows a comparison of glutamate binding sites in a 21-week-old human

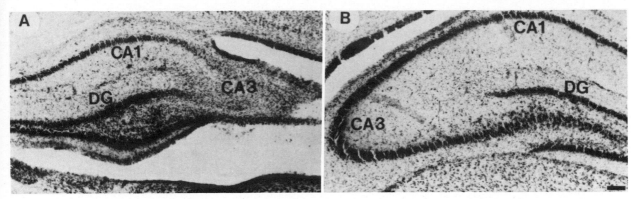

Fig. 12 Photomicrographs of Nissl-stained formalin-fixed sections of hippocampus from a 12-day-old rat which had been injected into the corpus striatum with 1 μl containing 0.1 μmol quisqualic acid at 7 days of age. (A) On the side of injection the tissue adjacent to the lateral ventricle is necrotic and CA_3 and CA_4 are disrupted. The opposite side (B) is intact. Bar = 100 μm; CA, cornu ammonis; DG, dentate gyrus. (From Silverstein et al., 1986b).

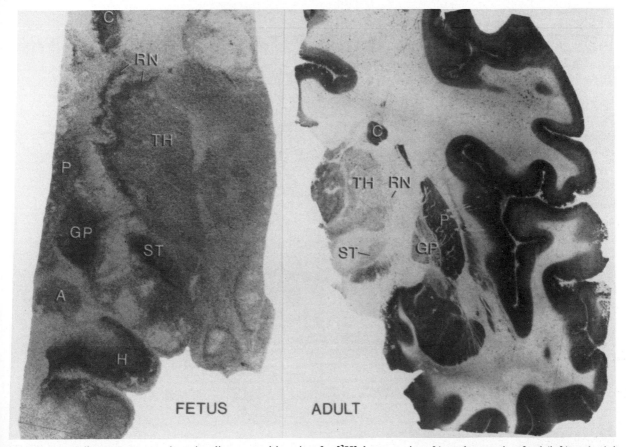

Fig. 13 Autoradiograms prepared to visualize recognition sites for [³H]glutamate in a 21 week gestation fetal (left) and adult (right) human postmortem brain. The autoradiograms were prepared as described in Greenamyre et al. (1987). Note high densities of binding in globus pallidus (GP), reticular nucleus of the thalamus (RN) and subthalamic nucleus (ST) in fetal brain with low densities of binding sites in adults. Other abbreviations: C, caudate nucleus; TH, thalamus; P, putamen; A, amygdala; H, hippocampus. (From Barks et al., 1987.)

fetal brain compared with a similar region from an adult brain using in vitro receptor autoradiography. For these studies, slide-mounted frozen sections were washed and incubated at 2 °C for 45 min in 50 nM Tris-HCl buffer containing CaCl$_2$ and 27 nM [^{3}H]glutamate, using a previously reported protocol (Greenamyre et al. 1987). Inclusion of calcium in the buffer enhances binding to quisqualate-preferring sites. Comparison of the fetus and adult demonstrates transient

regions of glutamate recognition site expression in globus pallidus, subthalamic nucleus and reticular nucleus of the thalamus. We also observed transient dense expression in the substantia innominata/basal nucleus region in one fetal brain. Transient expression of kainate receptors has also been observed in the human hippocampus (Represa et al., 1986).

Autoradiographic studies in the fetus have also demonstrated that the potential sites of action of

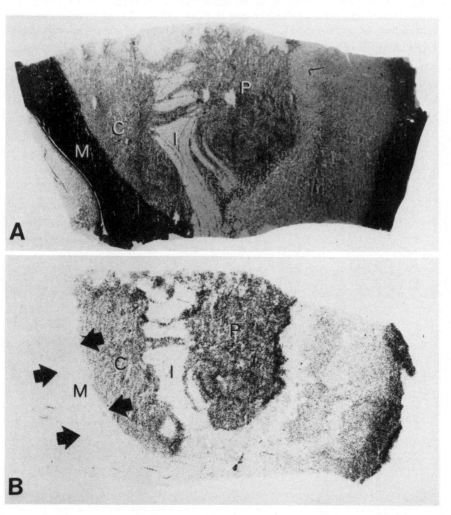

Fig. 14 Adjacent coronal frozen sections through a 21-week-old fetal brain stained for Nissl substance (A) and prepared for visualization of [^{3}H]glutamate recognition sites (B), as described above. Area of dense Nissl staining in A is germinal matrix (M), which does not contain [^{3}H]glutamate binding sites in autoradiogram (arrows). Glutamate binding sites are present in immature caudate (C) and putamen (P) and a patchy pattern of binding is apparent. (From Barks et al., 1987.)

glutamate neurotoxins may be distinct from those for mitotic toxins (Fig. 14). Glutamate recognition sites and recognition sites for other transmitters we have studied are not expressed in the germinal matrix, where mitotic disrupters exert their actions. If the appearance of recognition sites correlates with neurotoxicity, then these observations suggest that immature neurons are not vulnerable until they have migrated into their target areas and undergone initial differentiation.

Pharmacological studies using [^{3}H]glutamate displaced with quisqualate suggest that several regions expressing these sites (e.g., globus pallidus) contain predominantly high affinity quisqualate-preferring sites. However, the newborn hippocampus also contains substantial populations of NMDA-preferring sites and this type becomes more numerous throughout development. Autoradiographic studies of glutamate receptors indicate considerable regional segregation of receptor subtypes. More information is needed to understand the shifting relationships between these receptor subtypes during development. These sites are potential targets for glutamate analog neurotoxins and also may be functionally relevant to normal brain development. Frieder and Grimm (1987) demonstrated that prenatal monosodium glutamate causes long lasting cholinergic and adrenergic changes in the developing brain. The recognition sites described are possible targets mediating these effects. This work suggests a number of issues which deserve further exploration.

Analogies with human disorders

A variety of human brain disorders may be produced by mechanisms which disrupt dividing and/or differentiating neurons. Microcephaly is a relatively common outcome from early fetal insult (e.g., viral infections). Reduced neuronal replication in the neuroepithelium is one defect associated with Down's syndrome (Ross et al., 1984). Recent evidence suggests that synaptic neurotoxicity may play an important role in brain injury from hypoxia-ischemia, hypoglycemia and status epilepticus (Johnston and Silverstein, 1986; Rothman and Olney, 1987). Hypoxia-ischemia stimulates neurotransmitter turnover in immature brain and causes temporary paralysis of the high affinity glutamate uptake site (Silverstein et al., 1986a). Regions of the immature brain enriched in glutamate receptors are selectively vulnerable to hypoxic-ischemic injury. Glutamate receptor blockers prevent neuronal damage from hypoxia-ischemia in vivo and in vitro (Rothman and Olney, 1987; McDonald et al., 1987). Intrauterine hypoxia may cause a variety of neurological disorders and it is probable that some of its effects may be mediated by disruption of neurons bearing excitatory synapses. If this mechanism is an important one in humans, administration of toxic glutamate analogs to fetuses may produce animal models for some of these disorders.

Conclusions

Toxins disrupt developing neurocircuitry by interacting with target macromolecules in the brain. Certain selective mitotic disruptors briefly interact with nucleic acids and kill dividing neurons but leave differentiating neurons intact. Synaptic neurotoxins have the potential to ablate selected post-mitotic neurons which have acquired functional synapses. Recent work has provided new insights into the sites and actions of these two types of toxins. These chemical tools are useful for modelling fetal brain abnormalities and understanding relationships between abnormal circuitry and behavior.

Drugs and toxins disrupt brain development by targeting key molecules which direct brain formation. Study of animal models which produce selective neuropathologic, neurochemical or behavioral abnormalities is likely to provide insight into the molecular basis of brain development. Study of behavioral teratology is an important end in itself, but the analysis becomes more powerful when combined with insights into the morphologic and biochemical nature of disrupted

442

synaptic circuitry. The models presented in this review deserve further examination with these thoughts in mind. Replicating DNA in the germinal matrix of the embryonic brain and nascent synapses stimulated by toxic excitatory amino acids form two important groups of targets susceptible to developmental toxins. Improving understanding of the molecular nature of these events should allow a finer resolution of mechanisms of neurotoxicity.

These observations also underline the axiom that the developing brain is quantitatively and qualitatively unique. Brain maturation is characterized not only by acquisition of neurons and support elements but reorganization and loss of certain elements. Just as replicating neurons are absent in the adult brain, certain neurotransmitter circuits appear to be pruned in the course of development. No doubt, some of these evanescent circuits serve critical but temporary roles at appropriate stages for normal progression of brain and behavioral development. They also provide targets for teratogens which disrupt the fetal brain.

References

Adlard, B.P.F. and Dobbing, J. (1975) Maze learning by adult rats after inhibition of neuronal multiplication in utero. *Pediat. Res.*, 9: 139–142.

Adlard, B.P.F., Dobbing, J. and Sands, J. (1975) A comparison of effects of cytosine arabinoside and adenine arabinoside on some aspects of brain growth and development in the rat. *Br. J. Pharmacol.*, 54: 33–39.

Altman, J. (1966) Autoradiographic and histological studies of postnatal neurogenesis. *J. Comp. Neurol.*, 128: 431–474.

Altman, J. (1969) Autoradiographic and histologic studies of postnatal neurogenesis. III. Dating the time of production and onset of differentiation of cerebellar microneurons in rats. *J. Comp. Neurol.*, 135: 269–294.

Angevine, J.B. and Sidman, R.L. (1961) Autoradiographic studies of cell migration during histogenesis in the cerebral cortex of the mouse. *Nature*, 192: 766–768.

Balduini, W., Abbraccio, M.P., Lombardelli, G. and Cattabeni, F. (1984) Loss of striatal neurons after methylazoxymethanol acetate treatment in pregnant rats, *Dev. Brain Res.*, 15: 133–136.

Balduini, W., Cimino, M., Lombardelli, G., et al. (1986) Microencephalic rats as a model for cognitive disorders, *Clin. Neuropharmacol.*, 9: 58–518.

Barks, J., Sims, K., Greenamyre, T., Silverstein, F. and Johnston, M. (1988) Distribution of neurotransmitter receptors in human fetal brain, *Neurosci. Lett.*, 84: 131–136.

Beaulieu, M. and Coyle, J.T. (1981) Effects of fetal methylazoxymethanol acetate lesion on the synaptic neurochemistry of the adult rat striatum, *J. Neurochem.*, 37: 878–887.

Beaulieu, M. and Coyle, J.T. (1982) Fetally-induced noradrenergic hyperinnervation of cerebral cortex results in persistent down regulation of beta receptors, *Dev. Brain Res.*, 4: 491–494.

Calabresi, P. and Parks, R.E. (1980) Chemotherapy of neoplastic diseases. In *The Pharmacologic Basis of Therapeutics*, A. Goodman and L. Gilman (Eds.), Macmillan, New York, pp. 1249–1313.

Calvet, M., Drian, M. and Privat, A. (1974) Spontaneous electrical patterns in cultured Purkinje cells grown with an antimitotic agent. *Brain Res.*, 79: 285–290.

Cannon-Spoor, H.E. and Freed (1984). Hyperactivity induced by prenatal administration of MAM: association with altered performance on conditioning tasks. *Pharmacol. Biochem. Behav.*, 20: 189–193.

Campochiaro, P. and Coyle, J.T. (1978) Ontogenetic development of kainate neurotoxicity: correlates with glutamate innervation. *Proc. Natl. Acad. Sci. USA.*, 75: 2025–2029.

Chabner, B.A., Myers, C.E. and Oliverio, V.T. (1977) Clinical pharmacology of anticancer drugs. *Semin. Oncol.*, 4: 165–191.

Chema, S.H. and Lauder, J.M. (1983) Infrapyramidal mossy fibers in the hippocampus of methylazoxymethanol acetate induced microencephalic rats. *Dev. Brain Res.*, 9: 411–415.

Cook, T.M. and Crutcher, K.A. (1986) Intrahippocampal injection of kainic acid produces significant pyramidal cell loss in neonatal hippocampus of rats, *Neuroscience*, 18: 79–92.

Das, G.D. and Pfaffenroth, P. (1972) Effects of ethylnitrosourea on the development of the brain. *Experientia*, 28: 1076–1077.

DeBarry, J., Gombos, G., Klupp, T. and Hamori, J. (1987) Alteration of mouse cerebellar circuits following methylazoxymethanol treatment during development: immunohistochemistry of GABAergic elements and electron microscopic study, *J. Comp. Neurol.*, 261: 253–265.

Druckrey, H.S., Ivankovic, S. and Preussman, R. (1966) Teratogenic and carcinogenic effects in the offspring after a single injection of ethylnitrosourea to pregnant rats. *Nature*, 210: 1378–1379.

Fischer, M.H., Welker, C. and Waisman, H.A. (1972) Generalized growth retardation in rats induced by prenatal exposure to methylazoxymethanol acetate. *Teratology*, 5: 223–232.

Fishaut, J.M., Connor, J.D. and Lampert, P.W. (1974) Comparative effects of arabinosyl nucleosides upon the postnatal growth and development of the rat. *Pediatr. Res.*, 8: 825–829.

Frieder, B. and Grimm, V.E. (1987) Prenatal monosodium glutamate causes long-lasting cholinergic and adrenergic changes in various brain regions. *J. Neurochem.*, 48: 1359–1365.

Giurgea, C., Greinde, M.G., Preat, S., Puigdevall, J. (1982) Piracetam compensation of MAM-induced behavioral deficits in rats. In S. Corkin, K. Davis, J. Gravdin, E. Usdin and R. Wurtman (Eds.), *Alzheimers Disease, a Report of Progress*, Raven Press, New York, pp. 281–290.

Greenamyre, J.T., Penney, J.B., Young, A.B., Hudson, C., Silverstein, F.S. and Johnston, M.V. (1987) Evidence for a transient perinatal glutamatergic innervation of globus pallidus. *J. Neurosci.*, 7: 1022–1030.

Grondin, G., Sharkey, T., Jones, M., Sculthorpe, A. and Taylor, W. (1975) Postnatal cerebellar hypoplasia and dysfunction following methylazoxymethanol acetate treatment. *Proc. Soc. Exp. Biol. Med.*, 148: 156–159.

Haddad, R.K., Rabe, A. and Dumas, R. (1972) Comparison of effects of methylazoxymethanol acetate on brain development in different species. *Fed. Proc.*, 31: 1520–1523.

Haddad, R., Rabe, A. and Dumas, R. (1979) Neuroteratogenicity of methylazoxymethanol acetate: behavioral deficits of ferrets with transplacentally induced lissencephaly. *Neurotoxicology*, 1: 171–189.

Haddad, R.K., Rabe, A., Laqueur, G.L., Spatz, M. and Volsamis, M.M. (1969) Intellectual deficit associated with transplancentally induced microcephaly in the rat. *Science*, 163: 88–90.

Hallas, B.H. and Das, G.D. (1979) An aberrant nucleus in the telencephalon following administration of ENU during neuroembryogenesis. *Teratology*, 19: 159–164.

Hicks, S.P. and D'Amato, C.J. (1968) Cell migrations to isocortex in the rat. *Anat. Rec.*, 160: 619–634.

Johnston, M.V., Carman, A.B. and Coyle, J.T. (1981) Effects of fetal treatment with methylazoxymethanol acetate at various gestational dates on the neurochemistry of the adult cortex of the rat. *J. Neurochem.*, 36: 124–128.

Johnston, M.V. and Coyle, J.T. (1979) Histological and neurochemical effects of fetal treatment with methylazoxymethanol on the rat neocortex in adulthood. *Brain Res.*, 170: 135–155.

Johnston, M.V. and Coyle, J.T. (1980) Ontogeny of neurochemical markers for noradrenergic, GABAergic and cholinergic neurons in neocortex lesioned with the methylazoxymethanol acetate. *J. Neurochem.*, 34: 1429–1441.

Johnston, M.V. and Coyle, J.T. (1982) Cytotoxic lesions and the development of transmitter systems. *Trends Neurosci.*, 5: 153–156.

Johnston, M.V. and Silverstein, F.S. (1986) New insights into mechanisms of neuronal damage in the developing brain. *Pediatr. Neurosci.*, 12: 87–89.

Johnston, M.V., Grzanna, R. and Coyle, J.T. (1979) Methylazoxymethanol treatment of fetal rats results in abnormally dense noradrenergic innervation of neocortex. *Science*, 203: 369–371.

Johnston, M.V., Haddad, R., Carman-Young, A. and Coyle, J.T. (1982) Neurotransmitter chemistry of lissencephalic cortex induced in ferrets by fetal treatment with methylazoxymethanol acetate. *Dev. Brain Res.*, 4: 285–291.

Jones, E.G., Valentino, K.L. and Fleshman, J.W. (1982) Adjustment of connectivity in rat neocortex after prenatal destruction of precursor cells of layers II–IV. *Dev. Brain Res.*, 2: 425–431.

Jones, M.A. and Gardner, E. (1976) Pathogenesis of methylazoxymethanol-induced lesions in the postnatal mouse cerebellum. *J. Neuropathol. Exp. Neurol.*, 35: 413–444.

Jonsson, G. (1980) Chemical neurotoxins as denervation tools in neurobiology. *Ann. Rev. Neurosci.*, 3: 169–187.

Jonsson, G. and Hallman, H. (1982) Effects of prenatal methylazoxymethanol treatment on the development of central monoamine neurons. *Dev. Brain Res.*, 2: 513–530.

Kasubuchi, Y., Wakaizumi, S., Shimada, M. and Kusunoki, T. (1977) Cytosine arabinoside-induced transplacental dysgenetic hydrocephalus in mice. *Teratology*, 16: 63–70.

Langman, J. and Cardell, L. (1977) Cell degeneration and recovery of the fetal mammalian brain after a chemical insult. *Teratology*, 16: 15–30.

Langman, J. and Shimada, M. (1971) Cerebral cortex of mouse after a prenatal chemical insult. *Am. J. Anat.*, 132: 355–374.

Langman, J., Shimada, M. and Rodier, P. (1972) Floxuridine and its influence on postnatal cerebellar development. *Pediatr. Res.*, 6: 758–764.

Lovell, K.L., Goetting, M.G. and Jones, M.Z. (1980) Regeneration in the cerebellum following methylazoxymethanol-induced destruction of the external germinal layer. *Dev. Neurosci.*, 3: 128–139.

Matsumoto, H., Spatz, M. and Laqueur, G.L. (1972) Quantitative changes with age in the DNA content of methylazoxymethanol-induced microcephalic rat brain. *J. Neurochem.*, 19: 297–306.

Matsutani, T., Nagayoshi, M., Tamaru, M. and Tsukada, Y. (1980) Elevated monoamine levels in the cerebral hemispheres of microencephalic rats treated prenatally with methylazoxymethanol or cytosine arabinoside. *J. Neurochem.*, 34: 950–956.

McDonald, J.W., Silverstein, F.S. and Johnston, M.V. (1987) MK-801 protects the neonatal brain from hypoxic-ischemic damage. *Eur. J. Pharmacol.*, 140: 359–361.

Mohammed, A.K., Jonsson, G., Sundstrom, E., Minor, B.G., Soderberg, U. and Archer, T. (1986) Selective attention and place navigation in rats treated prenatally with methylazoxymethanol. *Dev. Brain Res.*, 30: 145–155.

Moran, T.H., Sanberg, P.R., Antuono, P.G. and Coyle, J.T. (1986) Methylazoxymethanol acetate (MAM) cortical hypoplasia alters the pattern of stimulation induced behavior in neonatal rats. *Dev. Brain Res.*, 27: 235–242.

Nagata, Y. and Matsumoto, H. (1969) Studies on methylazoxymethanol: methylation of nucleic acids in the fetal rat brain. *Proc. Soc. Exp. Biol. Med.*, 132: 383–385.

Nathanson, N., Cole, G.A. and VanderLoos, H. (1969) Heterotopic cerebellar granule cells following administration of cyclophosphamide to suckling rats. *Brain Res.*, 15: 532–536.

Olney, J. (1969) Brain lesion, obesity and other disturbances in mice treated with monosodium glutamate. *Science*, 164: 719–721.

Olney, J. (1971) Glutamate induced neuronal necrosis in the infant mouse hypothalamus: an electron microscopic study. *J. Neuropathol. Exp. Neurol.*, 30, 75.

Olson, J.M.M., Greenamyre, J.T., Penny, J.B. and Young, A.B. (1987) Autoradiographic localization of cerebellar excitatory amino acid binding sites. *Neuroscience*, in press.

Rabe, A. and Haddad, R.K. (1972) Methylazoxymethanol-induced microcephaly in rats: behavioral studies. *Fed. Proc.* 31: 1536–1539.

Represa, A., Tremblay, E., Schoevart, D. and Ben-Ari, Y. (1986) Development of high affinity kainate binding sites in human and rat hippocampi. *Brain Res.*, 384: 170–174.

Rodier, P.M. and Reynolds S.S. (1977) Morphological correlates of behavioral abnormalities in experimental congenital brain damage. *Exp. Neurol.*, 57: 81–93.

Rodier, P.M. (1977) Correlations between prenatally-induced alterations in CNS cell populations and postnatal function. *Teratology*, 16: 235–246.

Rodier, P.M. (1980) Chronology of neuron development: animal studies and their implications. *Dev. Med. Child. Neurol.*, 22: 252–545.

Ross, M.H., Galaburda, A.M. and Kemper, T.L. (1984) Downs syndrome: is there a decreased population of neurons? *Neurology*, 34: 909–916.

Rothman, S.M. and Olney, J.W. (1987) Excitotoxicity and the NMDA receptor. *Trends Neurosci.*, 10: 299–302.

Sanberg, P.R., Moran, T.H. and Coyle, J.T. (1987) Microencephaly: cortical hypoplasion induced by methylazoxymethanol. In J.T. Coyle (Ed.), *Animal Models of Dementia*, Alan Liss, New York, pp. 253–278.

Sanger, V., Yang, M. and Mickelson, O. (1972) Cycasin-induced central nervous system lesions in postnatal mice. *Fed. Proc.*, 1524–1529.

Schultze, B., Nowak, B. and Maurer, W. (1974) Cycle times of neural epithelial cells of various types of neurons in the rat. An autoradiographic study. *J. Comp. Neurol.*, 158: 207–218.

Seil, F.J., Leiman, A.L. and Woodward, W.R. (1980) Cytosine arabinoside effects on developing cerebellum in tissue culture. *Brain Res.*, 186: 393–408.

Shapiro, R. (1968) Chemistry of guanine and its biologically active significant derivatives. *Prog. Nucleic Acid Res. Biol.*, 8: 73–112.

Shimada, M. and Langman, J. (1970) Repair of the external granular layer of the hamster cerebellum after prenatal and postnatal administration of methylazoxymethanol. *Teratology*, 3: 119–134.

Silverstein, F.S., Buchanan, K. and Johnston, M.V. (1986a) Perinatal hypoxia-ischemia disrupts striatal high affinity 3H-glutamate uptake into synaptosomes. *J. Neurochem.*, 47: 1614–1619.

Silverstein, F.S., Chen, R. and Johnston, M.V. (1986b) The glutamate analogue quisqualic acid is neurotoxic in striatum and hippocampus of immature rat brain. *Neurosci. Lett.*, 71: 13–18.

Singh, S.C. (1977) Ectopic neurons in the hippocampus of the postnatal rat exposed to methylazoxymethanol during fetal development. *Acta Neuropathol.*, 40: 111–116.

Slevin, J.T., Johnston, M.V., Biziere, K. and Coyle, J.T. (1982) Methylazoxymethanol acetate ablation of mouse cerebellar granule cells: effects on synaptic neurochemistry. *Dev. Neurosci.*, 5: 3–21.

Spatz, M. and Laqueur, G.L. (1968) Transplacental chemical induction of microencephaly in two strains of rats. *Proc. Soc. Exp. Biol. Med.*, 129: 705–710.

Steiner, H.X., McBean, G.J., Kohler, C., Roberts, P.J. and Schwarcz, R. (1984) Ibotenate-induced neuronal degeneration in immature brain. *Brain Res.*, 307: 117–124.

Vorhees, C.V., Fernandez, K., Dumas, R.M. and Haddad, R.K. (1984) Pervasive hyperactivity and long-term learning impairments in rats with induced microcephaly from prenatal exposure to methylazoxymethanol. *Dev. Brain Res.*, 15: 1–10.

Watkins, J.C. and Olverman, H.J. (1987) Agonists and antagonists for excitatory amino acid receptors. *Trends Neurosci.*, 10: 265–272.

Zaczek, R. and Coyle, J.T. (1982) Excitatory amino acid analogues: neurotoxicity and seizures. *Neuropharmacology*, 21: 15–26.

Discussion

J.W. Olney: We have studied an hypoxic-ischemic model similar to the one you study but we are attempting to evaluate which brain regions are most sensitive and we do not find the globus pallidus very sensitive. Is this consistent with or contrary to your findings?

M.V. Johnston: We have found that glutamate (Glu) receptors measured autoradiographically in 7-day-old rats exposed to unilateral carotid ligation and hypoxia are disrupted in the globus pallidus as well as in selected regions of the caudate putamen and hippocampus (Silverstein et al., 1987). This is consistent with a sensitivity in this region. However, due to the cytological characteristics of the region, we found it difficult to quantitate the effect on the globus pallidus. We have noted that receptors expressed in the infant are predominantly of the quisqualate-preferring type.

J. W. Olney: In addition to the increased number of Glu receptors in globus pallidus, you found an increase in the capacity of the Glu uptake system. Would not the latter counter-balance the former with regard to vulnerability to hypoxic/ischemic damage?

M. V. Johnston: We indeed found that hypoxia-ischemia reversibly blocks Glu uptake. This step is important for mediation by excitatory amino acids damage (Silverstein et al., 1986).

J. W. Olney: If many of the Glu receptors through which Glu destroys neurons during neonatal hypoxia/ischemia are quisqualate receptors, how do you explain the ability of the *N*-methyl-D-aspartate (NMDA) antagonist, MK-801, to prevent such damage? Even if the NMDA/ionophore complex is totally blocked, Glu can kill neurons via quisqualate receptors which MK-801 does not block.

M. V. Johnston: We are investigating this issue. We found that MK-801 is strongly protective against damage from hypoxia-ischemia and NMDA in 7-day-old rats and partially protective against neurotoxicity of quisqualate in 1-day-old rat pups (McDonald et al., 1987; McDonald and Johnston, unpublished). This is consistent with some interaction between quisqualate and the NMDA type cation channel (Jahr and Stevens, 1987).

J. Sweeney: When MK-801 is given before onset of ischemic damage or 1.5 h after onset, you have total protection. However, not when given at the onset of the damage. Can you explain this discrepancy? Are you proposing a 2-stage model of destruction?

M. V. Johnston: MK-801 in our experiments was given either at the beginning of hypoxia *and* 1.25 h after the beginning, or simply at the beginning *or* at 1.25 h. Protocols for which it was given *both* at the beginning and end or at 1.25 h were fully neuroprotective against hypoxia-ischemia (McDonald et al., 1987). A dose at the beginning was only partially neuroprotective. We assume that the late dose was very effective in blocking events causing permanent injury and the early dose was not necessary. We have not hypothesized a 2-stage model but think there is a threshold effect (Silverstein and Johnston, 1984).

H. Sterz: I wonder if it is possible to use methylazoxymethanol as a time probe in order to produce specific extraneuronal lesions in organs, e.g., in heart or aortic arches that are dependent on neurogenic imput for correct development?

M. V. Johnston: This is a very interesting question that deserves exploration. I am not aware of studies of these effects. Though the treated animals are overtly healthy, we have not examined their hearts or blood vessels in detail.

R. Balazs: First of all I want to express my appreciation for your elegant studies. We have come to similar conclusions to yours on the basis of the analysis of a different system. We have recently obtained evidence that excitatory amino acid transmitters besides their possible neurotoxic action also serve transiently a trophic role (Balazs, Ch. 28, this volume). Here I should only like to mention that the responses of cerebellar granule cells to the stimulation of the NMDA-preferring subtype of Glu receptors depend on the maturational stage of the cells. In particular, NMDA promotes the survival in culture of the relatively immature granule cells. These are the counterparts of granule cells at the end of their migration when they became innervated by the mossy fibers, a great proportion of which is glutamatergic. This trophic phase is followed by a transient period when, as shown by Garthwaite and Garthwaite (1986), NMDA is toxic to the cells and finally in the adult the cells are resistant to NMDA. It is plausible that the granule cell/mossy fiber partnership is not unique in this respect and that at least some of the redundant projections in the developing brain may serve such a transient trophic function.

M. V. Johnston: We are presently exploring the ontogeny of Glu receptor subtypes and their connection with Glu ion channels and second messenger systems in the developing brain. In addition to our observation that Glu receptors are present in certain regions in the fetus and neonate and disappear at later times, we also noted shifts in receptor subtypes, for example from quisqualate-preferring receptors to NMDA-preferring receptors in certain regions during development period (Greenamyre et al., 1987). A shift in receptor subtypes and changing connections with ionic channels and second messengers such phosphoinositide (PI) turnover might be expected to alter the functional impact of receptor stimulation. I suspect that these phenomena are the basis for the very interesting results you have reported. We have found that exposure to an hypoxic-ischemic insult alters the apparent coupling between quisqualate type Glu receptors and PI turnover (Chen et al., 1987). Twenty-four hours after an hypoxic-ischemic insult in 7-day-old rat pups, the PI response to quisqualate is increased in slices. As shown by Nicoletti et al. (1986), Glu-stimulated turnover is markedly higher in the neonatal brain compared with the adult. In contrast with quisqualate, NMDA is relatively inactive in stimulating PI turnover but of course it is quite active in opening ionic channels and producing cell death. The contribution of quisqualate PI turnover to cell death following insults such as hypoxia-ischemia is presently unknown. Based on the function of inositol phosphates in other systems to increase intracellular calcium and evoke gene expression (Whitman et al., 1986), it is possible that Glu-stimulated PI turnover might serve as a trophic signal in the developing brain. Therefore, although the details of these relationships are far from clear, it seems to be reasonable to hypothesize that marked shifts in the functional impact of Glu are likely to be related to the biochemical shifts already observed in the developing brain.

446

References

Garthwaite, G. and Garthwaite, J. (1986) In vitro neurotoxicity of excitatory amino acid analogues during cerebellar development. *Neuroscience*, 17: 755–767.

Chen, C.K., Silverstein, F.S., Fisher, S.K., Statman, D. and Johnston, M.V. (1987) Perinatal hypoxia-ischemia enhances quisqualic acid and stimulated phosphoinositide (PPI) turnover. *J. Neurochem.*, in press.

Greenamyre, T., Peureg, J.B., Young, A.B., Hudson, C., Silverstein, F.S. and Johnston, M.V. (1987) Evidence for transient perinatal glutamatergic innervation of globus pallides. *J. Neurosci.*, 7: 1022–1030.

Jahr, C.E. and Stevens, C.F. (1987) Glutamate activates multiple single channel conductances in hippocampal neurons. *Nature*, 325: 522–525.

McDonald, J.W., Silverstein, F.S. and Johnston, M.V. (1987) MK-801 protects the neonatal brain from hypoxic-ischemic damage. *Eur. J. Pharmacol.*, 140: 359–361.

Nicoletti, F., Iadarola, M.J., Wroblewski, J.T. and Costa, E. (1986) Excitatory amino acid recognition sites coupled with inositol phospholipid metabolism: development changes and interactions with alpha1-adrenoreceptors. *Proc. Natl. Acad. Sci. U.S.A.*, 83: 1931–1935.

Silverstein, F.S. and Johnston, M.V. (1984) Effects of hypoxia-ischemia on monoamine metabolism in the immature brain. *Ann. Neurol.*, 15: 342–347.

Silverstein, F.S., Buchanan, K. and Johnston, M.V. (1986) Hypoxia-ischemia disrupts striatal high affinity 3H-glutamate uptake into synaptosomes. *J. Neurochem.*, 47: 1614–1619.

Silverstein, F.S., Torke, L., Barks, J. and Johnston, M.V. (1987) Hypoxia-ischemia produces focal disruption of glutamate receptors in developing brain. *Dev. Brain Res.*, 34: 33–39.

Whitman, M., Fleischman, L., Chahwala, S.B., Cantley, L. and Losoff, P. (1986) Phosphoinositide, mitogenesis, and oncogenesis. In J.W. Patrey (Ed.), *Phosphoinositides and Receptor Mechanisms*, Alan R. Liss, New York, pp. 197–217.

G.J. Boer, M.G.P. Feenstra, M. Mirmiran, D.F. Swaab and F. Van Haaren
Progress in Brain Research, Vol. 73
© 1988 Elsevier Science Publishers B.V. (Biomedical Division)

CHAPTER 28

Metabolic imbalance and nerve cell damage in the brain

Robert Balázs

Medical Research Council, Developmental Neurobiology Unit, 1 Wakefield Street, London WC1N 1PJ, UK

Introduction

Insults of various kinds, such as interference with the supply of oxygen and glucose, sustained seizure activity and brain trauma, may compromise survival of nerve cells in the CNS. In this review there is no room to consider the different conditions separately, rather an attempt will be made to extract mechanisms which seem to be common. This is evidently an over-simplification, as the different disorders have, besides common features, specific characteristics which must be taken into account and will influence treatment. There are excellent reviews and proceedings of symposia which may be consulted for more detailed information (e.g. Hossmann et al., 1977; Siesjö, 1981; Siesjö and Agardh, 1983; Siesjö and Wieloch, 1985; Nemoto, 1985; Inaba et al., 1985; Schwarcz and Ben-Ari, 1986). Finally, although this meeting is devoted to neuroteratology, the survey will not focus on the developing CNS. The implications are, however, most relevant and it should be noted that haemorrhagic/ischaemic lesions in the brain in the perinatal period are a major cause of intellectual and physical handicap in the child.

Vulnerability of the brain

This is related to the fact that although the brain is one of the great energy-consumer organs of the body, it lacks substantial energy stores. Thus the brain constitutes only about 2% of the body weight, yet it accounts for approximately 20% of the total oxygen uptake (for reviews see Balázs, 1969; Siegel et al., 1981; Siesjö and Agardh, 1983). It should be noted, however, that there are substantial regional differences: e.g. in the rat, glucose utilization in terms of labelled deoxyglucose uptake is about 0.4 μmol/g/min in the corpus callosum and 2 μmol/g/min in the inferior colliculus (Sokoloff et al., 1977). It is well documented that the brain normally derives almost all its energy from the aerobic oxidation of glucose, although ketone bodies may, in part, act as substitutes in special circumstances such as during the suckling period in the rat and in prolonged starvation in man (e.g. Balázs, 1969; Siegel et al., 1981). If the supply of oxygen and/or glucose is compromised, the substrate reserves in the brain are only sufficient to meet requirements for a very limited time (e.g. Balázs, 1969; Siesjö, 1981; Siesjö and Agardh, 1983). The breakdown of energy homeostasis results in immediate biochemical and morphological alterations throughout the CNS, but it should be emphasized that even if the energy supply is restored in time to prevent death, lasting pathological changes may occur which are usually preferentially localized to relatively well-defined parts of the brain (for review see Siesjö, 1981; Siesjö and Agardh, 1983). Such areas are the cerebral cortex, the hippocampus (pyramidal cells in layers 3 and 5–6, and in CA1 and CA3–4, respectively) and the cerebellar cortex (the inhibitory interneurones and Purkinje cells, although the latter are relatively spared in hypoglycaemia).

Biochemical consequences of severe metabolic stress

The exhaustion of the brain energy reserves, which, for example in hypoglycaemia, seems to occur when the glucose concentration in the blood falls to about 1 mM, is associated with a decrease of cerebral ATP levels from 3 to about 0.5 μmol/g, when the EEG becomes isoelectric and coma sets in (Siesjö and Agardh, 1983). Prior to this, the progressive reduction in the energy supply is accompanied by clinical signs, including behavioural changes, and overt coma may be preceded or accompanied by convulsions, which may contribute to the exhaustion of the endogenous substrates. The maintenance of the energy-dependent transmembrane ion gradients is compromised under these conditions, resulting in a decrease in the intracellular activity of K^+ and an increase in that of Na^+. Depolarization leads to an influx of Ca^{2+} through voltage-sensitive Ca^{2+} channels (VSCC), which is instrumental in the presynaptic release of transmitters, including, in particular, excitatory amino acids (EAA) (see below) even under conditions when the increase in extracellular K^+ prevents the firing of action potentials (e.g. Sykova, 1983). EAA may further aggravate the situation by stimulating the influx of Na^+ and Ca^{2+} (Mayer and Westbrook, 1987). Elevated cytosolic Ca^{2+} may activate proteinases and phospholipases (PLase) (see e.g. Siesjö, 1981). The resulting increase in free fatty acids together with the elevated $[Na]_i$ leads to the mobilization of Ca^{2+} from mitochondria and the endoplasmic reticulum, thus further augmenting cytosolic free Ca^{2+} levels (Siesjö and Wieloch, 1985). The liberation of arachidonic acid from phospholipids activates eicosanoid production (Fig. 1). Reactions in these pathways generate free radicals which, under pathological conditions, may also be formed in excess through other routes.

In the section below some of the changes which seem to be critical in inducing cell damage as a result of the metabolic imbalance will be discussed.

Redistribution of monovalent ions

During total cerebral ischaemia the intracellular uptake of Na^+ greatly exceeds the release of K_i^+ (at 1 h 139 vs. 64 meq/l; Hossmann et al., 1977). This is accompanied by an uptake of Cl^- and H_2O from the extracellular fluid causing a reversible shrinkage of the extracellular space from about 20 to 9%. K^+ released from nerve cells is mainly taken up by astrocytes, which also accumulate Cl^- and H_2O (Siesjö and Wieloch, 1985). Swelling of astrocytes is indeed one of the earliest signs of interference with the energy supply to the brain (see below), and this may further hinder the transport of substrates from the blood to the nerve cells. Swelling of neuronal structures, especially of dendrites, is also evident (Siesjö and Wieloch, 1985). At this stage, the alterations are still more or less reversible. In ischaemia, osmotically active substances, especially cations, are generated in the tissue, so that during reperfusion significant uptake of Cl^- and H_2O from the blood may cause further swelling (Hossmann, 1985). After prolonged ischaemia, a new phenomenon is manifested: the blood-brain barrier becomes permeable to macromolecules (see below: Eicosanoids) and the extracellular space starts to increase. The oedema is now associated with protein extravasation and the developing cyst signifies the stage of irreversible cell damage.

Elevation of free cytosolic calcium ions

It has long been suspected that elevated free $[Ca^{2+}]_i$ may cause cell degeneration, and the hypothesis has been put forward forcefully for such a role of Ca^{2+} in brain damage (Siesjö, 1981). The proposal is that metabolic stress can cause an increase in free cytosolic calcium as a result of Ca^{2+} entry from the extracellular fluid through the depolarization-activated VSCC and also through receptor-linked channels (e.g. associated with a subtype of EAA receptors). Ca^{2+} extrusion from the cells and the storage of Ca^{2+} require energy, which is in short supply. The toxic effect of elevated free $[Ca^{2+}]_i$ is believed to be mediated through the activation of proteinases and PLase. The increase in free fatty acids will further augment $[Ca^{2+}]_i$ by mobilization from cytoplasmic stores, and the effect is aggravated by the activation of eicosanoid formation, free radical generation and peroxidation of cell constituents.

Oxygen-derived free radicals

It has been known for some time that free radicals can cause tissue damage under certain conditions (e.g. oxygen toxicity, radiation exposure, vitamin E deficiency, carbon tetrachloride poisoning; Varon, 1973). However, the hypothesis put forward by Demopoulos et al. (1980), that excessive generation of free radicals may underlie cell injury as a result of ischaemia or CNS trauma, has been a conceptually new proposal.

There are many cellular reactions that involve *controlled* free radical formation, including those of the electron transport chain, the hydroxylation reactions of the endoplasmic reticulum and the initial steps in eicosanoid formation (Chance et al., 1979). Demopoulos et al. (1980) have suggested that free radical formation may occur when O_2 is deficient by uncoupling the electron transport chain. As a result coenzyme Q, which is at the transition from two to one electron transfer in the chain, may undergo auto-oxidation in the hydrophilic portion of the inner mitochondrial membrane, leading to the production of the superoxide radicals ($^{\cdot}O_2^-$). It seems that the really dangerous free radicals are not the superoxide, but the hydroxy radicals ($^{\cdot}OH$) and the singlet oxygen ($^1O_2$). These are formed by the metal-catalysed interaction of $^{\cdot}O_2^-$ with H_2O_2 catalysed by superoxide dismutase (SOD).

A different mechanism involving extravasation of blood was proposed for free radical damage occurring in CNS trauma (Demopoulos et al., 1980). Iron compounds such as hematin can accelerate the auto-oxidation of unsaturated lipids by 5 orders of magnitude.

Molecular damage due to free radicals may involve DNA, RNA, proteins and lipids. Polyunsaturated fatty acyl (PUFA) chains in membrane phospholipids are especially good substrates for peroxidative and metal-catalysed free radical reactions. These are initiated by the abstraction of an allylic H^+ from PUFA, followed by a rearrangement of the double bonds (conjugation) and the formation of peroxide radicals through the addition of oxygen. The interaction with another PUFA generates hydroperoxides, while the abstraction of H^+, e.g. from another PUFA, sets in motion the propagation of peroxidation. The consequences to the membrane structure are damaging: in contrast to the unsaturated bonds in PUFA, which are bent at an angle of $123°$, most of the double bonds are in the unbent configuration after peroxidation (Varon, 1973). The compaction of the membrane is further exaggerated by cross-linking adjacent lipid fatty acyl groups or proteins. The affected fatty acids finally fragment to form malondialdehyde and fluorescent products. The resulting change in the lipid composition and in viscosity may have severe consequences for the functioning of membrane enzymes and transport systems as well as receptor-mediated reactions.

It should be pointed out that there are important defence mechanisms against free radicals. These include enzymes removing free radicals such as SOD, catalases and peroxidases (in the brain the latter are most significant), as well as non-enzymatic antioxidants (α-tocopherol, ascorbate, sulphur-containing and phenolic amino acids). Furthermore, although it is firmly established that, in certain conditions, free radicals are involved in pathogenesis (see above), the evidence for their contribution to ischaemic brain damage is inconclusive. Extensive studies from the labora-

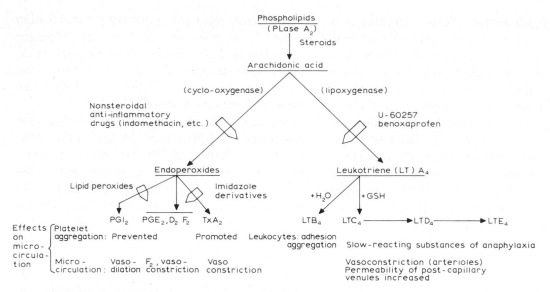

Fig. 1 Scheme of formation of eicosanoids: prostaglandins (PG), thromboxanes (Tx) and leukotrienes (LT). Certain critical enzymes are given in brackets, and some of the main inhibitors are also indicated. For more detailed information see Samuelsson (1983) and Wolfe (1982).

tory of Siesjö (1981) failed to detect the occurrence of enhanced lipid peroxidation in ischaemia. However, investigations from this group confirmed the observations of Myers (1979) indicating that the outcome of prolonged periods of ischaemia or hypoxia is significantly better in fasted than in fed animals, the difference being attributed to acidosis, which was pronounced in the latter group. Acidosis may exaggerate free radical damage as a result of the formation of the protonated form of superoxide radicals, which is a more lipid-soluble and stronger oxidant than $\cdot O_2^-$, and of the release of protein-bound iron and consequently an increased rate of peroxidation (Siesjö et al., 1985).

Eicosanoids

An important pathway of free radical generation is the formation of eicosanoids from arachidonic acid (Fig. 1). However, it is probably even more important that many of these substances are potent agents which influence cellular processes through second-messenger systems (cyclic nucleotide formation and Ca^{2+} mobilization), sensitize tissues to the effects of other mediators, but most significantly in the present context may have a powerful influence on cerebral microcirculation. The rate-limiting step in this cascade of reactions is the liberation of arachidonic acid from phospholipids activated by the elevation of $[Ca^{2+}]_i$, which may occur as a consequence of metabolic insults. It has been found that trauma, hypoxia, hypoglycaemia, ischaemia and status epilepticus result in a rapid increase in the content of free arachidonic acid and in stimulation of prostaglandin synthesis (for review see Wolfe, 1982). The cyclo-oxygenase pathway leads to the formation of prostacyclin (PGI_e), other prostaglandins (PG) and thromboxanes (Tx). PGI_2, the principal product in cerebral blood vessels and capillaries, causes vasodilation and prevents platelet aggregation. TxA_2 is a very potent constrictor of cerebral vessels and it promotes platelet aggregation. The lipoxygenase pathway (Samuelsson, 1983) produces leukotrienes (LT) which enhance the adhesion to the vessel walls of leukocytes and induce their aggregation (leukotriene B4, LTB_4). The cysteinyl derivatives of leukotrienes, of which LTD_4 is the most potent, cause vasoconstriction and increase the permeability of postcapillary venules. Thus these substances are important regulators of microcirculation – with PGI_2 promoting while Tx as well as LT cause interference with microcirculation. Fig. 1 shows some of the major inhibitors of these pathways which have also been used in therapy. Corticosteroids inhibit eicosanoid formation by inducing the synthesis of a protein inhibitor of PLase activity. Cyclo-oxygenase is inhibited by non-steroidal anti-inflammatory drugs, while a prostacyclin derivative, U-60257, and benoxaprofen block LT formation. With respect to cerebral pathological mechanisms, the inhibition of the synthesis of PGI_2 by lipid peroxidation products may be significant. It has been suggested that alterations in the balance of PGI_2 vs. Tx and LT may interfere with microcirculation and the retention of the proteins by the blood vessels, thus contributing to irreversible ischaemic brain damage (Demopoulos et al., 1980).

Excitatory amino acids (EAA)

The foundations of the recent interest in the possibility that EAA are involved in nerve cell injury caused by energy imbalance have been laid by the identification of these amino acids as abundant excitatory transmitters (e.g. Curtis and Watkins, 1960). The conceptual advance, linking the neuroexcitatory effects of EAA with their neurotoxic action, has been made by Olney et al. (1971), while the experimental approach was facilitated by the discovery and the synthesis of EAA transmitter receptors agonists and antagonists (Watkins and Evans, 1981).

Briefly, the current proposal is that in ischaemia, hypoxia, hypoglycaemia and as a result of sustained epileptic seizures, an excess of EAA is released which has a neurotoxic effect through over-stimulation of neurones. One of the major approaches in testing this proposal involved the use of EAA transmitter antagonists. It has been found that neuronal damage in the hippocampus or the caudate nucleus caused by

ischaemia (Simon et al., 1984) or by hypoglycaemia (Wieloch, 1985) could be prevented by focal administration of antagonists, which interact selectively with the N-methyl-D-aspartate (NMDA) -preferring EAA receptors, such as 2-amino-5-phosphonovalerate (APV) or 2-amino-7-phosphonoheptanoate (APH). Furthermore, a role for EAA transmitters in epilepsy has been indicated by the powerful anticonvulsant properties of EAA receptor antagonists in a wide range of animal models of epilepsy (Schwarcz and Meldum, 1985). Moreover, the involvement of synaptically released EAA in neuronal injury due to metabolic stress has been indicated by the observation that the removal of the corticostriatal or corticohippocampal glutamatergic input protects the striatum against hypoglycaemia (Wieloch et al., 1985) or the hippocampus against ischaemic damage (Pulsinelli, 1985).

Model systems for metabolic stress

Effect of anoxia on cerebellar slices

Now I will consider in vitro model systems, such as brain slices and cultured neural cells, which have certain advantages in elucidating mechanisms since, by limiting the influence of compounding secondary effects, the experimental conditions can be better controlled than in vivo. We decided to examine the effect of anoxia and ischaemia using rat cerebellar cortical slices, since we established methods for obtaining preparations which during incubation retained excellent structural preservation and biochemical as well as electrophysiological competence (e.g. Garthwaite et al., 1979; Crepel et al., 1981). The experimental question was whether synaptic failure, believed to be a major feature of the electric changes in transmission noted in hypoxia, reflects defects in presynaptic performance (Bosley et al., 1983). The neurochemical approach to investigate synaptic function was to examine Ca^{2+}-dependent stimulus-coupled transmitter release. In the cerebellar cortex the major excitatory and inhibitory transmitters are Glu/Asp and GABA,

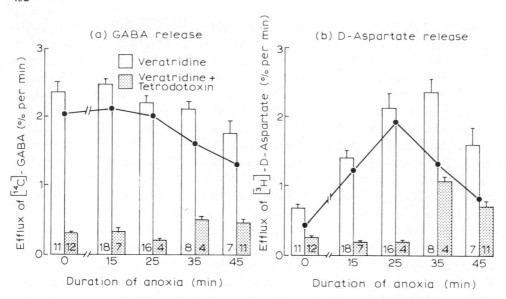

Fig. 2 Effect of anoxia (95% N_2/5% CO_2) on depolarization-induced [^{14}C]GABA (a) and D-[^{3}H]ASP release (b) from prelabelled hand-cut adult cerebellar slices. The mean $\pm$ S.E. (n indicated at the base of the bars) of the fractional release rate is given. Closed circles represent the stimulus-coupled release (the difference in efflux caused by 100 μM veratridine in the absence and the presence of 1 μM TTX). Note that evoked release of [^{14}C]GABA is not affected by 25 min of anoxia, while that of D-[^{3}H]Asp is markedly increased (from Bosley et al., 1983.)

respectively (Krnjevic, 1982). Therefore, the release from prelabelled slices of [^{14}C]GABA and D-[^{3}H]Asp (a metabolically relatively stable analogue of Glu and Asp) was induced by depolarization with either elevated K^+ or veratridine at different times after exposure of the tissue to anaerobic conditions, in both the presence and the absence of glucose (anoxia and 'ischaemia', respectively).

The intriguing observation was that anoxia, associated with a severe depression of ATP levels, may persist for a long time before adverse effects on presynaptic performance become detectable. Thus, evoked release of [^{14}C]GABA was not reduced during 25 min of anoxia, while surprisingly that of D-[^{3}H]Asp was markedly increased (Fig. 2). Morphological studies showed that in anoxia the earliest changes can be detected in glial cells (swelling), while nerve terminals are by far the most resistant (Figs. 3 and 4). This is consistent with the long preservation of neurochemical processes associated with transmitter release. However, the finding that the evoked release of D-[^{3}H]Asp is significantly greater in anoxia than in controls implies the operation of additional factors.

The increase in the D-[^{3}H]Asp release in anoxia was not due to a depression of amino acid

Fig. 3 Light micrographs of cerebellar slices incubated in glucose-containing Krebs-medium aerobically (a) or anaerobically for 10 min (b) and 30 min (c), and for 5 min of ischaemia (d). Note the good preservation in (a), the marked swelling of the radial fibres of the Bergmann glia in (b) and of the glial endfeet under the pia (arrows) in (c). Purkinje cells are little affected after 10 min in 95% N_2/5% CO_2, but they are swollen or pyknotic (arrowheads) after 30 min. Granule cell nuclei start to swell by 10 min of anoxia. Vacuolation is evident throughout the cerebellar cortex by 30 min (c), when most of the inhibitory interneurones are markedly swollen or pyknotic. After 5 min of ischaemia, vacuolation and glial swelling are evident in the molecular layer and granule cells start to become enlarged. Scale bar = 100 μm. (from Bosley et al., 1983.)

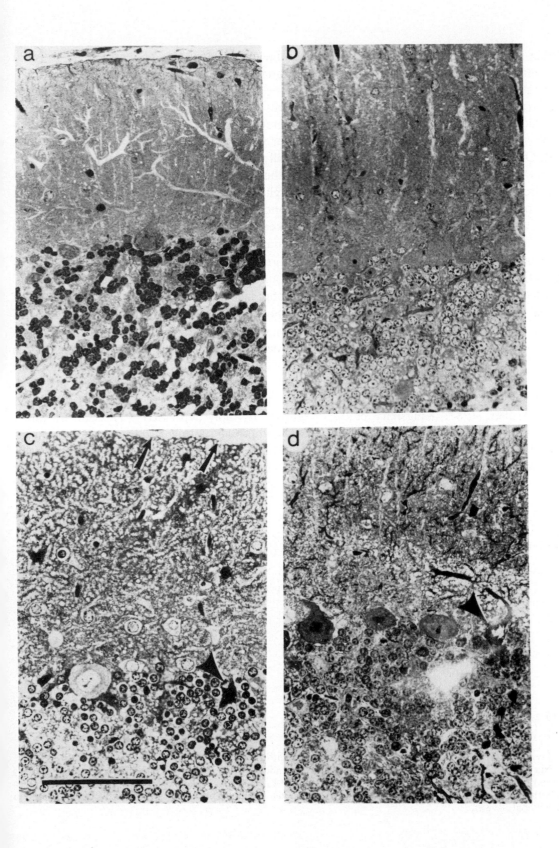

reuptake. Table 1 shows that evoked D-[^{3}H]Asp release was virtually unaffected by threo-3-hydroxy aspartate (T3HA), a potent inhibitor of acidic amino transport (Balcar and Johnston, 1972). Reuptake was a significant process accounting for about 40% of the total released D-Asp in both O_2 and N_2 atmosphere. However, the experiments with T3HA revealed that anoxia resulted in a dramatic increase in D-Asp efflux, predominantly originating from tetrodotoxin insensitive 'extrasynaptic' sites.

Findings on the stimulated release of endogenous amino acids were consistent with those obtained with the exogenous amino acids. Only four endogenous amino acids exhibited stimulus-coupled release in cerebellar slices: Glu, Asp, GABA and Gly. Although Gly is apparently not a transmitter in the cerebellum (Krnjevic, 1982), it may have a role in transmission by potentiating responses elicited by the stimulation of the NMDA-preferring subtype of Glu receptors (Johnson and Ascher, 1987; Kingsbury et al., 1988). Anoxia for 25 min resulted in an increase of veratridine-induced release of only one of the amino acids. This was Glu; however, it is noteworthy that the increase – compared with the

aerobic slices – was only about 50% vs. 4–6-fold elevation of D-[^{3}H]Asp release.

The difference in the findings with the endogenous and exogenous EAA facilitated a better understanding of the effects of anoxia on transmitter release. In cerebellar slices, D-[^{3}H]Asp is initially taken up to a greater extent by glia than by other structures (Wilkin et al., 1982). We found that glia are more vulnerable than nerve terminals to anoxia (cf. Fig. 3), when D-Asp efflux is markedly increased from non-synaptic (thus presumably glial) structures (Table 1, release in the presence of tetrodotoxin (TTX) and T3HA). It would appear that glia are not only morphologically but also metabolically compromised, since of all the endogenous amino acids only the efflux of Gln, which reflects cellular Gln levels, was markedly reduced in anoxia. Moreover, it is known that Gln synthetase (GS) is almost exclusively localized in astrocytes in the CNS (e.g. Patel et al., 1982, and refs. therein). Decreased Gln levels imply depressed ATP concentrations in the glial compartment (Gln synthesis requires ATP). The maintenance of the transmembrane Na^+ gradient, which is crucial for acidic amino acid transport, is energy-dependent. Thus, it is

TABLE 1

Increase of stimulated D-[^{3}H]aspartate release in anoxia is not due to inhibition of the reuptake of the amino acid

	D-[^{3}H]Asp efflux (% of tissue D-[^{3}H]Asp per min)					
	Control			Anoxia		
	T3HA		D-Asp reuptake	T3HA		D-Asp reuptake
	−	+		−	+	
Veratridine	0.59	0.94	0.35	2.13	3.68	1.55
Veratridine + TTX	0.27	0.49	0.22	0.18	1.93	1.75
Evoked release	0.32	0.45		1.95	1.75	

Slices preloaded with D-[^{3}H]Asp were incubated in an atmosphere of either 95% O_2/5% CO_2 (control) or 95% N_2/5% CO_2; exposure to anoxia was for 20 min before stimulation. Concentrations added to the basal medium (Krebs Henseleit solution) were 100 μM veratridine, 1 μM tetrodotoxin (TTX) and 500 μM threo-3-hydroxy-D,L-aspartate (T3HA). TTX and T3HA were present during both the unstimulated and the stimulated release periods. Estimates are the means of 4–16 experiments (data taken from Bosley et al., 1983).

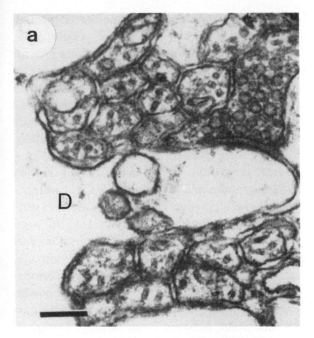

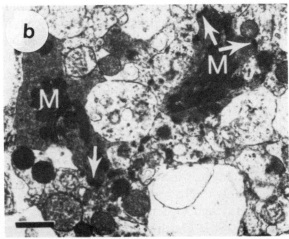

Fig. 4 (a) Electronmicrographs showing the badly swollen dendrite of a Purkinje cell (D) after 30 min of anoxia. However, the parallel fibre synapse on the dendritic spine is intact and contains a normal complement of synaptic vesicles. In addition, the ultrastructural appearance of the parallel fibres is similar to the controls. (b) Cerebellar glomerulus after 10 min of ischaemia. The mossy fibre rosettes (M), especially the mitochondria, are relatively well preserved, while the dendritic digits of the granule cells and their mitochondria are badly swollen. Scale bars 0.2 μm in (a) and 1 μm in (b). (From Bosley et al., 1983).

unlikely that the sites of the massive reuptake of D-Asp which takes place in anoxic slices (Table 1) were the astrocytes. It is more feasible that uptake occurred preferentially into nerve terminals, which are relatively spared in anoxia (Fig. 4). Such a redistribution of D-[^{3}H]Asp may account for the striking increase observed in the synaptic release of this substance during anoxia (Fig. 2). Similarly, anoxia might lead to the redistribution of endogenous Glu, although the relative increase in synaptic concentration may be less marked than in the case of D-[^{3}H]Asp, as the initial cellular distribution of Glu is not biased so much in favour of the glia. This may be a factor contributing to the relatively smaller rise in stimulated release of endogenous Glu than exogenous D-[^{3}H]Asp. The unaltered release of GABA during 25 min anoxia (Fig. 2) is consistent with the view that, in comparison with other structures, both the uptake of exogenous GABA and the concentration of endogenous GABA are high in nerve terminals under normal conditions.

This study (Bosley et al., 1983) demonstrated a selective increase in evoked Glu release in the anoxic brain tissue. This process may continue after the EEG becomes isoelectric, when it would depend on elevated [K$^+$]$_e$, rather than on the invasion of the terminals by action potentials. The hyperactivity of glutamatergic synapses under conditions of oxygen deprivation is not peculiar to the cerebellum or the experimental conditions used in this work. It has been observed that K$^+$-induced release of labelled Glu is increased from cerebral cortical slices in anoxia (Arnfred and Hertz, 1971). Furthermore, the increase in the amplitude of the deep tendon reflexes during hypoxia in vivo seems to be caused by an increase in EPSP size, which, in turn, is likely to be the result of an increased synaptic output of the relevant transmitter, i.e. Glu (Kristein, 1951). Finally, Benveniste et al. (1984), using intrahippocampal microdialysis, have observed a selective in vivo increase in the extracellular content of Glu (8-fold), Asp (3-fold) and Tau (2.6-fold) as a result of 10 min of complete cerebral ischaemia. In view of the neurotoxicity of EAA (Olney, Chapter 18 of this volume) and the relatively selective vulnerability in hypoxia of neurones which are thought to receive glutamatergic synaptic input, it can be concluded that hyper-release of Glu may be involved in neuronal damage in conditions which compromise energy production in the brain (Bosley et al., 1983; see also Benveniste et al., 1984).

Neural tissue culture

The view of the involvement of EAA in causing neuronal damage in anoxia has recently been supported by studies on cultured nerve cells. Rothman (1983) has observed that young nerve cells in dispersed hippocampal cultures (up to 2 days in vitro, DIV) are resistant to anoxia, while more mature neurones (at least 14 DIV) die after the same exposure. However, the death of mature neurones could be prevented, using either a high concentration of Mg^{2+}, which interferes with transmitter release and also selectively blocks the NMDA receptor-linked ion channel, or a wide-spectrum EAA receptor antagonist, γ-D-gluta-mylglycine (DGG) (Rothman, 1984). In agreement with these indications, exposure of the cultures to Glu or Asp resulted in the destruction of mature neurones (Rothman, 1984; Choi, 1985). Furthermore, the difference between young and mature neurones in their sensitivity to EAA is similar to that in their sensitivity to anoxia (Choi et al., 1987).

Excitatory amino acids during development: maturational stage-dependent trophic or toxic action

The dependence of the effect of EAA on the stage of maturation of nerve cells is highlighted in the developing cerebellum. We recognized this while studying mechanisms underlying the survival requirement in culture of granule cells taken from 6–8-day-old rat cerebellum (P6–8) for K^+-induced depolarization (Lasher and Zagon, 1972). It was observed that the effect of depolarization

in promoting cell survival is mediated through stimulated Ca^{2+} entry via VSCC (Gallo et al., 1987). The most convincing evidence was provided after it was discovered that granule neurones are endowed with VSCC, at which the potency of organic Ca^{2+} effectors, especially dihydropyridines (DHP), is as high as in muscle tissue (Kingsbury et al., 1986; Kingsbury and Balázs, 1987; see also Carboni et al., 1985). DHP Ca^{2+} agonists were able to replace elevated K^+ in rescuing granule cells (Fig. 5), while Ca^{2+} antagonists blocked the effect of depolarization on normal survival (Gallo et al., 1987). The vital question was, however, what is the physiological process that is mimicked by the K^+-induced Ca^{2+} entry into the granule cells? The critical information was that the survival dependence on depolarization develops in culture within a narrow time-span, between 2 and 4 DIV. Comparison of the maturation of the cells in culture with the development of the postmitotic granule cells in vivo led to the formulation of a hypothesis implicating the afferent input first received by granule neurones from the mossy fibres at the end of their migration as providing the trophic influence in vivo that is mimicked by depolarization in vitro (Gallo et al., 1987). Many of the mossy fibres are glutamatergic (Somogyi et al., 1986), and granule cells possess EAA receptors, including the NMDA subtype, which gates ion channels permeable not only to Na^+ and K^+, but also to Ca^{2+} (Cull-Candy and Ogden, 1985; Cull-Candy and Usowicz, 1987; Garthwaite et al., 1986; Mayer and Westbrook, 1987). Thus the hypothesis predicts that stimulation of NMDA receptors should sustain the survival of cerebellar granule cells under conditions (low medium-K^+) which otherwise result in the degeneration of these cells.

We have now tested this hypothesis (Balázs and Jørgensen, 1987; Balázs et al., 1988a,b) and Fig. 6 shows the dramatic influence of NMDA in promoting the survival of the cerebellar granule cells. The effect of NMDA was specific: it was inhibited by the selective receptor antagonist APV and by blocking the NMDA-receptor-linked ion

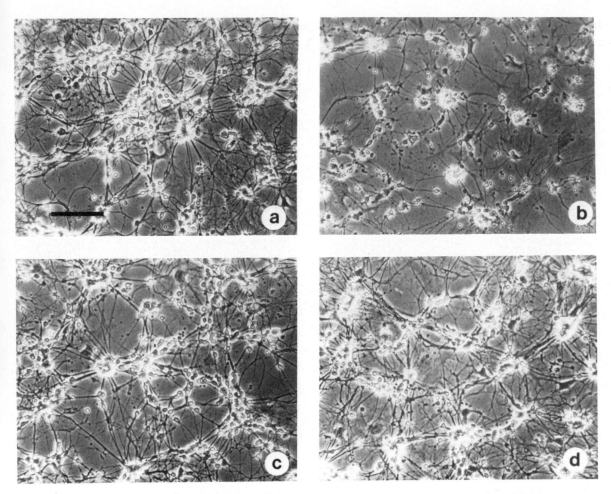

Fig. 5 Ca^{2+} agonsists can replace elevated K^+ in promoting the survival of cerebellar granule neurones. Cultures from rat cerebella (P6–8) were grown for 8 DIV in media containing K^+ at 25 mM (a) or 15 mM (b–d). The Ca^{2+} agonist (+)-(S)-202 791 was added at a concentration of 1×10^{-6} M (c) and 5×10^{-8} M (d) at 2 DIV. Scale bar, 100 μm. (From Gallo et al., 1987).

channel with MK-801 (Balázs, Hack and Cotman, unpublished observation). Furthermore, the potency and the efficacy of NMDA depended on the concentration of K^+, reflecting the voltage dependence of the blockade by Mg^{2+} of the receptor-linked ion channel (Nowak et al., 1984). Control experiments showed that the survival of cells secured by 25 mM K^+ was not compromised either by AVP or by NMDA. The findings indicate that (a) the critical trophic influence is Ca^{2+} entry: if this is brought about by opening the voltage-sensitive channels (by elevated K^+),

the blockade of the NMDA receptors and thus the receptor-linked Ca^{2+} conductance have no effect on survival. Furthermore, (b) NMDA exerts no toxic action on granule cells derived from P6–8 rat cerebella and cultured for 7–10 days. This behaviour is unusual for a neurone possessing EAA receptors since, as described above, there is extensive evidence that both in vivo and in vitro EAA may exert toxic actions on nerve cells. In particular, the detailed investigations by Garthwaite and colleagues have shown that in cerebellar slices, depending on the

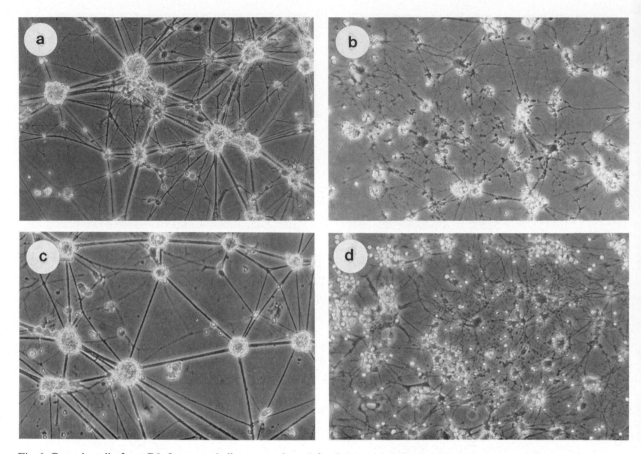

Fig. 6 Granule cells from P6–8 rat cerebella were cultured for 7 days. (a) Cell grown in a 10% fetal calf serum-containing medium in the presence of 25 mM K⁺ are preserved, but (b) degenerate when the K⁺ concentration is 10 mM. (c) Addition of 140 μM NMDA to sister cultures in 10 mM K⁺ rescues the cells. (d) This effect is blocked by the NMDA receptor antagonist, APV (140 μM).

developmental stage of the tissue, NMDA can induce granule cell degeneration (e.g. Garthwaite and Garthwaite, 1986a; Garthwaite et al., 1986b, 1987).

The trophic effect of NMDA on granule cells has become detectable in our studies, mainly because of certain properties of the culture which was used. The procedure of the dissociation of cerebellar tissue from P6–8 rat cerebellum, combined with certain manipulations of the culture conditions, initially results in the preferential selection for immature granule cells. Most of these cells would still carry on replicating in vivo, but in vitro they immediately start to differentiate. As a consequence, the culture is primarily composed of a cohort of more or less synchronously differentiating granule neurones. Thus transient effects which are dependent on the stage of maturation of the cells, and would easily be masked in the whole tissue, become clearly detectable. The trophic influence of the stimulation on the NMDA receptor is such a transient event in the life of the granule cells.

Combining the information on the toxic action of NMDA in cerebellar slices (Garthwaite and Garthwaite, 1986) with the trophic action of NMDA in granule cell cultures (Balázs et al., 1987, 1988a), we propose the following scenario for EAA receptor stimulation-mediated events in the cerebellum during development (Table 2).

TABLE 2

The effect of NMDA depends on the maturational state of cerebellar granule cells

Maturational state of granule cells	Effect of NMDA		
	Depolarization[a]	Trophic[b]	Toxic[c]
External granule cells	?	–	–
Postmitotic, migrating granule cells	?	–	–
Internal granule cells just arrived and innervated	?	+	–
differentiating	+	–	+
fully differentiated	±	–	–

[a] From Garthwaite et al., 1986, 1987.
[b] Balázs and Jørgensen, 1987; Balázs et al., 1987.
[c] Garthwaite and Garthwaite, 1986.
Effect elicited, + ; not detected, – ; weak, ± ; not known, ?

Granule cells are not sensitive to EAA until the end of their migration, when they first receive synaptic input from the mossy fibres. It is suggested that granule cells taken from P6–8 rat cerebellum after 2 days in culture are the in vitro counterparts of these newly innervated neurones. This is the stage of development when, according to our in vitro findings, NMDA receptor stimulation exerts a trophic influence on granule cells. Garthwaite and Garthwaite (1986), studying the toxic effect of EAA in cerebellar slices, have observed that only the differentiating granule cells are vulnerable to NMDA, although those in the upper region of the internal granule cell layer (IGL) are not adversely affected. These are the cells which have just arrived in the IGL, and according to our proposal NMDA is a trophic rather than a toxic factor for these cells. As the maturation of the cells progresses, NMDA becomes toxic to the cells. Finally, fully differentiated granule cells are not sensitive to NMDA: they are not vulnerable and, in contrast to the younger differentiating cells which are destroyed by NMDA, this EAA elicits only very weak depolarizing responses from the adult granule cells (Garthwaite et al., 1986, 1987).

Concerning the mechanisms of EAA action, results on cerebellar slices and dispersed cultures show that in both the trophic and the toxic effect, transmembrane Ca^{2+} entry plays a vital role. Observations on hippocampal cultures and incubated retina indicate the possible involvement of extracellular Na^+ and Cl^- in EAA-induced neuronal degeneration (Rothman and Olney, 1986; however, see Garthwaite and Garthwaite, 1986b). Recent findings by Choi (1987) are consistent with the view expressed in a review by Rothman and Olney (1986) that the immediate and the somewhat delayed toxic effects are exerted respectively by Na^+/Cl^- and Ca^{2+}.

We obtained evidence indicating that the survival-promoting effect of depolarization-induced Ca^{2+} entry is mediated through reactions involving calmodulin (Gallo et al., 1987). Certain properties of the Ca^{2+}-calmodulin-dependent protein kinase II make this enzyme a good candidate for mediating the trophic effect (for refs. see Gallo et al., 1987). Increased Ca^{2+} entry through the NMDA-receptor-linked channel may have led to trophic changes through the same route. NMDA receptors have been suggested as playing a role in plasticity in the mature CNS (Morris et al., 1986; Collingridge and Bliss, 1987) and also – though evidence is very limited – in the developing brain (Singer et al., 1986; Rauschecker and Hahn, 1987). It is plausible therefore that trophic influences mediated through the stimulation of NMDA receptors by synaptically released EAA are not unique to the cerebellar granule cells, but are manifested – depending on the developmental stage – in many nerve cell classes throughout the nervous system. During development, nerve cells make abundant projections, even to areas which they do not innervate in the adult (Purves and Lichtman, 1985). It is generally considered that this is a reflection of one of the principal strategies of the developing nervous system, this being to generate a surplus of cells, fibres and synapses in order to ensure that the proper connections are made. These redundant projections may, however, fulfil a functional role by providing, at the right time, a trophic influence on their transient synaptic partners.

Therapeutic implications

The realization that the liberation of excess EAA may be involved in causing neuronal damage in metabolic stress has obvious therapeutic implications. The possibilities have already been indicated in studies on experimental animals. Thus EAA antagonists are able to ameliorate brain damage in ischaemia and hypoglycaemia and can prevent seizures in experimental epilepsy (e.g. Meldrum et al., 1987). In these studies, EAA antagonists have been used, including the selective NMDA-receptor antagonists, APV and APH, whose penetration into the brain is limited. However, the discovery that dissociative anaesthetics and σ-opioids are powerful blockers of the NMDA-receptor-linked ion channels has now provided a new generation of drugs which may be administered systemically (Kemp et al., 1987). Results are already forthcoming to show that brain damage caused by metabolic insults can be prevented by their application, although further work must still be done to ensure the development of drugs which do not elicit undesirable psychotomimetic effects. Concerning the potential use of such agents in the treatment of perinatal brain damage, the trophic action of EAA transmitters on developing nerve cells must also be taken into account. Furthermore, with respect to the success of treatment, the question of how long after the insult cellular injury is still reversible has become most relevant. In this context, it is also worth mentioning that animal experiments suggest that even the adult mammalian CNS has some capacity for repair (e.g. Haber et al., 1983), and that a better understanding of factors which are essential to the survival of particular nerve cells may facilitate the prevention of irreversible damage after injury (Varon et al., Chapter 29 of this volume).

It is evident from this review that in addition to EAA other factors are also involved in the pathological effects of metabolic stress, and that the complex nature of these disorders must be taken into consideration in order to provide effective treatment.

Summary

The following changes, which seem to be critical in inducing cell damage in the CNS as a result of metabolic imbalance, due to insufficient supply of O_2 and/or glucose or overstimulation (sustained seizures), were considered: (1) perturbation of the K^+-, Na^+- and Cl^--transmembrane gradients, (2) elevation of cytosolic free Ca^{2+}, (3) excessive generation of free radicals and peroxidation of cellular constituents, (4) imbalance in the generation of particular eicosanoids, and (5) excessive liberation of excitatory amino acids (EAA).

Observations on the effects of EAA in model systems in vitro were presented in more detail, since the relatively well-controlled experimental conditions may facilitate the better understanding of mechanisms underlying the neurotoxic action of EAA. Recent observations indicating that EAA during development may also have a trophic influence were described and it was emphasized that the effect of EAA (trophic or toxic or eliciting no response) depends on the stage of maturation of the nerve cells.

Promising results from animal experiments indicate that information on mechanisms involved in cell injury induced by metabolic stress in the brain has important therapeutic implications.

Acknowledgements

The important contribution from my laboratory to the work included in this review, particularly by Mac Bosley, Vittorio Gallo, Bob Gordon, Niki Hack, Ann Kingsbury and Peter Woodhams, is acknowledged. I am grateful to Ole Jørgensen (Psychochemistry Institute, Copenhagen, Denmark) for his permission to give a relatively detailed account of our joint studies, prior to full publication. I am indebted to Carl Cotman, John Garthwaite and Silvio Varon for most helpful discussions.

References

Arnsfred, T. and Hertz, L. (1971) Effects of potassium and glutamate on brain cortex slices: Uptake and release of glutamic and other amino acids. *J. Neurochem.*, 18: 259–265.

Balázs, R. (1969) Carbohydrate metabolism. In A. Lajtha (Ed.), *Handbook of Neurochemistry, Vol. 3*, Plenum Press, New York, pp. 1–36.

Balázs, R. and Jørgensen, O. S. (1987) A new trophic function of excitatory transmitter amino acids. *Neuroscience*, 22: S41.

Balázs, R., Hack, N. and Jørgensen, O.S. (1988a) Stimulation of *N*-methyl-D-aspartate receptor has a trophic effect on differentiating cerebellar granule cells. *Neurosci. Lett.*, in press.

Balázs, R., Jørgensen, O.S., Hack, N., Gallo, V., Kingsbury, A. and Cotman, C. (1988b) Role of excitatory amino acids in the development of cerebellar granule cells. In G. Huether (Ed.), *Amino Acid Availability and Brain Function in Health and Disease*, Springer, Berlin, in press.

Balcar, V.J. and Johnston, C.A.R. (1972) The structural specificity of a high affinity uptake of L-glutamate and L-aspartate in rat brain slices. *J. Neurochem.*, 19: 2657–2666.

Benveniste, H., Drejer, J., Schousboe, A. and Diemer, N.H. (1984) Elevation of the extracellular concentrations of glutamate and aspartate in rat hippocampus during transient cerebral ischemia monitored by intracerebral microdialysis. *J. Neurochem.*, 43: 1369–1374.

Bosley, T.M., Woodhams, P.L., Gordon, R.D. and Balazs, R. (1983) Effects of anoxia on the stimulated release of amino acid neurotransmitters in the cerebellum in vitro. *J. Neurochem.*, 40: 189–201.

Carbini, E., Wojcik, W.J. and Costa, E. (1985) Dihydropyridines change the uptake of calcium induced by depolarization into primary cultures of cerebellar granule cells. *Neuropharmacology*, 24: 1123–1126.

Chance, B., Sies, H. and Boveris, A. (1979) Hydroperoxide metabolism in mammalian organs. *Physiol. Rev.*, 59: 527–605.

Choi, D.W. (1985) Glutamate neurotoxicity in cortical cell culture is calcium dependent. *Neurosci. Lett.*, 58: 293–297.

Choi, D.W. (1987) Ionic dependence on glutamate neurotoxicity. *J. Neurosci.*, 7: 369–379.

Choi, D.W., Maulucci-Gedde, M. and Kriegstein, A.R. (1987) Glutamate neurotoxicity in cortical cell culture. *J. Neurosci.*, 7: 357–368.

Collingridge, G.L. and Bliss, T.V.P. (1987) NMDA receptors – their role in long-term potentiation. *Trends Neurosci.*, 10: 288–293.

Crepel, F., Dunjal, S.S. and Garthwaite, J. (1981) Morphological and electrophysiological characteristics of rat cerebellar slices maintained in vitro. *J. Physiol.*, 316: 127–138.

Cull-Candy, S.G. and Ogden, D.C. (1985) Ion channels activated by L-glutamate and GABA in cultured cerebellar neurones of the rat. *Proc. R. Soc. (London)*, 224B, 367–373.

Cull-Candy, S.G. and Usowicz, M.M. (1987) Multiple conductance channels activated by excitatory amino acids in cerebellar neurones. *Nature*, 325: 525–528.

Curtis, D.R. and Watkins, J.C. (1960) The excitation and depression of spinal neurones by structurally related amino acids. *J. Neurochem.*, 6: 117–141.

Demopoulos, H.B., Flamm, E.S., Pietronigro, D.D. and Seligman, M.L. (1980) The free radical pathology and the microcirculation in the major central nervous system disorders. *Acta Physiol. Scand. Suppl.*, 492: 91–119.

Gallo, V., Kingsbury, A., Balázs, R. and Jørgensen, O.S. (1987) The role of depolarization in the survival and differentiation of cerebellar granule cells in culture. *J. Neurosci.*, 7: 2203–2214.

Garthwaite, J., Woodhams, P.L., Collins, M.J. and Balázs, R. (1979) On the preparation of brain slices: morphology and cyclic nucleotides. *Brain Res.*, 173: 373–377.

Garthwaite, G. and Garthwaite, J. (1986a) In vitro neurotoxicity of excitatory amino acid analogues during cerebellar development. *Neuroscience*, 17: 755–767.

Garthwaite, G. and Garthwaite, J. (1986b) Neurotoxicity of excitatory amino acid receptor agonists in rat cerebellar slices: dependence on calcium concentration. *Neurosci. Lett.*, 66: 193–198.

Garthwaite, J., Garthwaite, G. and Hajos, F. (1986) Amino acid neurotoxicity: relationship to neuronal depolarization in rat cerebellar slices. *Neuroscience*, 18: 449–460.

Garthwaite, G., Yamini, B.Jr. and Garthwaite, J. (1987) Selective loss of Purkinje and granule cell responsiveness to *N*-methyl-D-aspartate in rat cerebellum during development. *Dev. Brain Res.*, 36: 288–292.

Haber, B., Perez-Polo, J.R., Hashim, G.A. and Giffrida-Stella, A.M. (Eds.) (1983) *Nervous System Regeneration*, A.R. Liss, New York.

Hossmann, K.-A., Sakaki, S. and Zimmerman, V. (1977) Cation activities in reversible ischemia of the cat brain. *Stroke*, 77–81.

Hossmann, K.-A (1985) The pathophysiology of ischemic brain swelling. In Y. Inaba, I. Klatzo and M. Spatz (Eds.), *Brain Edema*, Springer, Berlin, pp. 367–384.

Inaba, Y., Klatzo, I. and Spatz, M.. (Eds.) (1985) *Brain Edema*, Springer, Berlin.

Johnson, J.W. and Ascher, P. (1987) Glycine potentiates the NMDA response in cultured mouse brain neurones. *Nature*, 325: 529–531.

Kemp, J.A., Forster, A.C. and Wong, E.H.F. (1987) Noncompetitive antagonists of excitatory amino acid receptors. *Trends Neurosci.*, 10: 294–298.

Kingsbury, A., Gallo, V. and Balázs, R. (1986) Dihydropyridine Ca^{2+} agonists are potent stimulators of Ca^{2+} uptake and transmitter release in cultured cerebellar granule cells. *Biochem. Soc. Trans.*, 14: 1136–1137.

Kingsbury, A. and Balázs, R. (1987) Effect of calcium agonists and antagonists on cerebellar granule cells. *Eur. J. Pharmacol.*, 140: 275–283.

Kingsbury, A., Gallo, V. and Balázs, R. (1988) Stimulus-coupled transmitter release of amino acids from cerebellar granule cells in culture. *Brain Res.*, in press.

Kristein, L. (1951) Early effects of oxygen lack and carbon dioxide excess on spinal reflexes. *Acta Physiol. Scand. Suppl.*, 80: 1–54.

Krnjevic, K. (1982) GABA and other transmitters in the cerebellum. In S.L. Palay and V. Chan-Palay (Eds.), *The Cerebellum – New Vistas*, Springer, Berlin, pp. 533–549.

Lasher, R.S. and Zagon, I.S. (1972) The effect of potassium on neuronal differentiation in cultures of dissociated newborn rat cerebellum. *Brain Res.*, 41: 428–488.

Lucas, D.R. and Newhouse, J.P. (1957) The toxic effect of sodium-L-glutamate on the inner layers of retina. *AMA Arch. Ophthalmol.*, 58: 193–201.

Mayer, M.L.A. and Westbrook, G.L. (1987) The physiology of excitatory amino acids in the vertebrate central nervous system. *Prog. Neurobiol.*, 28: 197–276.

Meldrum, B.S., Evans, M.C., Swan, J.A. and Simon, R.P. (1987) Protection against hypoxic/ischemic brain damage with excitatory amino acid antagonists. *Med. Biol.*, 65: 153–157.

Morris, R.G.M., Anderson, E., Lynch, G.S. and Baudry, M. (1986) The selective impairment of learning and blockade of long-term potentiation by N-methyl-D-aspartate receptor antagonists, AP5. *Nature*, 319: 774–776.

Myers, R.E. (1979) Lactic acid accumulation as a cause of brain edema and cerebral necrosis resulting from oxygen deprivation. In R. Korobkin and G. Guilleminault (Eds.), *Advances in Perinatal Neurology*, Spectrum Publishers, New York, pp. 85–114.

Nemeto, E.M. (1985) Brain ischemia. In A. Lajtha (Ed.), *Handbook of Neurochemistry, Vol. 9*, 2nd edn., Plenum Press, New York, pp. 553–588.

Nowak, L., Bregestovski, P., Ascher, P. and Herbet, A. (1984) Magnesium gates glutamate-activated channels in mouse central neurones. *Nature*, 307: 462–465.

Olney, J.W., Ho, O.L. and Rhee, V. (1971) Cytotoxic effect of acidic and sulphur containing amino acids on the infant mouse central nervous system. *Exp. Brain Res.*, 14: 61–76.

Patel, A.J., Hunt, A., Gordon, R.D. and Balázs, R. (1982) The activities in different neural cell types of certain enzymes associated with the metabolic compartmentation of glutamate. *Dev. Brain Res.*, 4: 3–11.

Pulsinelli, W.A. (1985) Deafferentiation of the hippocampus protects CA1 pyramidal neurons against ischemic injury. *Stroke*, 16: 144.

Purves, D. and Lichtman, J.W. (1985) *Principles of Neural Development*, Sinauer Assoc. Inc. Publ., Sunderland, MA.

Rauschecker, J.P. and Hahn, S. (1987) Ketamine-xylazine anaesthesia blocks consolidation of ocular dominance changes in kitten visual cortex. *Nature*, 236: 183–185.

Rothman, S.M. (1983) Synaptic activity mediates death of hypoxic neurons. *Science*, 220: 536–537.

Rothman, S.M. (1984) Synaptic release of excitatory amino acid neurotransmitters mediates anoxic neuronal death. *J. Neurosci.*, 4: 1884–1891.

Rothman, S.M. and Olney, J.W. (1986) Glutamate and the pathophisiology of hypoxic-ischemic brain damage. *Ann. Neurol.*, 19: 105–111.

Samuelsson, B. (1983) Leukotrienes: mediators of immediate hypersensitivity reactions and inflammation. *Science*, 220: 568–575.

Schwarcz, R. and Meldrum, B. (1985) Excitatory amino acid antagonists provide a therapeutic approach to neurological disorders. *Lancet*, i, 140–143.

Schwarcz, R. and Ben-Ari, Y. (Eds.) (1986) *Excitatory Amino Acids and Epilepsy*, Plenum Press, New York.

Siegel, G.J., Albers, R.W., Agranoff, B.W. and Katzman, R. (1981) *Basic Neurochemistry*, Little Brown and Co., Boston.

Siesjö, B.K. (1981) Cell damage in the brain: a speculative hypothesis. *J. Cereb. Blood Flow Metab.*, 1: 155–185.

Siesjö, B.K. and Agardh, C.D. (1983) Hypoglycemia. In A. Lajtha (Ed.), *Handbook of Neurochemistry*, 2nd edn., Little Brown and C., Boston.

Siesjö, B.K. and Wieloch, T. (1985) Cerebral metabolism in ischemia: neurochemical basis for therapy. *Br. J. Anaesth.* 57: 47–62.

Siesjö, B.K., Béndek, G., Koide, T., Westerberg, E. and Wieloch, T. (1985) Influence of acidosis on lipid peroxidation in brain tissues in vitro. *J. Cereb. Blood Flow Metab.*, 5: 253–258.

Simon, R.P., Swan, J.H., Griffith, T. and Meldum, B.S. (1984) Blockade of N-methyl-D-aspartate receptors may protect against ischemic damage in the brain. *Science*, 226: 850–852.

Singer, W., Kleinschmidt, A. and Bear, M.F. (1986) Infusion of an NMDA antagonist disrupts ocular dominance plasticity in kitten striate cortex. *Soc. Neurosci. Abstr.*, 12: 786.

Sokoloff, L., Reivich, M., Kennedy, C., Des Rosiers, M.H., Patlak, C.S., Pettigrew, K.D., Sakurada, O. and Shinohara, M. (1977). The [^{14}C]deoxyglucose method for the measurement of local cerebral glucose utilization: theory, procedure, and normal values in the conscious and anaesthetized albino rat. *J. Neurochem.*, 28: 897–916.

Somogyi, P., Halasy, K., Somogyi, J., Storm-Mathiesen, J. and Ottoson, O.P. (1986) Quantification of immunogold labelling reveals enrichment of glutamate in mossy and parallel fibre terminals in cat cerebellum. *Neuroscience*, 19: 1045–1050.

Sykova, E. (1983) Extracellular K$^+$ accumulation in the central nervous system. *Prog. Biophys. Mol. Biol.*, 42: 135–189.

Varon, S. (1973) Symposium on Free Radical Pathology, 1973. *Fed. Proc.*, 32: 1859–1908.

Wieloch, T. (1985) Hypoglycemia-induced neuronal damage prevented by an *N*-methyl-D-aspartate antagonist. *Science*, 230: 681–683.

Wieloch, T., Engelsen, B., Westerberg, E. and Auer, R. (1985) Lesion of the glutamatergic cortico-striatal projections in the rat ameliorate hypoglycemic brain damage in the striatum. *Neurosci. Lett.*, 58: 25–30.

Wilkin, G. P., Garthwaite, J. and Balázs, R. (1982) Putative acidic amino acid transmitters in the cerebellum. II. Electron microscopic localization of transport sites. *Brain Res.*, 244: 69–80.

Wolfe, L. S. (1982) Eicosanoids: prostaglandins, thromboxanes, leukotrienes and other derivatives of carbon-20 unsaturated fatty acids. *J. Neurochem.*, 38: 1–14.

Discussion

D. F. Swaab: In spite of all the mechanisms that may damage the neurons in hypoxic situations, it is still possible to transplant neurons. How do you explain this and what, according to your idea, is the factor that is responsible for *permanent* damage?

R. Balázs: Successful transplants are usually obtained from fetal tissue and it is known that fetal nerve cells are, in general, resistant to hypoxia. However, we must also consider the possibility that nerve cells are not as vulnerable as we have thought hitherto and if the proper conditions are provided they could escape degeneration. As I mentioned in my talk we are just at the beginning in the identification of such factors, which may also vary depending on cell types, but studies in which the adult brain was lesioned indicated that for certain nerve cells at least partial protection can be provided, for example by treatment with nerve growth factor or gangliosides.

J. W. Olney: It is an important question whether the excitatory amino acids (EAA) released during hypoxia are released exclusively from the synaptic (transmitter) pool. If so, it is possible that only certain EAA receptor sub-types are being hyperstimulated and protection may be achieved with antagonists specific for such receptors. However, if the release is indiscriminate from the metabolic as well as the transmitter pool, all EAA receptor sub-types will be flooded with EAA and protection may be difficult to achieve except with broad-spectrum antagonists that block all EAA receptors. How do you interpret your findings – are the EAA being released from the transmitter or metabolic compartment or both?

R. Balázs: From both. Stimulus-coupled release of glutamate (or D-aspartate) was increased in anoxia, which also caused, as indicated by the effect of the uptake inhibitors, a great rise in the leakage of D-aspartate from non-synaptic sites.

M. Mirmiran: You have shown that occupation of NMDA receptors might have trophic or degenerative effects depending on the stage of development. Could this account for a different sensitivity to hypoxia of the immature versus mature nervous system?

R. Balázs: It seems that nerve cells in certain parts of the brain are less vulnerable to certain EAA analogues in the immature animal than in the adult. Thus there is some correlation at least between the vulnerability of cells to EAA and the sensitivity to hypoxia. I doubt, however, that the trophic effects would contribute to the greater tolerance of the immature brain to hypoxia. The trophic phase of the cellular response to NMDA is transient and it is likely that there is a coexistence of nerve cells in different stages of maturation in the whole CNS during development. Thus the 'trophic' responders would be masked in the whole tissue.

H. J. Romijn: What is the time-span during maturation in which the cerebellar granule cells are vulnerable to NMDA receptor stimulation, that is, in between the trophic phase and the phase during which uncoupling of the receptor to the channel takes place?

R. Balázs: Differentiating granule cells seem to be vulnerable to NMDA. Since granule cell generation is a protracted process it is difficult to define precisely the age when the sensitivity becomes manifest. Garthwaite and Garthwaite (1986) have found that in the rat cerebellum the responses of granule cells to NMDA are marked at P8 and P14, but they are as weak at P21 as in the adult.

Reference

Garthwaite, G. and Garthwaite, J. (1986) In vitro neurotoxicity of excitatory amino acid analogues during cerebellar development. *Neuroscience*, 17: 755–767.

G.J. Boer, M.G.P. Feenstra, M. Mirmiran, D.F. Swaab and F. Van Haaren
Progress in Brain Research, Vol. 73
© 1988 Elsevier Science Publishers B.V. (Biomedical Division)

CHAPTER 29

Humoral and surface-anchored factors in development and repair of the nervous system

Silvio Varon, Brigitte Pettmann and Marston Manthorpe

Department of Biology, M-001, School of Medicine, University of California, San Diego, La Jolla, CA 92093, USA

Introduction

The nervous system, like any other body organ or system, represents a society of living cells, interacting with one another as well as with other body elements. This chapter will attempt to articulate a proposition which contains two components. First, that the behaviors of an individual neural cell, be it neuronal or glial, are largely regulated by its microenvironment – i.e., humoral signals from the extracellular fluid and anchored signals from the extracellular matrix or neighboring cell surfaces. Secondly, that changes in these extrinsic signals provide the cues that direct neural development, modulate the functional performance of adult neurons and glia, and often underlie the course if not the onset of neural pathologies. Concepts and information will be discussed here mainly in the context of neural development, as appropriate to the theme of this book but also because most of the data available (hence of the hypotheses inspired by them) are in fact derived from developing organisms and cells.

In this chapter, we shall focus largely on the regulation of neuronal survival (neuronotrophic agents) and neurite extension (neurite promoting agents). Most of the progress achieved in these areas was made possible by the development and utilization of neural cell cultures and we shall start, therefore, with a brief review of the concepts underlying the use of neural cells in vitro. And,

because validation of in vitro work rests in the final analysis with in vivo relevance, we will finish with a section on in vivo models demonstrating the presence and possible roles of neuronotrophic and neurite promoting agents in the repair of adult mammalian neural tissue.

For more comprehensive coverage of the neurobiological issues to be discussed, the reader is referred to a number of review articles, which may also prove instructive about the evolving nature of questions and answers (Levi-Montalcini, 1966, 1982; Varon, 1975a; Varon and Somjen, 1979; Varon and Adler, 1980; Thoenen and Barde, 1980; Varon et al., 1984a, 1987a; Manthorpe et al., 1986a; Le Douarin, 1982).

Regulatory signals and neural development

Proliferation, migration and differentiation are major morphogenetic processes which developing neural tissue shares with other tissues. Neural development involves additional processes, such as elongation of axons and dendrites (neurites), selective synapse formation, and neuronal cell death. These morphogenetic processes and their controls are best illustrated by the neural crest and its derivative cells, one component of the nervous system which has been investigated in great detail (Le Douarin, 1982).

The neural crest forms dorsally to the neural tube at the time of the latter's closure. From the trunk segment of the neural crest (the cephalic segment gives rise to many different derivatives), cells proceed immediately to migrate away in two main streams. The dorsal stream generates pigment cells that disperse in the skin. The ventral stream gives rise to both neurons and glia in most peripheral ganglia: the sensory dorsal root ganglia, the mainly noradrenergic sympathetic ganglia, the cholinergic ciliary ganglia, and the cholinergic enteric ganglia – as well as to the chromaffin cells of the adrenal medulla. The neural crest precursors of all these ganglionic cell populations have to migrate over pre-defined routes and receive along the way and/or at their final location the instructions needed to acquire their final positions and functional identities. Specifically, neuronal precursors must: (i) desegregate from the starting neural crest location, (ii) migrate along the appropriate routes, (iii) proliferate on the way and at their final location, (iv) stop their migration and resegregate into ganglionic clusters, (v) advance from neuroblasts to neurons, i.e. become permanently postmitotic, (vi) select the right transmitter mode, (vii) extend axons toward the correct innervation territory, (viii) make the proper synapses with their presumptive target cells, (ix) be instructed to die or survive, and (x) undergo additional differentiation steps – among other obligations.

Each of those steps must require a series of extrinsic signals, many of them involving the cells which a neuron will innervate and the glial cells with which it may associate. Much of the neurobiological research of recent years has been directed to the recognition and characterization of molecular signals underlying some of these processes. Several 'growth factors' have been found competent to stimulate the proliferation of glial cells from peripheral (PNS) and central (CNS) neural tissues, but practically nothing has yet been learned about the control of neuroblast proliferation or its arrest. On the other hand, considerable progress in the chemistry of extracellular matrix components and – to a lesser extent – cell surface constituents has provided some insight into two other morphogenetic processes, cell migration and neurite elongation. The main impetus toward molecular neurobiology, however, has come from Levi-Montalcini's discovery, nearly 50 years ago, of a special protein called Nerve Growth Factor (NGF).

It was known, at that time, that an innervation territory influences the number and size of the neurons addressing it. For example, early removal of a limb in the chick embryo leads to the near destruction of the spinal cord motor neurons destined to innervate that limb and, conversely, early implantation of an additional limb bud causes increased numbers and sizes of the corresponding spinal motor neurons (Prestige, 1970; Hamburger and Oppenheim, 1982). Bueker (1948) implanted, into a 2-year-old chick embryo, pieces of mouse sarcoma as an additional territory for sensory innervation by dorsal root ganglionic neurons. He observed hypertrophy of the dorsal root ganglia, and concluded that the sarcoma graft mimicked the implantation of an extra limb bud. Levi-Montalcini and Hamburger (1951), however, drew a different conclusion from similar experiments. They noticed that the sarcoma implant elicited neuritic overgrowth and neuronal hypertrophy from sympathetic as well as dorsal root ganglia, but not from the motor spinal cord. They proposed that the sarcoma graft may supply a humoral 'factor' which could reach via the bloodstream these two types of ganglion and act selectively on their neurons. Levi-Montalcini soon obtained two distinct pieces of evidence in support of a molecular agent responsible for the effects; (i) the same ganglionic effects could be elicited by sarcoma tissue grafted to the chorioallantoic membrane of the chick embryo, where it could become well-vascularized but could not be reached by the growing nerve fibers, and (ii) dorsal root ganglia and sympathetic ganglia would also respond in vitro to an extract of the mouse sarcoma graft. The 'Nerve Growth Factor' (or NGF for short) was born. The rest is history (Levi-Montalcini, 1966; Varon, 1975a; Greene and Shooter, 1980; Thoenen and Barde,1980;

among many other review articles).

Three main effects have been traditionally attributed to NGF: (1) promotion of neuritic outgrowth (hence its name), (2) support of neuronal survival and maintenance (a 'trophic' role), and (3) increased synthesis of transmitter-producing enzymes (specifically, the tyrosine hydroxylase controlling the production of noradrenaline in the sympathetic ganglia). Each of these three effects has inspired searches for other agents or factors which would be capable of regulating the same functions in NGF-sensitive or in other neurons.

In vitro approaches

Several types of neural culture have been and continue to be used for neurobiological investigations, each with its own advantages and restrictions (Varon, 1975b; Varon et al., 1983). Explant cultures involve pieces of tissue (or small 'organs' like ganglia) suitably anchored to a culture substratum. They come closest to preserving the cellular composition and organization of the original tissue, at least for some time, but allow direct visualization and access only to those cells that will migrate out of the main explant. Dissociation of a tissue into a cell suspension is the starting step for several other types of culture. The mixed cell suspension can be re-aggregated into clumps of a chosen size, inside which the cells will 'sort-out' with time in vitro to reconstruct a tissue-like organization – an excellent opportunity to study processes of cell migration, guidance and recognition. Alternatively, the mixed cell suspension can be seeded onto suitable surfaces (the culture 'substratum') to generate monolayer cultures, where individual cells can be inspected by microscopy in the living state or after fixation. Even more effectively, the mixed cell suspension can be fractionated by a variety of means to yield purified or enriched subpopulations which can then be cultured in isolation or after controlled recombination, providing the same advantages of a monolayer culture plus the opportunity to inves-

tigate heterotypic cell interactions. Lastly, clonal cell lines derived from specific tumors provide 'immortal' and proliferative populations which can be most readily grown to the numbers and mass needed for biochemical as well as other investigations.

Like the in vivo society, cultured cells are under continued influences from their microenvironment – here, under some degree of control by the investigator. A given neuron, for example, will be affected by its extracellular fluid (the culture medium), its extracellular matrix (the culture substratum), and all the other cells in the culture either by direct contacts or via modifications imposed by them on medium and substratum (Fig. 1). Because these cell-derived contributions occur from the very beginning, the medium and substratum compositions can only be 'defined' in terms of what the investigator uses to set up the culture and not what microenvironment the cultured cell will eventually see. The cell population seeded into the culture will also change very rapidly. Some of the seeded cells may be nonviable, while others may have difficulty in attaching to the substratum. Moreover, some cell types may progressively die, while others (e.g. glia, fibroblasts) may proliferate and take over the culture. Obviously, the outcome of a given culture

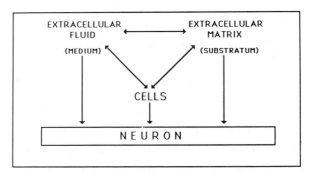

Fig. 1 Extrinsic influences on neuronal cells. The performances of a neuron depend on signals received from culture medium and substratum, as well as from other cells (neurons, non-neurons). The cells also modify the medium and substratum.

depends not only on its cellular composition but also on the composition and renewal of the initial culture medium and, although less widely recognized until recently, of the initial culture substratum.

Tissue and cell cultures from different sources have used a variety of 'basal' media comprising minerals, amino acids, vitamins and, occasionally, other small molecular weight substances. Basal media have been further supplemented with biological fluids (serum, ascites fluid, embryo extracts) of unknown composition, in an effort to approximate the rich humoral microenvironment that must occur in vivo. These complex culture media have two major disadvantages for molecular investigations: (i) their undefined composition does not permit one to assign observed cell responses to specific medium molecules, and (ii) the biological supplements may comprise inhibitory as well as stimulatory ingredients. Accordingly, efforts have been made in the last decade to design chemically defined medium supplements with which to replace serum supplementation without overt loss of cell performance (Barnes and Sato, 1980). Like basal media and biological supplements, these chemically defined supplements have largely been aimed at the 'growth' of non-neural cells (i.e. the numerical increase of a proliferative cell population). The same concepts, however, have been recently applied to maintenance and/or growth of neural cell cultures.

The N2 mixture – made up of insulin, transferrin, putrescine, progesterone and selenite – was originally designed to replace serum for the proliferative growth of neuroblastoma cells, a clonal line of sympathetic neuroblastic tumor cells (Bottenstein and Sato, 1979). The N1 mixture (differing from the N2 only by a lower concentration of transferrin) was then shown to replace serum also with regard to the maintenance of postmitotic neurons from embryonic dorsal root ganglia (Bottenstein et al., 1980) and a variety of other PNS and CNS neurons (Skaper et al., 1979). Not all five N1 ingredients are needed by neurons collected from different tissues or at different ages

(cf. Varon et al., 1987a). All neurons tested thus far appear to require insulin, with transferrin the second most needed ingredient and selenium a distinct third. The N1 or N2 mixtures are also beneficial for several glial cell cultures but need different additions for the actual growth of different glial cell types (e.g. Michler-Stuke and Bottenstein, 1982; Saneto and deVellis, 1987).

Culture substrata were initially viewed as passive surfaces for cell attachment and migration. It has become increasingly clear, however, that substrata profoundly affect (i) the quality and not only the extent of cell attachment, as well as the cell shape, (ii) the association among cocultured cells, and the desegregation-resegregation processes at the two ends of cell migration, (iii) the ability of most cells to proliferate, (iv) the ability of neurons to extend neurites, and (v) various transport and metabolic activities of a cell. Substratum properties, of course, will also depend on the cell population involved and the medium used and will change under their influence with time in culture. Tissue culture plastic is increasingly used for neural cultures only after being precoated with polycationic substances (polyornithine, polylysine, polyarginine) and/or extracellular matrix (ECM)-related materials (collagen, fibronectin, laminin, etc.). Polycations confer better adhesiveness, so that seeded cells will attach rapidly without the opportunity to cluster. ECM-related materials have both general and specific biological properties that are themselves under vigorous investigation.

Monolayer cultures of purified neural cells are particularly suited to measurement of biological activities of experimental agents introduced into the medium or pre-applied to the substratum. Fig. 2 shows two neuronal cultures, a 1-day-old culture of embryonic day 8 (E8) chick ciliary ganglionic neurons and a 5-day-old culture of E8 chick forebrain neurons. Such well-dispersed cultures allow direct counts (before or after fixation) of (i) viable neurons (attaching within a few hours from seeding), (ii) surviving neurons (after 1 or several days in culture) and (iii) neurons display-

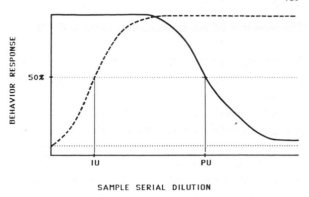

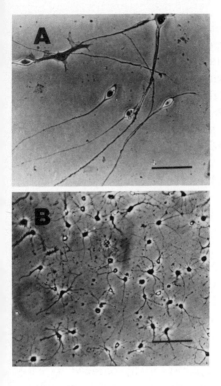

Fig. 3 Dose-response ('titration') curves for agents supporting neural cell behaviors in dispersed cell cultures. Solid line: serial dilution of a promoting agent. Broken line: serial dilution of an inhibitory agent. Fold-dilutions yielding half-maximal effects represent the 'titer' of the original sample.

Fig. 2 Low-density cultures of PNS and CNS neurons. (A) E8 chick ciliary ganglion neurons, 24 h. (B) E8 chick forebrain neurons, 5 days. Bars: 100 (A) and 120 (B) μm.

ing neuritic outgrowth (e.g., two or more cell body diameter lengths). Immunocytochemical staining of surface antigens or intracellular antigens (after appropriate permeabilization) can permit additional evaluations of (iv) neuronal subsets present in the culture or (v) antigenic changes following developmental or experimental modulations. Autoradiographic techniques can reveal changes in biosynthetic activities (e.g. labeling of cell nuclei with radio-thymidine in proliferative cells). Biochemical evaluations of cell content (extracts) or cell-released materials ('conditioned' medium) are also possible, although they may demand larger numbers of cultured cells.

Fig. 3 illustrates a typical 'titration' curve for bioactive experimental agents (Manthorpe et al., 1981a). One first chooses the appropriate test cell population and culture conditions so that the performance under study will not occur unless an effective agent is experimentally supplied. The sample containing the putative agent is introduced and serially diluted into microwells, which then receive identical aliquots of test cells and are incubated for the desired time. The degree of cell performance allows one to determine the half-maximal effect (whether stimulatory or inhibitory in nature) and the corresponding fold-dilution represents the number of activity units per ml of original (undiluted) sample. In fact, it is not unusual with crude test materials to obtain titration curves that display both the inhibitory (rising curve) and promoting (falling curve) features, suggesting that two opposing influences are present in the test material at concentrations such that the inhibitory influence is diluted out before the promoting one (Manthorpe et al., 1982).

One must stress that practically all the neural cultures investigated as bioassay systems (or for other purposes) thus far have been derived from prenatal or perinatal tissues. Consequently, the resulting information applies to developing neural cells and can encourage only speculations with regard to older cell properties.

The concept of neuronotrophic factors (NTFs)

Nerve growth factor has served – and continues to serve – as the prototype for a postulated family of specific proteins, generally designated neuronotrophic or neurotrophic factors (NTFs) and presumed to secure survival, functional maintenance, and growth and/or repair capabilities for selected populations of neurons (Varon, 1977; Varon and Adler, 1980). Information from the NGF studies suggests that (i) NTFs are generated and released by the innervation territories of the responsive neurons, (ii) they are taken up by axonal terminals and retrogradely transported to the neuronal cell bodies, and (iii) they exert their trophic action at the cell body level. Cultured glial cells, from both PNS and CNS sources, have also been found to produce NTFs (Varon and Manthorpe, 1982; Manthorpe et al., 1986a). It is generally presumed that the NTFs are released by the source cells into their humoral microenvironment to diffuse and bind to specific receptors on the surfaces of the target neurons. Recent findings (see further on) now suggest the alternative that the target neuron receptors may recognize NTFs presented to them in a surface-bound state – thereby providing an opportunity for spatial restriction (hence differential availability) of the NTF.

The concept of innervation territories as sources of NTFs also draws on an important morphogenetic event, the so-called developmental neuronal death. The early neuronal population undergoes partial cell death at the very time at which its axons have reached and interact with their innervation territory (Cowan et al., 1984). The extent of this developmental neuronal death was found to reflect the size of territory available for innervation. Three interesting questions were raised from such observations: (1) the initial neuronal population does not require the existence of the innervation territory for either survival or axonal growth, since both are optimal even if the territory has been ablated at an early time; (2) the neurons acquire a new 'vulnerability' at the time when their axons would encounter their innervation territory, once again regardless of the actual presence of the latter; and (3) availability of the innervation territory is essential for the survival of at least part of the neuronal population. It is this last point which prompted the hypothesis that the neurons which survive are those that manage to obtain a required trophic factor from the innervated tissue.

A test of this hypothesis became possible in the case of ciliary ganglionic (CG) neurons – an investigation which has led to the identification and purification of a new factor, ciliary neuronotrophic factor or CNTF (Manthorpe and Varon, 1985). CG neurons innervate the intrinsic musculature of the eye. In the chick embryo, CG neurons become postmitotic by E5, extend their axons into the eye by E8–10, and half of them die between E10 and E15. The neuronal death is greatly increased by early (E2) ablation of the eye primordium, and substantially reduced by early implantation of an additional eye primordium. Cultures were set up with E8 chick CG neurons and used as bioassays for the CNTF that should be extractable from the eye tissues. Trophic (i.e. survival-promoting) activity for these CG neurons was found (i) to be highly concentrated in eye, as compared to whole embryo, extracts, (ii) to reside mainly in the choroid–ciliary body–iris subcomponents of eye tissue – the specific innervation territories for CG neurons, and (iii) to reach their highest specific levels there over the E8–E15 developmental period. The chick eye CNTF was purified and found to be an acidic, 21–23 kDa monomeric protein (Barbin et al., 1984a) – quite different from the NGF protein (a very basic, 25 kDa dimeric protein). Nevertheless, the new CNTF proved to have trophic competence also for dorsal root and sympathetic ganglionic neurons – traditional targets for the NGF trophic action (see also further on).

Interestingly, more recent work has shown that CNTF is also quite abundant in most, if not all, peripheral nerve tissues of adult rats, which has raised the possibility of CNTF production by

Schwann cells in vivo. The rat nerve CNTF has also been purified (Manthorpe et al., 1986b) and found to have properties nearly identical to those of the chick CNTF. Yet another neuronotrophic factor, brain-derived neuronotrophic factor or BDNF, has been purified from adult pig brain and described as a basic, 13 kDa protein similar to NGF and acting specifically on DRG, but not on sympathetic or parasympathetic neurons (Barde et al., 1982).

Neuronotrophic factors and the Na$^+$, K$^+$ pump

The traditional targets for NGF are neurons from embryonic dorsal root (DRG) or sympathetic ganglia and the PC12 clonal line derived from an adrenal chromaffin cell tumor – all three types of target cell being neural crest derivatives. All these cells display at their surfaces two sets of specific NGF-binding sites, or 'receptors' (cf. Greene and Shooter, 1980). Type I receptors have a very high affinity (K_d = 10^{-11} M) and slow dissociation properties, are trypsin-stable and Triton X-100-resistant, and display in SDS gels an apparent molecular mass of 140–150 kDa. Type II receptors have lower affinity (K_d = 10^{-9} M) but faster dissociation properties, are trypsin-labile and Triton X-100-soluble, and have been assigned an apparent molecular mass of 80–100 kDa. Monoclonal antibodies have been raised against the much more abundant Type II receptors and may not cross-react with Type I receptors. The 10^{-11} M K_d range of Type I receptor binding affinity fits well with the 10^{-11} M ED$_{50}$ range at which NGF exerts its neuronotrophic and neurite promoting activities.

Once NGF binds to its receptors on the target cell, it must initiate sequences of events which ultimately lead to the gross cell responses observed – neuronal survival and neurite extension, among them. Very little is yet known about such intermediate events. A parsimonious view, illustrated in Fig. 4, would suggest that the same receptor type and the same initial sequence of events are involved in both of these responses, bringing

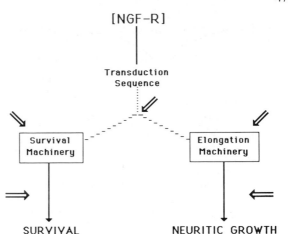

Fig. 4 Schematic representation of NGF modes of action. Encounter with its receptor (NGF-R) leads to a sequence of rapid events which will activate cellular machineries required for survival or neuritic growth. Arrows = other extrinsic influences apply at different steps of the overall sequence.

into action whatever cell machineries specifically underlie each of these two cell behaviors. The process also requires the availability of other extrinsic influences responsible for regulating each of these machineries (Varon and Skaper, 1980). Neuronal cell suspensions or monolayer cultures from E8 chick DRG proved to be an effective model system with which to investigate events occurring within minutes of NGF presentation and essential for the subsequent, NGF-supported viability of the neurons. Investigations of this model system have revealed that NGF-deprived neurons undergo a loss of nutrient transport capabilities that can be traced back to similarly reversible losses of transmembrane Na$^+$ gradients and, ultimately, of Na$^+$, K$^+$ pump activity (Varon and Skaper, 1983).

Fig. 5 illustrates the changes that monovalent cations undergo during deprivation and re-administration of NGF to DRG or sympathetic neurons. Intracellular K$^+$ drops and intracellular Na$^+$ rises to match their respective extracellular levels over the first 6 h of trophic deprivation, and NGF restores the original intracellular ionic concentrations within minutes of its delayed administration (Fig. 5 top). The restoration involves coupled Na$^+$ and K$^+$ transport, is sensitive to

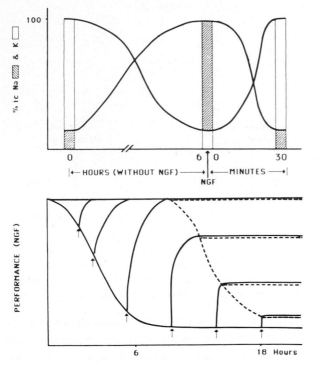

Fig. 5 NGF controls the Na$^+$, K$^+$ pump as well as the viability of target neurons. (top) NGF deprivation causes loss of K$^+$ and accumulation of Na$^+$ over a 6 h period, while re-administration of NGF reverses both events within minutes via pump reactivation. (bottom) Delayed supply of NGF restores both pump (solid lines) and viability (broken lines) fully if within 6 h before cell death begins.

external K$^+$ and internal Na$^+$ concentrations, requires energy, and is blocked by ouabain – the known characteristics of an operating Na$^+$, K$^+$ pump. If trophic deprivation is continued, neuronal death will occur several hours later, with a progression that parallels the earlier loss of Na$^+$, K$^+$ pump performance (Fig. 5 bottom). Conversely, re-administrations of NGF with different delays restore pump and viability to equal extents – fully over the first 6–8 h, decreasingly over the next 10 h (Fig. 5 bottom). The same strict correlation between the earlier performance of the pump and the later viability of the neurons is displayed if (i) both are reduced by reduced NGF concentrations or (ii) pump activity is directly restricted (ouabain, lower external K$^+$) despite maximal NGF levels (Varon and Skaper, 1983; Skaper and Varon, 1983a).

Another remarkable correlation between pump competence and neuronal survival is found when ganglionic neurons of different embryonic ages are examined (Skaper and Varon, 1983b). As illustrated in Fig. 6 (top), chick DRG neurons become maximally responsive to NGF at E8, at which time they are fully dependent on NGF for both pump and survival competence. With increasing age, both dependences on NGF decline progressively but always in strict parallel with each other, until by about E16 NGF-deprived neurons operate their pump and survive equally well as those receiving exogenous NGF. One must stress that dependence on an NTF and responsiveness to it are not synonymous, as the older neurons will still acknowledge the presence of NGF by other behaviors.

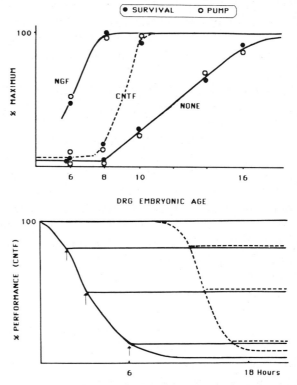

Fig. 6 (top) Dependence on trophic factors by DRG neurons decreases with embryonic ages, and in strict correlation, for Na$^+$, K$^+$ pump (○) and viability (●). (bottom) Delayed supply of CNTF prevents further losses of pump (solid lines) and viability (broken lines) but does *not* reverse them.

Fig. 6 (top) also shows the age-related responses of DRG neurons to another trophic factor, CNTF. Both pump performance and survival receive parallel support from CNTF, but only starting between E8 and E10 (and to the extent that they remain dependent on a trophic support). CNTF, however, differs markedly from NGF in one crucial respect, illustrated in Fig. 6 (bottom). Delayed presentations of CNTF stop further declines of pump performance and neuronal viability, but fail to restore any loss already incurred with regard to the pump and, consequently,the later cell survival. Additional studies have shown that certain phorbol esters are capable of replacing both NGF and CNTF for the survival of their respective target neurons (Montz et al., 1985). Delayed presentation of phorbol esters to trophic factor-deprived neurons will also stop further losses of pump competence and viability but fails to restore any previous loss, just as the presentation of CNTF did (cf. Fig. 6 bottom) and in contrast with the effects of NGF (cf. Fig. 5 bottom) (Skaper et al., 1986).

From these and other data, one can begin to build a model of what molecular regulations may be involved in the trophic support of neuronal survival, which is schematically illustrated in Fig. 7. Phorbol esters are known to mimic diacylglycerol (DAG) for the stimulation of protein kinase C (PKC: a Ca^{2+}-, DAG- and phospholipid-dependent kinase). Several agents, interacting with their own cell surface receptors, promote the phosphatidylinositide pathway (PI) which raises intracellular DAG (and Ca^{2+}) levels and thus stimulates PKC. The close similarity between the phorbol ester and the CNTF effects on DRG neurons, therefore, suggests that CNTF operates via PI pathway and PKC stimulation to promote the phosphorylation of proteins which will prevent (but not reverse) pump and viability losses. NGF is, in fact, reported to stimulate the PI pathway (Contreras and Guroff, 1987) and may, thus, also protect pump and viability via the PKC mechanism. However, NGF is also capable of stimulating cyclic AMP levels (Skaper and

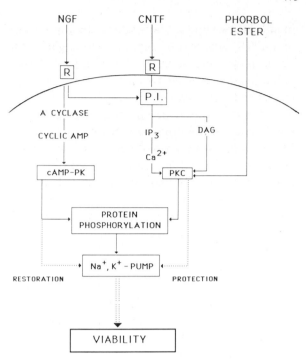

Fig. 7 Diagrammatic model for biochemical events underlying the pump- and survival-support by NGF, CNTF and phorbol esters. Abbreviations: R = corresponding receptors, A Cyclase = adenylate cyclase, cAMP-PK = cyclic AMP-dependent protein kinase, PI = phosphatidylinositide, IP_3 = inositoltriphosphate, DAG = diacylglycerol, PKC = protein kinase C.

Varon, 1981), hence cyclic AMP-dependent protein kinases, and it may be that there lies the distinctive ability of NGF to reverse and not merely stop the loss of pump performance. Several research groups are investigating NGF effects on protein phosphorylation in PC12 cells and are beginning to recognize NGF-promoted phosphoproteins that reflect PKC or cyclic AMP-dependent kinases (Togari and Guroff, 1985; Cremins et al., 1986).

Neuronal survival and control of free radicals

NGF, CNTF and BDNF are all neuronotrophic protein factors recognized or selected for their impact on specified PNS neurons. A search for CNS-addressing neuronotrophic agents is hampered by the cellular heterogeneity of CNS tissues in at least two major ways. One is that many cells in a CNS culture (neurons as well as glia) could serve as internal sources of NTFs for others, a difficulty that can be partially avoided by using low-density cultures of enriched neuronal cells. The other is that wide-spectrum trophic agents (i.e. agents addressing most neurons) are readily recognized, but very small subsets of neurons requiring specific trophic support could only be visualized by use of cell-specific markers. Nevertheless, studies of prenatal chick and rat CNS neuronal cultures have already yielded some intriguing contributions (Varon et al., 1987c; Chau et al., 1988).

Spinal cord and brain neurons, under culture conditions where they do not survive for even 24 h, will be maintained for at least a few days with media conditioned by Schwann or astroglial cell cultures (Manthorpe et al., 1982; Barbin et al., 1984b; Varon et al., 1984b). The trophic activity of these glia-conditioned media resides with low molecular weight agents, rather than with protein factors. Investigations of PNS as well as CNS neurons led to the recognition that the main trophic agent involved was pyruvate (Skaper et al., 1984; Selak et al., 1985). Fig. 8 (top) illustrates some of these points by way of traditional titration curves. Despite the use of a laminin substratum (see further on) and the N1 supplement, a traditional basal medium such as Eagle's basal medium (EBM) will fail to support CNS neuronal survival. After its conditioning by astroglial cells (ACM), EBM will become competent with a newly acquired trophic titer of about 3 trophic units (TU)/ml. Another basal medium, Dulbecco's modified Eagle's medium (DMEM), supports CNS neurons without prior conditioning, with a titer of about 10 TU/ml. EBM does not contain pyruvate, while DMEM does at 1 mM concentrations. EBM supplemented with 1 mM pyruvate acquires the same trophic competence as DMEM. And a similar acquisition of pyruvate by EBM occurs in the course of its conditioning by astroglial cells, to about one third of the pyruvate concentration and trophic titer of fresh DMEM

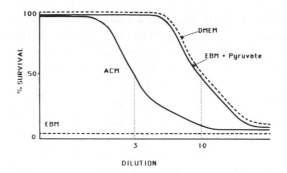

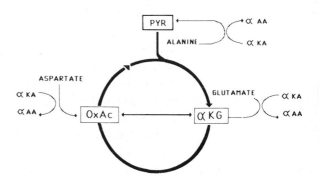

Fig. 8 Dependence on pyruvate of the survival of prenatal CNS neurons. (top) Eagle's basal medium (EBM, bottom line) lacks pyruvate and fails to support neuronal survival. EBM 'conditioned' by astroglial cells (ACM) acquires some pyruvate and provides corresponding support. EBM supplemented with 1 mM pyruvate matches for trophic support the Dulbecco's modified Eagle's medium (DMEM) which itself contains 1 mM pyruvate. (bottom) Pyruvate can be replaced in its survival-supporting role by α-ketoglutarate (αKG) or oxaloacetate (OxAc), or by any α-amino acid (αAA) transaminating to those tricarboxylic acid cycle participants in the presence of α-ketoacid (αKA) acceptors.

It appeared, therefore, that the CNS neurons in these cultures required pyruvate rather than glucose (present in all media) for their survival.

The trophic requirement for pyruvate could also be met if one supplied pyruvate-free cultures with (i) α-ketoglutarate or oxaloacetate, but not any other tricarboxylic cycle intermediates, or (ii) those amino acids which can transaminate to pyruvate (alanine), α-ketoglutarate (glutamate and glutamine) or oxaloacetate (aspartate and asparagine) – the latter condition also requiring the supply of α-ketoacids as amino-group acceptors (Facci et al., 1985, 1986). The relationships among these several compounds, illustrated in Fig. 8 (bottom), suggest that the trophic requirement for pyruvate concerns the generation of energy needed for neuronal survival.

An independent line of investigations has led to the recognition that (i) CNS neurons could also be maintained (in the absence of pyruvate or its surrogate molecules) by protein factors present in PNS or CNS wound fluids (Manthorpe et al., 1982) and (ii) such a trophic protein abounded in red blood cells (Williams et al., 1985). Purification of the trophic protein from human red blood cells led to its identification with catalase (Walicke et al., 1986). Catalase could substitute for pyruvate for all the CNS and PNS neurons that had previously revealed total or partial dependences on pyruvate (Chau et al., 1988). The known function of catalase is to break down hydrogen peroxide and thus reduce its availability to generate hydroxyl free radicals ($^{\cdot}OH$), known to be the most dangerous among the water-soluble peroxides (see Fig. 9, top). Inhibitors of the enzymatic activity of catalase also blocked its trophic competence and, conversely, other substances known for their anti-oxidant properties also provided support for the neuronal survival (Walicke et al., 1986; Chau et al., 1987). Lastly, the ability of catalase to support neuronal survival in the absence of pyruvate required the presence of glucose in a dose-dependent fashion and involved conferring on the neurons the ability to consume glucose through their tricarboxylic acid cycle (Chau et al., 1988).

Fig. 9 illustrates some of the features of a regulatory model suggested by the findings just reviewed. Oxygen and hydroxyl radicals ($^{\cdot}O_2^-$; $^{\cdot}OH$), whether exogenously or endogenously generated, will lead to a peroxidation block of the glucose-to-pyruvate pathway, hence of energy production from glucose. Exogenous pyruvate will bypass the block, while catalase and other antioxidants will either prevent or correct the block itself. The different extents to which neu-

rons from different embryonic tissues depend on pyruvate or catalase suggest that these neurons also differ in the degree to which they are susceptible to peroxidation damage of their glucose pathway – a difference which might characterize them in vivo as well as in vitro and at adult as well as developmental ages. Other functions, besides energy production, may also be attacked by an excess of free radicals – particularly those involving membrane lipids. An attractive speculation would thus extend the model to include as one role of traditional neuronotrophic factors the enhancement of neuronal defenses against peroxidation damage (Varon et al., 1987c; Perez-Polo and Werrbach-Perez, 1985).

Such speculations are in agreement with a more general concept of modern cell biology concerning free radicals, cell damage and cell senescence (e.g. Pryor, 1982; Fridovich, 1983; Bors et al., 1984; Cutler, 1985). Of particular in-

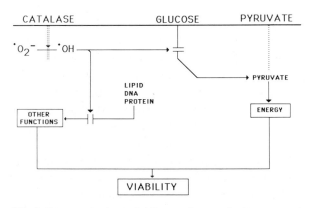

Fig. 9 Diagrammatic model for catalase and pyruvate equivalent competence to support the survival of prenatal neurons in vitro. Oxygen radicals ($^{\cdot}O_2^-$) generate hydroxyl radicals ($^{\cdot}OH$) via production of H_2O_2. A peroxidative block on the glucose-to-pyruvate pathway could be prevented by catalase or bypassed by exogenous pyruvate. Peroxidative damage may also affect other functions required for neuronal viability.

terest in our own context is that free radical damage may be involved in specific neuropathological situations in humans, for example, retinal phototoxicity, post-ischemic brain injury, brain aging processes, and neurodegenerative diseases such as Alzheimer's and Parkinson's (Vitorica et al., 1984; Halliwell and Gutteridge, 1985; Bannon et al., 1984; among others). Also encouraging are some observations that NGF increases the resistance of neuroblastoma cells to the free-radical-mediated cytotoxicity of 6-hydroxydopamine (Tiffany-Castiglioni and Perez-Polo, 1981), possibly by increasing the cell production of catalase and dismutases (Perez-Polo and Werrbach-Perez, 1985). Perhaps along similar lines may be a recent finding that NGF stimulates cognitive functions in aged rats (Gage et al., 1986).

Neurite regulation and extracellular matrix

Some of the early experiments using CG neurons to probe for ciliary neuronotrophic factors revealed the existence of factors, distinct from the neuronotrophic ones, whose special competence was to anchor themselves to polycationic (and other) substrata and confer on them the ability to stimulate neuritic outgrowth (Collins, 1978; Varon et al., 1979; Adler and Varon, 1980; Davis et al., 1985b). Fig. 10 illustrates the different behaviors of ciliary ganglionic neurons when cultured with both the trophic and the neurite promoting factors (A: survival + neurites) or with only one (B: survival but no neurites) or the other (C: initial neurite outgrowth, but no survival). These polycation-binding neurite promoting factors (PNPFs) were present in media conditioned by several cell cultures including glial ones (Adler et al., 1981), contained carbohydrate moieties (Adler et al., 1983), and stimulated neuritic outgrowth from CNS as well as PNS neurons (Manthorpe et al., 1983; Barbin et al., 1984b).

The anchorage-dependence and carbohydrate content of these PNPFs directed subsequent investigations to purified constituents of extracellular matrix (ECM). Laminin, one of the ECM glycoproteins tested, proved to be a most potent neurite promoter (Baron van Evercooren et al., 1982; Manthorpe et al., 1983; Wewer et al., 1983). The neurite promoting region of the laminin molecule appears restricted to the distal

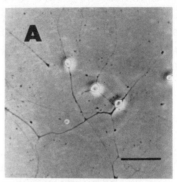
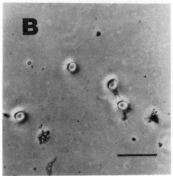
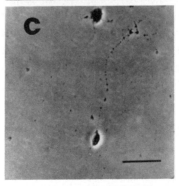

Fig. 10 Distinctive influences of neuronotrophic and neurite promoting factors. E8 chick ciliary ganglion neurons were cultured for 24 h in the presence of (A) both neuronotrophic and neurite promoting agents, (B) only the neuronotrophic support or (C) only the neurite promoting factor. Magnification bar = 200 μm.

portion of its long arm (Edgar et al., 1984; Engvall et al., 1986). Purification of PNPF from Schwannoma-conditioned medium led to the demonstration that (i) it owed its neurite promoting activity to its laminin content, but (ii) the laminin was packaged with proteoglycans (also ECM constituents) in such a way as to be resistant to inactivation by anti-laminin antibodies and to interferences by serum components (Manthorpe et al., 1981b; Davis et al., 1985a,b, 1987c).

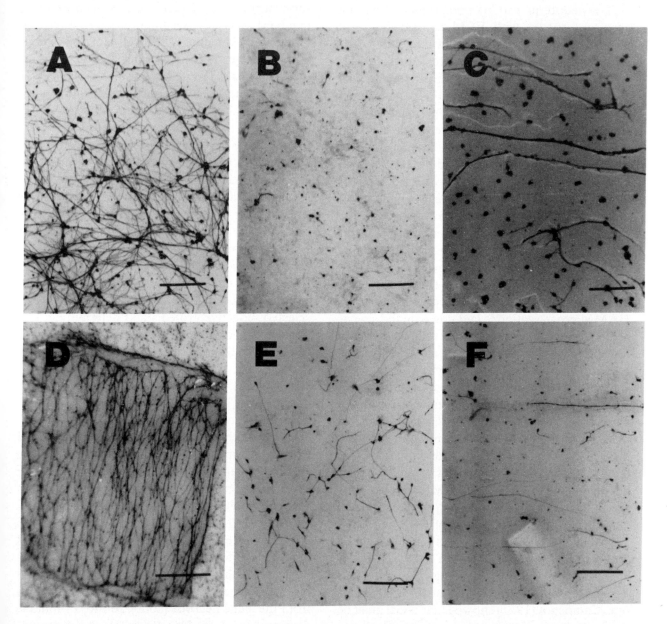

Fig. 11 Human or rat membrane matrix promotes neuritic growth of PNS and CNS neurons in vitro. A–D, E8 chick ciliary ganglion neurons; E,F, E4 chick spinal cord neurons. Random (A) or oriented (D) neurite growth is supported by the basement membrane but not the stromal (B) face of the matrix, and follows basement membrane (laminin immunoreactive) profiles on cross-sections of folded matrix (C). Magnification bars: 200 (C), 450 (A,B,E,F) and 1000 (D) μm.

Similar involvements of laminin and/or proteoglycans have been reported for other PNPFs, from media conditioned by corneal endothelial (Lander et al., 1985) or PC12 cells (Matthew and Patterson, 1983).

The neurite promoting competence of culture substrata coated with ECM constituents, and laminin in particular, prompted attempts to demonstrate a similar neurite promoting competence in naturally assembled ECM itself. One such preparation was obtained from human placental amnion membrane by lysing and removing its epithelial cell layer (Davis et al., 1987a,b). The resulting human amnion membrane matrix (HAMM) can be laid down on a nitrocellulose paper strip and tested as a culture substratum for PNS and CNS neurons. Some of those cultures, as well as cultures using a similar preparation (RAMM) from rat amnion membranes (Manthorpe et al., 1987), are illustrated in Fig. 11. Massive neurite outgrowth is promoted on the basal membrane face (A) but not the stroma face (B) of a HAMM preparation. If a HAMM cross-section is laid down on the side as a substratum, neurites will grow only on the basal membrane portion of it and grossly coincide with its laminin-immunoreactive profile (C). In some HAMM or RAMM preparations, neuritic growth is highly oriented in parallel bundles (D). Spinal cord and other CNS neurons grow extensive neurites on a RAMM substratum (E, F). Note the lack of species specificity, with human or rat matrix being equally competent on chick or rat test neurons. HAMM and RAMM preparations are now being investigated as potential 'bridge' materials for the regeneration of PNS and CNS axons across a lesion gap in adult mammals (e.g. Davis et al., 1987a; Manthorpe et al., 1987).

Nerve growth factor has long been viewed as a neurite promoting factor as much as a trophic one. Campenot (1977) showed that NGF must be available at the growth cone locale for neurites to grow or even be maintained. Gundersen and Barrett (1980) were able to alter the orientation of growth cones by imposing local NGF gradients.

Greene and Tischler (1976) and many others have demonstrated the ability of NGF to elicit neuritic outgrowth from PC12 cells which had never before expressed that property (cf. Greene and Shooter, 1980). In all cases, as with the neuronal survival function of NGF, it has been assumed that NGF operates as a humoral agent. A recently developed technique, called 'cell-blot', has forced a provocative re-assessment of that assumption (Carnow et al., 1985; Pettmann et al., 1987). In this technique, NTF-containing materials (e.g. extracts from chick eye or rat nerve for CNTF, or from mouse submaxillary gland for NGF) are electrophoresed on an SDS gel (to separate different proteins largely according to size) and then electrophoretically blotted onto nitrocellulose strips. The nitrocellulose strips are then used as substrate for the culturing of probe neurons (e.g. CG neurons for CNTF, E8 DRG neurons for NGF) with media lacking the NTF, and the surviving neurons are stained with MTT, a vital dye that is taken up and modified only by living cells. This technique is particularly useful in identifying selected bioactive proteins and determining their molecular properties without having first to isolate them from a crude source material (Rudge et al., 1987).

Fig. 12 shows fields of nitrocellulose blots comprising CNTF or NGF bands isolated first by SDS-PAGE. Very few CG or DRG neurons survive outside the trophic factor bands (a,b). E8 CG neurons survive only on a CNTF band (c), while E8 DRG neurons are supported only by an NGF band (d). Neurons from E10 DRG, which can receive trophic support by either factor (cf. Fig. 6A), will survive on either blotted protein (e,f). However, the use of an antibody against neurofilament protein in place of the MTT vital dye reveals that NGF, in contrast to CNTF, is also able to elicit a vigorous neurite outgrowth from the same neurons (compare Fig. 12 f and e, respectively). It is clear, therefore, that neuronotrophic factors can express both their survival promoting (trophic) and their neurite promoting (when applicable) competences from a substra-

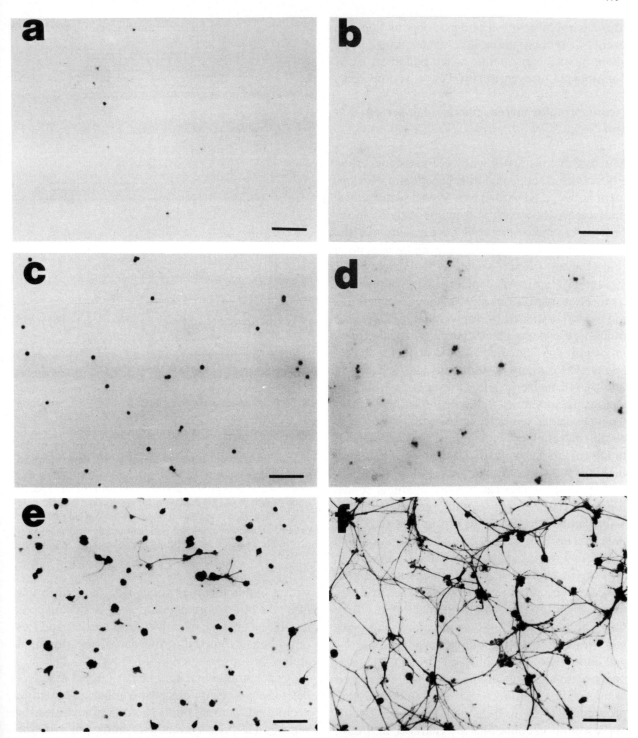

Fig. 12 Neuronal survival and neurite outgrowth visualized by a 'cell blot' technique. Chick embryo neurons were cultured for 48 h on nitrocellulose blots of electrophoresed CNTF or NGF, with no trophic factors in the culture medium. a–d = MTT staining; e,f = neurofilament protein immunostaining. Survival of E8 chick ciliary ganglion or DRG neurons occurs only on the blotted bands of their respective trophic factor CNTF (c) or NGF (d), but not on other regions of the blot (a,b). E10 DRG neurons can be supported by either CNTF (e) or NGF (f) bands, but respond with vigorous neurite growth only to NGF (f).

tum-anchored position and not only as humoral agents. It remains to be investigated whether the same factors can operate when bound to ECM components or even to surfaces of 'source' cells.

Neuronotrophic factors and the adult nervous system

Much of the past work with NTFs has concerned PNS neurons, collected during perinatal development and studied with in vitro model systems. For many years, however, and increasingly so in recent times, neuroscientists have entertained the notion that NTFs may play a much more general role (Varon, 1975c; Apple, 1981; Varon et al., 1984a, 1987a,b). An expanded 'neuronotrophic hypothesis' has proposed that adult CNS neurons in vivo are sustained by appropriate NTFs just as much as developing PNS neurons are in vitro or in vivo. If so, neuronotrophic deficits may be responsible for many dysfunctions and/or death of adult CNS neurons, and interventions with exogenous factors may facilitate repair or protect against further damage. It seems fitting to conclude this chapter with a brief survey of NTF involvements in two experimental in vivo models of PNS and CNS regeneration in the adult rat.

Fig. 13 illustrates the silicone chamber model for nerve regeneration (Lundborg et al., 1982a,b; Varon and Williams, 1986; Williams et al., 1987). A sciatic nerve is mobilized and cut proximally to its bifurcation, a 2 mm piece of nerve is discarded, and the proximal and distal stumps are inserted into the two ends of a silicone tube to define an empty, 10-mm-long chamber space (Fig. 13A). One month later a nerve structure will have regenerated across this interstump gap, and axons will continue to grow into and through the distal nerve segment to reach and reinnervate their end organs. Regeneration across the chamber proceeds with a well-defined sequence (B): (i) nerve stump exudate fills the chamber in 1 day; (ii) a co-axial fibrin matrix coalesces out of the fluid materials within 1 week; (iii) cells migrate from both stumps into this matrix and populate it

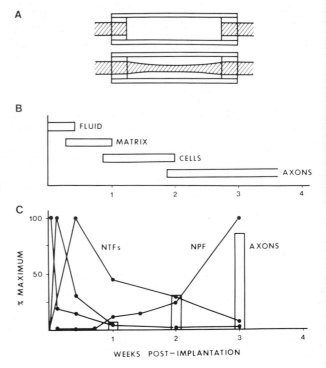

Fig. 13 Neuronotrophic (NTFs) and neurite promoting (NPFs) factors in a silicone chamber model for peripheral nerve regeneration in the adult rat. (A) Schematic representation of the chamber: proximal and distal stumps of a transected sciatic nerve are inserted into the opposite ends of a silicone tube, leaving a 10-mm-long gap ('chamber') through which a nerve regenerate will form within one month. (B) Sequential appearance of various components of the regeneration progress. (C) NTFs for the main neuronal contributors to a sciatic nerve appear and peak early, whereas NPFs develop later in conjunction with cell immigration and predict the advance of regenerating axons into the chamber.

with a circumferential population of perineurial-like cells and a core population of Schwann cells and blood vessels, over the next 2 weeks; and (iv) only then, axons will grow out of the proximal stump and myelination will follow.

The chamber fluid has been examined at different time points for neuronotrophic and neurite promoting factors (Fig. 13C). NTF activities for sensory (DRG), sympathetic and spinal motor neurons appear in that order in the chamber fluid, peak within the first few days and decline to a low but sustained level thereafter (Longo et al., 1983).

On the other hand, PNPF activity in the fluid and laminin immunoreactivity in the structure only appear after cell immigration has occurred, and axonal advance proceeds in precise temporal coincidence with their increases (Longo et al., 1984). While the findings were only correlative, they did provide a first demonstration of the occurrence and temporal modulation of such factors in traumatic repair circumstances of an adult mammalian nerve.

Axonal regeneration usually fails in the CNS of adult mammals. Aguayo and collaborators (1982) have shown that CNS axons do regenerate for considerable distances if supplied with a peripheral nerve segment in which to grow. Peripheral nerve may be a positive terrain because of its contents of NTFs and NPFs (cf. Varon, 1977). A septo-hippocampal model system has been developed to test these hypotheses (Varon et al., 1987d). The hippocampal formation receives much of its cholinergic innervation from the medial septum and diagonal band nuclei, largely via the fimbria/fornix tract. A crucial set of observations has recently linked cholinergic CNS neurons with NGF. NGF is produced and available in the hippocampal tissue and can be retrogradely transported from there to the septal cholinergic cell bodies (Korsching et al., 1985, 1986). Medial septum cholinergic neurons display immunoreactive and NGF-binding NGF receptors (Taniuchi et al., 1986). NGF causes an increase in choline acetyltransferase (ChAT) in these neurons both in vitro and in vivo (Hefti et al., 1984, 1985). One could, therefore, hypothesize that: (i) complete transection of the fimbria/fornix would interrupt the delivery to the medial septum cholinergic neurons of their putative trophic factor, NGF; (ii) the resulting trophic deprivation should lead to deterioration and even death of these neurons; and (iii) administration of exogenous NGF should substantially prevent the fimbria/fornix-induced damage to the septal cholinergic neurons. Recent work from several laboratories has proven that such is indeed the case (Hefti, 1986; Williams et al., 1986; Kromer, 1987).

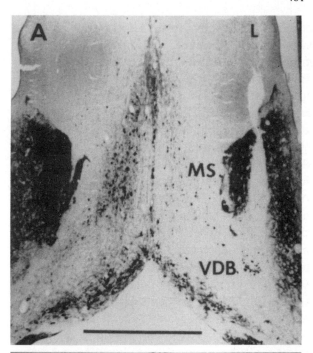

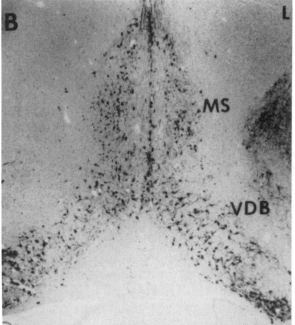

Fig. 14 Coronal sections of adult rat brain, stained for choline acetyltransferase and showing cholinergic neurons in the medial septum (MS) and vertical limb of the diagonal band (VDB). (A) Unilateral transection (left side of photograph) of the fimbria/fornix causes the disappearance of stainable neurons on the same side. (B) Neuronal loss is prevented by continuous infusion of NGF into the ipsilateral ventricle. Magnification bar = 1 mm.

Fig. 14 displays coronal sections from adult rats which received a unilateral, complete fimbria/fornix transection and were continuously infused with or without NGF for 14 days into the ipsilateral ventricle. The sections are immunostained for ChAT, thereby providing for the detection of cholinergic neurons as ChAT-positive cells. Contralaterally to the fimbria/fornix lesion (left sides), ChAT-positive neurons are well identified in numbers practically matching those of an unoperated animal. On the side of the lesion and with only vehicle infusion (A), about 80% of the ChAT-positive neurons in the medial septum are no longer detectable. In dramatic contrast, the lesion side of NGF-treated animals (B) continues to display a nearly full population of ChAT-positive cells. Such experiments provide unequivocal evidence of a strong trophic competence of NGF for these adult CNS cholinergic neurons. A question that remains to be fully addressed, however, is whether the cells 'lost' after axotomy are actually dead and NGF protects them against this death, or whether the axotomized cells have lost their ChAT (and acetylcholinesterase) contents and NGF, in preventing such a loss, maintains their visibility by immunostaining (cf. Hagg et al., 1987).

Further investigations of NTF roles in the adult CNS will probably proceed in two distinct directions (cf. Varon et al., 1987b,d). One, along the lines of the model just described, should (i) further define the action of NGF (and other agents) on the 'acute' damage imparted by the experimental, mechanical lesion, (ii) attempt to 'bridge' the lesion gap with neurite-promoting or even NTF-carrying prosthetic materials (e.g. the already discussed HAMM), and (iii) evaluate by electrophysiological and behavioral means any functional regeneration following hippocampal re-innervation. The other, along the more general lines of the neuronotrophic hypothesis, should (i) seek alternate ways to impart chronic as well as acute lesions, (ii) explore non-experimental chronic deficits, such as may occur in aged animals, and (iii) evaluate whether interventions with exogenous NTFs might lead to sufficient improvements to warrant some future investigation of clinical applications to a human patient.

Summary and concluding remarks

Functional neuroteratology, the theme of this Summer School, necessarily focuses on defects of neural circuits resulting from fetal exposure to noxious influences and leading to dysfunction of neural behaviors or of body functions that are neurally controlled. Neural circuitry defects may involve normally established networks which fail to perform because of inappropriate intra-network communications, and many presentations at this meeting have properly emphasized potential defects in neurotransmission – presynaptic generation and release of neurotransmitters, postsynaptic receptors and transduction mechanisms. On the other hand, the neuroteratological defect may reflect the defective construction of a neural circuit, that is, disrupted regulation of neuronogenesis (neuroblast proliferation, neuronal cell death), neuritogenesis (elongation and directional guidance of axons and dendrites) and/or synaptogenesis (specific connectivity, selection of transmitter mode, functional synapse formation). It is this second area – regulation or disregulation of the genesis of neural circuitry – that has been addressed in this chapter.

We have reviewed here current knowledge and concepts concerning several classes of specific proteins which control neuronal survival and functional maintenance (neuronotrophic factors) and/or neuritic growth and guidance (neurite promoting factors). Both types of factor may address a target neuron either from its humoral environment (extracellular fluid) or after anchorage to neighboring structures (extracellular matrix, local cell surfaces). We have seen that both types of factor operate not only during neural development but also with regard to the maintenance and repair capabilities of the adult neuron, and thus serve as crucial 'physiological' control elements in the generation and maintenance of functional circuitry. It appears reasonable, therefore, to postulate that teratogenic agents may achieve their final consequences through the disruption of such control systems; the production and delivery of these factors from innervation territories and glial cell partners and/or their reception and response machineries in the target neurons. This postulation arises from our neurobiological knowledge rather than from the actual recognition of neuroteratological situations explicitly involving such factors. It is, therefore, intended to draw attention to possible rather than actual involvements of these factors in functional neuroteratology. There are, nevertheless, a few aspects touched upon in this chapter which may have a more obvious bearing on the main theme of this Summer School.

(a) Disruption of NGF supply. Systemic administration of antiserum against NGF to neonatal mice leads to the permanent destruction of their peripheral sympathetic systems, the so-called immunosympathectomy (cf. Levi-Montalcini, 1966, 1982; Greene and Shooter, 1980). Administration of NGF itself to a pregnant rodent dam induces formation of anti-NGF antibodies which causes in the early fetuses destruction of both dorsal root and sympathetic ganglionic neurons (Johnson et al., 1986). Such obvious examples of functional neuroteratology, however, result from experimental manipulations and there is no clear example to date of naturally occurring interferences with NGF or other neuronotrophic factor availability. Attempts to establish unequivocally NGF disturbances in familial disautonomia (a genetic disease involving damage to several peripheral ganglia) have not been successful, thus far (Breakefield and Combi, 1987).

(b) Free radicals and neuronal death. We have seen that prenatal CNS (and, to a lesser extent, PNS) neurons in monolayer cultures are particulary susceptible to peroxidation damage, which affects their ability to utilize glucose as an energy source and thus leads to neuronal death. Peroxi-

dation damage may result from an increased generation of free radicals (cf. Balasz, Chapter 28 of this volume), a reduction in cellular mechanisms for antioxidant defense, or an inadequate turnover/replacement of the damaged cell components – leading to the speculation that neuronotrophic factors may provide protection against free radical attack. Here, too, there is experimental but no naturally occurring evidence for such a view. The cytotoxicity of 6-hydroxydopamine on catecholaminergic neurons (cf. Kostrzewa, Chapter 26 of this volume) is mediated through free radical generation, and the protection offered by NGF to sympathetic neurons in such an experimental situation appears to involve an increased production by the neurons of catalase and superoxide desmutases (Perez-Polo and Werrbach-Perez, 1985).

(c) NGF and CNS cognitive functions. We have recently demonstrated that exogenously supplied NGF reduces cognitive deficits in aged rats (Gage et al., 1986; Fischer et al., 1987), presumably through its trophic action on cholinergic neurons in the basal forebrain. Functional neuroteratology clearly includes early defects in memory processing and learning, which in turn may reflect irregularities in the development and/or function of CNS cholinergic components. The observation that NGF is a critical regulator of CNS cholinergic function is a recent one, and little information is yet available on its impact (or the consequences of interfering with it) with regard to pre- and perinatal development of cognitive behaviors. Nevertheless, it would seem reasonable to view these types of study as a future avenue for important advances.

Acknowledgements

This work was partially supported by grants BNS-85-01766 and BNS-86-17034 from NSF, grant NS-16349 from NIH. B.P. is a Chargé de Recherche at the INSERM.

484

References

Adler, R. and Varon, S. (1980) Cholinergic neuronotrophic factors: V. Segregation of survival- and neurite-promoting activities in heart conditioned media. *Brain Res.*, 188: 437–448.

Adler, R., Manthorpe, M., Skaper, S. D. and Varon, S. (1981) Polyornithine-attached neurite-promoting factors (PNPFs): culture sources and responsive neurons. *Brain Res.*, 206: 129–144.

Adler, R., Manthorpe, M. and Varon, S. (1983) Lectin reactivity of PNPF, a polyornithine-binding neurite-promoting factor. *Dev. Brain Res.*, 6: 69–75.

Aguayo, A., Davis, S., Richardson, P. and Bray, G. (1982) Axonal elongation in peripheral and central nervous system transplants. *Adv. Cell. Neurobiol.*, 3: 215–234.

Appel, S. H. (1981) A unifying hypothesis for the cause of Amyotrophic Lateral Sclerosis, Parkinsonism and Alzheimer disease. *Ann. Neurol.*, 10: 499–505.

Bannon, M. J., Goedert, M. and Williams, B. (1984) The possible relation of glutathione, melanin and 1-methyl-4-phenyl-1,2,5,6-tetrahydropyridine (MPTP) to Parkinson's Disease. *Biochem. Pharmacol.*, 33: 2697–2698.

Barbin, G., Manthorpe, M. and Varon, S. (1984a) Purification of the chick eye Ciliary Neuronotrophic Factor (CNTF). *J. Neurochem.*, 43: 1468–1478.

Barbin, G., Selak, I., Manthorpe, M. and Varon, S. (1984b) Use of central neuronal cultures for the detection of neuronotrophic agents. *Neuroscience*, 12: 33–43.

Barde, Y.-A., Edgar, D. and Thoenen, H. (1982) Purification of a new neurotrophic factor from mammalian brain. *EMBO J.*, 1: 549–553.

Barnes, D. and Sato, G. (1980) Methods for growth of cultured cells in serum-free medium. *Anal. Biochem.*, 102: 255.

Baron Van Evercooren, A., Kleinman, H. K., Ohno, S., Marangos, P., Schwartz, J. P. and Dubois-Dalcq, M. E. (1982) Nerve Growth Factor, laminin and fibronectin promote neurite growth in human fetal sensory ganglia cultures. *J. Neurosci. Res.*, 8: 179–194.

Bors, W., Saran, M. and Tait, D. (Eds.) (1984) *Oxygen Radicals in Chemistry and Biology*, deGruyter, Berlin.

Bottenstein, J. E. and Sato, G. (1979) Growth of a neuroblastoma cell line in serum-free supplemented medium. *Proc. Natl. Acad. Sci. USA*, 76: 514–517.

Bottenstein, J. E., Skaper, S. D., Varon, S. and Sato, G. H. (1980) Selective survival of neurons from chick embryo sensory ganglionic dissociates using defined, serum-free supplemented medium. *Exp. Cell Res.*, 125: 183–190.

Breakefield, X. O. and Combi, F. (1987) Molecular genetic insights into neurological diseases. *Annu. Rev. Neurosci.*, 10: 535–594.

Bueker, E. D. (1948) Implantation of tumors in the hind limb field of the embryonic chick and developmental response of the lumbosacral nervous system. *Anat. Record*, 102: 369–390.

Campenot, R. (1977) Local control of neurite development by nerve growth factor. *Proc. Natl. Acad. Sci. USA*, 74: 4516–4519.

Carnow, T. B., Manthorpe, M., Davis, G. E. and Varon, S. (1985) Localized survival of ciliary ganglionic neurons identifies neuronotrophic factor bands on nitrocellulose blots. *J. Neurosci.*, 5: 1965–1971.

Chau, R. M. W., Skaper, S. D. and Varon, S. (1988) Peroxidative block of glucose utilization and survival in CNS neuronal cultures. *Neurochem. Res.*, 13: 611–616.

Collins, F. (1978) Induction of neurite outgrowth by a conditioned-medium factor bound to the culture substratum. *Proc. Natl. Acad. Sci. USA*, 75: 5210–5213.

Contreras, M. L. and Guroff, G. (1987) Calcium-dependent Nerve Growth Factor-stimulated hydrolysis of phosphoinositides in PC12 cells. *J. Neurochem.*, 48: 1466–1472.

Cowan, C. W., Fawcett, J. W., O'Leary, D. D. M. and Stanfield, B. B. (1984) Regressive events in neurogenesis. *Science*, 225: 1258–1265.

Cremins, J., Wagner, J. A. and Halegoua, S. (1986) Nerve Growth Factor action is mediated by cyclic AMP and Ca^{++}/phospholipid-dependent protein kinases. *J. Cell Biol.*, 103: 887–893.

Culter, R. G. (1985) Peroxide-producing potential of tissues: inverse correlation with longevity of mammalian species. *Proc. Natl. Acad. Sci. USA*, 82: 4798–4802.

Davis, G. E., Manthorpe, M., Engvall, E. and Varon, S. (1985a) Isolation and characterization of rat schwannoma neurite promoting factor: evidence that the factor contains laminin. *J. Neurosci.*, 5: 2662–2671.

Davis, G. E., Varon, S., Engvall, E. and Manthorpe, M. (1985b) Substratum-binding neurite promoting factors: relationships to laminin. *Trends Neurosci.*, 8: 528–532.

Davis, G. E., Blaker, S. N., Engvall, E., Varon, S., Manthorpe, M. and Gage, F. H. (1987a) Human amnion membrane serves as a substratum for growing axons in vitro and in vivo. *Science*, 236: 1106–1109.

Davis, G. E., Engvall, E., Varon, S. and Manthorpe, M. (1987b) Human amnion membrane as a substratum for cultured peripheral and central nervous system neurons. *Dev. Brain Res.*, 33: 1–10.

Davis, G. E., Klier, F. G., Engvall, E., Cornbrooks, C., Varon, S. and Manthorpe, M. (1987c) Association of laminin with heparan and chondroitin sulfate-bearing proteoglycans in neurite-promoting complexes from rat Schwannoma cells. *Neurochem. Res.*, 12: 909–921.

Edgar, D., Timpl, R. and Thoenen, H. (1984) The heparin-binding domain of laminin is responsible for its effects on neurite outgrowth and neuronal survival. *EMBO J.*, 3: 1463–1468.

Engvall, E., Davis, G. E., Dickerson, K., Ruoslahti, E., Varon, S. and Manthorpe, M. (1986) Mapping of domains in human laminin using monoclonal antibodies; localization of the neurite-promoting site. *J. Cell Biol.*, 103: 2457–2465.

Facci, L., Skaper, S. D. and Varon, S. (1985) Specific replacements of pyruvate for trophic support of central and peripheral nervous system neurons. *J. Neurochem.*, 45: 926–934.

Facci, L., Skaper, S. D. and Varon, S. (1986) Transaminase of glutamate to citric acid cycle intermediates in cultured neurons correlates with the ability of oxoacids to support neuronal survival in vitro. *Biochem. J.*, 234: 605–610.

Fischer, W., Wictorin, K., Björklund, A., Williams, L. R., Varon, S. and Gage, F. H. (1981) Amelioration of cholinergic neuron atrophy and spatial memory impairments in aged rats by Nerve Growth Factor. *Nature*, 329: 65–68.

Fridovich, I. (1983) Superoxide radical: an endogenous toxicant. *Annu. Rev. Pharmacol. Toxicol.*, 23: 239–257.

Gage, F. H., Wictorin, K., Fisher, W., Williams, L. R., Varon, S. and Björklund, A. (1986) Chronic intracerebral infusion of Nerve Growth Factor (NGF) improves memory performance in cognitively impaired aged rats. *Soc. Neurosci. Abstr.*, 12: 1580.

Greene, L. A. and Shooter, E. M. (1980) The Nerve Growth Factor: biochemistry, synthesis, and mechanism of action. *Annu. Rev. Neurosci.*, 3: 353–402.

Greene, L. A. and Tischler, A. S. (1976) Establishment of a noradrenergic clonal line of rat adrenal pheochromocytoma cells which respond to nerve growth factor. *Proc. Natl. Acad. Sci. USA*, 73: 2424–2428.

Gundersen, R. W. and Barrett, J. N. (1980) Characterization of the turning response of dorsal root neurites toward nerve growth factor. *J. Cell Biol.*, 87: 546–554.

Hagg, T., Vahlsing, H. L., Manthorpe, M. and Varon, S. (1987) Delayed intraventricular NGF infusion reverses axotomy-induced loss of medial septum ChAT-positive neurons. *Soc. Neurosci. Abstr.*, 13: 922.

Halliwell, B. and Gutteridge, J. M. C. (1985) Oxygen radicals and the nervous system. *Trends Neurosci.*, 8: 22–26.

Hamburger, V. and Oppenheim, R. N. (1982) Naturally occurring neuronal death in vertebrates. *Neurosci. Comment.*, 1: 39–55.

Hefti, F. (1986) Nerve Growth Factor promotes survival of septal cholinergic neurons after fimbrial transections. *J. Neurosci.*, 6: 2155–2162.

Hefti, F., Dravid, A. and Hartikka, J. (1984) Chronic intraventricular injections of Nerve Growth Factor elevate hippocampal choline acetyltransferase activity in adult rats with partial septo-hippocampal lesions. *Brain Res.*, 293: 305–311.

Hefti, F., Hartikka, J. J., Eckenstein, F., Gnahn, H., Heumann, R. and Schwab, M. (1985) Nerve Growth Factor increases choline acetyltransferase but not survival or fiber outgrowth of cultured fetal septal cholinergic neurons. *Neuroscience*, 14: 55–68.

Johnson, E. M. Jr., Rich, K. M. and Yip, H. K. (1986) The role of NGF in sensory neurons in vivo. *Trends Neurosci.*, 9: 33–37.

Korshing, S., Auburger, G., Heumann, R., Scott, J. and Thoenen, H. (1985) Levels of nerve growth factor and its mRNA in the central nervous system of the rat correlate with cholinergic innervation. *EMBO J.*, 4: 1389–1393.

Korshing, S., Heumann, R., Thoenen, H. and Hefti, F. (1986) Cholinergic denervation of the rat hippocampus by fimbrial transection leads to a transient accumulation of nerve growth factor (NGF) without change in mRNA NGF content. *Neurosci. Lett.*, 66: 175–180.

Kromer, L. F. (1987) Nerve Growth Factor treatment after brain injury prevents neuronal death. *Science*, 235: 214–216.

Lander, A. D., Fujii, D. K. and Reichardt, L. F. (1985) Laminin is associated with the 'neurite outgrowth promoting factors' found in conditioned media. *Proc. Natl. Acad. Sci. USA*, 82: 2183–2189.

Le Douarin, N. M. (1982) *The Neural Crest*, Cambridge University Press, Cambridge, UK.

Levi-Montalcini, R. (1966) The Nerve Growth Factor: its mode of action on sensory and sympathetic neurons. *Harvey Lect.* 60: 217–259.

Levi-Montalcini, R. (1982) Developmental neurobiology and the natural history of Nerve Growth Factor. *Annu. Rev. Neurosci.*, 5: 341–361.

Levi-Montalcini, R. and Hamburger, V. (1951) Selective growth stimulating effects of mouse sarcoma on sensory and sympathetic neurons systems of the chick embryo. *J. Exp. Zool.*, 116: 321–362.

Longo, F. M., Skaper, S. D., Manthorpe, M., Williams, L. R., Lundborg, G. and Varon, S. (1983) Temporal changes in neuronotrophic activities accumulating in vivo within nerve regeneration chambers. *Exp. Neurol.*, 81: 756–769.

Longo, F. M., Hayman, E. G., Davis, G. E., Ruoslahti, E., Engvall, E., Manthorpe, M. and Varon, S. (1984) Neurite promoting factors and extracellular matrix components accumulating in vivo within nerve regeneration chambers. *Brain Res.*, 309: 105–117.

Lundborg, G., Gelberman, R. H., Longo, F. M., Powell, H. C. and Varon, S. (1982a) In vivo regeneration of cut nerves encased in silicone tubes: growth across a six millimeter gap. *J. Neuropath. Exp. Neurol.*, 41(4): 412–422.

Lundborg, G., Longo, F. M. and Varon, S. (1982b) Nerve regeneration model and trophic factors in vivo. *Brain Res.*, 232: 157–161.

Manthorpe, M. and Varon, S. (1985) Regulation of neuronal survival and neuritic growth in the avian ciliary ganglion. In G. Guroff (Ed.), *Growth and Maturation Factors, Vol. 3*, J. Wiley & Sons, New York, pp. 77–117.

Manthorpe, M., Skaper, S. D. and Varon, S. (1981a) Neuronotrophic factors and their antibodies: in vitro microassays for titration and screening. *Brain Res.*, 230: 295–306.

Manthorpe, M., Varon, S. and Adler, R. (1981b) Neurite-promoting factor in conditioned medium from RN22 schwannoma cultures: bioassay, fractionation and properties. *J. Neurochem.*, 37: 759–767.

Manthorpe, M., Longo, F. M. and Varon, S. (1982) Comparative features of spinal neuronotrophic factors in fluids collected in vitro and in vivo. *J. Neurosci. Res.*, 8: 241–250.

Manthorpe, M., Engvall, E., Ruoslahti, E., Longo, F. M., Davis, G. E. and Varon, S. (1983) Laminin promotes neuritic regeneration from cultured peripheral and central neurons. *J. Cell Biol.*, 97: 1882–1890.

Manthorpe, M., Rudge, J. and Varon, S. (1986a) Astroglial cell contributions to neuronal survival and neuritic growth. In S. Fedoroff and A. Vernadakis (Eds.), *Astrocytes, Vol. 2*, Academic Press, New York, pp. 315–376.

Manthorpe, M., Skaper, S. D., Williams, L. R. and Varon, S. (1986b) Purification of adult rat sciatic nerve ciliary neuronotrophic factor. *Brain Res.*, 367: 282–286.

Manthorpe, M., Danielsen, N., Vahlsing, H. L., Pettmann, B., Davis, G. E., Engvall, E. and Varon, S. (1987) Rat amnion membrane is a growth-promoting surface for cultured peripheral and central neurons. *Soc. Neurosci. Abstr.*, 13: 1484.

Matthew, W. D. and Patterson, P. H. (1983) The production of a monoclonal antibody that blocks the action of a neurite outgrowth-promoting factor. *Cold Spring Harbor Symp. Quant. Biol.*, 48: 625–631.

Michler-Stuke, A. and Bottenstein, J. (1982) Proliferation of glial-derived cells in defined media. *J. Neurosci. Res.*, 7: 215–228.

Montz, H. P. M., Davis, G. E., Skaper, S. D., Manthorpe, M. and Varon, S. (1985) Tumor-promoting phorbol diester mimics two distinct neuronotrophic factors. *Dev. Brain Res.*, 23: 150–154.

Perez-Polo, J. R. and Werrbach-Perez, K. (1985) Effects of Nerve Growth Factor on the in vitro responses of neurons to injury. In J. Eccles and M. R. Dimitrijevic (Eds.), *Recent Achievements in Restorative Neurology, Vol. 1*, S. Karger, Basel, pp. 321–337.

Pettmann, B., Varon, S. and Manthorpe, M. (1987) Visualization of nerve growth factor biological activities by a cell-blot technique using ganglionic neurons as probes. *Soc. Neurosci. Abstr.*, 13: 1608.

Prestige, M. C. (1970) Differentiation, degeneration and the role of the periphery: quantitative considerations. In F. O. Schmitt (Ed.), *The Neurosciences: Second Study Program*, Rockefeller University Press, pp. 73–82.

Pryor, W. A. (Ed.) (1982) *Free Radicals in Biology, Vol. 5*, Academic Press, New York.

Rudge, J., Davis, G., Manthorpe, M. and Varon, S. (1987) An examination of ciliary neuronotrophic factors from avian and rodent tissue extracts using a blot and culture technique. *Dev. Brain Res.*, 32: 103–110.

Saneto, R. P. and deVellis, J. (1987) The use of primary oligodendrocyte and astrocyte cultures to study glial growth factors. In J. R. Perez-Polo (Ed.), *Handbook of Nervous System and Muscle Factors*, CRC Press, Boca Raton, FL, in press.

Selak, I., Skaper, S. D. and Varon, S. (1985) Pyruvate participation in the low molecular weight trophic activity for CNS neurons in glia-conditioned media. *J. Neurosci.*, 5: 23–28.

Skaper, S. D. and Varon, S. (1981) Mutually independent cyclic AMP and sodium responses to Nerve Growth Factor in embryonic chick dorsal root ganglia. *J. Neurochem.*, 37: 222–228.

Skaper, S. D. and Varon, S. (1983a) Control of the Na^+, K^+-pump by Nerve Growth Factor is essential to neuronal survival. *Brain Res.*, 271: 263–271.

Skaper, S. D. and Varon, S. (1983b) Ionic behaviors and Nerve Growth Factor dependence in developing chick ganglia. II. Studies with neurons of dorsal root ganglia. *Dev. Biol.*, 98: 257–264.

Skaper, S. D., Adler, R. and Varon, S. (1979) A procedure for purifying neuron-like cells in cultures from central nervous tissues with a defined medium. *Dev. Neurosci.*, 2: 233–237.

Skaper, S. D., Selak, I., Manthorpe, M. and Varon, S. (1984) Chemically defined requirements for the survival of cultured 8-day chick embryo ciliary ganglion neurons. *Brain Res.*, 302: 281–290.

Skaper, S. D., Montz, H. P. M. and Varon, S. (1986) Control of Na^+, K^+-pump activity in dorsal root ganglionic neurons by different neuronotrophic agents. *Brain Res.*, 386: 130–135.

Taniuchi, M., Schweizer, J. B. and Johnson, E. M. (1986) Nerve growth factor receptor molecules in rat brain. *Proc. Natl. Acad. Sci. USA*, 83: 1950–1954.

Thoenen, H. and Barde, Y.-A. (1980) Physiology of nerve growth factor. *Physiol. Rev.*, 60: 1284–1335.

Tiffany-Castiglioni, E. and Perez-Polo, J. R. (1981) Stimulation of resistance to 6-hydroxydopamine in a human neuroblastoma cell line by Nerve Growth Factor. *Neurosci. Lett.*, 26: 157–161.

Togari, A. and Guroff, G. (1985) Partial purification and characterization of a Nerve Growth Factor-sensitive kinase and its substrate from PC12 cells. *J. Biol. Chem.*, 260: 3804–3811.

Varon, S. (1975a) Nerve Growth Factor and its mode of action. *Exp. Neurol.*, 48 (3, part 2): 75–92.

Varon, S. (1975b) Neurons and glia in neural cultures. *Exp. Neurol.*, 48 (3, part 2): 93–134.

Varon, S. (1975c) In vitro approaches to the study of neural tissue aging. In G. Maletta (Ed.), *Survey of the Aging Nervous System*, DHEW Pub. (NIH) 74-296: pp. 59–76.

Varon, S. (1977) Neural growth and regeneration: a cellular perspective. *Exp. Neurol.*, 54: 1–6.

Varon, S. and Adler, R. (1980) Nerve growth factors and control of nerve growth. *Curr. Topics Dev. Biol.*, 16: 207–252.

Varon, S. and Manthorpe, M. (1982) Schwann cells: an in vitro perspective. *Adv. Cell. Neurobiol.*, 3: 35–95.

Varon, S. and Skaper, S.D. (1980) Short-latency effects of Nerve Growth Factor: an ionic view. In E. Giacobini, A. Vernadakis, A. Shahar (Eds.), *Tissue Culture in Neurobiology*, Raven Press, New York, pp. 333–347.

Varon, S. and Skaper, S.D. (1983) The Na$^+$, K$^+$-pump may mediate the control of nerve cells by Nerve Growth Factor. *Trends Biochem. Sci.*, 8: 22–25.

Varon, S. and Somjen, G. (1979) Neuron-glia interactions. *Neurosci. Res. Prog. Bull.*, 17: 1–239.

Varon, S. and Williams, L.R. (1986) Peripheral nerve regeneration in a silicone model chamber: cellular and molecular aspects. *Peripheral Nerve Repair Regeneration*, 1: 9–25.

Varon, S., Manthorpe, M. and Adler, R. (1979) Cholinergic neuronotrophic factors: I. Survival, neurite outgrowth and choline actyltransferase activity in monolayer cultures from chick embryo ciliary ganglia. *Brain Res.*, 173: 29–45.

Varon, S., Adler, R., Manthorpe, M. and Skaper, S.D. (1983) Culture strategies for trophic and other factors directed to neurons. In S.E. Pfeiffer (Ed.), *Neuroscience Approached through Cell Culture, Vol. 2*, CRC Press, Boca Raton, FL, pp. 53–77.

Varon, S., Manthorpe, M. and Williams, L.R. (1984a) Neuronotrophic and neurite promoting factors and their clinical potentials. *Dev. Neurosci.*, 6: 73–100.

Varon, S., Skaper, S.D., Barbin, G., Selak, I. and Manthorpe, M. (1984b) Low molecular weight agents support survival of cultured neurons from the CNS. *J. Neurosci.*, 4: 654–658.

Varon, S., Manthorpe, M., Davis, G.E., Williams, L.R. and Skaper, S.D. (1987a) Growth Factors. In S.G. Waxman (Ed.), *Functional Recovery in Neurological Disease, Advances in Neurology, Vol. 47*, Raven Press, New York, pp. 493–521.

Varon, S., Manthorpe, M., Williams, L.R. and Gage, F.H. (1987b) Neuronotrophic factors and their involvements in the adult CNS. In R.D. Terry (Ed.), *Aging and the Brain*, Raven Press, New York, pp. 259–285.

Varon, S., Skaper, S.D. and Manthorpe, M. (1987c) Trophic and toxic mechanisms in neuronal survival. In A. Vernadakis (Ed.), *Model Systems of Development and Aging in the Nervous System*, M. Nijhoff, Boston, MA, pp. 299–317.

Varon, S., Williams, L.R. and Gage, F.H. (1987d) Exogenous administration of neurotrophic factors in vivo protects central nervous system neurons against axotomy induced degeneration. In F.J. Seil, E. Herbert and B.M. Carlson (Eds.), *Neural Regeneration, Progress in Brain Research, Vol. 71*, Elsevier, pp. 191–201.

Vitorica, J., Machado, A. and Satrustegui, J. (1984) Age-dependent variations in peroxide-utilizing enzymes from rat brain mitochondria and cytoplasm. *J. Neurochem.*, 42: 351–356.

Walicke, P., Varon, S. and Manthorpe, M. (1986) Purification of a human red blood cell protein supporting the survival of cultured CNS neurons, and its identification as catalase. *J. Neurosci.*, 6: 1114–1121.

Wewer, U., Albrechtsen, R., Manthorpe, M., Varon, S., Engvall, F. and Ruoslahti, E. (1983) Human laminin isolated in a nearly intact, biologically active form from placenta by limited proteolysis. *J. Biol. Chem.*, 258: 12654–12660.

Williams, L.R., Selak, I., Skaper, S.D., Manthorpe, M. and Varon, S. (1985) Central nervous system-directed neuronotrophic activity present in red blood cells. *Brain Res.*, 336: 99–105.

Williams, L.R., Varon, S., Peterson, G., Wictorin, K., Fischer, W., Bjorklund, A. and Gage, F.H. (1986) Continuous infusion of Nerve Growth Factor prevents basal forebrain neuronal death after fimbria-fornix transection. *Proc. Natl. Acad. Sci. USA*, 83: 9231–9235.

Williams, L.R., Danielsen, N., Muller, H. and Varon, S. (1987) Exogenous matrix precursors promote functional regeneration across a 15 mm gap within a silicone chamber in the rat. *J. Comp. Neurol.*, 264: 284–290.

Discussion

A.J. Patel: You suggested two secondary messengers for the action of nerve growth factor (NGF), namely, cyclic AMP and inositol phosphatide. Do you think all actions of NGF, including that on a number of cholinergic cells, are mediated by either of these two mechanisms? Our preliminary results would suggest that the effect of NGF on central cholinergic cells does not use the above-mentioned secondary messenger systems.

S. Varon: Cyclic AMP and phosphatidyl inositide products are two of the recognized messengers of NGF among several others. The only one linked to a functional response (such as the Na/K pump) is the protein kinase C-related mechanism (Togari and Guroff, 1985; Gremins et al., 1986). Many of the protein phosphorylation mechanisms, however, cross-interact, and some may well be bypassed to achieve the same effect.

H.J. Romijn: Is the formation of free radicals the main reason that nerve cells in tissue culture obtain most of their energy from the glycolytic pathway instead of the Krebs cycle, a situation opposite to what is the case in vivo? Anticipating your answer: why can nerve cells not synthesize their own catalase?

S. Varon: Your speculation is a plausible one. Note, however, that our CNS cultures which would burn glucose through the Krebs cycle when protected by exogenous catalase (or other anti-oxidants such as vitamin E) do not find their glycolytic pathway adequate for survival. We do not know that neurons *cannot* synthesize their own catalase, only that prenatal neurons in culture do not have *sufficient* endogenous anti-oxidant protection. Human neuroblastoma cells under NGF do increase their catalase content, according to Perez-Polo and Werrbach-Perez (1985).

A. Dekker: ACTH-like peptides and gangliosides have been shown to have an inhibiting effect on protein kinase C (Aloyo et al., 1983; Kim et al., 1986). These compounds also have a positive effect on axonal regeneration (Strand and Smith, 1980; Ledeen, 1984). Can you explain the difference with the *positive* effect of NGF on kinase C?

S. Varon: NGF and other compounds can act via numerous mechanisms. That gangliosides do not increase protein kinase C activity means that there are other pathways by which growth can be stimulated. Moreover, the neuritogenic effect of NGF has not yet been traced to an NGF-induced protein kinase C stimulation.

W. H. Gispen: I liked your scheme for the role of protein kinases in the trophic effects of neuronotrophic factors. I would like to note here that a major phosphoprotein in the growth cone membrane is identical to the growth-associated protein GAP43 or B50 which is a major substrate to protein kinase C in the nervous system (De Graan et al., 1986). However, what is the evidence that the Na^+/K^+ pump is regulated in its activity by the kinase you imply in NGF action?

S. Varon: Phorbol esters, best known to operate via activation of protein kinase C, prevent the loss of Na^+/K^+ pump activity (and viability) that develops in young dorsal root ganglion neurons when deprived of NGF (Montz et al., 1985). It appears plausible (though not proven) that NGF and ciliary neuronotrophic factor (CNTF) impart the same protection via a similar stimulation of protein kinase C (Skaper et al., 1986), and NGF has been shown to activate the inositide phosphate pathway that leads to protein kinase C stimulation (Contreras and Guroff, 1987). Not known is how NGF (but not CNTF or phorbol esters) *reverses* early losses of pump and viability, since here protein kinase C does not appear to be involved (no success by phorbol esters; Skaper et al., 1986). We speculate that NGF activates other kinases for the reversal effect. These could for example be cyclic AMP-dependent ones, since NGF does raise cAMP in these neurons (Skaper and Varon, 1981).

R. Balazs: While talking about possible mechanisms associated with the action of growth factors it may be worth mentioning recent observations on PC12 cells, although these are transformed nerve cells (Greenberg et al., 1985; Morgan and Curran, 1986). In these cells very soon after exposure to NGF a set of genes, including proto-oncogenes, becomes transiently expressed, while after a significant delay another set of genes is expressed. At least one of the gene products, that of *c-fos*, is a protein which is located in the nucleus and is known to attach to DNA. It may therefore be involved in the regulation of transcription processes.

S. Varon: Stimulation of proto-oncogenes may be important for the regulation not only of proliferative behaviors in

growing cells (including PC12 cells) but also of differentiated behaviors in stationary or in postmitotic cells like neurons. Those gene products which operate in a nuclear location would indeed be expected to regulate transcription processes, while others which can operate from the cytoplasm (e.g. tyrosine kinase) can regulate translation or post-translational events. This is a promising area of investigation for neuronotrophic and neurite-promoting factors, as well as the 'growth' factors such as epidermal growth factor (EGF), platelet-derived growth factor (PDGF), insulin-like growth factors (IGFs), etc.

References

Aloyo, V.J., Zwiers, H. and Gispen, W.H. (1983) Phosphorylation of B-50 protein by calcium activated phospholipid-dependent protein kinase and B-50 protein kinase. *J. Neurochem.*, 41: 649–653.

Contreras, M.L. and Guroff, G. (1987) Calcium-dependent Nerve Growth Factor-stimulated hydrolysis of phosphoinositides in PC12 cells. *J. Neurochem.*, 48: 1466–1472.

Cremins, J., Wagner, J.A. and Halegoua, S. (1986) Nerve Growth Factor action is mediated by cyclic AMP and Ca^{++}/phospholipid-dependent protein kinases. *J. Cell Biol.*, 103: 887–893.

De Graan, P.N.E., Oestreicher, A.B., Schrama, L.H. and Gispen, W.H. (1986) Phosphoprotein B-50: localization and function. In W.H. Gispen and A. Routtenberg (Eds.), *Phosphoproteins in Neuronal Function, Progress in Brain Research, Vol. 69*, Elsevier, Amsterdam, pp. 37–50.

Greenberg, M.E., Greene, L.A. and Ziff, E.B. (1985) Nerve growth factor and epidermal growth factor induce rapid transient changes in proto-oncogene transcription in PC12 cells. *J. Biol. Chem.*, 260: 1401–1410.

Kim, J.Y.H., Goldenring, J.R., De Lorenzo, R.J. and Yu, R.K. (1986) Gangliosides inhibit phospholipid-sensitive Ca^+-dependent kinase phosphorylation of rat myelin basic proteins. *J. Neurosci. Res.*, 15: 159–166.

Ledeen, R.W. (1984) Biology of gangliosides: neurotogenic and neuronotrophic properties. *J. Neurosci. Res.*, 12: 147–159.

Montz, H.P.M., Davis, G.E., Skaper, S.D., Manthorpe, M. and Varon, S. (1985) Tumor-promoting phorbol diester mimics two distinct neuronotrophic factors. *Dev. Brain Res.*, 23: 150–154.

Morgan, J.I. and Curran, T. (1986) Role of ion flux in the control of *c-fos* expression. *Nature*, 322: 552–555.

Perez-Polo, J.R. and Werrbach-Perez, K. (1985) Effects of Nerve Growth Factor on the in vitro responses to neurons to injury. In: J. Eccles and M.R. Dimitrijevic (Eds.), *Recent Achievements in Restorative Neurology, Vol. 1*, S. Karger, Basel, pp. 321–337.

Skaper, S.D. and Varon, S. (1981) Mutually independent cyclic AMP and sodium responses to Nerve Growth

Factor in embryonic chick dorsal root ganglia. *J. Neurochem.*, 37: 222–228.

Skaper, S.D., Montz, H.P.M. and Varon, S. (1986) Control of Na$^+$,K$^+$ pump activity in dorsal root ganglionic neurons by different neuronotrophic agents. *Brain Res.*, 386: 130–135.

Strand, F.L. and Smith, C.M. (1980) LPH, ACTH and motor systems. *Pharmacol. Ther.*, 11: 509–533.

Togari, A. and Guroff, G. (1985) Partial purification and characterization of a Nerve Growth Factor-sensitive kinase and its substrate from PC12 cells. *J. Biol. Chem.*, 260: 3804–3811.

G.J. Boer, M.G.P. Feenstra, M. Mirmiran, D.F. Swaab and F. Van Haaren
Progress in Brain Research, Vol. 73
© 1988 Elsevier Science Publishers B.V. (Biomedical Division)

CHAPTER 30

Gangliosides as cell adhesion factors in the formation of selective connections within the nervous system

Robert E. Baker

Netherlands Institute for Brain Research, Meibergdreef 33, 1105 AZ Amsterdam ZO, The Netherlands

Introduction

Gangliosides are glycosphingolipids, containing sialic acid, which are normal constituents of all plasma membranes in vertebrate cells, but which are particularly enriched in neural tissues. Gangliosides consist of a hydrophobic ceramide portion which is embedded in the outer leaflet of the plasma membrane, and a hydrophilic oligosaccharide chain extending into the extracellular environment (Fig. 1). The hydrophobic portion of the molecule may participate in signal transduction across the membrane (Brady and Fishman, 1979) while the hydrophilic oligosaccharide chains are believed to be involved in intercellular recognition and/or adhesion (Brady and Fishman 1979; Holmgren et al., 1980; Ledeen, 1985). About 20 different gangliosides have been currently identified, differing from one another in the composition of both their oligosaccharide chains and ceramide. The most commonly used classification of individual gangliosides is currently based on the number and location of the sialic acid residues (Svennerholm, 1980).

Gangliosides are synthesized in the Golgi apparatus of the cell body through the sequential addition of single saccharide units and sialic acid to the ceramide moiety (Tettamanti et al., 1987). Once synthesized, gangliosides are transferred via rapid axoplasmic flow to the nerve terminals (see Ledeen, 1985). There does not appear to be any preferential transport of a given ganglioside, all species transporting at the same rate in both the CNS and PNS (Aquino et al., 1987). Ganglioside insertion into the neural membrane can occur throughout the neuron, suggesting that there may not be a selective preference for any given part of the cell (see Gammon et al., 1985; Mirsky et al., 1978). However, other studies have indicated a preferential accumulation of gangliosides at the nerve terminals (Hansson et al., 1977; Seyfried et al., 1983, 1984).

In addition to anterograde transport, retrograde transport has been shown to occur (Aquino et al., 1987) with simultaneous migration of all species. Degradation also proceeds in a step-wise manner, individual hexose sugars being split from the parent molecule within lysosomes of the cell body (Sandhoff et al., 1987).

During development there are striking changes in the concentration and pattern of gangliosides within neurons throughout the nervous system. These developmental changes occur as consecutive phenomena associated with neural genesis, differentiation, maturation (i.e., synaptogenesis) and myelination (see Brunngraber, 1979; Dreyfus et al., 1980; Rosner, 1977, 1982). All of the major gangliosides are present in all of the neural tissues

492

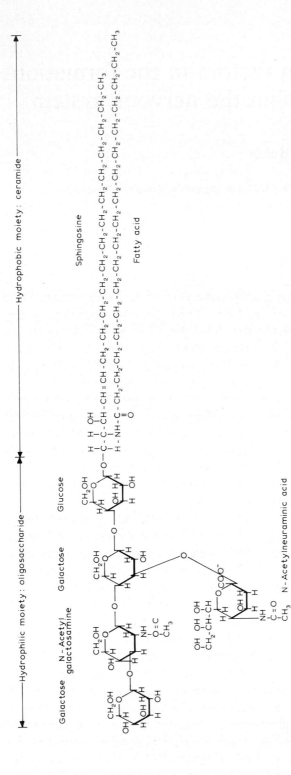

Fig. 1. Structure of the GM1 ganglioside showing the hydrophobic ceramide moiety and the hydrophilic oligosaccharide chain with its sialic acid residue. With the permission of Raven Press.

examined to date, though there are regional differences in pattern and concentrations (Kracun et al., 1984).

Gangliosides as membrane receptors

There have been numerous observations linking plasma membrane gangliosides with the function of surface binding sites. Probably the most exhaustively studied receptor is the monosialoganglioside GM1, which has been shown to selectively bind cholera toxin (Cuatrecasas, 1973; Hansson et al., 1977; Moss et al., 1976; Van Heyningen, 1974). Cells lacking GM1 in their membranes do not bind any significant amounts of cholera toxin, whereas cells containing incorporated (exogenously supplied) GM1 do interact with the toxin. Tetanus toxin also appears to selectively bind to gangliosides, though it has not been established whether the binding is selectively restricted to a given species (Yavin and Habig, 1984; though see Critchley et al., 1982).

Hormones may also selectively bind to plasma membrane gangliosides. Mullin et al. (1976) demonstrated apparent binding of thyroid stimulating hormone to GD1b. Van Heyningen (1974) suggested that serotonin selectively binds to a mixture of gangliosides. However, if the experimental tissue strips were first treated with sialidase, which removes the sialic acid residues from the oligosaccharide chains of glycoproteins and glycolipids, no selective binding occurs. Vengris et al. (1976) and Besancon and Ankel (1974) demonstrated that GM2 and GT1 gangliosides increased adhesion of human interferon to ganglioside-deficient transformed mouse cell lines, whereas GM1 and GD1a were without effect. A recent review by Hakomori (1987) has indicated that GM3 and GM1 may selectively promote or inhibit the phosphorylation of fibroblast, growth factor and epidermal and platelet-derived growth factor. Finally, Holmgren et al. (1980) showed that Sendai virus evinced high affinities for gangliosides with disialic acid residues on a terminal galactose sugar.

Given the developmental changes in ganglioside composition throughout the CNS, their location on the plasma membrane at crucial cell surfaces, and their role in recognition and adhesion, it can be safely assumed that gangliosides are critical factors in normal neural development. The question we must now ask is which of these developmental processes are most influenced by internal and/or external changes in the environment and to what extent. And finally, what long-term neural consequences may result from interfering with the proper sequencing of ganglioside production?

Neuronotrophic properties of gangliosides

Gangliosides as a class of compounds exert a wide range of neuronotrophic effects, i.e., promotion of survival and/or metabolism. One of the first reports of such a neuronotrophic effect came from a series of experiments reported by Agnati et al. (1983a,b) who demonstrated that retrograde degeneration following nigrostriatal lesions in rats was partly counteracted by chronic treatment with purified GM1. In these experiments a partial hemitransection of the dopaminergic tract in the rat was performed. Daily intraperotineal injections of GM1 resulted in a significant preservation of neurons as evidenced by elevated striatal tyrosine hydroxylase activity (Fig. 2; Toffano et al., 1983). Ganglioside-treated animals also had longer dendrites in the striatum indicating that the treatment induced collateral sprouting from the remaining dopaminergic axons.

Since these initial studies were reported a number of lesioned systems of the CNS have been reported (see Ledeen, 1984). Ganglioside treatment also appears to protect cholinergic (Wojcik et al., 1982) adrenergic and serotonergic (Jonsson et al., 1984) systems from the degenerative effects of mechanical and chemical lesioning. Intraperitoneal injections of GM1 ganglioside prior to surgery have also been shown to protect rat hippocampal slices from ATPase decay following removal to recording chambers (Bianchi et al.,

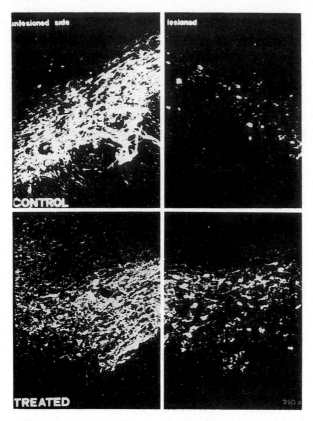

Fig. 2. Fluorescence microphotographs from a coronal brain section showing dopamine cell bodies in the medial part of the substantia nigra of the intact side (left two photographs) and of the lesioned side (right two photographs) of a partially hemitransected rat after saline (top) or GM1-treatment (bottom). Photographs were kindly supplied by G. Toffano.

1986; Gorio et al., 1985) suggesting that even healthy neurons may be primed to respond favorably to exogenously presented gangliosides.

How gangliosides evoke this sparing effect is unknown, but it may be linked to complex events associated with the metabolic machinery of the neuron. Exogeneous gangliosides can be directly incorporated into neural membranes (see Ghidoni et al., 1986), where they exert a number of actions, including: (i) activation of Na,K-ATPase system which is of importance in membrane ion conductance (Karpiak et al., 1986; Leon et al., 1981), (ii) activation of membrane kinase systems and subsequent protein phosphorylation (Goldenring

et al., 1985; Hakomori, 1987), (iii) modulation of transmitter receptors (Agnati et al., 1983a,b; Hakomori et al., 1986) (iv) involvement in neurotransmission through interaction with synaptic membranes and transmitter release (see Rahmann and Probst, 1986; Tettamanti et al., 1985; Wieraszko and Seifert, 1986), (v) modulation of membrane receptor molecules (Bremer et al., 1984; Hakomori, 1987) and (vi) activation of various enzyme systems (Agnati et al., 1983b; Roisen et al., 1981; Toffano et al., 1983; Wojcik et al., 1982). At the moment it is unclear whether gangliosides enhance, trigger or permit the activation of the neuronal metabolic machinery associated with survival and regeneration.

Altered biosynthesis of gangliosides

Numerous articles and reviews have been reported in the literature concerning the changes in synthesis of gangliosides that occur under pathological conditions (see O'Brien, 1983). I shall, therefore, only briefly summarize these observations. Broadly speaking, ganglioside abnormalities are associated with two types of pathological conditions: ganglioside storage disease (gangliosidosis) and oncogenetically transformed cells. In the former, some five types of storage disorders have been reported, with GM1 and GM2 gangliosidosis being the most commonly observed. These storage disorders are characterized by progressive mental and motor deterioration, with an early death. Each disease appears to be transmitted as an autosomal recessive trait. The structure of the ganglioside associated with these disorders is identical to that of the normal ganglioside species, though the levels of the affected species may be many times that of normal tissues. The cause of GM1 and GM2 gangliosidosis is due to the absence of degradation enzymes in the lysosome. A number of animal models occur for GM1 gangliosidosis, the most frequently reported being feline GM1 gangliosidosis, which results from similar enzyme deficiencies described in humans. Such animal mutants can serve as experimental models for therapy, which currently includes cloning of the gangliosidase genes for replacement therapy (O'Brien, 1983).

Virtually nothing has been reported on the effects drugs and/or chemicals may have on the production of gangliosides in vivo or in vitro. Several reports are now in the literature regarding the effect alcohol has on gangliosides. It has been shown that as little as a single intoxicating dose of alcohol can decrease the total amount of ganglioside present in several major brain regions in the adult rat (Klemm and Foster, 1986). The immediate effect of alcohol intoxication is proposed to be a disorientation of the gangliosides in the plasma membrane resulting in an alteration of receptor and enzyme characteristics of the entire plasma membrane. It has been proposed that changes in ganglioside composition in the presence of alcohol may be causally involved in the development of long-term tolerance and/or addiction in the adult. However, there does not appear to be any significant alteration of the ganglioside association with myelin in rat pups born to alcohol-exposed dams, though the level of GM1 was consistently decreased in the experimental group (Gnaedinger et al., 1984; also see Vrbashi et al., 1984). It was not shown whether gangliosides other than GM1 were affected by these exposures. It is not known, therefore, whether rat pups born to mothers chronically exposed to intoxicating levels of alcohol during the crucial periods of ganglioside change-overs suffer from deficiencies in ganglioside profiles within any given area of the brain, or if there are long-term anatomical, behavioral or physiological consequences to such exposure. Given the changes in ganglioside production which occur at sensitive stages of neural development, any interference in the normal sequencing of these changes may well result in severe neurological dysfunction at later stages of development.

A variety of cloned mouse cell lines have been used to study the effects of carcinogenic agents on the modulation of gangliosides (see Fishman and Brady, 1976). Such cells are transformed from their normal state into cells which lack growth restraints, have reduced growth nutrient requirements and are morphologically distinct from normal cells when exposed to carcinogens. In general, however, cloned mouse cell lines have been used only to examine the relationship of gangliosides to the transformation processes. Transformed cell lines lack the more complex gangliosides usually as a result of a decrease in the activity of glycosyltransferases. There are, instead, significant increases in the monosialogroups (in particular GM2 and GM3 gangliosides). These plasma membrane ganglioside increases are also observed to occur in a variety of tumor cells, and in the serum of rats afflicted with Morris hepatoma (Skipski et al., 1975).

Neuritogenic properties of gangliosides

Curiously enough it was observations made on cortical neurons in humans and cats suffering from ganglioside storage diseases that pointed to one of the most obvious effects gangliosides exert on neurons (Purpura and Suzuki, 1976; Purpura and Baker, 1978). The accumulation of unmetabolized gangliosides results in significant alterations in neural morphology, invariably a pathological enlargement of the cell body (see Walkley, 1987). In addition, in many cases this cellular ballooning is accompanied by the formation of a meganeurite between the soma and initial segment of the axon from which synaptic and secondary neurites are often seen to sprout (Fig. 3). Normal appearing, functional synapses can form on these ectopic spines (Karabelas and Walkley, 1985) demonstrating that a rearrangement of synaptic networks is occurring in response to the stored gangliosides. Since the ectopic synaptic spines and neurites occurred in mature neurons, the stored gangliosides were thought to exert a neuritogenic effect.

Shortly after these observations were reported, a number of studies appeared demonstrating the neuritogenic properties of exogenously supplied mixtures of purified bovine gangliosides on cul-

496

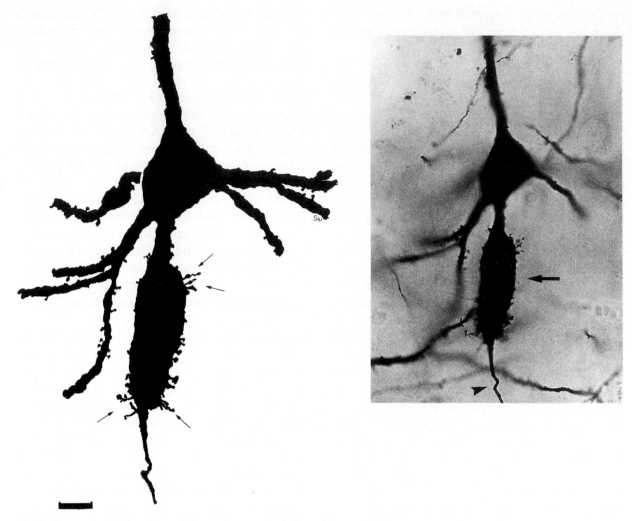

Fig. 3. Camera lucida drawing and photomicrograph of a layer III pyramidal neuron of neocortex in feline GM1 gangliosidosis. A prominent meganeurite is present which has displaced the initial segment of the axon distally (arrow and arrowhead, respectively, in photomicrograph). Small neuritic and spine like processes cover the meganeurite surface (arrows, camera lucida drawing). Calibration bar equals 10 μm and applies to the drawing as well. Figure kindly supplied by S.U. Walkley.

tures of primary neural tissues and neuroblastoma cell lines (Dreyfus et al., 1981; Hauw et al., 1981; Morgan and Seifert, 1979; Roisen et al., 1981). In all cases, within 48 h of exposure there was an enhanced outgrowth and elongation of neurites in these tissues (Fig. 4). Similar results have now been reported by a number of laboratories (see Ledeen, 1984) using a variety of neural cell types and neuroblastoma cell lines. The neuritogenic effect has been shown to reside in the gangliosides

themselves (Byrne et al., 1983), with most major species evincing high levels of neuritogenic activity. In the case of primary dorsal root ganglion (DRG) cultures the neuritogenic effects can be enhanced by the simultaneous addition of nerve growth factor (Doherty et al. 1986; Leon et al., 1984; Varon et al., 1986).

The first in vivo indication that gangliosides may facilitate repair within the CNS occurred 11 years ago (Ceccarelli et al., 1976) with the report-

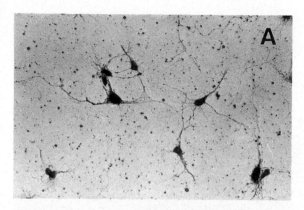

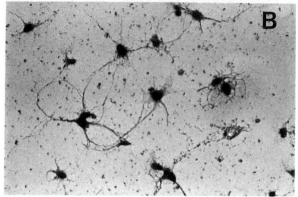

Fig. 4. Photomicrographs of chick cerebral neurons grown in vitro. A. In control medium. B. In control medium plus 10^{-6} M mixed gangliosides. Photographs were kindly supplied by H. Dreyfus.

ed enhanced recovery of function following lesions in the nerve supplies to the nictitating membrane of the cat. Both presynaptic and post-synaptic (cholinergic and adrenergic, respectively) lesions were made and functional recovery evaluated by measuring the contraction of the nictitating membrane following direct stimulation of the sympathetic trunk. Both cholinergic and adrenergic reinnervation was enhanced in animals which received intraperitoneal injections of a mixture of brain cortex gangliosides. Since 1976 numerous reports in the literature have shown gangliosides to be effective in the repair of many types of central and peripheral lesions (see Ledeen, 1984). In many of these studies there is an increase in the number of regenerating axons

coupled with a more rapid return of innervation in ganglioside-treated animals than seen in controls. This suggests that enhanced outgrowth is occurring as well as increased numbers of fibers.

Gangliosides as specifying agents

In all of the lesion studies utilizing behavior as the means for assessing reinnervation, it is remarkable that the behavioral repertoire are normal and that even learned behaviors can be retained (Ceccarelli et al., 1976; Fass and Ramirez, 1984; Karpiak, 1983; Sabel et al., 1984). These results suggest that selective regeneration is occurring. None of these studies, however, specifically addressed the question of selective reinnervation as a result of the ganglioside treatment.

A few reports from the literature suggest that gangliosides may indeed be involved in the formation of selective interneuronal connections. In the first study Obata et al. (1977) described the effect of glycolipid additions to the culturing medium on the development of neuromuscular junctions in co-cultures of embryonic chick skeletal muscle and spinal cord. Their results showed that only globoside and the GM1 ganglioside significantly increased the formation of neuromuscular junctions in this model.

In the second, Marchase (1977) utilized dissociated dorsal and ventral halves of embryonic chick retinae which had been radiolabelled and allowed to adhere to organotypic explants of optic tectum. The results of these interactions showed preferential adhesion by ventral retina to dorsal tectum and dorsal retina to ventral tectum, a schema which occurs in vivo. Protease and glycosidase treatment of these tissues determined that preferential adhesiveness of the tissues depended on interactions between proteins and terminal *N*-acetylgalactosamine residues located as a double gradient across both tissues. That is, adhesion of central retina to dorsal tectum depended on proteins located on the retina and *N*-acetylgalactosamine on the tectum. The reverse is true for dorsal retina and ventral tectum:

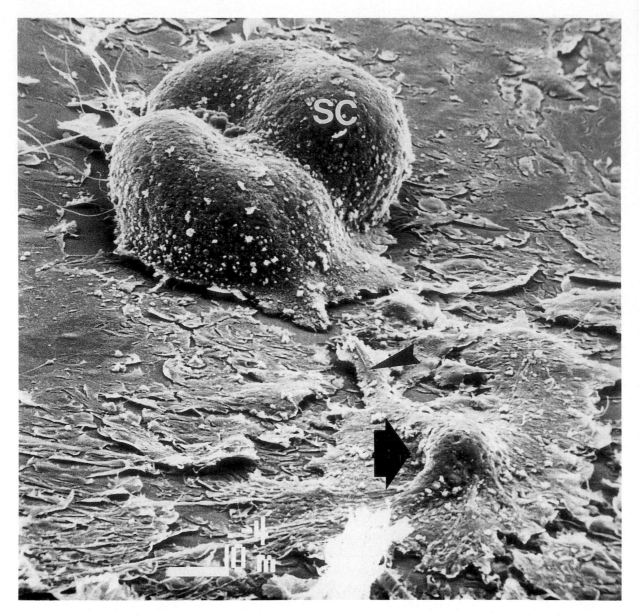

Fig. 5. Scanning electron micrograph of spinal cord-dorsal root ganglion (SC-DRG) organotypic explant grown for 27 days in vitro in a galactose-supplemented serum-free medium. The DRG (arrow) has migrated away from the cord. A bundle of sensory afferent fibers connects the DRG with the cord explant (arrow head).

N-acetylgalactosamine located on the retinal cells and proteins on the tectum.

The molecule which was concentrated dorsally in both retina and tectum appears to require a terminal *N*-acetylgalactosamine for adhesion to occur and was not affected by protease treatment.

The ganglioside GM2 was proposed as a molecule fitting these qualifications, though no gradient of GM2 could be detected in either tissue. However, lecithin vesicles coated with GM2 preferentially adhered to the ventral tectal surfaces. The protein was suggested to be UDP-galactose: GM2 galactosyltransferase, which was 30-times more concentrated in ventral retina compared with dorsal retina.

Further evidence that cell surface carbohydrates in the embryonic chick retinotectal system are involved in selected cell-cell adhesion has been provided by Blackburn et al. (1986). Neural retinal cells rapidly and specifically adhere to ganglioside-coated surfaces, the adhesion being specific for the carbohydrate moiety of the ganglioside. The extent of adhesion varied with the species of ganglioside coating and with the age of the retinal tissues. While all gangliosides exhibited adhesive affinity for the retinal cells, the strength of adhesion varied from ganglioside to ganglioside. Retinal cells were approximately three-times more strongly attracted to GM2 (the most adhesive of the gangliosides tested) than to GM1.

In both of the above retinal studies the entire retina was used. However, only the retinal ganglion cells project beyond the retina and synapse with tectal neurons in vivo. It has not been established whether retinal ganglion cells also exhibit the selectivity observed above. Another in vitro model system has been used in our laboratory over the past several years. This model consists of organotypic explants of fetal mouse spinal cord-dorsal root ganglia (SC-DRG; Fig. 5) and has been shown to be useful in determining factors underlying long-term selective interneuronal connectivity.

Gangliosides and specification within an in vitro model

Crain and Peterson (1974, 1981) pioneered the SC-DRG model and showed that mature cultures evinced a selected restriction of the sensory afferents to dorsal cord regions. These results are similar to the in vivo localization of DRG afferents (see Fitzgerald, 1985; Smith, 1983; Stelzner,

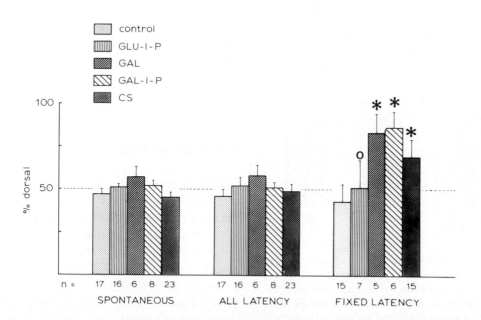

Fig. 6. Bar graph showing the distribution of bioelectric activities in spinal cord-dorsal root ganglion explants chronically exposed to a variety of hexose-sugar additives. Spontaneous and all-latency responses were equally distributed across the dorsal and ventral aspects of the cord while the location of the fixed-latency responses (denoting sensory afferent endings within the cord) were significantly located in the dorsal regions of the cord. * = differs significantly from 50% and control values; ○ = differs significantly from galactose-1-phosphate values.

1972). Our earlier work (Baker et al., 1982) demonstrated that, in the presence of a serum-supplemented medium, the sensory afferents evinced a significant dorsal cord preference over the entire culturing period, and that the only developmental change observed was the dropping out of fibers which entered the explant ventrally. The surprising finding, however, was that the omission of serum from the medium resulted in the subsequent loss of the dorsal cord preferences by the DRG afferents: they terminated equally in the dorsal and the ventral halves of the cord. We concluded that some factor(s) present in the serum was responsible for the selectivity observed in the former culture series. The question then be-

came what factor or factors were responsible for the selectivity.

A series of experiments using SC-DRG were carried out over the past several years from which we have established conditions under which selectivity can be returned to explants grown in a serum-free medium. In the first such study, the effects of galactose (both as D(+)galactose and as galactose-1-phosphate) on the localization of DRG terminals (determined electrophysiologically) was studied (Baker et al., 1983). The results of these additions showed that galactose-grown cultures displayed significant dorsal cord preferences by the DRG sensory afferents (Fig. 6). Galactose was not present in any of the media used to make up our serum-free medium and was chosen due to its presence in the oligosaccharide chains of a variety of nerve cell plasma membrane components, but in particular, the oligosaccharides of all gangliosides.

In a companion study, the addition of an unknown mixture of gangliosides to our chemically defined medium (CDM) was examined (Baker, 1983). The distribution of fixed latency points terminating within the dorsal regions of the cord explants was significantly higher in the ganglioside-grown cultures compared with control cultures and similar to those reported for galactose-grown explants (Fig. 7).

Gangliosides, bioelectric activity and selectivity

Centrally generated spontaneous bioelectric activity (SBA) also plays an important role during the development of SC-DRG connections. There may be an optimal level of functional activity necessary for selectivity to be expressed in this model (Corner et al., 1987). Explants grown in the presence of tetrodotoxin (TTX) (Baker et al., 1984) or elevated Mg^{2+} (Baker et al., 1986) show significant reductions in the level of spontaneous or evoked discharges in the cord. Under these conditions, explants which normally would show selectivity develop nonselective afferent projection patterns (Baker, 1985). This suggests

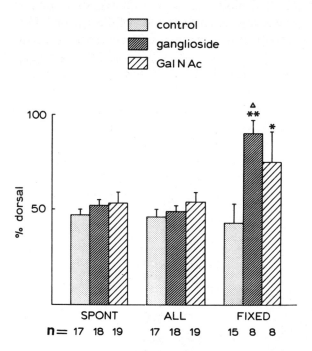

Fig. 7. Bar graph showing the distribution of bioelectric activities in spinal cord-dorsal root ganglion explants exposed to a mixture of gangliosides and N-acetylgalactosamine (Gal NAc). The spontaneous and all-latency responses were equally distributed across the dorsal and ventral aspects of the cord while the location of the fixed-latency points were significantly located in the dorsal regions of the cord in the experimental groups. * = less than $P < 0.05$ (with respect to control value); ** = less than $P < 0.005$ (with respect to controls); $\triangle$ = $P < 0.0005$ with respect to the 50% level.

that, as in the retinotectal system (Freeman, 1977; Reh and Constantine-Paton, 1985; Schmidt and Tieman, 1985), SBA is required for the proper wiring of the developing cord-DRG network.

In the case of galactose-grown SC-DRG explants the afferent selectivity for dorsal cord was dependent upon the presence of SBA within the cord (Baker, 1985). Histological localization of HRP-filled fibers revealed that explants chronically exposed to tetrodotoxin (TTX), even with the addition of galactose, showed a significant loss of dorsal cord selectivity (Table 1). TTX disrupts a variety of metabolic functions which are dependent on SBA (Bergey et al., 1981; Edwards and Grafstein, 1984; Goldenring et al., 1985; Riccio and Matthews, 1985), which may include formation and/or transportation of gangliosides to distant areas of the neuron. (Chronic depolarization of cerebellar neurons in vitro, on the other hand, significantly increases the synthesis of several ganglioside species; Hinrichs et al., 1987).

TABLE 1

Dorsal root ganglion fiber distribution within spinal cord explants chronically exposed to tetrodotoxin (TTX) while grown in a galactose (gal)- and ganglioside (gang)-supplemented serum-free medium

	n	total number fibers	%D	%DM
galactose group	8	19 ± 5	87 ± 6	
gal-TTX group I	13	16 ± 4	54 ± 8^a	
gal-TTX group II	11	24 ± 5	69 ± 5	41 ± 12
gang-TTX group	10	10 ± 2^b	89 ± 9^b	84 ± 11^b

%D represents a comparison between the number of horse radish peroxidase-stained fibers located in the dorsal half of the cord vs those in the ventral half; %DM considers only those fibers radiating away from the two dorsolateral most compartments and represents fiber growth in the dorsomedial cord vs the ventral half of the explant. Data are mean $\pm$ S.E.M.
[a] $P < 0.05$ compared with gal group.
[b] $P < 0.01$ compared with gal-TTX group II.

The addition of mixed gangliosides to the CDM resulted in a slight, but significant, reduction in the number of points from which evoked potentials could be obtained, suggesting that these compounds may have activity-suppressing characteristics on spinal neurons in vitro (Baker, 1983). These suspicions were confirmed in a recent study which showed a near cessation of SBA recorded in the presence of a growth medium containing GM1 (Baker, 1987). In the former report, however, the SC-DRG evinced selective projection patterns, which even the total abolition of SBA by TTX addition failed to erase (Baker and Van der Togt, 1986; Table 1). This led us to conclude that something in the ganglioside mixture was able to by-pass the requirement for function in the formation of selective connections, perhaps through the direct involvement of the gangliosides themselves. These data further implicate gangliosides as an important factor in intercellular recognition.

All of the experiments mentioned above employed an unknown mixture of commercially available gangliosides, thereby begging the question of whether the mixture itself is required for sensory afferent selectivity, or whether, as in their neuritogenic abilities (Byrne et al., 1983) all gangliosides are equally capable of eliciting the observed preferences for dorsal cord. We have only recently determined that not all gangliosides can foster selectivity: SC-DRG explants grown in GM1-supplemented medium fail to develop dorsal cord preferences (Baker and Gaasbeek Janzen, in preparation). Exogenous additions of GM1, however, significantly reduce SBA in the cord explant (Baker, 1987) which may, in turn, interfere with the very same processes giving rise to the nonselectivity observed in galactose-grown cultures silenced by TTX (Baker, 1985).

Concluding remarks

The topics reviewed and data presented corroborate the central role gangliosides play in many aspects of normal and abnormal neuronal development. There is now ample documentation in the recent literature that these compounds can hasten the repair and/or long-term changes in synaptic organization. Our own studies focus on the ability of gangliosides to influence the selectivity of connections in an in vitro model system. While we have not been able to point to a given species or combination of species of gangliosides as **the** selectivity/adhesion factor, several observations are suggestive of the direction. In several ganglioside-storage diseases GM1 and GM2 accumulation elicit atypically located neurites and spine formation in a variety of neural cell types. Oncogenic transformed cell lines also show significant increases in GM1, GM2 and GM3 (Fishman and Brady, 1976). At least GM1 (and probably GM2) has been shown to be a binding site molecule in its own right, while GM1 and GM3 are involved in phosphorylation of growth factor receptors. GM1, GM2 and GM3 are also implicated as selectivity/adhesion molecules in the visual system and neuromuscular junction. Preliminary analysis of ganglioside profiles in SC-DRG explants grown in media which do or do not support selective sensory afferent selectivity suggests that GM2 and GM3 are not present in the nonselective cultures, but are only present in those evincing selectivity (Baker, Guerold and Dreyfus, in preparation). GM2, GM3 and GD3 are gangliosides believed to be associated with undifferentiated membranes occurring in actively dividing and/or fetal plasma membranes. Although GM3 is heavily concentrated in glial cells (see Dreyfus et al., 1980) all three species are normally found in immature neuronal tissues both in vivo and in vitro. Their levels decrease with maturation and may even be missing in mature neurons. While increased depolarization of cerebral neurons in vitro leads to an increase in GM1, GM2, GM3 and GD3, the suppressive effects of TTX and GM1 on SBA in organotypic cord explants with subsequent decreases in GM2 and GM3 probably accounts for the lack of selectivity observed in cultures exposed to these media. GM2 and GM3 are thought to be gangliosides associated with nondifferentiated, mobile membranes (see Tettamanti et al., 1987; Toffano et al., 1983). Given these data, studies are being undertaken to examine what role these monosialogangliosides play in the formation of sensory afferent connections in SC-DRG explants.

The mechanisms by which gangliosides are involved in synaptic transmission are not yet fully understood. Gangliosides as a class of compounds exhibit a great affinity for divalent cations, and in particular for Ca^{2+} (Tettamanti et al., 1985). Thus, gangliosides may facilitate the localization of Ca^{2+} at the synapse where its involvement in synaptic transmission can occur. The addition of exogenous gangliosides to the growth medium may enhance Ca^{2+} localization via their direct incorporation into neural membranes (see Ghidoni et al., 1986). Moreover, there are selected affinities between different gangliosides and different transmitter and receptor molecules (see Agnati et al., 1983a,b; Cumar, 1978; Hollman and Seifert, 1986; Wieraszko and Seifert, 1986) depending on the area of the CNS being studied. These affinities might, in turn, result in the prolonged opening of Ca^{2+} channels with local transmitter release and/or increased membrane fluidity (Tettamanti et al., 1985) dependent on the spectrum of gangliosides present at the synapse.

It is not known whether any given ganglioside or group of gangliosides may be an instructive agent(s) in the formation of selective interneuronal connections within any given area of the developing CNS. With all neurons producing the same species of gangliosides (albeit in slightly different quantities) and following similar developmental sequelae, it is difficult to imagine how gangliosides could label any given neuron or group of neurons with the membrane characteristics necessary to attract and hold a given population of terminals charging in for space at the table. The answer may lie in the amply demonstrated and selective manner in which a given, purified ganglioside differentially elicits metabolic, neurotransmissive and membrane receptor responses from different types of neurons at various stages of development. Organotypic SC-DRG explants have proven to be a dependable model system on which the effects of ganglioside administration can be monitored over extended periods in vitro. While we have not been able to provide data demonstrating what events gangliosides induce which result in the formation of selective connections in this system, we believe the stage is now set for future studies which may define the cellular conditions required for long-term neuron-neuron associations.

Summary

Gangliosides are a family of glycosphingolipids present throughout vertebrate tissues, but which are particularly abundant in nervous tissues. The location, structure and physico-chemical properties of gangliosides make them well suited for playing a key role in the formation and maintenance of interneural connections. The various actions by gangliosides on neurons are briefly discussed. While little is currently known about the action of chemicals and/or drugs on the formation of ganglioside profiles during critical stages of neural development, studies indicate that long-term addiction or tolerance may be associated with perturbations in ganglioside composition within neural membranes. Studies have shown that the introduction of exogenous mixtures of gangliosides can hasten the in vivo repair of neural lesions. This is accomplished by a sharp increase in the production and elongation of neurites. Behavioral and functional studies suggest this repair is selective. In vitro studies have validated the in vivo observations regarding increased neuritogenesis and elongation in a variety of neural tissues. Recent work using organotypic explants of fetal mouse spinal cord-dorsal root ganglia (SC-DRG) has provided evidence that gangliosides induce the formation of selective sensory afferent projection patterns within the cord, even in the absence of bioelectric activity. We have now shown that there are qualitative and quantitative shifts in the types of gangliosides present in SC-DRG explants when grown in media which foster selective afferent projection patterns. These data suggest that gangliosides are involved in the formation of selective interneuronal connections.

References

Agnati, L.F., Benfenati, F., Battistini, N. Caviocchioli, L., Fuxe, K. and Toffano, G. (1983a) Selective modulation of H-3-spiperone labelled 5-HT receptors by subchronic treatment with the ganglioside GM1 in the rat. Acta Physiol. Scand., 117: 311–314.

Agnati, L.F., Fuxe, K., Calza, L. Benfenati, F. Caviocchioli, L., Toffano, G. and Goldstein, M. (1983b) Gangliosides increase the survival of lesioned nigral dopamine neurons and favor the recovery of dopaminergic synaptic function in striatum of rats by collateral sprouting. Acta Physiol. Scand., 119: 347–363.

Aquino, D.A., Bisby, M.A. and Ledeen, R.W. (1987) Bidirectional transport of gangliosides, glycoproteins and neutral glycosphingolipids in the sensory neurons of rat sciatic nerve. Neurosciences, 20: 1023–1029.

Baker, R.E. (1983) Effects of gangliosides on the development of selective afferent connections within fetal mouse spinal cord explants. Neurosci. Lett., 41: 81–84.

Baker, R.E. (1985) Horseradish peroxidase tracing of dorsal root ganglion afferents within fetal mouse spinal cord explants chronically exposed to tetrodotoxin. Brain Res., 334: 357–360.

Baker, R.E. (1987) Effects of gangliosides on spontaneous bioelectric activity in organotypic spinal cord explants in vitro. Med. Sci. Res., 15: 541–542.

Baker, R.E. and van der Togt, C. (1986) Gangliosides restore the specificity of afferent projection patterns in spinal cord explants chronically exposed to tetrodotoxin. Neurosci. Lett., 67: 285–288.

Baker, R.E., Habets, A.M.M.C., Brenner, E. and Corner, M.A. (1982) Influence of growth medium, age in vitro and spontaneous bioelectric activity on the distribution of sensory ganglion evoked activity in spinal cord explants. Dev. Brain Res., 5: 329–341.

Baker, R.E., Corner, M.A. and Kleiss, M. (1983) Effects of chemical additives on functional innervation patterns in mouse spinal cord-ganglion explants in serum-free medium. Neurosci. Lett., 41: 321–324.

Baker, R.E., Corner, M.A. and Habets, A.M.M.C. (1984) Effects of chronic suppression of bioelectric activity on the development of sensory ganglion evoked responses in spinal cord explants. J. Neurosci., 4: 1187–1192.

Baker, R.E., Corner, M.A., Lammertse, T. and Furth, E. (1986) Some functional effects of suppressing bioelectric activity in fetal mouse spinal cord-dorsal root ganglion explants. Exp. Neurol., 94: 426–430.

Bergey, G.K., Fitzgerald, S.C., Schrier, B.K. and Nelson, P.G. (1981) Neuronal maturation in mammalian cell cultures is dependent on spontaneous electrical activity. Brain Res., 207: 49–58.

Besancon, F. and Ankel, H. (1974) Binding of interferon to gangliosides. Nature, 252: 478–480.

Bianchi, R., Tanigro, D., Milan, F., Giudici, G. and Gorio, A. (1986) In vivo treatment with GM1 prevents the rapid decay of ATPase activities and mitochondrial damage in hippocampal slices. Brain Res., 364: 400–404.

Blackburn, C.C., Swank-Hill, P. and Schnaar, R.L. (1986) Gangliosides support neural retina cell adhesion. J. Biol. Chem., 261; 2873–2881.

Brady, P.O. and Fishman, P.H. (1979) Biotransducers of membrane-mediated information. Adv. Enzymol., 50: 303–323.

Bremer, E.G., Hakomori, S., Bowen-Pope, D.F. Raines, F. and Ross, R. (1984) Ganglioside-mediated modulation of cell growth, growth factor binding and receptor phosphorylation. J. Biol. Chem. 259: 6818–6825.

Brunngraber, E.G. (1979) Neurochemistry of Amino Sugars, C.C. Thomas, Springfield, IL U.S.A.

Byrne, M.C., Ledeen, R.W., Roisen, F.J., Yorke, G. and Sclafani, J.R. (1983) Ganglioside-induced neuritogenesis: verification that gangliosides are the active agents and comparison of molecular species. J. Neurochem., 41: 1214–1222.

Ceccarelli, B., Aporti, F. and Finesso, M. (1976) Effects of brain gangliosides on functional recovery in experimental regeneration and reinnervation. Adv. Exp. Med. Biol., 71: 275–293.

Corner, M.A., Habets, A.M.M.C. and Baker, R.E. (1987) Bioelectric activity is required for regional specificity of sensory ganglion projections to spinal cord explants cultured in vitro. Roux's Arch. Dev. Biol., 196: 133–136.

Crain, S.M. and Peterson, E.R. (1974) Enhanced afferent synaptic functions in fetal mouse spinal cord-sensory ganglion explants following NGF-induced ganglion hypertrophy. Brain Res., 79: 145–153.

Crain, S.M. and Peterson, E.R. (1981) Selective innervation of target regions within fetal mouse spinal cord and medulla explants by isolated dorsal root ganglia in organotypic co-cultures. Dev. Brain Res., 2: 341–362.

Critchley, D.R., Streuli, C.H., Kellie, S., Ansell, S. and Petel, B. (1982) Characterization of the cholera toxin receptor on BALB/c 3T3 cells as a ganglioside similar to, or identical with, ganglioside GM1. Biochem. J., 204: 209–219.

Cuatrecasas, P. (1973) Gangliosides and membrane receptors for cholera toxin. Biochemistry, 12: 3558–3566.

Cumar, F.A. (1978) Dopamine release from nerve endings induced by polysialogangliosides. Biochem. Biophys. Res. Commun., 84: 65–69.

Doherty, P., Dickson, J.G., Flanigan, T.P. and Walsh, F.S. (1986) Molecular specificity of ganglioside action on neurite regeneration in cell cultures of sensory neurons. In G. Tettamanti, R.W. Ledeen, K. Sandhoff, Y. Nagai and G. Toffano (Eds.), Gangliosides and Neuronal Plasticity, Liviana Press, Padova, pp. 335–346.

Dreyfus, H., Louis, J.C., Harth, S. and Mandel, P. (1980) Gangliosides in cultured neurons. Neuroscience, 5: 1647–1655.

Dreyfus, H., Harth, S. Massarelli, R. and Louis, J.C. (1981) Mechanisms of differentiation in cultured neurons: involvement of gangliosides. In M.M. Rapport and A. Gorio (Eds.), Gangliosides in Neurological and Neuromuscular Function, Raven Press, New York, pp. 151–170.

Edwards, D.L. and Grafstein, B. (1984) Intraocular injection of tetrodotoxin in goldfish decreases fast axonal transport of (H-3)glucosamine-labeled materials in optic axons. Brain Res., 299: 190–194.

Fass, B. and Ramirez, J.J. (1984) Effects of ganglioside treatments on lesion-induced behavioral impairments and sprouting in the CNS. J. Neurosci. Res., 12: 445–458.

Fishman, P.H. and Brady, P.O. (1976) Biosynthesis and function of gangliosides. Science, 194: 906–915.

Fitzgerald, M. (1985) The post-natal development of cutaneous afferent fibre input and receptive field organization in the rat dorsal horn. J. Physiol., 364: 1–18.

Freeman, J.A. (1977) Possible regulatory function of acetylcholine receptor in maintenance of retinotectal synapses. Nature, 269: 218–222.

Gammon, C.M., Goodrum, J.F., Toews, A.D., Okabe, A. and Morell, P. (1985) Axonal transport of glycoconjugates in the rat visual system. J. Neurochem. 44: 376–387.

Ghidoni, R., Trichera, M., Venerando, B., Fiorilli, A. and Tettamanti, G. (1986) Metabolism of exogenous GM1 and related glycolipids in the rat. In G. Tettamanti, R.W. Ledeen, K. Sandhoff, Y. Nagai and G. Toffano (Eds.), Gangliosides and Neural Plasticity, Liviana Press, Padova, pp. 183–200.

Gnaedinger, J.M., Norohna, A.B. and Druse, M.J. (1984) Myelin gangliosides in developing rats: the influence of maternal ethanol consumption. J. Neurochem., 42: 1281–1285.

Goldenring, R.J., Otis, L.C., Yu, R.K. and Delorenzo, R.J. (1985) Calcium/ganglioside-dependent protein kinase activity in rat brain membrane. J. Neurochem., 44: 1229–1234.

Gorio, A., Digregorio, F., Janigro, D., Milan, F., Vitadello, M. and Bianchi, R. (1985) Gangliosides have a decay preventing activity on neuronal membrane functions. In Neuronal Plasticity and Gangliosides, Fidia Research Series 8: 27.

Hakomori, S.I., Bremer, E. and Okada, Y. (1986) Ganglioside mediated modulation of growth factor receptor function. In G. Tettamanti, R.W. Ledeen, K. Sandhoff, Y.

Nagai and G. Toffano (Eds.), Gangliosides and Neuronal Plasticity, Liviana Press, Padova, pp. 201–214.

Hakomori, S.I. (1987) Ganglioside-mediated modulation of growth factor receptor function and cell adhesion. In H. Rahmann (Ed.), Gangliosides and Modulation of Neuronal Function, Springer-Verlag, Heidelberg, pp. 465–479.

Hansson, H.A., Holmgren, J. and Svennerholm, L. (1977) Ultrastructural localization of cell membrane GM1 ganglioside by cholera toxin. Proc. Natl. Acad. Sci. U.S.A., 74: 3782–3786.

Hauw, J.J., Fenelon, S., Boutry, J.M. And Escourolle, R. (1981) Effets des gangliosides sur la croissance de ganglions spinaux de cobaye en culture in vitro. Résultats préliminaires concernant une préparation de gangliosides de cortex cérébral de boeuf. C.R. Acad. Sci. Paris, 292: 569–571.

Hinrichs, U. Thomsen, S., Van Echten, G. and Sandhoff, J. (1987) Effect of veratrine on ganglioside biosynthesis in cerebellar cultures; In, H. Rahmann (Ed.), Gangliosides and Modulation of Neuronal Function, Springer-Verlag, Heidelberg, pp. 319–320.

Hollman, M. and Seifert, W. (1986) Gangliosides modulate glutamate receptor binding in rat brain synaptic plasma membranes. Neurosci. Lett., 65: 133–138.

Holmgren, J., Svennerholm, L., Elwing, H., Fredman, P. and Strannegard, O. (1980) Sendai virus receptor: proposed recognition structure based on binding to plastic-absorbed gangliosides. Proc. Natl. Acad. Sci. U.S.A., 77: 1947–1950.

Jonsson, G., Gorio, A., Hallman, H., Janigro, D., Kojima, H. and Zononi, R. (1984) Effect of GM1 ganglioside on neonatally neurotoxin induced degeneration of serotonin neurons in rat brain. Dev. Brain Res., 16: 171–180.

Karabelas, A.B. and Walkley, S.U. (1985) Altered patterns of evoked synaptic activity in cortical pyramidal neurons in feline ganglioside storage disease. Brain Res., 339: 329–336.

Karpiak, S.E. (1983) Ganglioside treatment improves recovery of alternation behavior after unilateral entorhinal cortex lesion. Exp. Neurol., 81: 330–339.

Karpiak, S.E., Shu Li, Y., Aceto, P. and Mahadik, S.P. (1986) Acute effects of gangliosides on CNS injury. In G. Tettamanti, R.W. Ledeen, K. Sandhoff, Y. Nagai and G. Toffano (Eds.), Gangliosides and Neuronal Plasticity, Liviana Press, Padova, pp. 407–414.

Klemm, W.R. and Foster, D.M. (1986) Alcohol, in a single pharmacological dose, decreases brain gangliosides. Life Sci., 39: 897–902.

Kracun, I., Rosner, H., Cosovic, C. and Stravljenic, A. (1984) Topographical atlas of the gangliosides of the adult human brain. J. Neurochem., 43: 979–989.

Ledeen, R.W. (1984) Biology of gangliosides: neuritogenic and neuronotrophic properties. J. Neurochem. Res., 12: 147–159.

Ledeen, R.W. (1985) Gangliosides of the neuron. Trends Neurosci., 8: 169–174.

Leon, A., Facci, L., Toffano, G., Sonnino, S. and Tettamanti, G. (1981) Activation of Na^+,K^+-ATPase by nanomolar concentrations of GM1 ganglioside. J. Neurochem., 37: 350–357.

Leon, A., Benvegnu, D., Dai Toso, R., Presti, D., Facci, L. Giorgi, O. and Toffano, G. (1984) Dorsal root ganglia and nerve growth factor: a model for understanding the mechanism of GM1 effects on neuronal repair. J. Neurosci. Res., 12: 277–287.

Marchase, R.B. (1977) Biochemical investigations of retinotectal adhesive specificity. J. Cell Biol., 75; 237–257.

Mirsky, R. Wendon, L.M.B., Black, P. Stolkin, C. and Bray, D. (1978) Tetanus toxin: a cell surface marker for neurones in culture. Brain Res. 148: 251–259.

Morgan, J.I. and Seifert, W. (1979) Growth factors and gangliosides: a possible new perspective in neuronal growth control. J. Supramol. Struct., 10: 111–124.

Moss, J., Fishman, P.H., Manganiello, V.C., Vaughn, M. and Brady, R.O. (1976) Functional incorporation of ganglioside into intact cells: induction of choleragen responsiveness. Proc. Natl. Acad. Sci. U.S.A., 73: 1034–1035.

Mullin, B.R., Fishman, P.H., Lee, G., Aloj, S.M., Ledley, F.D., Winand, R.J., Kohn, L.D. and Brady, R.O. (1976) Thyrotropin ganglioside interactions and their relationship to the structure and function of thyrotropin receptors. Proc. Natl. Acad. Sci. U.S.A., 73: 842–846.

Obata, K., Oide, M. and Handa, S. (1977) Effects of glycolipids on in vitro development of neuromuscular junction. Nature, 266: 369–371.

O'Brien, J.S. (1983) The gangliosides. In G.S. Stanbury (Ed.), The Metabolic Basis of Inherited Disease, McGraw-Hill, New York, pp. 945–969.

Purpura, D.P. and Suzuki, K. (1976) Distortion of neuronal geometry and formation of aberrant synapses in neuronal storage disease. Brain Res., 116: 1–21.

Purpura, D.P. and Baker, H.J. (1978) Meganeurite and other abberant processes of neurons in feline GM1 gangliosidosis. Brain Res., 143: 13–26.

Rahmann, H. and Probst, W. (1986) Ultrastructural localization of calcium at synapse and modulatory interactions with gangliosides. In G. Tettamanti, R.W. Ledeen, K. Sandhoff, Y. Nagai and G. Toffano (Eds.), Gangliosides and Neuronal Plasticity, Liviana Press, Padova, pp. 125–135.

Reh, T.A. and Constantine-Paton, M. (1985) Eye-specific segregation requires neural activity in three-eyed Rana pipiens. J. Neurosci., 5: 1132–1143.

Riccio, R.V. and Matthews, M.A. (1985) The effect of intraocular injection of tetrodotoxin on fast axonal transport of H-3-prodine and H-3-fuscose-labeled materials in the developing rat optic nerve. Neuroscience, 16: 1027–1039.

Roisen, F.J., Bartfeld, H., Nagele, R. and Yorke, G. (1981) Ganglioside stimulation of axonal sprouting in vitro. Science, 214: 577–578.

Rosner, H. (1977) Ganglioside, sialoglycoproteins and acetylcholinesterase of the developing mouse brain. Roux's Arch. Entwickl. Mech. Org., 183: 325–335.

Rosner, H. (1982) Ganglioside changes in the chicken optic lobes as biochemical indicators of brain development and maturation. Brain Res., 236: 49–61.

Sabel, B.A., Dunbar, G.L. and Stein, D.G. (1984) Gangliosides minimize behavioral deficits and enhance structural repair after brain injury. J. Neurosci. Res., 12: 429–443.

Sandhoff, K., Schwarzmann, G., Sarmientos, F. and Conzelmann, E. (1987) Fundamentals of ganglioside catabolism. In H. Rahmann (Ed.), Gangliosides and Modulation of Neuronal Function, Springer-Verlag, Heidelberg, pp. 231–250.

Schmidt, J.T. and Tieman, S.B. (1985) Eye-specific segregation of optic afferents in mammals, fish and frogs: the role of activity. Cell. Mol. Neurobiol., 5: 5–34.

Seyfried, T.N., Miyazawa, N. and Yu, R.K. (1983) Cellular localization of gangliosides in the developing mouse cerebellum: analysis using the weaver mutant. J. Neurochem., 41: 491–505.

Seyfried, T.N., Bernard, D.J. and Yu, R.K. (1984) Cellular distribution of gangliosides in the developing mouse cerebellum: analysis using the staggerer mutant. J. Neurochem., 43: 1152–1162.

Skipski, V.P., Katapodis, N., Prendergast, J.S. and Stock, C.C. (1975) Gangliosides in blood serum from normal rats and Morris hepatoma 5132tc bearing rats. Biochem. Biophys. Res. Commun., 67: 1122–1127.

Smith, C.L. (1983) The development and postnatal organization of primary afferent projections to the rat thoracic spinal cord. J. Comp. Neurol., 220: 29–43.

Stelzner, D.J. (1972) The normal postnatal development of synaptic endfeet in the lumbosacral spinal cord and of responses in the hindlimbs of the albino rat. Exp. Neurol., 31: 337–357.

Svennerholm, L. (1980) Ganglioside designation. Adv. Exp. Med; Biol., 125: 11-19.

Tettamanti, G., Sonnino, S., Ghidoni, R., Masserini, M. and Venerando, B. (1985) Chemical and functional properties of gangliosides. Their possible implication in the membrane-mediated transfer of information. In V. Degiorgio and M. Corti (Eds.), Physics of Amphiphiles: Micelles, Vesicles and Microemulsions, Ital. Soc. Phys., Milan, pp. 607–636.

Tettamanti, G., Ghidoni, R. and Trinchera, M. (1987) Fundamentals of brain ganglioside biosynthesis. In H. Rahmann (Ed.), Gangliosides and Modulation of Neuronal Function, Springer-Verlag, Heidelberg, pp. 191–204.

Toffano, G., Savioni, G., Moroni, F., Lombardi, G., Calza, L. and Agnati, L. (1983) GM1 ganglioside stimulates the regeneration of dopaminergic neurons in the central nervous system. Brain Res., 261: 163–166.

Van Heyningen, W.E. (1974) Gangliosides as membrane receptors for tetanus toxin, cholera toxin and serotonin. Nature, 249: 415–417.

Varon, S., Skaper, S.D. and Katoh-Semba, R. (1986) Neuritic responses to GM1 ganglioside in several in vitro systems. In G. Tettamanti, R.W. Ledeen, K. Sandhoff, Y. Nagai and G. Toffano (Eds.), Gangliosides and Neuronal Plasticity, Liviana Press, Padova, pp. 215–230.

Vengris, V.E., Reynolds, F.H., Jr., Hollenberg, M.D. and Pitha, P.M. (1976) Interferon action: role of membrane gangliosides. Virology, 72: 486–493.

Vrbashi, S.R. Grujic-Injoi, B. and Ristic, M. (1984) Phospholipid and ganglioside composition in rat brain after chronic intake of ethanol. J. Neurochem., 42: 1235–1239.

Walkley, S.U. (1987) Further studies on ectopic dendrite growth and other geometrical distortions of neurons in feline GM1 gangliosidosis. Neuroscience, 21: 313–331.

Wieraszko, A. and Seifert, W. (1986) Involvement of gangliosides in the synaptic transmission in the hippocampus and striatum of the rat brain. In G. Tettamanti, R.W. Ledeen, K. Sandhoff, Y. Nagai and G. Toffano (Eds.) Gangliosides and Neuronal Plasticity, Liviana Press, Padova, pp. 137–151.

Wojcik, M., Ulas, J. and Oderfeld-Nowak, B. (1982) The stimulating effect of ganglioside injections on the recovery of choline acetyltransferase and acetylcholinesterase activities in the hippocampus of the rat after septal lesions. Neuroscience, 7: 495–499.

Yavin, E. and Habig, W.H. (1984) Binding of tetanus toxin to somatic neural hybrid cells with varying ganglioside composition. J. Neurochem., 42: 1313–1320.

Discussion

W.H. Gispen: If one compares the role of neural cell adhesion molecules (NCAMs) to that of the ganglioside GM1 it is remarkable to note that in the NCAM the glycomoiety affects affinity of the cell-cell contact and in the ganglioside the glycomoiety, as your work suggests, promotes selectivity. This seems an intriguing difference. Given the fact that the GM1 molecule is also abundantly present in the neural tissue, do you expect a role for gangliosides in cell adhesion (and/or tissue damage repair mechanisms) in other tissues than the nervous system?

R.E. Baker: In fact both NCAM and gangliosides promote cell-cell adhesion and most probably in a similar way since it is indeed believed that both utilize the polysaccharide portions of their structures for recognition and adherence. While gangliosides have been put forward as a possible selectivity molecule (Marchase, 1977), no one has yet demonstrated any particular ganglioside to fulfill this role. What my own studies have shown is that there are differences in gangliosidic profiles in spinal cord/dorsal root ganglion (SC-DRG) explants which may be correlated with selective afferent projections. This would suggest that in some way these molecules may be involved in the process of selective cell-cell recognition. Obviously continued studies with our model system will be needed to resolve this fundamental question.

I am unaware of any studies utilizing exogenously supplied gangliosides to enhance the repair of damaged tissues other than those reported for the central and peripheral nervous system (e.g., Agnati et al., 1983a,b). However, as you've pointed out, since gangliosides are an integral component of all vertebrate plasma membranes, it would not be too surprising that an exogenously administered source would be beneficial to the repair of non-neural tissues as well.

S. Varon: Can there be ganglioside-recognizing protein activity as receptors for cell-cell recognition? Also, the SC-DRG system of Crain and Peterson (1974) showed differential recognition by DRG growth cones to ventral versus dorsal glial outgrowth from the cord.

R. E. Baker: There are ganglioside transfer proteins present in neural tissues (Gammon and Ledeen, 1985). This suggests that there could be a selective protein-ganglioside complex which, if present at the surface of the cell, might serve as a source of cell-cell recognition. However, I do not believe the specificity of the protein-ganglioside interaction has been firmly established yet. Indeed, there have been reports that DRG fibers are influenced by glia in the cord, but our own studies shed little light on this phenomenon. In chemical-defined (CDM) ventral DRG entrances occur. These remain throughout the culturing period suggesting that in this medium the route of ingrowth may not be affected by local cell types. However, in CDM there is much less glial outgrowth away from the cord explant but what glial elements remain within the cord explant, and how sensory afferents interact with them, are unknown at the present.

R. Balazs: In view of the interesting effect of galactose, may I ask you what is known about the production and metabolism of galactose in neural cultures?

R. E. Baker: To my knowledge nothing is known about the metabolism of galactose in neural tissues grown in vitro. Certainly nothing is known about the uptake and subsequent utilization of galactose in our own model, though we are, of course, anxious to trace metabolic pathways of this sugar in SC-DRG cultures.

R. Balazs: My other question is related to your finding that in the presence of galactose there is a marked increase in the amount of gangliosides GM2 and GM3 within the cultures. I vaguely remember these gangliosides are relatively concentrated only in glial cells; Could you comment on this?

R. E. Baker: We have preliminary data (Baker, Guerold and Dreyfus, unpublished observations) indicating a difference in ganglioside content in SC-DRG explants chronically exposed to galactose or galactose-free media. In the former cultures there were significant amounts of GM3, with smaller amounts of GM2, neither of which could be measured in the latter cultures. Whether either or both of these gangliosides are concerned with the selectivity seen in galactose-grown cultures would be pure speculation at this time. Seyfried et al. (1982) were unable to demonstrate significant amounts of GM2 or GM3 in mutant mouse cerebella, and since GM2 was not detected in mice showing active astrocytosis, it was assumed that these two compounds were only minor constituents of astrocytic membranes. Dreyfus et al. (1980), on the other hand, showed that both GM3 and GM2 were primarily located in embryonic chick glial cells grown in vitro, but that neurons also contained low levels of each ganglioside. Moreover, the level of GM2 in their neuronal cultures increased more than 3-fold between 5 and 7 days in vitro, which, in our experience using dissociated rat neocortical explants, is a period of initial synapse formation (Romijn et al., 1982). Monosialogangliosides have been suggested as selectivity factors in synapse formation in both the retino-tectal and neuromuscular systems (Marchase, 1977; Obata et al., 1977), and are implicated in many other growth-promoting conditions (e.g., Ledeen, 1984, 1985) as well as in repair of disease and in lesion studies (Ledeen, 1984, 1985). A considerable amount of work will be needed before we can determine whether these data are concerned with the selectivity observed in any of the models in current use.

References

Agnati, L. F., Benfenati, F., Battistini, N., Caviocchiolo, L., Fuxe, K. and Toffano, G. (1983a) Selective modulation of H-3-spiperone labelled 5-HT receptors by subchronic treatment with the ganglioside GM1 rat. Acta Physiol. Scand., 117: 311–314.

Agnati, L. F., Fuxe, K., Calza, L., Benfenati, F., Caviocchioli, L., Toffano, G. and Goldstein, M. (1983b) Gangliosides increase the survival of lesioned nigral dopamine neurons and favor the recovery of dopaminergic synaptic function in striatum of rats by collateral sprouting. Acta Physiol. Scand., 119: 347–363.

Crain, S. M. and Peterson, E. R. (1974) Enhanced afferent synaptic functions in fetal mouse spinal cord-sensory ganglion explants following NGF-induced ganglion hypertrophy. Brain Res., 79; 145–152.

Dreyfus, H., Louis, J. C., Harth, S. and Mandel, P. (1980) Gangliosides in cultured neurons. Neuroscience, 5: 1647–1655.

Gammon, C. M. and Ledeen, R. W. (1985) Evidence for the presence of a ganglioside transfer protein in brain. J. Neurochem., 44: 979–982.

Ledeen, R. W. (1984) Biology of gangliosides: neurotogenic and neuronotrophic properties. J. Neurochem., 12: 147–159.

508

Ledeen, R.W. (1985) Gangliosides of the neuron. Trends Neurosci., 8: 169–174.

Marchase, R.B. (1977) Biochemical investigations of retino-tectal adhesive specificity. J. Cell. Biol., 75: 237–258.

Obata, K., Oide, M. and Handa, S. (1977) Effects of glycoli-pids on in vitro development of neuromuscular junction. Nature, 226: 369–371.

Romijn, H.J., Habets, A.A.M.C., Mud, M.T. and Wolters, P.S. (1982) Nerve outgrowth, synaptogenesis and bioelec-tric activity in fetal rat cerebral cortex tissue cultured in serum-free, chemically defined medium. Dev. Brain Res., 2: 583–589.

Seyfried, T.N., Yu, R.K. and Miyazawa, N. (1982) Differen-tial cellular enrichment of gangliosides in the mouse cere-bellum: analysis using neurological mutants. J. Neurochem., 38: 551–559.

G.J. Boer, M.G.P. Feenstra, M. Mirmiran, D.F. Swaab and F. Van Haaren
Progress in Brain Research, Vol. 73
© 1988 Elsevier Science Publishers B.V. (Biomedical Division)

CHAPTER 31

Prenatal neurotransmitter programming of postnatal receptor function

Jeannette C. Miller and Arnold J. Friedhoff

Millhauser Laboratories of the Department of Psychiatry, New York University School of Medicine, New York, NY 10016, USA

Introduction

The biogenic amine transmitter systems in the brain have far-reaching regulatory influence on both motor and mental function. Biochemical studies in animals, and observations in humans, dating back to the early 1950s, provided the first evidence of a role for these systems in the mediation of behavior. For example, Woolley and Shaw (1954) speculated that serotonin might have a role in maintaining mental stability because the hallucinogenic drug LSD could be shown to act at peripheral serotonin receptors. About the same time, reserpine, which depletes transmitter storage vesicles of serotonin and the catecholamines dopamine (DA) and norepinephrine (NE) in the brain (Shore et al., 1955; Carlsson et al., 1957), was discovered to have an antipsychotic effect in man, and was also found to induce Parkinsonian-like extrapyramidal side-effects. By the end of the '50s, the metabolism of the catecholamines in the central nervous system (CNS) had been characterized and DA, in particular, was shown to be an important neurotransmitter in the basal ganglia of the extrapyramidal system (Bertler and Rosengren, 1959). Later, drugs that act on the serotonergic and noradrenergic systems were found to have antidepressant actions.

A role for DA in mediating certain mental functions has been inferred from the actions of neuroleptic drugs, and agents such as amphetamine, on the DA system (see Seeman, 1980, for review). These compounds can affect activity level, emotional responsivity and associative processing (Cole et al., 1966; Angrist et al., 1975). A role for NE and serotonin in mediating mood, level of arousal and sleep has been inferred from the actions of antidepressant drugs, agents whose biochemical activity resides in their inhibitory action on noradrenergic and serotonergic reuptake and on other presynaptic mechanisms (Charney et al., 1981; Sulser, 1983). Finally, the biogenic amines appear to play important roles in a variety of neuroendocrine functions (McEwen, 1982).

These far-ranging regulatory functions of the biogenic amine systems in the brain require that, during development, they be integrated with the systems they are destined to regulate, and that they be capable of meeting the demands imposed by a complex postnatal environment. The successful matching of a biological system with future environmental demands requires input, during development, from a number of sources. The input of the genes, whose adaptive value results from selective processes and probably other less well understood influences, is central; however, it is becoming increasingly clear that extragenetic influences play an important role in updating genetic information, and in specifying the way in which genetic information will be translated in a given individual (see Campbell and Perkins, Chapter 33 of this volume).

Genetic information, in the main, is ancient, and was selected in a world quite different from ours, both in chemical environment and in the requirements for survival and successful adaptation. The fetus is sheltered from both maternal chemicals and the influence of the outside world by the placenta, so that information about its contemporaneous environment must be transmitted to the fetus transplacentally. Prenatal maternal influences have been little studied but may play a crucial role in adaptation and adaptability in postnatal life. Immediately after conception, the principal source of embryonic RNA is from the maternal egg (Beaconsfield et al., 1980). Thus the first proteins may be of maternal origin. As development proceeds, the placenta acts to transfer much selected information from mother to child. Postnatally, biological adaptive mechanisms act in concert with learned coping strategies, to maintain stable behavioral function.

In the past, there has been interest primarily in prenatal factors producing structural teratology. The study of postnatal influences on development has been focused largely on nurturing factors. More recently, attention has been given to more subtle developmental influences on the functional aspects of the brain. As will be seen later, in the absence of observable structural teratology, changes in behavioral function can be produced by alteration in transmitter function. We have been interested in determining, through the use of pharmacological probes, to what extent information about the chemical environment of the outside world can cross the placenta and influence fetal brain development. Extragenetic information could be vitally important in fine-tuning an organism to its environment. One approach to the study of factors that may alter developmental patterns is to determine the way in which selective drugs affect development during different phases of prenatal life. One phase of great interest is that during which brain neurotransmitter systems develop specific target receptors.

In this review, we will discuss what is known about the development of three neurotransmitter systems in brain – the dopaminergic, noradrenergic and cholinergic muscarinic, with emphasis on studies that we and others have carried out on the effects of extragenetic influences on the development of receptors and receptor-mediated functions of these systems. From the findings of these studies, it will be seen that both receptor density and the ability of transmitter systems to make adaptive responses to changes in the biochemical environment are not fixed, but can be altered by prenatal intervention. These prenatal changes are reflected in modifications of postnatal behavior. In humans, prenatal influences could conceivably alter susceptibility to both mental and motor disorders and response to psychopharmacological agents (Friedhoff and Miller, 1983a).

Development of dopaminergic, beta-noradrenergic and cholinergic muscarinic neurotransmitter receptors

While numerous studies have been carried out on the development of the monoaminergic and cholinergic muscarinic systems in brain, almost all have focused on the ontogeny of presynaptic elements, for example, the transmitter itself, the transmitter-synthesizing enzymes and transmitter reuptake systems (Lauder and Bloom, 1974; Schlumpf et al., 1980; Coyle and Yamamura, 1976; Olson and Seiger, 1972; Coyle, 1974; Verney et al., 1982; Verney et al., 1984). It is known that these presynaptic elements are well-developed prior to birth; however, there is very little information on the development of receptor-mediated functioning. While there are a number of reports on the postnatal ontogeny of catecholaminergic and cholinergic muscarinic receptors (Hartley and Seeman, 1983; Harden et al., 1980; Pittman et al., 1980; Morris et al., 1980; Coyle and Yamamura, 1976; Kuhan et al., 1980; Ben-Barak and Dudai, 1979), few studies have been carried out on the development of these receptors prior to birth, a time when alterations in the chemical environment of the developing brain could have profound effects on later behavior.

Prenatal development of DA binding sites

An important aspect of receptor maturation is the development of pharmacological selectivity and the ability of the receptor protein to distinguish stereoisomers. The first evidence that a receptor protein is present on a cell surface is that the cell develops the ability to bind a substance destined to be its future ligand with greater affinity than that with which the substance is bound to the surrounding membrane.

We (Friedhoff and Miller, 1983b) investigated the prenatal ontogeny of DA binding sites by examining the kinetic properties and development of specificity of these sites beginning early in fetal development and continuing through birth. Sites showing some properties of a DA binding site can be found prior to gestational day (GD) 18 but not before GD 15. In Table 1, it can be seen that these sites bind [^{3}H]dopamine, which can be displaced

by dopaminergic compounds in a competitive manner; however, these sites also have crossover specificity with beta-noradrenergic, muscarinic compounds and serotonin, but not with alpha-adrenergic substances or amino acid transmitters. The rules that govern the cross-specificity of the developing receptor may be related to structural similarities among certain receptor types. In this regard, it is of much interest that beta-adrenergic and muscarinic receptors show significant homology in amino acid sequence as well as in hydrophobicity profile, suggesting that these two proteins derive from a common ancestor (Dixon et al., 1986; Kubo et al., 1986).

In Table 2, the fetal ontogeny of specific [^{3}H]spiroperidol (DA-D$_2$) binding sites is shown. Prior to GD 15 selective binding can be detected. Between GD 15 and GD 18, when the binding sites appear to lack true phenotypic specificity, specific [^{3}H]spiroperidol binding can be demonstrated but saturable kinetics are not observed. This period appears to be the time during which

TABLE 1

IC$_{50}$ values (μM) of drugs in displacing [^{3}H]dopamine or ^{3}H-QNB binding to fetal (GD 16–17) and adult rat brain homogenates

Drug	[^{3}H]Dopamine		^{3}H-QNB	
	Fetal	Adult	Fetal	Adult
Dopamine	0.9	0.001–0.38[a]	>10	>10[b]
L-Norepinephrine	0.6	0.25[a]	>10	>10[b]
Apomorphine	7.5	0.003–0.18[a]	>10	–
(+)-Butaclamol	0.9	0.160–0.29[a]	>10	–
Atropine	11.0	400	0.005	0.001–0.002[b]
Oxotremorine	35.0	494	0.640	0.500–0.800[b]
Scopolamine	–	–	0.006	0.001[b]
Nicotine	–	–	>10	>10[b]
Isoproterenol	0.7	>10	>10	>10[b]
Serotonin	10.0	≫10	≫10	–

The following drugs were ineffective on either [^{3}H]dopamine or ^{3}H-QNB binding at 10 μM in rat fetal brain: clonidine, GABA, glutamic acid, glycine and phentolamine. Specific [^{3}H]dopamine binding was defined as the difference between total binding at 1.0 nM and that determined in the presence of 5 μM (+)-butaclamol. Specific ^{3}H-QNB binding was defined as the difference between total binding at 0.5 nM and that determined in the presence of 1 mM oxotremorine.
[a] Adult data from Seeman (1980).
[b] Adult data from Yamamura and Snyder (1974).

TABLE 2

K_d (nM) and B_{max} (fmol/mg protein) for [^{3}H]spiroperidol and [^{3}H]quinuclidinylbenzilate (^{3}H-QNB) binding to fetal forebrain and adult rat brain membranes

Tissue	[^{3}H]Spiroperidol		^{3}H-QNB	
	K_d	B_{max}	K_d	B_{max}
Fetal (GD 13)	a	a	0.40	3.3
Fetal (GD 16)	b	b	1.11	76.7
Fetal (GD 18)	0.092	4.9	–	–
Fetal (GD 20)	0.180	11.5	0.07	164.9
Adult (striatum)	0.085	410.0	0.07	3230.0

[a] Specific [^{3}H]spiroperidol binding was not detectable.
[b] Specific binding detectable but not saturable. K_d and B_{max} for each radioligand were determined as previously described (Miller and Friedhoff, 1986b).

these binding sites are mutable, as will be seen later. Around GD 18, saturable binding kinetics can be demonstrated by Scatchard analysis (Friedhoff and Miller, 1983b). Bruinink et al. (1983) reported detectable receptors at GD 17.5 and saturable binding properties for [^{3}H]-spiperone binding to D_2 sites in fetal forebrain at GD 19.

Another subtype of DA receptor is the D_1, which is coupled to adenylate cyclase. Activation of this subtype by DA or DA agonists stimulates the production of cAMP (Kebabian et al., 1972). D_2 receptors, on the other hand, inhibit adenylate cyclase activity (Stoof and Kebabian, 1981). The ontogeny of D_1 receptor activity during fetal brain development has not been reported; however, a D_1 receptor-mediated increase in cAMP in chick retina at embryonic days 10–11 has been described (Ventura et al., 1984). In this species, retinal D_2 specific binding is detected later at embryonic days 17–18.

Both D_1 and D_2 binding sites develop a high degree of stereoselectivity even though DA itself has no asymmetrical carbon atoms and thus no stereoisomers. We examined the development of stereoselectivity of brain DA binding sites with the stereoisomers of butaclamol. The (+)-isomer is a therapeutically active drug with high affinity and selectivity for the D_2 receptor, while the (–)-isomer is therapeutically inactive and has low affinity for the D_2 binding site (Seeman, 1980). We have found that the recognition sites detected during GD 14.5–17.5 with [^{3}H]spiroperidol do not distinguish between the isomers of butaclamol. Offspring of rats treated during this period with either (+)- or (–)-butaclamol were found to have a significant reduction in D_2 binding sites postnatally. In vitro studies of the ability of the isomers of butaclamol to displace [^{3}H]spiroperidol from D_2 sites revealed that the D_2 binding site does not show stereoselectivity until GD 18.5 (Miller and Friedhoff, 1986a).

Prenatal development of muscarinic cholinergic receptors

The prenatal developmental pattern of muscarinic cholinergic receptors in brain has been extensively studied in human fetal tissue (Ravikumar and Sastry, 1985). Using [^{3}H]quinuclidinylbenzilate (^{3}H-QNB), a specific muscarinic receptor antagonist, Ravikumar and Sastry (1985) found that muscarinic binding sites appear at 16–18 weeks with slow development until 20 weeks followed by a lag phase of 4 weeks. Rapid receptor formation then occurs during the last trimester of fetal life. These investigators also observed a modulatory effect of GTP on ^{3}H-QNB binding in 16–18-week-old human fetal cortex, from which it seems that the receptor and the transducing elements appear simultaneously during ontogeny. We have studied the prenatal development of ^{3}H-QNB binding sites in rat forebrain (Friedhoff and Miller, 1983b). As can be seen in Table 2, specific, saturable binding can be demonstrated as early as GD 13. Furthermore, these binding sites exhibit the pharmacological specificity of mature muscarinic receptors early during fetal brain development (see Table 1).

Prenatal development of beta-noradrenergic binding sites

The postnatal developmental pattern of beta-adrenergic receptors has been previously characterized in the rat (Pittman et al., 1980). In the cerebral cortex, which contains mostly beta-adrenergic receptors, the total number of binding sites increases sharply between postnatal days 10 and 21. The temporal course of beta-receptor development does not appear to correlate with presynaptic ontogeny (Pittman et al., 1980). Bruinink et al. (1982) found that beta-adrenergic receptor binding can be detected early in fetal brain development. We have also carried out studies of the fetal development of beta-adrenergic receptors in rat forebrain. Although the data are preliminary, specific binding of the beta-antagonist [³H]dihydroalprenolol (³H-DHA) could be detected at GD 13.5 (10.4 fmol bound/mg protein). At GD 14.5, saturation kinetics can be demonstrated by Scatchard analysis ($K_d = 0.5$ nM; $B_{max} = 18.9$ fmol/mg protein). This is in marked contrast to the development of beta-adrenergic receptors in fetal heart, where low specific ³H-DHA binding is detectable at GD 13.5–17.5, but saturation kinetics cannot be shown until GD 18.5 ($K_d = 1.24$ nM; $B_{max} =$

21.2 fmol/mg protein). Our data on the appearance of saturable binding sites for beta receptors in the heart are in agreement with those reported earlier by Chen et al. (1979).

Effect of prenatal psychoactive drug exposure on postnatal receptor development and function

Drug effects on D_2 receptor development and DA activity

In the first study ever carried out showing that alteration of the availability of transmitter during fetal development can alter the number of target receptors, we showed that reducing DA at the receptor site prenatally, either by blocking the developing receptor with the neuroleptic drug haloperidol, or by blocking DA synthesis with α-methyl-*p*-tyrosine, produced a significant decrease in the number of D_2 receptors postnatally, as assessed with the specific D_2 antagonist [³H]spiroperidol (Rosengarten and Friedhoff, 1979; and see Table 3). The effect seen with prenatal haloperidol treatment has been replicated using another potent neuroleptic, (+)-butaclamol (Miller and Friedhoff, 1986a). The decrease in D_2 binding sites in striatum of offspring exposed prenatally to a neuroleptic is

TABLE 3

Specific binding of [³H]spiroperidol (fmol/mg protein) to striatal membranes of offspring of rat mothers subjected to various treatments

Treatment	Age				
	14 days	21 days	28 days	35 days	60 days
Saline	190.0 ± 12.1	199.2 ± 6.4	250.7 ± 9.3	241.0 ± 14.3	222.1 ± 12.4
Haloperidol	75.0 ± 5.0	80.7 ± 7.1	93.5 ± 10.7	155.0 ± 9.3	173.0 ± 9.2
	($P < 0.001$)	($P < 0.001$)	($P < 0.001$)	($P < 0.001$)	($P < 0.05$)
α-MT	60.0 ± 11.4	147.8 ± 7.1	247.8 ± 12.1		
	($P < 0.001$)	($P < 0.01$)	n.s.		

Data from Rosengarten and Friedhoff (1979).
Pregnant rats were given either haloperidol (2.5 mg/kg/day), α-methyl-*p*-tyrosine (α-MT), 50 mg/kg/day, or saline intraperitoneally on GDs 5–20. *P* values vs. saline controls.

TABLE 4

Striatal dopamine and metabolite levels at baseline and after acute haloperidol challenge in 30-day-old offspring exposed in utero to haloperidol

Treatment (n = 6/group)		Concentration (μg/g tissue $\pm$ S.E.)		
In utero	Challenge	DA	DOPAC	HVA
Saline	Saline	5.12 $\pm$ 0.45	1.68 $\pm$ 0.26	0.74 $\pm$ 0.05
Saline	Haloperidol	4.15 $\pm$ 0.32	3.13 $\pm$ 0.21	1.86 $\pm$ 0.12
Haloperidol	Saline	4.52 $\pm$ 0.36	1.52 $\pm$ 0.17	0.61 $\pm$ 0.05
Haloperidol	Haloperidol	4.11 $\pm$ 0.28	3.15 $\pm$ 0.19	1.87 $\pm$ 0.12

Data from Rosengarten et al. (1983b).
DOPAC = dihydroxyphenylacetic acid; HVA = homovanillic acid.

opposite to the effect observed in postnatal animals treated with neuroleptics (see Seeman, 1980, for review). For the postnatal period the adjustment of receptor concentration to the availability of transmitter is homeostatic in nature; that is, blocking receptors or otherwise decreasing access of dopamine results in an increase in receptor density. The decrement observed in these binding sites after prenatal intervention does not appear to be related to a general anti-maturational effect on nigrostriatal DA neurons inasmuch as neither DA nor its metabolites dihydroxyphenylacetic acid (DOPAC) and homovanillic acid (HVA) are altered by the prenatal neuroleptic treatment (see Table 4).

We later found that this effect could be confined to a critical period from GD 15 to 18 (Rosengarten et al., 1983b; and see Table 5). The changes produced by prenatal intervention, including those in the critical prenatal period, persist well into adulthood (Rosengarten and Friedhoff, 1979), so that although the total number of DA receptors increased during early postnatal life, receptor number in animals subjected to neuroleptic treatment during fetal life always remains somewhat behind that in their untreated counterparts. This critical period is interesting from another perspective as well, because it is then that receptors develop the specificity, stereo-

selectivity and kinetic properties of mature receptors (Miller and Friedhoff, 1986a). Before GD 15 these receptors can be characterized as a kind of protoreceptor, recognizing DA, but without the exquisite pharmacological selectivity that characterizes the mature receptor. By GD 17–18 they have all of the properties of their postnatal counterpart. Interestingly, after GD 17–18 the receptors are no longer mutable, and neuroleptics given after GD 17–18 do not modify the number of postnatal receptors (Miller and Friedhoff, 1986a; and Table 5).

TABLE 5

Effect of haloperidol treatment during discrete periods of gestation on postnatal [^{3}H]spiroperidol binding to striatal membranes of rats aged 15 days

Gestation period (days)	n	[^{3}H]Spiroperidol bound (pmol/g tissue $\pm$ S.E.)
Saline	15	5.37 $\pm$ 0.26
12–13	10	6.33 $\pm$ 0.40
13–14	8	6.13 $\pm$ 0.40
15–16	16	4.01 $\pm$ 0.22[a]
17–18	10	3.64 $\pm$ 0.35[a]
19–20	10	5.37 $\pm$ 0.32

Data from Rosengarten et al. (1983b).
[a] $P < 0.001$ vs. saline-treated group.

While prenatal D_2 antagonist treatment produces a decrement in D_2 binding sites, prenatal exposure to the precursor of DA, L-dopa, during the critical period results in a 27% increase in the number of striatal [^{3}H]spiroperidol binding sites measured postnatally. This effect of agonist exposure during fetal brain development on postnatal D_2 receptor number could not be shown if treatment occurred after GD 18 (Rosengarten and Friedhoff, unpublished data). Taken together, these findings of a differential effect of DA agonist/antagonist treatment, in utero, on D_2 receptor ontogeny have led us to speculate that the normal programming of DA receptor concentration during development is contingent upon exposure of developing neuronal cells to DA.

Functional effects of prenatal neuroleptic exposure

The decrement induced by prenatal intervention with a neuroleptic is more than just an adventitious effect of drug exposure. Dopamine-dependent behaviors such as apomorphine-induced stereotypy are also significantly reduced, even more than the number of receptors (Rosengarten and Friedhoff, 1979; Rosengarten et al., 1983a). An additional functional effect occurs through an alteration of the ability of the dopaminergic system to up-regulate postnatally, that is, to become supersensitive in response to post-synaptic dopamine receptor blockade by neuroleptics. In preliminary experiments, we found (Friedhoff and Rosengarten, unpublished results) that animals exposed prenatally to a neuroleptic do not show the normal increase in D_2 receptors when treated again as adults with a neuroleptic for 28 days. In naive rats, D_2 receptor number increases about 25% in response to one to four weeks of postnatal treatment with a neuroleptic (see Seeman, 1980, for review). Interestingly, prenatal exposure to a neuroleptic during the critical period *reduces* receptor number by a similar amount, about 25%. Because of this concordance of the number of absent receptors with the number of new receptors that appear in the supersensitive state we have considered the possi-

bility that the receptors which fail to emerge as a result of prenatal neuroleptic treatment are the same population that increases in response to postnatal blockade. We have speculated that the population of D_2 receptors which respond to chronic blockade or overstimulation, by respectively increasing or decreasing receptor number, may be a population distinct from that involved in the turnover of the normal complement of DA receptors. This could occur if those receptors that up-regulate or down-regulate are under different regulatory control at the genomic level than those involved in normal receptor turnover. We have little evidence to support this notion, as yet, although our preliminary observation, that animals exposed prenatally to a neuroleptic are unable to develop dopaminergic receptor supersensitivity, is consistent with this idea. The loss of the ability to up-regulate in response to chronic blockade may occur because the missing 25% are the up-regulatable population.

There are also reports from other investigators of functional teratological effects resulting from exposure to neuroleptics during ontogeny. Rats exposed to pimozide during nursing show deficits in conditioned avoidance response (Lundborg and Engel, 1974). Shalaby and Spear (1980) treated pregnant rats with haloperidol throughout gestation and postnatally until weaning. They found that control offspring at 7 weeks of age exhibit a suppression of locomotor activity in response to a low dose of the DA agonist apomorphine, while haloperidol-exposed offspring do not. Hull et al. (1984) have shown that prenatal haloperidol exposure during GD 7–21 results in a marked demasculinization effect on male rats, which, they hypothesize, occurs by an action of the drug on neurons that regulate sex behavior in the adult rat.

Edley (1983) reported a 22% increase in [^{3}H]spiperone binding accompanied by a 70% increase in [^{3}H]naloxone (opiate) binding sites in striatum of offspring of rat mothers treated with haloperidol from GD 15 until birth. We have consistently found a decrease in the number of D_2

receptors with haloperidol treatment administered after GD 15, but before birth. It is noteworthy that we have found an increase in D_2 binding sites in pups exposed immediately postnatally via drug given to their mothers and transmitted to the pups in the milk during nursing (Rosengarten and Friedhoff, 1979). Adventitious postnatal exposure could occur if prenatally exposed offspring are not cross-fostered with control mothers at birth.

One final functional implication of the prenatally induced decrement has to do with the relationship of the D_1 and D_2 receptor subtypes of the dopaminergic system. D_1 receptor concentration is significantly higher than the concentration of D_2 receptors in rat striatum (Seeman, 1980). D_1 activation of adenylate cyclase activity by DA agonists is inhibited by D_2 agonist stimulation (Stoof and Kebabian, 1981); therefore normal D_1 stimulation of cAMP formation is modulated by D_2 activity. Rosengarten et al. (1986), in studies of the behavioral consequences of manipulation of striatal D_1/D_2 activity, have found that an imbalance in the ratio of these activities, induced in vivo by administration of a low dose of a selective D_2 antagonist followed by a behavioral activating dose of a DA agonist, induces a behavioral syndrome referred to as repetitive jaw movements (RJM). This behavioral syndrome in rats may be mediated by mechanisms that are similar to those in human tardive dyskinesia, a debilitating extrapyramidal disorder seen in some patients after chronic treatment with neuroleptics. Spontaneous RJMs are observed in aged rats in which the differential decline with age, of D_2 vs. D_1 receptors, favors heightened D_1 activity. Spontaneous oral dyskinesia often develops in aged humans. In preliminary studies, Rosengarten and Friedhoff have found that prenatal treatment with D_2-selective drugs such as haloperidol, which produce a postnatal decrement in striatal D_2 binding sites, does not alter the number of D_1 sites. Thus rats exposed prenatally to haloperidol have an increase in D_1 relative to D_2 receptors and also exhibit spontaneous RJMs

after birth (Rosengarten and Friedhoff, unpublished results).

Drug effects on the muscarinic cholinergic system

In contrast to the dopaminergic system, the cholinergic system does not adapt to pharmacological alterations in the availability of acetylcholine during prenatal development. Prenatal as well as early postnatal exposure to the muscarinic antagonist atropine does not alter the number of striatal ^{3}H-QNB binding sites (See Table 6). The reason for the resistance of fetal muscarinic cholinergic receptors to alteration by cholinergic antagonists may be that these receptors achieve mature receptor kinetics at an early stage in fetal development (Friedhoff and Miller, 1983b). However, this system does change secondarily in concert with changes produced by dopaminergic antagonists (Miller and Friedhoff, 1986b). Haloperidol given on GD 14.5–17.5, which produces a decrement in D_2 receptors, also produces an increase in muscarinic receptors and in choline acetyltransferase (ChAT) activity (see Table 7). This, conceivably, could result from the fact that the dopaminergic system inhibits the release of acetylcholine in the striatum (Miller and Friedhoff, 1979). Inasmuch as the dopaminergic

TABLE 6

Effect of exposure in utero or early postnatal exposure to saline or atropine on specific ^{3}H-QNB binding (pmol/mg protein) to rat striatal membranes

Treatment	In utero[a]	Early postnatal[b]
Saline	0.59 ± 0.11 ($n = 9$)	1.33 ± 0.09 ($n = 8$)
Atropine	0.59 ± 0.14 ($n = 7$)	1.31 ± 0.13 ($n = 8$)

Specific ^{3}H-QNB binding was defined as the difference between total binding at 1.0 nM and that determined in the presence of 1 mM oxotremorine.
[a] Water or atropine (50 mg/kg) was administered p.o. to pregnant rats on GDs 5–20. Pups were killed at PN age 7.
[b] Neonates were injected i.p. daily with 50 mg/kg atropine or saline on PN days 2–12 and killed at PN age 17.

TABLE 7

Effect of in utero exposure to haloperidol on GD 14.5–17.5 on striatal ³H-SPIRO, ³H-QNB binding and on choline acetyltransferase (ChAT) activity in offspring at PN ages 14 and 32 days (means ± S.D.)

Treatment	Age (days)	n	³H-SPIRO binding (fmol/mg protein)	³H-QNB binding (fmol/mg protein)	Spec. act. (ChAT) (nmol/mg protein/h)
Vehicle	14	14	113.9 ± 20.3	584.0 ± 1.8	416.9 ± 16.4
Haloperidol	14	13	77.9 ± 27.4[d]	838.5 ± 25.9[a]	532.0 ± 9.2[a]
Vehicle	32	12	250.0 ± 6.4	928.0 ± 41.1	907.0 ± 14.3
Haloperidol	32	11	182.9 ± 50.8[c]	1283.0 ± 42.4[a]	1098.0 ± 20.3[b]

Significantly different from vehicle: [a] $P < 0.05$; [b] $P < 0.02$; [c] $P < 0.01$; [d] $P < 0.001$.
³H-SPIRO (spiroperidol) binding reflects specific binding to the dopamine (D_2) receptor, ³H-QNB (quinuclidinylbenzilate) binding reflects specific binding to muscarinic cholinergic receptors.
Data from Miller and Friedhoff (1986b).

system inhibits the cholinergic, a decrease in the number of D_2 receptors could disinhibit the cholinergic system, increase the release of acetylcholine, and alter the number of postsynaptic cholinergic sites. It seems unlikely, however, that this is the explanation, because functional dopaminergic-cholinergic interaction does not occur until the second week of postnatal life (Coyle and Campiochiaro, 1976). Alternatively, the increase in ³H-QNB binding sites may reflect an increase in presynaptic muscarinic sites, which might also be reflected in the observed increase in ChAT activity. If this were the case, one could speculate that an increased number of cholinergic cells may have developed in response to the fetal exposure to neuroleptic. This could also imply an antitrophic role for DA in the development of these interneurons, perhaps by inhibiting the secretion of NGF. This latter possibility is given some credence by the finding that NGF receptors are found in cholinergic neurons of the striatum (Hefti et al., 1986).

Drug effects on the beta-adrenergic system

Dreyfuss et al. (1977) previously showed that a beta-adrenergic antagonist, nadolol, is transferred across the placenta to the fetus, with significant amounts accumulating during early gestation up to day 16. Rosen et al. (1979) studied the effects of propranolol administered to pregnant rats on GD 8–21 and observed no significant differences between propranolol-treated and nontreated controls in litter size, birth-weight or stillbirths.

We have been interested in determining whether fetal programming during a critical period may be a generic phenomenon, involving many transmitter systems. Therefore, in addition to our studies of the effects of drugs on development of the DA system, we also investigated the effects of prenatal exposure to a beta-adrenergic antagonist on postnatal development of ³H-DHA binding sites. Our preliminary data show that propranolol given to pregnant rats on GD 12.5–16.5 produces a decrement in the number of beta-adrenergic binding sites in the postnatal heart, but an increase in the number of these receptors in the cerebral cortex (see Table 8). Based on our in vitro studies of the development of beta receptors in fetal heart, GD 12.5–16.5 falls during the vulnerable 'protoreceptor' period for beta receptors, and during this period the number of receptors decreases in response to an attenuation of ligand supply produced by the beta antagonist propranolol. In contrast, from our in vitro studies we have found that, in the cerebral cortex, by GD 12.5–16.5, the receptors have developed mature

TABLE 8

Effect of in utero exposure to propranolol on GD 12.5–16.5 on cortical and heart [³H]dihydroalprenolol (³H-DHA) binding sites in offspring at postnatal age 21 days (means ± S.D.)

Treatment	n	Cortex: ³H-DHA binding (fmol/mg protein)	Heart: ³H-DHA binding (fmol/mg protein)
Saline	8	90.4 ± 13.78	37.5 ± 10.5
Propranolol	8	113.2 ± 22.2[a]	25.3 ± 13.0[b]

Pregnant rats received daily i.p. injections of propranolol (30 mg/kg) or saline on GDs 12.5–16.5. Specific binding of the beta adrenergic antagonist ³H-DHA to cortical and heart membranes was determined in the presence of 1 μM propranolol.
[a] Significantly different from controls, $P < 0.05$.
[b] Not significantly different.

kinetics, and thus the number of receptors in the cortex increases in response to blockade by propranolol.

Summary and conclusions

By prenatal administration of pharmacological agents that alter transmitter supply to the emerging DA receptor, it has been found that receptor number can be altered. In contrast to postnatal animals, in which a reduction in transmitter supply results in a homeostatic increase in receptor density, the prenatal animal responds to similar conditions with a decrease in receptor density. These alterations in receptor density, through prenatal interventions, also have functional and behavioral consequences in the postnatal animal. There is a critical or sensitive period toward the end of gestation during which alterations in receptor number can be produced. During this period the DA binding site has partial properties of a receptor and has been termed a protoreceptor.

We also have preliminary evidence that there may be a vulnerable period during which a phenomenon, similar to that observed with the DA receptor, can be produced in the developing beta-adrenergic receptor system in the heart. Brain beta-adrenergic receptors may also be sensitive to prenatal intervention at an earlier point in gestation, inasmuch as treatment after GD 15, when the brain beta receptors have developed mature characteristics, produces an increase in the number of these binding sites postnatally.

Treatment with musarinic cholinergic agents during the last half of gestation failed to alter muscarinic binding sites in the brain; however, this system matures very early, so the critical period may occur in the first half of gestation. It is very interesting, from this standpoint, that the cholinergic system is central in primary information transfer in the brain. Its early maturation may reflect this central role, while the more plastic dopamine system may be more responsive to environmental influences on development, so that it can regulate muscarinic activity according to variable programs elaborated through the interaction of genetic and environmental factors.

Our findings have prompted us to propose that drugs such as haloperidol or propranolol simulate spontaneously occurring conditions that modify transmitter supply. We have not directly demonstrated that such alterations occur in the absence of drugs; however, it is conceivable that maternal neuropeptides, maternal hormones and maternally transmitted environmental chemicals could mediate such alterations. The extent to which particular chemicals or maternally derived substances cross the placenta in order to effect fetal receptor development has not been established. It may be, however, that, rather than thinking of the placenta as a barrier, it should be reviewed as a organ by which reduced amounts of a wide range of maternal chemicals are made available to the fetus so that it can adjust gene expression to the chemical realities of the contemporary world.

From the adaptive standpoint, the reduction in receptors that occurs when transmitter supply is reduced during the critical period of fetal development is antihomeostatic; however, just such an antihomeostatic response may make the most sense, from the adaptive standpoint, in the prenatal organism. The prenatal period, during which survival of the fetus is dependent on physiological support by the mother, is a time when the developing organism must devise means for integrating diverse developmental paths. During this period receptor number must be coordinated with transmitter supply. From the adaptive standpoint, when a developing cell, bearing dopamine receptors, senses that there is little dopamine in its surround, it need express fewer receptors in order to match receptor number to transmitter supply. When the animal is born, and obliged to survive via its own physiological and biochemical systems, homeostatic responses enhance the chance for survival. The function of homeostasis is to maintain physiological balance. This has clear survival value, inasmuch as the organism is surviving as it is, while new balances may threaten its existence. Thus, when dopamine supply is reduced in the postnatal animal the number of receptors increases, as a result of which net change in dopaminergic outflow is resisted.

We do not know what the mechanism is by which these prenatal programming responses occur. In the case of the dopaminergic system the primary messenger for initiating the response appears to be dopamine itself. Both dopamine receptor antagonists and dopamine synthesis inhibitors produce the programming response. Beyond this first message, the mechanism is unknown. Whether the number of receptor-bearing cells is reduced or only the density of receptors is not clear. This is an important question to pursue in future investigation.

Prenatal programming responses are of great interest to those concerned with biochemical and behavioral teratology. The effects of prenatal pharmacological intervention are also of interest from the standpoint of functional teratology of the brain (also see C. Kellogg, Chapter 14 of this volume); however, we have proposed that these drug effects may mimic normal adaptive shaping of development by information transfer across the placenta from maternal and environmental sources.

Acknowledgements

This research was supported in part by a New York University Biomedical Research Support Program, a grant from the Tourette Syndrome Association Permanent Research Fund to J.C.M. and by NIMH grant MH 08618 and NIMH Research Scientist Award 14024 to A.J.F.

References

Angrist, B., Thompson, H., Shopsin, B. and Gershon, S. (1975) Clinical studies with dopamine-receptor stimulants. *Psychopharmacologia*, 44: 273–280.

Beaconsfield, P., Birdwood, G. and Beaconsfield, R. (1980) *The Placenta*, Sci. Am., pp. 95–102.

Ben-Barak, H. and Dudai, Y. (1979) Cholinergic binding sites in rat hippocampal formation: properties and ontogenesis. *Brain Res.*, 166: 245–249.

Bertler, A. and Rosengren, E. (1959) Occurrence and distribution of dopamine in brain and other tissues. *Experientia*, 15: 10.

Bruinink, A., Lichtensteiger, W. and Schlumpf, M. (1982) Pre- and postnatal development of beta-adrenergic, dopaminergic, serotonergic and spirodecanone binding sites in rat forebrain. In *Drugs and Hormones in Brain Development Symposium*, Zurich, April 7–8. Abstracts, p. 19.

Bruinink, A., Lichtensteiger, W., Schlumpf, M. (1983) Pre- and postnatal ontogeny and characterization of dopaminergic D_2, serotonergic, S_2 and spirodecanone binding sites in rat forebrain. *J. Neurochem.*, 40: 1227–1236.

Carlsson, A., Rosengren, E., Bertler, A. and Nilsson, J. (1957) Effect of reserpine on the metabolism of catecholamines. In S. Garattini and V. Ghetti (Eds.), *Psychotropic Drugs*, Amsterdam, Elsevier, pp. 363–372.

Charney, D.S., Menkes, D.B. and Heninger, G.R. (1981) Receptor sensitivity and the mechanism of action of antidepressant treatment. *Arch. Gen. Psychiatry*, 38: 1160–1180.

Chen, F.M., Yamamura, H.I. and Roeske, W.R. (1979) Ontogeny of mammalian myocardial beta-adrenergic receptors. *Eur. J. Pharmacol.*, 58: 255–264.

Cole, J.O., Goldbert, S.C. and Davis, J.M. (1966). Drugs in the treatment of psychosis: controlled studies. In P. Solomon (Ed.), *Psychiatric Drugs*, Grune & Stratton, New York, pp. 153–180.

Coyle, J.T. (1974) Biochemical aspects of the catechol-aminergic neurons in the brain of the fetal and neonatal rat. In K. Fuxe, L. Olson and Y. Zooterman (Eds.), *Dynamics of Degeneration and Growth in Neurons*, Pergamon Press, New York, pp. 425–434.

Coyle, J.T. and Campochiaro, P. (1976) Ontogenesis of dopaminergic-cholinergic interactions in the rat striatum. *J. Neurochem.*, 27: 673–678.

Coyle, J.T. and Yamamura, H.I. (1976) Neurochemical aspects of ontogenesis of cholinergic neurons in the rat brain. *Brain Res.*, 118: 429–440.

Dixon, R.A.F., Kobilka, B.K., Strader, D.J., Benovic, J.L., Dohlman, H.G., Frielle, T., Bolanowski, M.A., Bennett, D.C., Rands, E., Diehl, R.E., Mumford, R.A., Slaten, E.E., Sigal, I.S., Caron, M.G., Lefkowitz, R.J. and Strader, C.D. (1986), Cloning of the gene and cDNA for mammalian beta-adrenergic receptor and homology with rhodopsin. *Nature*, 321: 75–79.

Dreyfuss, J., Shaw, J. and Miller, T.J. (1977) Nadolol: placental transfer and excretion in the milk of rats. *Toxicol. Appl. Pharmacol.*, 39: 275–282.

Edley, S.M. (1983) Effects of prenatal haloperidol on receptors in the developing rat striatum: opposite changes in naloxone and spiperone binding. *Neurosci. Abstr.*, 9(2): 874.

Friedhoff, A.J. and Miller, J.C. (1983a) Clinical implications of receptor sensitivity modification. *Annu. Rev. Neurosci.*, 6: 121–148.

Friedhoff, A.J. and Miller, J.C. (1983b) Prenatal psychotropic drug exposure and the development of central dopaminergic and cholinergic transmitter systems. In M. Schlumpf and W. Lichtensteiger (Eds.), *Drugs and Hormones in Brain Development, Monographs Neural Sciences*, Karger, Basel, pp. 91–98.

Harden, T.K., Wolfe, B.B., Sporn, J.R., Perkins, J.P. and Molinoff, P.B. (1980) Ontogeny of beta-adrenergic receptors in rat cerebral cortex. *Brain Res.*, 125: 99–108.

Hartley, E.J. and Seeman, P. (1983). Development of receptors for dopamine and noradrenaline in rat brain. *Eur. J. Pharmacol.*, 91: 391–397.

Hefti, F., Hartikka, J., Salvatierra, A., Weiner, W.J. and Mash, D.C. (1986) Localization of nerve growth factor receptors in cholinergic neurons of the human basal forebrain. *Neurosci. Lett.*, 69: 37–41.

Hull, E.M., Nishita, J.K., Bitran, D. and Dalterio, S. (1984) Perinatal dopamine-related drugs demasculinize rats. *Science*, 224: 1011–1013.

Kebabian, J.W., Petzold, G.L. and Greengard, P. (1972) Dopamine-sensitive adenylate cyclase in the caudate nucleus of the rat brain, and its similarity to the 'dopamine receptor'. *Proc. Natl. Acad. Sci. USA*, 69: 2145–2153.

Kubo, T., Fukuda, K., Mikami, A., Maeda, A., Takahashi, H., Mishina, M., Haga, T., Haga, K., Ichiyama, A., Kangawa, K., Kojima, M., Matsuo, H., Hirose, T. and Numa, S. (1986) Cloning, sequencing and expression of complementary DNA encoding the muscarinic acetylcholine receptor. *Nature*, 323: 411–416.

Kuhar, M.J., Birdsall, N.J.M., Burgen, A.S.V. and Hulme, E.C. (1980) Ontogeny of muscarinic receptors in rat brain. *Brain Res.*, 184: 375–383.

Lauder, J.M. and Bloom, F.E. (1974) Ontogeny of monoamine neurons in the locus coeruleus, raphe nuclei and substantia nigra of the rat. I. Cell differentiation. *J. Comp. Neurol.*, 155: 469–482.

Lundborg, P. and Engel, J. (1974) Learning deficits and selective biochemial brain changes in 4-week old offspring of nursing rat mothers treated with neuroleptics. In G. Sedvall, B. Uvnas and Y. Zotterman (Eds.), *Antipsychotic Drugs: Pharmacodynamics and Pharmacokinetics*, Pergamon Press, Oxford, pp. 261–169.

McEwen, B.S. (1982) Steroid hormone action in the brain: cellular and behavioral effects. In F.O. Schmitt, S.J. Bird and F.E. Bloom (Eds.), *Molecular Genetic Neuroscience*, Raven Press, New York, pp. 265–276.

Miller, J.C. and Friedhoff, A.J. (1979) Dopamine receptor-coupled modulation of the K^+-depolarized overflow of ^{3}H-acetylcholine from rat striatal slices: alteration after chronic haloperidol and alpha-methyl-*p*-tyrosine pretreatment. *Life Sci.*, 25: 1249–1256.

Miller, J.C. and Friedhoff, A.J. (1986a) Development of specificity and stereoselectivity of rat brain dopamine receptors. *Int. J. Dev. Neurosci.*, 4: 21–26.

Miller, J.C. and Friedhoff, A.J. (1986b) Prenatal neuroleptic exposure alters postnatal striatal cholinergic activity in the rat. *Dev. Neurosci.*, 8: 11–116.

Morris, M.J., Dausse, J.-P., Devynck, M.-A. and Meyer, P. (1980) Ontogeny of alpha$_1$ and alpha$_2$ adrenoreceptors in rat brain. *Brain Res.*, 190: 268–271.

Olson, L. and Seiger, A. (1972) Early prenatal ontogeny of central monoamine neurons in the rat: fluorescence histochemical observations. *Z. Anat. Entw. Gesch.*, 137: 301–316.

Pittman, R.N., Minneman, K.P. and Molinoff, P.B. (1980) Ontogeny of beta$_1$ and beta$_2$ receptors in rat cerebellum and cerebral cortex. *Brain Res.*, 188: 357–368.

Ravikumar, B.V. and Sastry, P.S. (1985) Muscarinic cholinergic receptors in human fetal brain: characterization and ontogeny of ^{3}H-quinuclidinylbenzilate binding sites in frontal cortex. *J. Neurochem.*, 44: 240–246.

Rosen, G.S., Lin, M., Spector, S. and Rosen, M.R. (1979) Maternal, fetal and neonatal effects of chronic propranolol administration in the rat. *J. Pharmacol. Exp. Ther.*, 208: 118–122.

Rosengarten, H. and Friedhoff, A.J. (1979) Enduring changes in dopamine receptor cells of pups from drug administration to pregnant and nursing rats. *Science*, 203: 1133–1135.

Rosengarten, H., Carr, K. and Friedhoff, A.J. (1983a) Persistent changes in CNS dopaminergic activity following prenatal exposure to neuroleptics. *Neurosci. Abstr.*, 9: 228.

Rosengarten, H., Friedman, E. and Friedhoff, A.J. (1983b) Sensitive periods to the neuroleptic effect of haloperidol to reduce dopamine receptors. In A.M. Guiffrida-Stella, B. Haber, G. Hashim and J.R. Perez-Polo (Eds.), *Nervous System Regeneration*, Alan Liss, New York, pp. 511–513.

Rosengarten, H., Schweitzer, J.W. and Friedhoff, A.J. (1986) Selective dopamine D_2 receptor reduction enhances a D_1 mediated oral dyskinesia in rats. *Life Sci.*, 39: 29–35.

Schlumpf, M., Shoemaker, W.J. and Bloom, F.E. (1980) Innervation of embryonic rat cerebral cortex by catecholamine-containing fibers. *J. Comp. Neurol.*, 192: 361–376.

Seeman, P. (1980) Brain dopamine receptors. *Pharmacol. Rev.*, 32: 228–313.

Shalaby, I.A. and Spear, L.P. (1980) Chronic administration of haloperidol during development: later psychopharmacological responses to apomorphine and arecoline. *Pharmacol. Biochem. Behav.*, 13: 685–690.

Shore, P.A., Silver, S.L. and Brodie, B.B. (1955) Interaction of reserpine, serotonin, and lysergic acid diethylamide in brain. *Science*, 122: 284–285.

Stoof, J.C. and Kebabian, J.W. (1981) Opposing roles of D-1 and D-2 dopamine receptors in efflux of cyclic AMP from rat neostriatum. *Nature*, 294: 366–368.

Sulser, F. (1983) Mode of action of antidepressant drugs. *J. Clin. Psychiatry*, 44: 14–20.

Ventura, A.J.M., Klein, W. and De Mello, F.G. (1984) Differential ontogenesis of D_1 and D_2 receptors in the chick embryo retina. *Dev. Brain Res.*, 12: 217–223.

Verney, C., Berger, B., Adrien, J., Vigny, A. and Gay, M. (1982) Development of rat cerebral cortex. A light microscopic immunocytochemical study using anti-tyrosine hydroxylase antibodies. *Dev. Brain Res.*, 5: 41–52.

Verney, C., Berger, B., Baulac, M., Helle, K.B. and Alvarez, C. (1984) Dopamine-beta-hydroxylase-like immunoreactivity in the fetal cerebral cortex of the rat: noradrenergic ascending pathways and terminal fields. *Int. J. Dev. Neurosci.*, 2: 491–503.

Woolley, D.W. and Shaw, E. (1954) A biochemical and pharmacological suggestion about certain mental disorders. *Science*, 119: 587–588.

Yamamura, H. and Snyder, S.H. (1974) Muscarinic cholinergic receptor binding in rat brain. *Proc. Natl. Acad. Sci. USA*, 71: 1725–1729.

Discussion

E. Fride: If you measure dopamine (DA) binding at a 'difficult' DA target area like the prefrontal cortex, which develops later than the nigro-striatal system, would you then come to a different conclusion concerning the vulnerable period?

J.C. Miller: The critical period for a neuroleptic on the developing prefrontal DA system may differ from that found for the nigro-striatal system. Unfortunately, we do not have sufficient data on the prefrontal system. The data that we do have indicate that they are unchanged by treatment during gestational days 15–17 (Rosengarten and Friedhoff, unpublished data). However, as you suggest, the D_2 receptors in the prefrontal cortex are significantly fewer in number than those in the striatum and are difficult to accurately characterize, even in the mature adult.

A.J. Patel: For a number of neurotransmitter receptors, you suggested K_d values to be about 100–1000-times higher at young embryonic ages in comparison with adult ages. Of course, one of the widely advocated interpretations is maturation of synapses. However, it is also possible that at embryonic ages, the proportion of proliferative cells is very high, so one may also hypothesize that proliferative cells have receptors with higher K_d than non-proliferative adult brain cells.

J.C. Miller: Yes, this is a plausible explanation.

T.A. Slotkin: Is it possible that haloperidol acts through inhibition of cell proliferation, as proposed by Patel and Lewis (Chapter 25 of this volume). Elimination of cells which would have expressed DA and acetylcholine (ACh) receptors would equally well explain your results.

J.C. Miller: Inasmuch as Patel and Lewis (Chapter 25) have shown that a neuroleptic can inhibit neuronal cell proliferation (at relatively high drug concentrations as compared to that used in our experiments) it is possible that this is one mechanism by which D_2 receptors are reduced rather than by an effect on dopamine cells. We have not examined the effect of prenatal haloperidol exposure on the number of dopaminergic or cholinergic cells found in the striatum postnatally. Reduction of cell number would not explain the effect seen on the cholinergic system, since choline acetyltransferase (ChAT) activity and cholinergic muscarinic binding sites (which are most likely presynaptic) are increased by prenatal neuroleptic exposure.

H.J. Romijn: What is the mechanism by which neurotransmitters are released during early development in order to set the numerical density of receptors on the postsynaptic element? Is spiking activity necessary or is it a passive release? If the latter is the case, would there be a shift during maturation of the neuron from passive to active spiking release?

J.C. Miller: There is no direct evidence, to my knowledge, on the mechanism of dopamine release during fetal neuronal development. It seems unlikely that active, depolarized release would occur before birth. At some point during early postnatal maturation of the neurons, a shift to active release occurs but I do not know when this is.

J.M. Lauder: In answer to the previous question regarding release mechanism in developing transmitter systems, I would just like to mention that transmitters seem to be spontaneously released from growth cones in a tonic fashion, which may relate to their proposed roles in development. How this may be regulated is unknown.

R. Balázs: It is interesting that you have found that the muscarinic receptors are apparently not affected by atropine. At least in vitro there is a marked down-regulation by agonists (Shifrin and Klein, 1980; Burgoyne and Pearce, 1981). It would be worth trying to examine the effect of agonists rather than antagonists in your experimental paradigm concerning the elevation of ChAT activity in the neuroleptic-treated animals. May it be that this is related to a compensatory increase in the enzyme activity subsequent to the reduction of DA-receptor binding sites?

J.C. Miller: We have not as yet tried cholinergic muscarinic agonists in our paradigm. Considering that the functional relationship of the dopaminergic system to that of the cholinergic system in striatum is an inhibitory one (Lehmann and Langer, 1983), one could suppose that as the cholinergic neurons are maturing, they become disinhibited by antagonism of D_2 receptors by haloperidol, resulting in more ChAT activity. However, there is no evidence that a direct inhibitory interaction is operating during fetal development. It is not known whether the D_2 receptor binding sites that are eliminated by the prenatal haloperidol treatment are postsynaptic or presynaptic, since the D_2 receptor subtype is localized to both elements.

C.K. Kellogg: Considering that the greatest increase in synaptogenesis in the striatum occurs around postnatal day 14–15 in the rat and reflects in large part the formation of cholinergic synapses, do you have any evidence that prenatal exposure to haloperidol may have altered the synaptogenesis?

J.C. Miller: No. We have not looked in depth at possible changes in the functional interaction between the dopaminergic and cholinergic system postnatally, which, if they occurred, might reflect altered synaptogenesis.

A. Dekker: Is there evidence for a differential sensitivity of pre- vs. postsynaptic receptors during development. If haloperidol blocks presynaptic receptors initially, it might increase the amount of DA released and a subsequent reduction in receptor number on the postsynaptic side. Later on haloperidol might induce postsynaptic supersensitivity.

J.C. Miller: Whether haloperidol affects the presynaptic vs. postsynaptic D_2 receptors differentially during development is unknown. Binding of haloperidol to postsynaptic receptors is likely to occur in any event and it is not established that, prenatally, blockade of presynaptic receptor results in an increase in DA release. Furthermore, in our paradigm we find that the presence of more DA, e.g. through giving the precursor, L-dopa, prenatally, rather than producing a reduction in receptor number, produces a marked increase (Rosengarten et al., 1983). This effect is opposite to that seen postnatally (Friedhoff et al., 1977). Furthermore, functional dopaminergic neurons, at least in the adult, respond in a very short time to neuroleptics by going into depolarization block, which decreases DA release (Bunney and Grace, 1978). To determine whether pre- vs. postnatal D-2 receptors are differentially sensitive during fetal brain development requires selective pre- vs. postsynaptic D_2-specific drugs.

M.V. Johnston: Is it possible that DA normally antagonizes growth of striatal cholinergic neurons, serving as a natural 'antitrophic factor'. Nerve growth factor (NGF) stimulates ChAT in growing striatal cholinergic neurons and it might synergistically stimulate more ChAT in your prenatally treated rats than in normal rats.

J.C. Miller: This is an interesting thought. If DA were to do so, one would suppose that DA normally inhibits the release of NGF in the developing striatum. One would expect then that rats exposed prenatally to L-dopa, where we know that D_2 receptors are increased (Rosengarten et al., 1983), show a decrement in ChAT activity. We do not know whether this is the case. In general, studies related to the possible involvement of NGF in the cholinergic effect seem to be important to carry out.

References

Bunny, W.S. and Grace, A.A. (1978) Acute and chronic haloperidol treatment: comparison of effects on nigral dopaminergic cell activity. *Life Sci.*, 23: 1715–1728.

Burgoyne, R.D. and Pearce, B. (1981) Muscarinic acetylcholine receptor regulation and protein phosphorylation in primary cultures of rat cerebellum. *Dev. Brain Res.*, 2: 55–63.

Friedhoff, A.J., Bonnet, K.A. and Rosengarten, H. (1977) Reveral of two manifestations of dopamine receptor supersensitivity by administration of L-dopa. *Res. Commun. Chem. Pathol. Pharmacol.*, 16: 411–423.

Lehmann, J. and Langer, S.Z. (1983) The striatal cholinergic interneuron: synaptic target of dopaminergic terminals? *Neuroscience*, 10: 1105–1120.

Rosengarten, H., Friedman, E. and Friedhoff, A.J. (1983) Sensitive periods to the neuroleptic effect of haloperidol to reduce dopamine receptors. In A.M. Guiffrida-Stella, B. Haber, G. Hashim and J.R. Perez-Polo (Eds.), *Nervous System Regeneration*, Alan Liss, New York, pp. 511–513.

Shifrin, G.S. and Klein, W.L. (1980) Regulation of muscarinic acetylcholine receptor concentration in cloned neuroblastoma cells. *J. Neurochem.*, 34: 993–999.

G.J. Boer, M.G.P. Feenstra, M. Mirmiran, D.F. Swaab and F. Van Haaren
Progress in Brain Research, Vol. 73
© 1988 Elsevier Science Publishers B.V. (Biomedical Division)

CHAPTER 32

Neuropeptide influences on the development of their receptors

Gail E. Handelmann

Central Nervous System Diseases Research, G.D. Searle & Company, AA5C, St. Louis, MO 63198, USA

Introduction

Neurotransmitters and neurohormones play a different role in the developing animal than they do in the adult. While in the adult they activate the cells of their target organs to perform various functions, in the immature organism they tend to organize the cells to develop into a functional unit. Such organizing influences during development have been established for several types of hormones, such as the gonadal steroid hormones (see e.g. Bermant and Davison, 1974, for review) and thyroxine (e.g. Eayres and Holmes, 1964). One important property of the mature tissue is its ability to respond to chemical signals, in the form of either hormones or neurotransmitters. In order for the brain or other organs to respond to input, receptors for various compounds must be located in appropriate sites and in appropriate densities. Within the brain, for example, receptors for a given neurotransmitter are distributed unequally in various regions. How is the number and type of receptor that a cell will express determined during the course of development? One hypothesis is that the presence of the hormone or neurotransmitter itself is an important signal.

The experiments described in this review were initiated to determine whether the neuropeptides, a relatively new class of neurotransmitters and hormones, play a role in development. The strategy adopted was to alter the levels of a particular neuropeptide in a developing animal, and then, when the animal was fully mature, to test it for perturbations in physiological systems in which the peptide is known to play a role. Neonatal albino rat pups were injected subcutaneously with either a neuropeptide or saline once daily during the first week after birth, a time of rapid growth of the brain and other organs in rats. The pups were cross-fostered, and each mother reared pups of both treatment groups. The pups were weaned on day 23, and behavioral and neurochemical observations were made when the rats were fully mature adults, at least 40 days of age.

Experiments involving the three neuropeptides vasopressin, substance P and [met]enkephalin are described. For each peptide, the findings indicate long-term developmental influences on behavior and sensitivity to the peptide administered, and that these effects are correlated with changes in the number of peptide receptors expressed.

Vasopressin

Vasopressin (VP) is a neuropeptide contained in the brain and pituitary. Two actions of pituitary VP have been identified in the periphery. One is to increase reabsorption of water in the kidney by acting on specific receptors located on the distal tubule and collecting duct of the nephron. The second is to cause vasoconstriction. The receptors of the vasculature appear to be of a different type, however, displaying pharmacological properties different from those of the renal receptor (Sawyer et al., 1981). VP contained in central neural pathways has also been proposed to be involved in memory processes (Van Wimersma Greidanus et al., 1983).

To determine whether VP might influence the development of systems in which VP plays a role, neonatal albino rat pups were injected with VP (4 or 40 μg/100 g body weight; 395 U/mg) on days 1–7 after birth. When the rats were mature, their daily urine volume and water intake were measured. Later the sensitivity of their kidneys and vasculature to the actions of VP was measured by physiological assays.

The rats injected as neonates with VP exhibited polyuria as adults, indicating a long-term effect on their ability to regulate water balance. The physiological assay indicated that their kidneys were less sensitive to VP, in that their urine-concentrating response to VP was attenuated (Handelmann et al., 1983). Neither the rats' blood pressure nor their hypertensive response to VP, however, was altered.

Similar effects on urinary function were achieved in Brattleboro rats, a strain in which the hypothalamus does not synthesize VP (Wright and Kutscher, 1977; Boer et al., 1984). It is interesting that polyuria was also produced in Wistar rats treated as neonates with a VP antagonist (Snijdewint and Boer, 1987). The kidney weights of the treated rats were severely reduced, however, suggesting a serious morphological defect, and therefore a different type of developmental effect.

The relative insensitivity of the VP-treated rats' kidneys to VP suggested a deficit in the VP receptor adenylate cyclase complex. VP receptors in the kidney are linked to adenylate cyclase, so that VP stimulation causes accumulation of cAMP. In the kidneys of rats treated as neonates with VP, the production of cAMP in response to VP was attenuated (Handelmann et al., 1983). The production of cAMP in response to calcitonin or parathyroid hormone was unaffected, however,

suggesting that the developmental influence of VP was selective for the VP receptor complex. The deficit in cAMP production could be due to a deficit in adenylate cyclase or in the VP binding site. We measured VP binding to the rats' kidneys, and found that the maximal binding capacity of the tissue was decreased (Handelmann and Sayson, 1984). The affinity of the binding sites for VP, however, was unchanged (Fig. 1).

As mentioned above, VP in central neural pathways has been proposed to play a role in memory processes. If the neonatal VP treatment altered VP receptor expression in the brain as it did in kidney, one might expect to find altered memory function in the treated rats. In one experiment, we tested the ability of the rats treated as neonates with VP to learn a complex spatial maze task, but found no difference in their rate of learning from that of saline-treated rats (Handelmann, unpublished data). Rats which had received VP antiserum as neonates in order to decrease endogenous VP concentrations, however, had memory impairments in both active and passive avoidance tasks (Moratella et al., 1987). These data indicate that abnormally low levels of VP present during development can have a long-term influence on the brain; whether these effects are also due to altered receptor expression will be of interest. Another point to be explored is whether the VP-treated rats exhibit altered memory function when tested in avoidance tasks.

These experiments indicate a long-lasting deleterious effect of VP on the development of VP binding sites in the kidney, an impairment of physiological significance for the animal. The effect of VP during the first neonatal week may be selective for the kidney, and for VP receptors within the kidney. Why VP receptors in the kidney and not the cardiovasculature were affected is unclear. Susceptibility to the developmental influence may be a function of the type of tissue (e.g. kidney vs. vascular tissue), the pharmacological properties of the receptors, or the developmental stage of the tissue or receptors at the time of the exposure to the peptide. There is apparently

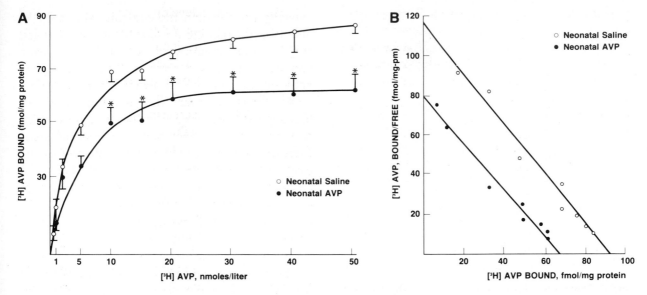

Fig. 1 (A) Specific binding of [³H]vasopressin (VP) to kidney slices from adult rats treated as neonates with VP (4 mg/100 g body weight) or saline. Treatments were made on days 1–7 after birth. * Significantly different from neonatal saline group (Student's test, $P < 0.05$). (B) Scatchard plot of the data in panel A. (Modified from Handelmann and Sayson, 1984). AVP, arginine-VP.

a critical period during development for the susceptibility to the influence of VP, as female rats treated after day 14 and male rats treated after day 20 did not exhibit impaired water balance (Handelmann, unpublished data).

Substance P

Substance P (SP) is a peptide with a wide distribution in the nervous system (see Jessell, 1983, for review) and several well-characterized physiological actions. SP appears to act as a neurotransmitter in the sensory afferents of the spinal cord, specifically the nociceptive afferents. SP is localized in neuronal cell bodies in spinal sensory ganglia which make synapses in the dorsal horn (Hökfelt et al., 1975). The peptide appears to be most potent in exciting spinal neurons which respond to noxious stimuli (Henry, 1976; Randic and Miletic, 1977). Injected into the spinal cord, SP produces behaviors indicative of sensation, such as scratching and biting (Hylden and Wilcox, 1980; Seybold et al., 1982). In addition,

SP and SP receptors are contained in brain regions thought to play a role in modulation of pain perception, such as the periaqueductal grey, dorsal raphe and locus coeruleus (Hökfelt et al., 1977; Jessell, 1982; Quirion et al., 1983). SP is also contained in nerves supplying the salivary glands, and acts directly to produce salivation (Chang and Leeman, 1970; Ekstrom and Wahlestedt, 1982). Finally, SP injected intravenously causes vasodilation (Bury and Mashford, 1977; Chahl and Walker, 1981).

In our experiments, neonatal rat pups were injected with SP (1 μg/pup/day) during the first week after birth. When the rats were mature, their sensitivity to mildly painful thermal stimulation was measured, using the conventional 'paw-lick' test. In addition, their sialogogic and cardiovascular responses to intravenous SP were measured.

Pain perception was altered in the rats treated as neonates with SP. The rats were more sensitive to the cutaneous stimulation than were the controls, especially when they had previous experience with the test situation (Fig. 2; Handel-

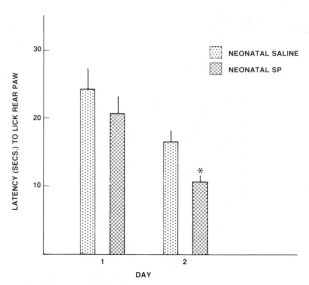

Fig. 2 Pain threshold of adult rats as measured by their latency to lick their rear paws when placed on a surface warmed to 50 °C. As neonates, the rats were treated with either substance P (1 mg/pup/day) or saline on days 1–7 after birth. * Significantly different from the neonatal saline group ($P < 0.05$, Student's t-test). (Modified from Handelmann et al., 1984).

capacity for SP than the controls, although the affinity of the binding sites for SP was unchanged (Fig. 3; Handelmann et al., 1987). Various brain regions also showed increased SP binding on autoradiographic analysis (Table 1; Handelmann et al., 1987), although the distribution of SP binding was not altered. Hindbrain regions which play a role in pain perception, such as the locus coeruleus and dorsal raphe, were affected by the treatment, while spinal cord was not. This is of particular interest, considering that the rats were most hyperalgesic after repeated exposure to the cutaneous stimulation, suggesting a role of central processing of the sensory information.

In summary, neonatal exposure to SP produced long-lasting effects on adult expression of SP receptors, which was correlated with increased sensitivity to SP and behavioral changes. Again the developmental influence was selective, as not all tissue containing SP receptors was affected.

Enkephalin and morphine

Opioid peptides, particularly those that interact with the mu subclass of opiate receptors, are known to play a role in pain perception. Administration of peptides or other compounds which bind to the mu receptors, such as morphine, elicit analgesia. Opioid peptide pathways and mu receptors are located in the dorsal horn of the spinal cord (Hokfelt et al., 1977; Lamotte et al., 1976), and in brain regions associated with pain perception. They are distributed in other brain regions as well, particularly those related to motor function (Herkenham and Pert, 1982).

In our experiments, neonatal albino rats were injected either with the peptide [met]enkephalin or with morphine (1 μg/pup/day) on days 1–7 after birth. When the rats were fully mature, their pain sensitivity was measured, again using the 'paw-lick' test. In addition, the motor development and adult motor behavior was assessed in the rats treated as neonates with morphine.

Rats injected as neonates with either [met]-

mann et al., 1984). These rats may therefore become more rapidly sensitized to pain or to situations in which they receive aversive stimulation. These rats' also salivated more in response to SP, suggesting that their salivary glands were more sensitive to the effects of SP than those of the control rats. Their cardiovascular responses to SP were unaltered (Handelmann et al., 1984).

These results indicated long-term effects of SP on the development of SP pathways. The fact that the SP-treated rats' salivary glands had become more sensitive to injected SP suggested a possible alteration in SP receptors in the glands. Similarly, the increase in pain sensitivity suggested that the transmission of sensory information was more efficient in these rats; they might have become more sensitive to endogenously released SP after sensory stimulation. Consequently, we measured SP binding to tissue from salivary glands, brain and spinal cord.

Salivary gland membranes from the rats treated as neonates with SP had a greater binding

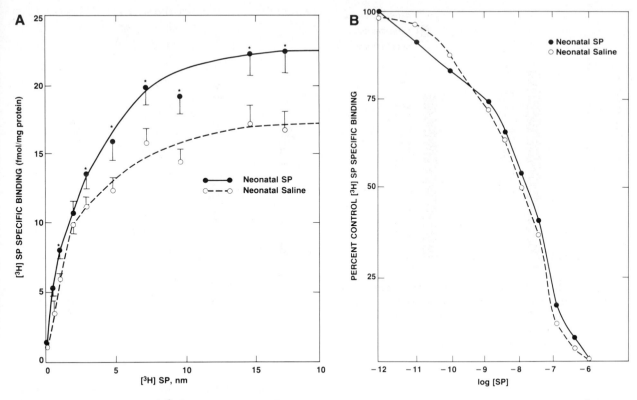

Fig. 3 (A) Specific binding of [³H]substance P to salivary gland membranes from adult rats. (B) Displacement of [³H]substance P binding from salivary gland membranes by unlabelled substance P, indicating that the affinity of the substance P binding is similar in the two groups (Modified from Handelmann et al., 1987).

TABLE 1

Autoradiographic measurement of substance P receptors in adult rat brain

Brain region	Optical density		
	Neonatal saline	Neonatal SP	% increase
Central grey	0.74 ± 0.01	0.83 ± 0.02	13
Dorsal raphe	0.81 ± 0.05	1.06 ± 0.03	31
Septo-fimbrial n.	0.44 ± 0.02	0.66 ± 0.02	50
Locus coeruleus	0.73 ± 0.04	1.10 ± 0.07	50
Dorsal tegmental n.	0.38 ± 0.02	0.59 ± 0.02	55
Hypoglossal n.	0.29 ± 0.02	0.50 ± 0.05	72

Pups were injected subcutaneously with either saline or SP (1 mg/pup) each day on postnatal days 1–7. From Handelmann et al. (1987).

enkephalin or morphine were less sensitive to cutaneous thermal stimulation than were saline-treated controls (Fig. 4). The difference was apparent on every test in the 'paw-lick' procedure, suggesting an elevation of their pain threshold. Similar effects on adult pain tolerance have been shown with perinatal administration of beta-endorphin (Sandman et al., 1979) and methadone (Zagon and McLaughlin, 1980). In addition, the rats injected with morphine showed a retarded rate of development of several motor reflexes (Handelmann and Dow-Edwards, 1985). As adults they had impaired motor coordination, as indicated by their ability to balance on a rotor-rod, and an unusual gait: their stride was longer and they tended to walk with their feet turned outward (Fig. 5; Handelmann and Dow-Edwards, 1985).

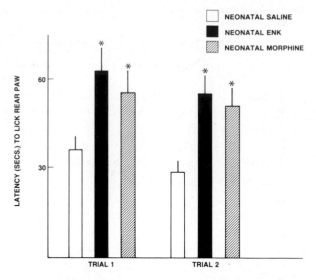

Fig. 4 Pain threshold of adult rats as measured by their latency to lick their rear paws when placed on a surface warmed to 50°C. Rats were treated on days 1–7 after birth with [met]enkephalin or morphine (1 mg/pup daily s.c.) or saline. *Significantly different from the neonatal saline group ($P < 0.05$, Student's test).

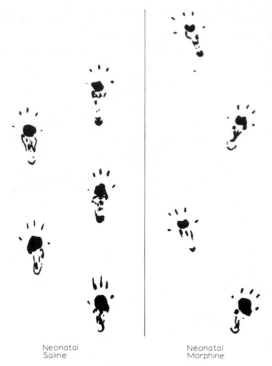

Fig. 5 Tracings of footprints of adult rats walking in a straight alley. The rats treated as neonates with morphine had greater stride lengths than the controls, and walked with their feet turned at an angle to the direction of the track.

Such alterations in behaviors in which the opioid peptides are known to play a role again suggested possible alterations in the function of opioid pathways. Mu and delta opiate receptors were measured in the brains of the morphine-treated rats by autoradiography when they were 180–360 days old. Increases in mu opiate binding, as measured with [³H]naloxone, were observed in the striatum and nucleus accumbens, structures known to be involved in motor function. No changes in delta opioid binding were observed in any brain region, suggesting a selective effect of the neonatal morphine treatment (Handelmann and Quirion, 1983). Because opiates inhibit neural activity in the striatum (Bradley and Brooks, 1984), we predicted that the increased number of opiate receptors might lead to a diminished basal level of activity in this area and, as a result, in other related brain areas, such as motor cortex. We measured metabolic activity, as indicated by local cerebral glucose utilization, in various brain regions of rats treated as neonates

with morphine. Significant reductions in the rate of glucose utilization were found in several motor areas, including the striatum, and also in several areas involved in pain perception, particularly the posterior and dorsomedial thalamic nuclei (Table 2; Handelmann and Dow-Edwards, 1985). This suggests that the alteration in opiate receptors results in decreased functional activity. As the stratium is important in motor coordination, changes in activity in this region may underlie the changes in coordination and gait in the morphine-treated rats. Similarly, the increased pain threshold exhibited by these rats may be due to altered functional activity in the thalamic nuclei responsible for the transmission of painful stimulation to the cortex.

In summary, neonatal opiate treatment had long-lasting effects on the expression of mu opiate

TABLE 2

Brain regions with altered rates of glucose utilization following neonatal morphine treatment

	Neonatal saline	Neonatal morphine
Motor areas		
Caudate-putamen	77 ± 2	53 ± 4
Globus pallidus	39 ± 3	29 ± 5
Motor cortex	68 ± 7	52 ± 4
Paramedian n.	44 ± 4	22 ± 3
Pain areas		
Posterior thalamus	76 ± 2	60 ± 4
Dorsomedial thalamus	84 ± 9	42 ± 5
Somatosensory cortex	72 ± 6	60 ± 2
Limbic areas		
Anteroventral thalamus	90 ± 2	74 ± 2
Lateral septum	42 ± 2	36 ± 1
Medial mammillary n.	83 ± 7	71 ± 2

Results are given as μmol/100 g/min; means ± S.E.M. significantly different at $P < 0.05$, Student's t-test. Modified from Handelmann and Dow-Edwards (1985).

receptors in rat brain, and also produced retarded motor development and later motor impairments, as well as altered pain sensitivity. The treatment led to decreased metabolic activity in brain regions in which receptors were elevated and in related areas.

Discussion

This series of experiments demonstrates that early exposure to neuropeptides has a long-term influence on the expression of neuropeptide receptors in the adult. This action occurs independently of changes in organ weight or neuropeptide content of the tissue. The developmental influence appears to be specific to receptors for the peptide or ligand administered. The change in receptor number is of physiological and behavioral significance for the animal (Table 3).

The neonatal peptide treatments had no effect on the distribution of peptide receptors, suggesting that only areas which would normally express the receptors are influenced. Within an area, however, it is not known whether the peptide acts to alter the number of cells expressing the receptors, or to alter the number of receptors expressed by each cell. The results of future experiments will allow us to decide between these two alternatives, and, hopefully, will suggest possible mechanisms by which peptides produce their long-term effects.

The effect on receptor number can be either an increase or decrease. The reason for the particular direction of change is unclear. It may have to do with the function of the peptide, the type of tissue (e.g. brain vs. kidney), or with the developmental stage of the tissue when the peptide is administered. In adults, up- or down-regulation of receptors

TABLE 3

Survey of effects of neonatal administration of three neuropeptides

	VP	SP	Opiates/opioid peptides
Behavioral and physiological changes	↓ urine concentration	↑ rate of sensitization to pain	↑ pain threshold, motor impairment
Sensitivity of target organs to peptide	↓ in kidney	↑ in salivary glands	
Change in receptor number	↓ in kidney	↑ in brain, salivary gland	↑ mu receptors in brain
Change in cyclic nucleotide formation	↓ in cAMP formation in kidney		

often occurs after changes in neurotransmitter or hormone levels (for reviews see Catt et al. 1979; Lesniak and Roth, 1976). The changes in receptor number are transient, however; when the ligand levels return to normal, so do receptor concentrations. The developmental influences on receptor number described here, however, persist well into adulthood, and probably for the life of the animal. Therefore, while it may be a phenomenon related to adult receptor regulation, the developmental regulation is likely to occur through a different mechanism, and direct comparison is not appropriate.

In our experiments, we have added neuropeptides to developing systems at a time when they are ordinarily exposed to such chemical influences. Do neuropeptides, released endogenously, normally play a role in development? It is possible that the amount of a neuropeptide present in the system during development might be an important clue to the developing system concerning the chemical environment in which it will eventually function. As such, regulation of receptor number at this stage by neuropeptides might be important in ensuring that the target tissue makes appropriate responses to the peptide during normal physiological events. In this way, the unique variations in the amount of a particular neuropeptide to which a young animal is exposed may lead to individual differences in any number of characteristics, such as the differences in pain threshold exhibited by rats in our experiments.

·The importance of such a regulatory mechanism in humans is apparent when it is considered that there are many situations in which a fetus or infant may be exposed to abnormal amounts of a neuropeptide. Neuropeptide levels are influenced by a large number of physiological and pharmacological events, and numerous drugs act by binding to neuropeptide receptors. For example, the use of opiate drugs by pregnant and nursing women is quite common, and children born to mothers who used heroin or methadone during pregnancy have been shown to have motor impairments. They perform poorly on perceptual-

motor tasks (Ramer and Lodge, 1975; Wilson et al., 1973, 1979), have poor fine-motor coordination (Wilson et al., 1981), and begin walking later than matched control children (Strauss et al., 1976). These findings suggest that exposure of children to opiates affects development of motor regions of the brain, by a mechanism similar to those we have found in rats. There are also conditions which produce high levels of VP which can be passed from a mother to her offspring. Inappropriate secretion of VP can be associated with tumors, hemorrhage and neurological, pulmonary and endocrine diseases (Bartter, 1977). In addition, a number of therapeutic drugs cause VP release, including analgesics, diuretics and tricyclic compounds (Bartter, 1977), and cigarette-smoking is a potent releaser of VP, through inhalation of nicotine (Husain et al., 1974; Seyler et al., 1986). These conditions might also produce deleterious effects on fetal or infant development.

There is evidence to suggest that other neuropeptides may have similar long-term effects on neural development. For example, neonatal treatment with MSH or ACTH had long-term effects on rats' performance of learning tasks (Beckwith et al., 1977; Champney et al., 1976; McGivern et al., 1987), which might result from altered expression of these neuropeptide receptors. In addition, other classes of neurotransmitters may play a similar role in regulating the developmental expression of their receptors (see Miller and Friedhoff, Chapter 31, and Kellogg, Chapter 14 of this volume). The results of future studies must determine whether all neurotransmitters act to regulate the development of their receptor systems. In particular, physiological and pharmacological conditions which alter neurotransmitters in pregnant or postpartum mothers, or in their children, need to be examined. In addition to conditions which radically alter the developing child's chemical environment, subtle environmental stimuli could alter the secretion of neurotransmitters and thereby produce physiological and behavioral differences between individuals which would form the basis of normal physiological and pathophysiological variations within a population.

References

Bartter, F.C. (1977) The syndromes of inappropriate secretion of antidiuretic hormones (SIADH). In A.B. Schwartz and H. Lyons (Eds.), *Acid-Base and Electrolyte Balance*, Grune and Stratton, New York.

Beckwith, B.E., Sandman, C.A., Hothersall, D. and Kastin, A.J. (1977) Influence of neonatal injections of alpha-MSH on learning, memory, and attention in rats. *Physiol. Behav.*, 18: 63–71.

Bermant, G. and Davison, J.M. (1974) *Biological Bases of Sexual Behavior*, Harper and Row, New York.

Boer, G.J., Kragten, R., Kruisbrink, J. and Swaab, D.F. (1984) Vasopressin fails to restore postnatally the stunted brain development in the Brattleboro rat, but affects water metabolism permanently. *Neurobehav. Toxicol. Teratol.*, 6: 102–109.

Bradley, P.B. and Brooks, A. (1984) A microiontophoretic study of the actions of mu, delta, and kappa opiate receptor agonists in the rat brain. *Br. J. Pharmacol.*, 83: 763–772.

Bury, R.W. and Mashford, M.C. (1977) Cardiovascular effects of synthetic substance P in several species. *Eur. J. Pharmacol.*, 45: 335–340.

Catt, K.J., Harwood, J.P., Aguilera, G. and Dufau, M.L. (1979) Hormonal regulation of peptide receptor and target cell responses. *Nature*, 280: 109–116.

Chahl, L.A. and Walker, S.B. (1981) Responses of the rat cardiovascular system to substance P, neurotensin, and bombesin. *Life Sci.*, 29; 2009–2015.

Champney, T.F., Sahley, T.L. and Sandman, C.A. (1976) Effects of neonatal cerebral ventricular injection of ACTH 1–9 and subsequent adult injections on learning in male and female albine rats. *Pharmacol. Biochem. Behav. 5, Suppl. 1*: 3–9.

Chang, M.M. and Leeman, S.E. (1970) Isolation of a sialogogic peptide from bovine hypothalamic tissue and its characterization as substance P. *J. Biol. Chem.*, 245: 4784–4790.

Eayres, J.T. and Holmes, R.L. (1964) Effect of neonatal hyperthyroidism on pituitary structure and function in the rat. *J. Endocrinol.*, 29: 71–81.

Ekstrom, J. and Wahlestedt, C. (1982) Supersensitivity to substance P and physalaemin in rat salivary glands after denervation or decentralization. *Acta Physiol. Scand.*, 115: 437–446.

Handelmann, G.E. and Dow-Edwards, D. (1985) Modulation of brain development by morphine: effects on central motor systems and behavior. *Peptides*, 6, Suppl. 2: 29–34.

Handelmann, G.E. and Quirion, R. (1983) Neonatal exposure to morphine increases opiate binding in the adult forebrain. *Eur. J. Pharmacol.*, 94: 357–358.

Handelmann, G.E. and Sayson, S.C. (1984) Neonatal exposure to vasopressin decreases vasopressin binding sites in the adult kidney. *Peptides*, 5: 1217–1219.

Handelmann, G.E., Russell, J.T., Gainer, H., Zerbe, R. and Bayorh, M. (1983) Vasopressin administration to neonatal rats reduces antidiuretic response in adult kidneys. *Peptides*, 4: 827–832.

Handelmann, G.E., Selsky, J.H. and Helke, C.J. (1984) Substance P administration to neonatal rats increases adult sensitivity to substance P. *Phys. Behav.*, 33: 297–300.

Handelmann, G.E., Shults, C.W. and O'Donohue, T.L. (1987) A developmental influence of substance P on its receptor. *Int. J. Dev. Neurosci.*, 5: 11–16.

Henry, J.L. (1976) Effects of substance P on functionally identified units in cat spinal cord. *Brain Res.*, 114: 439–451.

Herkenham, M. and Pert, C.B. (1982) Light microscopic localization of brain opiate receptors: a general autoradiographic method which preserves tissue quality. *J. Neurosci.*, 2: 1129–1143.

Hökfelt, T., Kellerth, J.-O., Nilsson, G. and Pernow, B. (1975) Substance P: localization in the central nervous system and in some primary sensory neurons. *Science*, 190: 889–890.

Hökfelt, T., Ljungdahl, A., Terenius, L., Elde, R. and Nilsson, G. (1977) Immunohistochemical analysis of peptide pathways possibly related to pain and analgesia: enkephalin and substance P. *Proc. Natl. Acad. Sci. USA*, 74: 3081–3085.

Husain, M.K., Frantz, A.G., Ciarochi, F. and Robinson, A.G. (1975) Nicotine-stimulated release of neurophysin and vasopressin in humans. *J. Clin. Endocrinol. Metab.*, 41: 1113–1117.

Hylden, J.L.K. and Wilcox, G.L. (1980) Intrathecal morphine and substance P in mice: pain and analgesia. *Fed. Proc.*, 39: 761.

Jessell, T.M. (1982) Pain. *Lancet*, ii: 1084–1088.

Jessell, T.M. (1983) Substance P in the nervous system. In L.L. Iversen, S.D. Iversen and S.H. Snyder (Eds.), *Handbook of Psychopharmacology, Vol. 16*, Plenum, New York, pp. 1–105.

Lamotte, C., Pert, C. and Snyder, S.H. (1976) Opiate receptor binding in primate spinal cord: distribution and changes after dorsal root section. *Brain Res.*, 112: 407–412.

Lesniak, M.A., and Roth, J. (1976) Regulation of receptor concentration by homologous hormones. *J. Biol. Chem.*, 251: 3720–3729.

McGivern, R.F., Rose, G., Berka, C., Clancy, A.N. and Sandman, C.A. (1987) Neonatal exposure to a high level of ACTH 4–10 impairs adult learning performance. *Pharmacol. Biochem. Behav.*, 27: 133–142.

Moratella, R., Borrell, J., Sanchez-Franco, F. and Del Rio,

J. (1987) Neonatal administration of vasopressin anti-serum induces long-term deficits on active and passive avoidance behavior in rats. *Behav. Brain Res.*, 23: 231–237.

Quirion, R., Shults, C.W., Moody, T.W., Pert, C.B., Chase, T.N. and O'Donohue, T.L. (1983) Autoradiographic distribution of substance P receptors in rat central nervous system. *Nature*, 303: 714–716.

Ramer, C.M. and Lodge, A. (1975) Neonatal addiction: a two-year study. Part I. Clinical and developmental characteristics of infants of mothers on methadone maintenance. *Addict. Dis.*, 2: 227–234.

Randic, M. and Miletic, V. (1977) Effect of substance P on cat dorsal horn neurons activated by noxious stimuli. *Brain Res.*, 128: 164–169.

Sandman, C.A., McGivern, R.F., Berka, C., Walker, J.M., Coy, D.H. and Kastin, A.J. (1979) Neonatal administration of beta-endorphin produces 'chronic' insensitivity to thermal stimuli. *Life Sci.*, 25: 1755–1760.

Sawyer, W.H., Grzonka, Z. and Manning, M. (1981) Neurohypophysial peptides. Design of tissue-specific agonists and antagonists. *Mol. Cell. Endocrinol.*, 22: 117–134.

Seybold, V.S., Hylden, J.L.K. and Wilcox, G.L. (1982) Intrathecal substance P and somatostatin in rats: behaviors indicative of sensation. *Peptides*, 3: 49–54.

Seyler, L.E., Pomerleau, O.F., Fertig, J.B., Hunt, D. and Parker, K. (1986) Pituitary hormone response to cigarette smoking. *Pharmacol. Biochem. Behav.*, 24: 159–162.

Snijdewint, F.G.M. and Boer, G.J. (1987) Neonatal treatment of Wistar rats with vasopressin-antagonist dP[Tyr(Me)²]AVP inhibits body and brain development and induces diabetes insipidus. *Neurobehav. Toxicol. Teratol.*, 8: 213–217.

Strauss, M.E., Starr, R.H., Ostera, E.M., Chavez, C.J. and Stryker, J.C. (1976) Behavioral concomitants of prenatal addiction to narcotics. *J. Pediat.*, 89: 842–846.

Van Wimersma Greidanus, T.B., Van Ree, J.M. and DeWeid, D. (1983) Vasopressin and memory. *Pharmacol. Ther.*, 20: 437–458.

Wilson, G.S., Desmond, M.M. and Verniaud, W.M. (1973) Early development of infants of heroin-addicted mothers. *Am. J. Dis. Child.*, 126: 457–462.

Wilson, G.S., McCreary, R., Kean, J. and Baxter, J.C. (1979) The development of preschool children of heroin-addicted mothers: a controlled study. *Pediatrics*, 63: 135–141.

Wilson, G.S., Desmond, M.M. and Wait, R.B. (1981) Follow-up of methadone-treated and untreated narcotics-dependent women and their infants: health, developmental, and social implication. *J. Pediat.*, 98: 716–722.

Wright, W.A. and Kutscher, C.L. (1977) Vasopressin administration in the first month of life: effects on growth and water metabolism in hypothalamic diabetes insipidus rats. *Pharmacol. Biochem. Behav.*, 6: 505–509.

Zagon, I.S. and McLaughlin, P.J. (1980) Protracted analgesia in young and adult rats maternally exposed to methadone. *Experientia*, 36: 329–330.

Discussion

C.K. Kellogg: Evidence has been reported indicating that the particular peptide characteristic of neurons may be influenced by the environment of those neurons during development. Do you have any evidence that altering the neural environment pharmacologically during development may influence the peptidergic characteristic of neurons?

G.E. Handelmann: We have no evidence to suggest that the neonatal peptide treatments influence the peptidergic phenotype of neurons.

J.W. Olney: I would like to compliment you on this very elegant series of studies. Is anything known about the developmental period when peptides can penetrate blood-brain barriers and enter brain in the human?

G.E. Handelmann: The timing of maturation of the human blood-brain barrier is a controversial issue at present. The best evidence, however, indicates that levels of plasma proteins are high in CSF during the perinatal period, and that adult levels are reached after six months of age (Adinolfo, 1985). This would suggest that the CNS is accessible to peptides during both pre- and postnatal development in humans.

G.J. Boer: You have found lasting effects of early vasopressin (VP) exposure on kidney receptor setting and we and others have reported this for the Brattleboro rat strain too (Wright and Kutscher, 1977; Boer et al., 1984). However, in our recent studies with Wistar rats we failed to see this induction of polyurea with early treatment of 10 μg VP per day for the first 2 weeks (Snijdewint and Boer, 1988). What do you think can be an explanation for these discrepancies in outcome?

G.E. Handelmann: We do not yet understand all of the variables which are important to this phenomenon. Without reviewing your procedures, it is difficult to pinpoint what the critical differences might be. The previous studies, however, were performed using Osborn-Mendel, Sprague-Dawley or Brattleboro rats. Perhaps there is some difference in the process of kidney maturation in the Wistar rats which causes them to respond differently from the other strains.

T.A. Slotkin: Physiological responses to receptor stimulation can occur with very few receptor sites (assessed by binding). We have found a good urine-concentrating response to DDAVP prior to day 7. Could you comment on this?

G.E. Handelmann: The kidney does appear to be responsive to VP during the early neonatal period. Our hypothesis is that the concentration of VP during this period acts to determine an appropriate number of VP receptors to be expressed in the tissue, but probably does not play a role in the initial appearance of the receptors. An interesting question related to this issue is whether the receptor regulation is mediated simply by the ligand binding to the receptor, or whether the physiological consequences of the binding are required. If the latter is the case, then the time of the appearance of the receptors would be less important to the regulation than the timing of the receptor coupling to second messengers, etc.

W. Lichtensteiger: You showed that neonatal treatment with a peptide (i.e., the agonist) resulted in an increased number of substance P and naloxone binding sites, but decreased the number of VP sites. Do you think that this is due to the difference in the tissue analysed (VP sites in the kidney, the others in the brain) or to a different principle of regulation?
G. E. Handelmann: It is possible that the direction of the effect on receptor number is related to the type or function of the tissue (e.g. kidney vs. brain), to the pharmacology of the receptor, or to the maturational stage of the tissue at the time of the peptide administration. There is not enough evidence at present to choose among these alternatives, although this is a central issue which needs to be resolved.

References

Adinolfo, M. (1985) The development of the human blood-CSF-brain barrier. *Dev. Med. Child Neurol.*, 27: 532–537.

Boer, G.J., Kragten, R., Kruisbrink, J. and Swaab, D.F. (1984) Vasopressin fails to restore postnatally the stunted brain development in the Brattleboro rat, but affects water metabolism permanently. *Neurobehav. Toxicol. Teratol.*, 6: 103–109.

Schultberg, M., Foster, G.A., Gage, F.H., Björklund, A. and Hökfelt, T. (1986) Coexistence during ontogeny and transplantation. In T. Hökfelt, K. Fuxe and B. Pernow (Eds.) *Coexistence of Neuronal Messengers – A New Principle in Chemical Transmission, Progress in Brain Research, Vol. 68*, Elsevier, Amsterdam, pp. 129–145.

Snijdewint, F.G.M. and Boer, G.J. (1988) Neonatal treatment with vasopressin-antagonist dP[Tyr(Me)^2]AVP, but not with vasopressin antagonist d(CH$_2$)$_5$[Tyr(Me)^2]AVP, inhibits body and brain development and induces polyuria in the rat. *Neurotoxicol. Teratol.*, submitted.

Wright, W.A. and Kutscher, C.L. (1977) Vasopressin administration in the first month of life: effects on growth and water metabolism in hypothalamic diabetes insipidus rats. *Pharmacol. Biochem. Behav.*, 6: 505–509.

G.J. Boer, M.G.P. Feenstra, M. Mirmiran, D.F. Swaab and F. Van Haaren
Progress in Brain Research, Vol. 73
© 1988 Elsevier Science Publishers B.V. (Biomedical Division)

CHAPTER 33

Transgenerational effects of drug and hormonal treatments in mammals: a review of observations and ideas

John H. Campbell and Penny Perkins

Department of Anatomy, School of Medicine, University of California, Los Angeles, CA 90024, USA

Introduction

The consequences of disturbing neuroendocrine systems of young developing animals persist for various lengths of time. Short-term acute effects are the easiest to study. However, changes which outlast the presence of an injected drug or altered hormone level are no less important. A teratogen acting in utero can damage an animal for life. Even more enduring changes carry over from a stressed animal to its offspring. Insults to a female which perturb her progeny are well known. These 'maternal effects' present little problem for the imagination although those resulting from treatments made very early in the mother's life imply some lasting deficits in her reproductive functions. More unexpected are effects which continue to grandoffspring and great-grandoffspring of treated animals.

This article is concerned with disturbances to several neuroendocrine systems of young animals having the following remarkable combination of consequences:
1. Experimentally treating a young animal induces characteristic abnormalities which persist into adulthood.
2. Crossing treated males to normal females gives offspring with altered phenotype.
3. Abnormalities carry over to multiple generations (usually demonstrated in F2 progeny of treated females).
4. Some of the transmitted alterations coincide with known functions of the perturbed neuroendocrine system or with the changes that the treatment induced in the parent animal.

Transgenerational effects of hormone or drug exposure lie at the intersection of genetics and physiology and have different meanings for the two disciplines. Endocrinologists are interested in their physiological significance for the individual neuroendocrine system or for neuroendocrine systems in general. They design studies to describe the transmitted alterations. The geneticist is troubled by their contradiction of the long-standing, basic principles of Mendelian inheritance. Transgenerational effects are suggestive of Lamarckian inheritance or the transmission of acquired characteristics from parent to offspring. The geneticist's overriding concern is whether a study proves the heresy to be real, and if so, what new genetic mechanisms must be acknowledged. Physiological descriptions of the transmitted condition, for him, are secondary. Unfortunately, designing a study toward one of these objectives often weakens it for the other.

In order to include both perspectives we will describe some of the more notable induced carry-over effects, discuss the technical problems for their genetic verification and review the possible mechanisms which underlie them.

Terminology

Two special notations will be used to avoid certain ambiguities in the literature. Physiologists have counted generations of animals from various starting points. When a pregnant animal is injected with a drug her offspring have been called the 'F0', 'F1' and even 'second' generation. In this paper the animals exposed to the experimental conditions in utero are the starting generation. Their progeny, the grandoffspring of the original pregnant animal, constitute the F1 generation. We will designate them F*1 to emphasize this counting scheme which differs from the usage in some of the original reports. Offspring of the F*1 individuals are F*2. If a male animal is treated and subsequently bred, or if a female is treated *before* mating, it will be described as F0 and its offspring will be of the F*1 generation. The important fact to emphasize is that F*1 animals were not conceived at the time of treatment, although their gametes or gamete progenitors were extant.

Offspring of treated animals have been bred mainly by two regimes. Crossing female descendants of treated animals with normal males for repeated generations will be called *outcrossing* and generate a *maternal line*. In contrast, breeding experimental line males and females together at each generation will be *incrossing*. The main difference between the two regimes is that only one parent can transmit the acquired trait in the former while both can contribute the altered influence in the latter. Also, outcrossing dilutes the original genetic heritage from the treated parent at each generation.

Examples of transgenerational effects

We begin this section of examples with a caveat. Each case reviewed is substantially more complex than its brief description here. The interested

reader should consult the original cited articles for further details and interpretations.

Thyroid

Thyroid hormones play key roles in both development and adult metabolism. Injecting a single dose of thyroxine into newborn rats will permanently depress the circulating levels of that hormone and of thyroid stimulating hormone (TSH) (Bakke and Lawrence, 1966; Gellert et al., 1971). Moreover, if neonatally treated female rats are bred their F*1 and F*2 descendants will also have low TSH levels, as well as other alterations.

Removing the thyroid glands of a pregnant rat also alters the control of TSH for multiple outcrossed maternal generations (Bakke et al., 1975; Fujii et al., 1985). Undisturbed levels of TSH are normal in F*1, F*2 and F*3 animals but their response to injections of TSH-releasing hormone or to removal of the thyroid is muted.

In experiments originally intended as controls, Bakke et al. (1975) removed the thyroids of male rats prior to mating with normal females. Unexpectedly, their F*1 progeny had enlarged pituitaries and thyroids, lowered TSH levels (although the drop did not reach statistical significance in their data) and significant changes in various other developmental, physiological and morphological characteristics of one sex or the other.

Thyroxine levels are stabilized in a complex way by feedback loops between the thyroid, pituitary and hypothalamus. These controls have been called the 'thyrostat', as an analogy with a thermostat for maintaining constant temperature. Bakke et al. (1975) propose that the set point of an animal's thyrostat is established during a critical perinatal period on the basis of the prevailing hormonal environment. This setting then persists for the life of the animal. From this model they suggest that their experimental animals transmitted altered thyrostat settings to subsequent generations. Physically, these settings might correspond to the numbers of receptors for TRH on the thyrotroph cells of the pituitary.

Insulin

The etiology of insulin diseases is complex and confused. Offspring of female diabetics are born with enlarged islets of Langerhans and increased incidents of macrosomia and congenital deformities (Jackson, 1960; Neel, 1962). Diabetes also interferes with male gametogenesis (Oksanen, 1975) and there are poorly supported suggestions that it affects offspring of men (Jackson, 1954; but see Rubin, 1958). At least nine groups of workers have treated animals with diabetogenic drugs, such as alloxan, and examined their descendants. All except for Gept (1965) have reported transgenerational effects of one kind or another to persist for the duration of their studies (Bartelheimer and Kloos, 1952; Baranov and Sokoloverova, 1966; Okamoto, 1965; Ohno, 1969; Foglia et al., 1970; Spergel et al., 1971; Aerts and Van Assche, 1977; Milner and Sheffrin, 1982).

In the first long-term study, Okamoto (1965) chemically destroyed the beta cells of male and female rats, guinea pigs and rabbits one month before mating. The F*1 progeny developed fewer beta cells per islet. Pituitaries and adrenals also were histologically affected. Some of the offspring in turn were injected with alloxan and the deficiency was exaggerated further in the next generation. The progressive cell decrease from this experimental regime eventually led to overt

TABLE 1

Condition of beta cells and incidence of diabetes in descendents of serially diabetized Wistar rats

	Pancreatic beta cells			Number of animals	
	No. of cases	Beta cells per islet	Cell size (μm)	Examined	With diabetes
Normal controls					
	33	66.3	110.3	30	0
Both parents with alloxan diabetes					
F1	13	48.3	107.0	28	0
F2	4	33.4	100.4	5	0
F3	3	24.6	94.9	5	0
F4	1	20.8	91.8	8	0[a]
F5	1	17.9	89.1	14	12 severe[b] 2 mild[c]
Fathers with alloxan diabetes crossed with normal females					
F1	25	58.5	107.7	22	0
F2	4	53.2	101.9	16	0
F3	4	44.7	94.2	7	0
F4	4	37.6	91.9	9	0
F5	4	29.4	80.7	11	0
F6	4	20.8	85.2	17	0[a]
F7	4	16.6	79.3	20	17 severe[b] 3 mild[c]

From the data of Okamoto (1965).
[a] Sometimes slight and intermittent.
[b] Severe or persistent.
[c] Intermediate or transient.

diabetes without drug treatment (see Table 1). Diabetes erupted among F*5 animals when both mothers and fathers were injected at each generation and in the F*7 generation if only males were treated. Ohno (1969) confirmed these findings in a smaller parallel study and Foglia et al. (1970) found that surgically removing the pancreases of six generations of female rats produced glucose intolerance in the seventh generation.

Spergel et al. (1971, 1975) and Goldner and Spergel (1972) used a simpler paradigm in a study involving one thousand rats. They injected subdiabetogenic doses of alloxan into one generation of preweanling rats and mated the animals among themselves and to normal controls. The progeny from treated males mated with normal females statistically were less glucose-tolerant than normal, as were those from exposed females crossed with normal males. The F*1 animals were pooled and incrossed for six more generations without further treatment. Glucose tolerance progressively deteriorated. By the fifth generation some rats were overtly diabetic and the others were unusually sensitive to administered alloxan.

Morphine

Morphine stimulates endorphin receptors involved in a diversity of neural, hormonal, immunological and developmental functions. Injecting narcotics into neonatal rats slows development and leads to permanent defects in nervous system structures, behavior and responses to hormonal stresses (Smith et al., 1977; Glick et al., 1977; Sonderegger and Zimmermann, 1978; Sonderegger et al., 1979a)

These same types of abnormality also appear among the F*1 offspring (Smith and Joffe, 1973; Joffe et al., 1978; Friedler, 1974, 1978; Friedler and Cochin, 1972; Friedler and Wheeling, 1979; Sonderegger et al., 1979b; Zimmermann and Sonderegger, 1980). Fig. 1 compares two 7-day-old offspring of a morphine-treated male inbred mouse with an age-matched control from our laboratory. The two F*1 pups weighed half as much as normal and obviously were behind in

their development. Such carryover effects are highly sporadic, however, and vary markedly in degree from one litter or individual to another.

Zimmermann and Sonderegger (1980) found that most progeny of neonatally narcotized female rats grew abnormally slowly. The rats eventually caught up with controls in size but retained a higher tolerance to pain, a characteristic that mimics direct exposure to morphine. A few F*1 progeny had permanent extreme deficiencies. They were smaller, lacked pain sensation and maintained their hind limbs tonically in full extension. Two such females successfully conceived but delivered their F*2 pups stillborn over a two-day-period.

Parathyroid

The parathyroid is a key regulator of calcium ion levels in the blood, acting on kidneys, bone and other organs. Fujii (1978) removed the glands from pregnant rats on day 5 of gestation and incrossed the resulting offspring. Blood calcium levels were significantly depressed for at least four generations and responded substantially less

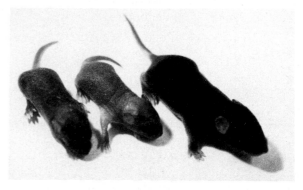

Fig. 1 Delayed growth of the F1 offspring of a male mouse treated neonatally with morphine. The two pups on the left were sired by an inbred C57BL/6 male mouse which had been injected twice daily for 21 days after birth with increasing amounts of morphine to a final dosage of 8 mg/kg body weight. The father of the control on the right was injected with saline. The two male parents were bred with normal C57BL/6 females on the same day and the pups were photographed 7 days after birth.

when the parathyroids were removed from these animals. Also, F*2 rats were killed by smaller quantities of intravenous calcium chloride than controls ($LD_{50} \approx 26$ mg/kg vs. ≈ 33 mg/kg for normals; Fujii et al., 1980). By the seventh incrossed generation, blood calcium levels had reverted to normal but gonadal alterations remained (Fujii and Yamamoto, 1983). The ovaries senesced late in aged F*7–9 females and testosterone levels declined less with age in the males.

Few effects of parathyroid stress have been shown to pass through the male line. F*3 males of Fujii's incrossed parathyroidectomized line sired apparently normal progeny with control females (Fujii and Morita, 1978). Unfortunately, the reciprocal *outcross* of F*3 females to control males was not reported for comparison. Also, Fujii and Morita (1978) saw no transgenerational consequences of removing the parathyroids from adult male rats, possibly because the animals become aspermic within three months. However, grafting extra parathyroid glands onto adult male rats did affect the male F*1 offspring (Sakamoto and Fujii, 1980). Testes matured early in F*1 males, with testosterone levels elevated 2–4 fold at three weeks of age. Concomitantly, testosterone-dependent somatic organs were smaller, indicating a decrease in tissue sensitivity to the hormone.

Suppression of insect diapause by LSD

A well known hormonally regulated process of insects is pupal diapause, the delayed emergence of the adult from the pupa. The butterfly *Pieris brassicae* produces several broods a year. The last of the season overwinter as resting pupae in response to the short day lengths of autumn. Injecting lysergic acid (LSD) into the caterpillars counteracts this photoperiodic signal and its effects linger for multiple generations (Vuillaume and Berkaloff, 1974). Table 2 records that 78% of *P. brassicae* reared under short-day laboratory conditions diapaused. Twenty μg of LSD dropped this incidence to 18%. It also affected

the three subsequent generations. Exposure of even one male or female grandparent to LSD significantly decreased the likelihood that an F*2 pupa would diapause. Injecting LSD into both parents, as caterpillars, is lethal to offspring. These F*1 progeny die either at the end of the pupal stage or as malformed imagos.

LSD appears to induce two superimposed changes in offspring. Besides suppressing their diapause it makes them more resistant. F*1 caterpillars tolerate twice the normal lethal dose of LSD.

Carryover effects on immunity and development

In addition to hormone dysfunctions, perinatal disturbances of the immune system and organogenesis reportedly can also affect descendants of males for multiple generations. However, these claimed carryover effects are controversial.

Early in this century biologists induced carryover changes in morphology of various organisms, especially unicellular forms. A notable case in

TABLE 2

Effects of LSD on *P. brassicae*

Progeny generation	% of pupae which diapause[a]		LD_{50}
	Not treated	+ 20 μg LSD[b]	
Parental	78	18	35 μg
First			
A ♂(*) × ♀(n)	99	100	60 μg
B ♂(*) × ♀(*)	25	97	
C ♂(*) × ♀(n)	79	48	
Second			5–10 μg
♂ from A × ♀(n)	45		
♀ from B × ♂(n)	57		
Third			5–10 μg

Data abstracted from Vuillaume and Berkaloff (1974).
[a] Each percentage figure represents 60–378 individuals.
[b] Injected into 5th instar larva.
*, parent injected with LSD.
n, normal parent.

mammals involved defects from injecting anti-lens antiserum into pregnant rabbits (Guyer and Smith, 1918; 1920). Some offspring exposed in utero were born with malformed eyes and they transmitted eye defects in the sporadic manner expected for a recessive genetic trait. The abnormalities grew more and more pronounced over the course of five incrossed generations, rather than dying out (resembling the case of Spergel's rats treated with alloxan; see above). Several physiologists tried to repeat these experiments. However, they were unable to prepare antisera that were teratogenic and therefore could not follow the inheritance of induced eye defects. For a perceptive evaluation of these and other early studies, the reader is referred to Detlefsen (1925).

Inheritance of immunity has been studied more recently. It is well accepted that an immunized mother can transmit antibody molecules or lymphocytes to her progeny through the placenta or milk supply (Auerback and Clark, 1975). More unexpectedly, it was found that inoculating *male* neonatal mice with antigens also modifies the immune response of offspring (Gorczynski and Steele, 1980, 1981; Gorczynski et al., 1983; Steele, 1984). Cellular as well as soluble antigens and both immunizing and tolerizing schedules were effective. Up to half of the F*1 and F*2 descendants of tolerized mice were tolerant or partially tolerant to that antigen. Several other investigators have observed other, less spectacular male carryover effects (Guttman and Aust, 1963; Mullbacher et al., 1983) but attempts directly to replicate Gorczynski and Steele's results so far have failed (Brent et al., 1981, 1982; Smith, 1981; Nisbett-Brown and Wegmann, 1981; McLaren et al., 1981). The discrepancies have been analysed in detail by Steele (1981b and Steele et al., 1984) and his critics (Lewin, 1981; Brent, 1981). It seems likely to us that the immune system can transmit alterations across generations although not necessarily by the frankly Lamarckian mechanism proposed by Steele (1981a). See, for example, the complex findings of Gorczynski et al. (1983).

Other more restricted transgenerational effects

Effects of a variety of other parental treatments carry over to a narrower range of offspring. Some have been documented only among the first generation from treated males (see listing in Soyka and Joffe, 1980; also Adams et al., 1982). Others cross multiple generations but only through female lines (see examples in Caspari, 1948; Jinks, 1964; Svetlof and Korsakova, 1972; Denenberg and Rosenberg, 1967; Wehmer et al., 1970; Barnett, 1973; Ratner and Tchuraev, 1978; Zamenhof and Marthens, 1978; Beach et al., 1982) or through asexual cycles (see Goldschmidt, 1938; Csaba and Lantos, 1977). A third type of effect progressively intensifies from generation to generation while the animals are maintained in the inducing environment (Lints and Lints, 1965; Koloss, 1966; Mampell, 1968; Kahn, 1982; Wallace et al., 1983). Some of these cases eventually may turn out to include the full range of hereditary properties of the examples reviewed above (especially those of Mampell, 1968, and Fried and Charlebois, 1979). Others may be inherently simpler.

Mampell (1966) has advised that transgenerational effects may be far more prevalent than generally believed. We concur. Physiologists and endocrinologists can expect to discover substantially more examples if they examine the offspring of their experimental animals. We likewise agree with Barnett (1973) that cumulative carryover effects 'should be looked for, and recorded when found, even when they are extremely inconvenient to the experimenter and cannot be explained.' The same is true for observed absences of carryover effects, despite the difficulty of reporting 'negative' findings.

Difficulties for verifying induced transgenerational effects

Carryover effects as described above are complex and present a number of difficulties for experimental verification. The most important are the following.

1. Sporadic occurrence of altered progeny among the offspring of stressed animals. Some parental treatments affect only a portion of offspring. There are several possible reasons. The alteration might have variable expressivity in offspring, as seems to be the case for DDM induced by morphine. A few F*1 individuals exceed a threshold between a minor and major degree of affliction. Alternatively, an experimental treatment might induce an alteration in only some germ line cells of an animal. A low or variable incidence of affected progeny does not in itself cast doubt on the reality of a carryover effect but it can create serious problems for demonstrating and characterizing them. Any adequate study of a sporadic carryover effect should precisely describe the incidence of affected offspring, attempt to identify the factors which influence that incidence and present an experimental protocol that maximizes it.

2. Quantitative alterations. All variations are 'quantitative' in a purist sense, but some are large enough that affected and unaffected individuals can be distinguished unambiguously. Unfortunately, some carryover effects are not that great. They can be demonstrated by comparing distribution curves of measurements for progeny from experimental and control crosses but some or many individual animals cannot be unmistakably identified as affected or normal (e.g. Steele, 1984). Statistical analysis of distributions within a population is a valid analytic technique. However, geneticists simply will not accept statistical tests on the tails of distribution curves, or modest shifts in means as proof for biological phenomena as radical as 'Lamarckian inheritance' (Brent, 1981). Too many alternative possible explanations are no less believable. A foremost goal of a methodology must be to dichotomize cleanly affected and non-affected animals. This is especially important for studies which continue into subsequent generations.

3. Variations among strains. Phenotypic traits that are subject to modification by conditions experienced by parents or earlier ancestors can be expected to vary from one strain or substrain of animals to another. This makes it difficult to ensure that different laboratories (especially at different times) are working with equivalent animals. In fact, laboratories trying to replicate others' studies often obtain significantly different results. The differences observed among the more than half-dozen studies on progeny of various animals with chemical diabetes are a good example. Presumably, variation among strains has a genetic basis as is the case in plants. Some varieties of flax are susceptible to experimental induction of hereditary alterations called genotrophs while others are not (Cullis, 1977). Plant breeders have found it possible and informative to characterize the basis for this difference through crosses of 'plastic' and 'nonplastic' varieties by standard genetic procedures. It is not necessary for an experimental procedure to be effective for all strains or species, but a treatment must give reproducible results in some animals available to other laboratories.

4. Unintentional selection. Selection changes the characteristics of animals from one generation to another. It turns out to be very difficult to eliminate the *possibility* of this factor intruding in multigenerational experiments. Prenatal death, variation in litter size, failure of some pairs of animals to mate or conceive and even choosing which animals to breed for the next generation all can cause artifacts if they are biased toward the character under study. Such bias is distinctly possible for a neuroendocrine alteration. Cryptic selection is particularly capable of increasing or decreasing the intensity of carryover effects during the course of a multigenerational study (Guyer and Smith, 1920; Korec, 1981; Spergel et al., 1975).

It is important to realize that natural selection cannot be eliminated from an experiment. The best that one can do is estimate its total possible effect from litter size variation, amounts of perinatal death and so forth and compare the 'worst case' magnitude with experimental findings. Protocols for untreated control lines should be designed very carefully to indicate the possible effects of selection.

A very different level of selection distorts the literature. Scientists naturally publish data which is statistically significant and ignore negative findings. If twenty people examine the progeny of experimentally stressed male animals, one is expected to find them to differ from controls by a 'statistically significant' amount ($P < 0.05$). If only this 'significant' observation is reported the literature will become skewed.

Examining twenty traits in one study presents the same problem. Obviously, investigators must examine various inducing regimes, look at a variety of phenotypic measures, and even test subsets of data for significance: transmission from females only, progeny of the treated males, total numbers of animals vs. numbers of litters in which defects show up and so forth. Unfortunately it is usually impossible to tell from an article how many possible parameters the statistically verified ones correspond to. We suggest that investigators use separate standards to evaluate the confidence of two aspects of their findings: (A) how solidly the observations show that a treatment did induce changes in succeeding generations; the usual significance level of 0.05 is far too loose here: and (B) what syndrome of changes is carried over. Conventional measures of significance are appropriate for this purpose.

5. *Inadequately defined genetic background of the experimental animals.* Most transgenerational studies of drug and hormonal treatments have been conducted on inadequately characterized strains of animals. Because geneticists are skeptical of purported Lamarckian inheritance, this field has been left mainly to physiologists. These latter scientists naturally design studies around the logic of their field instead of genetic paradigms. For example, Goldner and Spergel (1972)

deliberately chose outbred animals for their studies of the transmission of latent diabetes because 'A non-inbred strain of rat... more closely resembles the genetic state of the human population than does the inbred animal, brother-sister mated for more than twenty generations. Any genetic information gleaned from such an inbred strain could be applied only with difficulty to the understanding of human diabetes mellitus.' More extreme problems arise for a carryover process which operates only in genetically obscure species (such as insect diapause). Ultimately, inheritance must be related to contemporary genetics. That paradigm is to relate genetic phenomena to the base sequence of a DNA molecule. Geneticists will fully accept induced carryover effects only when the DNA responsible for them is isolated. This goal is becoming more and more realistic. However, it is feasible only in genetically standard organisms.

6. *Subjective measures.* Neuroendocrines have sophisticated functions. Some can be observed only with complex assay systems or technical expertise. In particular, judgement is required to conduct and interpret some behavioral tests. Such tests are valid, and indeed underlie whole fields of research. Yet geneticists will reject demonstrations of the inheritance of acquired characters by assay methods that have a possible subjective component or seem more complex than necessary. They demand that at least one transmitted characteristic be completely objective, such as body weight, a simple count or a measurement that anyone can make.

7. *Nonspecificity of effects.* Some transgenerational changes have no obvious relationship to the disturbed neuroendocrine system. Their ad hoc character makes these persisting changes more difficult to believe and less interesting than specific changes. It is primarily their similarity to the short-term disturbances that induced them that distinguishes carryover effects from ordinary mutation. The preceding paragraph describes the

reasons for tracing changes in generalized characteristics, such as body weight, because they are objective and unambiguous. However, it is necessary *also* to demonstrate specific changes in progeny if they occur. This is important even if it requires specialized analytic procedures that may be complicated and not wholly precise. One generally useful and objective indicator of specificity is an altered sensitivity of progeny to the drug or treatment used to induce the change in the parent. Exposing animals to LSD, alloxan, morphine and tolerizing antigens makes their descendants more sensitive to those particular agents.

Mechanisms

Induced carryover effects have been compared to Lamarckian inheritance of acquired characters. The essential difference is that Lamarckism presumes that acquired modifications in phenotype automatically carry over to progeny as an innate, primary feature of inheritance. In contrast, the carryover effects of stress to neuroendocrine systems must be ascribed to special mechanisms that individual neuroendocrine systems have happened to evolve (Campbell, 1982). Without those evolved specializations, insults to an animal would be confined strictly to that individual. Whether these mechanisms evolved in order that experiential information can be usefully transmitted to progeny (as suggested for glucose regulation by Goldner and Spergel, 1972) or whether transmission is merely a byproduct of elaboration that a system evolved for other functions is an open question.

The artificially induced transgenerational changes in studies reviewed above are obviously maladaptive, but this may be misleading. Presumably the adaptive purpose for a carryover mechanism would be to pass along fine adjustments of a thyrostat, a glucosestat, calcium regulation, tendency to diapause, tolerance to an antigenic specificity or developmental rate. It is easy to believe that tuning any of these properties in an animal of one generation according to the slight imbalances experienced by its parents could be useful. However to demonstrate carryover effects, experimentalists must abuse these systems to degrees far beyond any functional meaning. Nudging the thyrostat setting of mice by amounts that could be adaptive would be experimentally unnoticeable. Thus, the gyrations induced by addicting baby mice to morphine or extirpating the thyroid are irrelevant to the issue of adaptiveness of carryover mechanisms.

An adaptive genetic explanation for induced carryover effects must answer two separate questions. One concerns the type of change made in the structure of the gene. The other is how a neuroendocrine imbalance triggers that genetic change to take place. Thirty years ago both problems seemed intractable. In the words of Waddington (1957), 'It seems to be the opinion of nearly all recent authors, with the exception of Lysenko and his followers in Russia, that the lack of conclusive evidence for such effects and the difficulty of envisaging even in theory a mechanism by which they might operate, justify one in completely rejecting this theory.' Fortunately, the enormous progress in genetics over the past 30 years has overturned this situation.

Before the DNA revolution, genes were considered to be abstract units of sacred information, transcendental to the physical world except for rare, spontaneous, random and blind mutations. We now have a more realistic material view (Campbell, 1982, 1983). Genes are biological molecules and, like all components under the control of cells, are substrates for enzymes. Cells have enzymes to catalyse many deliberate sorts of alterations in gene structure, including inversions, transpositions, duplications, base pair substitutions, and corrections of one gene according to the sequence of another. Each of these types of alteration is known to produce transgenerational changes in variable characteristics of lower organisms or plants. It would fall well within precedents set by other species for any of them to underlie carryover effects in a neuroendocrine system of mammals. Identifying the type of DNA alteration responsible for a particular carryover effect, the gene involved and (eventually) the enzymatic pathway that catalyses that change, amounts to a conventional, if ambitious, program in molecular genetics.

The more challenging puzzle is how a neuro-endocrine imbalance induces a germ cell to change its genome. The Weismann barrier between the soma and germ-line is formidable and certainly most experiences of the soma have no effect whatsoever on heredity (Weismann, 1893). It is this barrier and not the presumed inviolability of the structure of gene molecules which makes carryover effects in animals surprising. In fact, text books on cell biology describe without reserve examples of induced carryover effects in organisms which do not separate somatic and germ lines, such as bacteria, single-celled protista and plants (e.g. Alberts et al., 1983). We also accept labile gene changes which occur 'spontaneously' in metazoans because they do not imply a communication between the soma and germ-line (Belyaev et al., 1981a; but see Belyaev et al., 1981b).

Various investigators have suggested that drugs and hormone imbalances exert effects on progeny by acting on germinal cells. According to Guyer and Smith (1920) 'Ever since the discovery of the existence of such special internal secretions as hormones and chalones doubtless every biologist has thought of the possibility and many have expressed the idea that such substances might be concerned in some way in transmitting the results of somatic modifications to the germ, although, to our knowledge, no one has yet supplied a plausible explanation of how somatogenic [traits] are converted into blastogenic modifications by such means.'

Our increased understanding of hormones make this speculative activity of neuroendocrines increasingly plausible. It is becoming apparent that most neuroendocrines have multiple target tissues and functions. Some are broadcast throughout the bloodstream as endocrines while at the same time secreted regionally to regulate adjacent cells as paracrines and even produced ultralocally by cells to stimulate themselves as autocrines. Also, many are used simultaneously to regulate and coordinate somatic physiology (as hormones), the nervous system (as neurotransmitters and neuromodulators), the immune system (as immune regulators) and development (as trophic and tropic agents). We have suggested (Campbell, 1982) that it is more meaningful to call these chemical messengers 'cybernins'; conveyers of information, rather than 'hormones', 'neuroendocrines', 'neuroimmunoendocrines', 'hormone-like growth factors' and other like terms which emphasize individual physiological roles. Cybernins carry out their functions in an integrated fashion. A major emphasis in contemporary endocrinological research is to demonstrate that a cybernin known to regulate one aspect of physiology also functions in other areas and that these roles are interwoven. Any cell potentially can tap into a cybernin circuit merely by expressing on its surface receptors for that messenger molecule. Some cybernins are indeed perceived by many different cell types. We have included in this review examples of carryover effects from the immune system and from development, despite their more speculative status, in order to emphasize the scope of the cybernin system.

An intriguing extension of the cybernin concept is that these same molecules also regulate the genetic system. By this perspective cybernins would signal germ-line cells in the same general way that they do other targets. They would bind to specific cell surface receptors (presumably expressed from the same gene as in many or all target cells) and initiate the same pattern of intracellular and genetic activities as in other cells (Campbell and Zimmermann, 1982).

It is suggestive that most treatments which induce transgenerational effects also produce long-lasting somatic changes in the treated animal. One injection of thyroxine or insulin into a neonate alters TSH or glucose regulation for the life of the animal (Bakke et al., 1975; Csaba, 1980). An obvious possible basis for this persistance is that signals from hormone receptors induce specific changes in DNA structure which are stable through chromosomal replication and cellular division.

We have proposed the term *automodulation* for the case in which cell surface receptors regulate the enzymatic alteration of their own genes (Campbell, 1982; Campbell and Zimmermann, 1982; Fig. 2). The definitive example in mammals occurs as part of the immune response. B lymphocytes of the immune system synthesize immunoglobulin molecules and plant them on their outer membranes as cell surface receptors for antigens. When these receptors are stimulated they send signals to the cell nucleus to induce specific enzymatic alterations in the structure of the immunoglobulin genes. These change the receptor's subsequent responses to stimuli.

Automodulation is a plausible mechanism for permanently setting levels of hormones during critical periods in development, such as for the thyrostat. Moreover it would allow changes to cross generations with no extra physiological machinery beyond that evolved to mediate the somatic functions. Inheritance of thyrostat settings would only require the genes activated at the critical perinatal period in the thyrotroph cell also to be expressed at that time in germ-line cells.

There is no direct evidence for gene automodulation in germ-line cells. However, the physiology of these cells is poorly known. The most obvious prediction of the model is that germinal cells have receptors for various neuroendocrines. Interestingly, receptors have been detected on *Xenopus* or mouse eggs for acetylcholine, adrenaline, 5-hydroxytryptamine and dopamine (Kusano et al., 1977), progesterone and insulin (El-Etr et al., 1979, 1980; but see Wallace and Misulovan, 1980), and purines (Lotan et al., 1982). Germinal cells of males are harder to study than large oocytes but circumstantial evidence suggests that they too carry receptors for cybernins. For example spermatogenic cells in

mouse testes synthesize endorphins. If these cybernins have autocrine functions, as Kilpatrick and Millette (1986) suggest, then male germ-line cells would have morphine receptors. Also, deficiencies in a variety of hormones arrest sperm production (including, by the way, insulin and parathyroid hormone, Oksanen, 1975; Fujii and Morita, 1978). It would be interesting to test egg cells systematically for receptors for the whole range of hormones, cell growth factors, neuromodulators etc. that have been discovered in mammals.

Automodulation in germinal cells would directly explain why injecting drugs into animals changes the sensitivity of their offspring to those

RECEPTOR GENE AUTOMODULATION

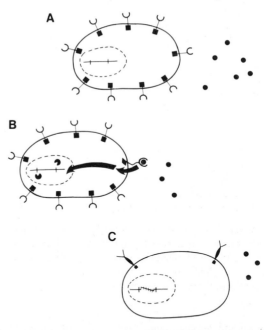

Fig. 2 Model for automodulation of a hormone receptor gene. A. A cell is shown with hormone receptors in its membrane and the receptor gene in the nucleus. B. Upon binding the hormone an activated receptor signals a set of specific nuclear enzymes to rearrange the structure of the receptor gene. C. The modified gene changes the cell's responsiveness to the hormone. Automodulation might affect the number of receptors on the cell membrane, their binding properties or the signal that they generate when activated.

TABLE 3

Suggested mechanisms for induced carryover effects

Suggested mechanism	Ref.
A. Effects transmitted by males and through multiple generations	
Automodulation	1
Direct genetic transformation: uptake of DNA from soma by germ cells	2
Transfer of genetic material from affected somatic tissue to germ cells by a vector	3
Mutation	4
'Paramutation' as a presumed heritable 'restraint on gene expression without altering structural DNA'	5
Combination of two mechanisms: one in males, the other for multiple female generations	–
Contrived data or artifact	6, 7
B. Male transmission through a single generation	
Damage to the sperm by a drug	8
Change in component of sperm besides DNA	9
Transmission of a drug through semen	10
Change in a component of semen other than sperm e.g. hormone, antibody, or lymphocyte	8
Methylation of DNA at specific sites	–
Altered coital activity of male	8
C Transmission through multiple female generations	
Self-perpetuating alteration in:	
a cellular organelle	11, 12
the uterus or placenta or milk supply	13
the immune system (auto-antibodies)	14
a neuroendocrine system	15
behavior	16
Changes in the numbers of copies of:	
extrachromosomal genetic elements	17
extranuclear intracellular particles	18
genes in multigene families	19, 20
Altered heritable pattern of gene regulation	21
Integration of an episome which can be in either a cytoplasmic or chromosomal state	22
D. Progressive change while animals are kept under inducing conditions	
Artifact from improved rearing conditions instituted over the course of the study	23
Progressive loss of virulence of an endemic pathogen or change in a symbiont organism	24, 25
Progressive depletion of an essential dietary nutrient	26
Extra replication of heterochromatin	27
Selection	28

1. Campbell and Zimmermann, 1982.
2. Kanazawa and Imai, 1974.
3. Steele, 1981.
4. Detlefsen, 1925.
5. Spergel et al., 1971.
6. Koestler, 1971.
7. Huxley and Carr-Saunders, 1923.
8. Joffe, 1979.
9. McLaren, 1979.
10. Lutwak-Mann et al., 1967.
11. Jinks, 1964.
12. Caspari, 1948.
13. Zamenhof et al., 1972.
14. Goldsmith et al., 1973.
15. Aerts and Van Assche, 1979.
16. Denenberg and Rosenberg, 1967.
17. Bucheton and Picard, 1978.
18. Mampell, 1968.
19. Cullis, 1977.
20. Ritossa, 1976.
21. Bussey and Fields, 1974.
22. Barigozzi et al., 1962.
23. Agar et al., 1954.
24. Barnett, 1961.
25. Mampell, 1965.
26. Wallace et al., 1983.
27. Beardmore et al., 1975.
28. Waddington, 1952.

compounds. As another detail, Kusano et al. (1977) have called attention to the substantial variation in the presence and abundance of receptors for particular neuroendocrines among batches of *Xenopus* eggs. Perhaps germinal cells vary in which receptor systems are active, or which are active at a particular time. A stochastic element in receptor expression would agree with the sporadic carryover effects seen among the progeny of animals exposed to certain cybernin stimuli.

Gene automodulation is only one of several proposed mechanisms for induced carryover effects. Kanazawa and Imai (1974) have suggested that DNA is transferred from soma to germinal cells in a process resembling transformation in bacteria. Steele (1981a) believes that a retrovirus vector carries genetic information to the testes from stimulated antibody-producing cells. He has elaborated his model for the immune system but it could be further developed to apply to endocrine organs. Such direct flows of nucleic acid from the body to the germ-line would correspond to a true Lamarckian process.

Another class of explanations for male transmission depends on components other than DNA of sperm (such as a patch of membrane possibly with cybernin receptors or a 'cytoplasmic' structure). As a pertinent example, Sastry et al. (1982) have detected enkephalin (as immunoreactivity) in mature spermatozoa. Extracellular agencies are also possible. Gorczynski et al. (1983) showed that immunologically tolerant male mice seem to transmit some factor to female mates inducing them in turn to transmit hyporesponsiveness maternally to their progeny. This factor might be lymphocytes or antibody molecules in both sexes.

Table 3 catalogues a number of suggestions for how drug influences might be transmitted through one sex or the other. These ideas are germane because several of them might be superimposed to produce the full range of carryover effects seen in the examples described above. For example, hyperparathyroidism might change calcium metabolism through multiple generations in female

lines by one mechanism and testosterone levels in descendants of males by another. A particular possibility that must be kept in mind is that a drug which induces an automodulation process might also alter uterine or placental function as an entirely independent secondary action. A second subsidiary mechanism could explain why F*1 animals sometimes differ from those of the F*2 generation (as in the cases of thyroxine and LSD exposure described above). Because transgenerational effects of physiological manipulations are outside conventional orthodoxy it is generally felt that they must be rare. This may be a wrong perception. The alternative is that there are many possible ways for events in one generation to affect the next, ranging from trivial to sophisticated. As a complex multifunctional trait adaptively evolves it tends to accumulate associations with other genes that may affect progeny. As physiology becomes more integrated many traits may interact with ones that affect offspring.

Nonspecific carryover effects

A final question with a major bearing on mechanism is the degree of specificity of the transgenerational effects induced by stress. Presumably the carryover effects described here are specific. Diabetogeneic drugs induce glucose intolerance and thyroidectomy disrupts thyroxine balance in progeny. However, the consequences of these treatments may overlap more than the literature suggests. Blood glucose levels have not been measured in progeny of hypothyroid animals nor have studies of induced diabetes included response times of F*1 animals placed on a hot plate. Endocrinologists naturally concentrate their attention on traits in progeny related to the cybernin that they are studying.

Various investigators have found that the most obvious carryover effect of neonatal morphine exposure is a delay in postnatal maturation. Retarded postnatal weight gain also carries over from thyroidectomy, protein deprivation and certain subdiabetic regimes. There are two plausible reasons for these overlaps. One is that various stresses trigger a common response mechanism. Organisms do have generalized stress-response systems. One that extends taxonomically from bacteria to higher animals was defined originally as heat shock responses but now is known to be stimulated by a variety of stresses (Hammond et al., 1982). Animals, plants and bacteria all have been found to respond to certain general stresses by enzymatically changing DNA sequences in their chromosomes (Echols, 1981; McClintock, 1984; Strand and McDonald, 1985).

The existence of a common carryover mechanism for a variety of neuroendocrine stresses is an attractive idea. It probably cannot account for all of the effects discussed above. However, from a medical point of view induction of a DDM syndrome by a variety of neuroendocrine imbalances could be substantially more important than more restricted carryover responses.

A second possible reason for stresses on different hormone systems to induce similar effects on progeny is that cybernin circuits are highly interrelated to one another. They modulate and regulate the sensitivity of cells to each other. Many, if not most, cybernins also act on other cybernin-producing cells. Instead of representing independent communication channels between pairs of tissues cybernins are locked into a network which, at least indirectly, links most together. Alterations in one cybernin component will cascade through the network producing secondary and tertiary effects on an ever-widening array of characters. For example, alloxan-induced diabetes disturbs LHRH and thereby gonadotrophins which in turn alter sex steroids (Cusan et al., 1980). Drug interventions at different points in the network might ramify to a common cybernin system that has evolved the machinery to affect offspring generations. In the progeny a limited number of transmitted changes might again expand to a range of phenotypic properties.

Immunologists have realized the fundamental roles of network properties in the operation of the immune system. The connectivity among cybernins gives it a network capacity as well. However, the cybernins are richer in diversity and function than immune molecules and their potential range of network properties is commensurately larger. The complexities reported for transgenerational effects probably can be understood only by a network level of integration of development, immunity and neuroendocrine regulation with inheritance.

Summary

Hormonal stresses at critical periods during development can lead to long-lasting, even permanent, abnormalities in adult hormone levels. Evidently the steady-state values of certain endocrine control circuits are set in part on the basis of hormone levels about the time of birth instead of being rigidly programmed genetically. This developmental flexibility might allow adapted hormone levels of a mother to be impressed upon her fetal offspring as an epigenetic 'maternal effect'. Two features of the carryover effects in several endocrine systems suggest even more elaborate underlying mechanisms, possibly even involving induced changes in gene structure. These disturbances can persist for multiple generations and be passed on by male as well as female parents.

This article reviews the most notable carryover effects reported in the literature, discusses the difficulties of interpreting their descriptions, and catalogues the rather extensive set of mechanisms that have been proposed to explain transgenerational effects of one sort or another.

Acknowledgement

Supported by funds from the Biomedical Research Support Grant through the School of Medicine, UCLA.

References

Adams, P.M., Fabricant, J.D. and Legator, M.S. (1982) Active avoidance behavior in the F1 progeny of male rats exposed to cyclophosphamide prior to fertilization. *Neurol. Toxicol.*, 4: 531–534.

Agar, W.E., Drummond, F.H., Tiegs, O.W. and Gunson, M.M. (1954) Fourth (final) report on a test of McDougall's Lamarckian experiment on the training of rats. *J. Exp. Biol.*, 31: 307–321.

Aerts, L. and Van Assche, F.A. (1977) Rat foetal endocrine pancreas in experimental diabetes. *J. Endocrinol.*, 73: 339–346.

Aerts, L. and Van Assche, F.A. (1979) Is gestational diabetes an acquired condition? *J. Dev. Physiol.*, 1: 219–225.

Alberts, B., Bray, D., Lewis, J., Raff, M., Roberts, K. and Watson, J.D. (1983) *Molecular Biology of the Cell*, Garland Pub., New York.

Auerbach, R. and Clark, S. (1975) Immunological tolerance: Transmission from mother to offspring. *Science*, 189: 811–813.

Bakke, J.L. and Lawrence, N. (1966) Persistent thyrotropin insufficiency following neonatal thyroxine administration. *J. Lab. Clin. Med.*, 67: 477–482.

Bakke, J.L., Lawrence, N.L., Bennett, J. and Robinson, S. (1975) Endocrine syndromes produced by neonatal hyperthyroidism, hypothyroidism, or altered nutrition and effects seen in untreated progeny. In D.A. Fisher and G.N. Burrow (Eds.), *Perinatal Thyroid Physiology and Disease*, Raven Press, New York, pp. 79–112.

Baranov, V.G. and Sokoloverova, I.M. (1966) Experimental model of latent diabetes mellitus in rats and factors promoting transition to overt diabetes. *Fed. Proc. Trans. Suppl.*, 25: T55–T58.

Barigozzi, C., Halfer, C. and Sgorbati, G. (1962) Melanotic tumours of drosophila: a partially Mendelian character. *Heriditas*, 17: 561–575.

Barnett, S.A. (1961) Some effects of breeding mice for many generations in a cold environment. *Proc. R. Soc. B*, 155: 115–135.

Barnett, S.A. (1973) Maternal processes in the cold-adaptation of mice. *Biol. Rev.*, 48: 477–508.

Bartelheimer, H. and Kloos, K. (1952) Die Auswirkung des experimentellen Diabetes auf Graviditat und Nachkommenschaft. *Z. Gesamte Exp. Med.*, 119: 246–265.

Beach, R.S., Gershwin, M.E. and Hurley, L.S. (1982) Gestational zinc deprivation in mice: persistence of immunodeficiency for three generations. *Science*, 218: 469–471.

Beardmore, J.A., Lints, F. and Al-Baldawi, A.L.F. (1975) Parental age and heritability of sternopleural chaeta numbers in *Drosophila melanogaster*. *Heredity*, 34: 71–82.

Belyaev, D.K., Ruvinsky, A.O. and Borodin, P.M. (1981a) Inheritance of alternative states of the fused gene in mice. *J. Hered.*, 72: 107–112.

Belyaev, D.K., Ruvinsky, A.O. and Trut, L.N. (1981b) Inherited activation-inactivation of the star gene in foxes. *J. Hered.*, 72: 267–274.

Brent, L. (1981) Lamarck and immunity: the tables unturned. *New Scientist*, 90: 493.

Brent, L., Rayfield, L.S., Chandler, P., Fierz, W., Medawar, P.B. and Simpson, E. (1981) Supposed Lamarckian inheritance of immunological tolerance. *Nature*, 290: 508–512.

Brent, L., Chandler, P., Fierz, W., Medawar, P.B., Rayfield, L.S. and Simpson, E. (1982) Further studies on supposed Lamarckian inheritance of immunological tolerance. *Nature*, 295: 242–244.

Bucheton, A. and Picard, G. (1978) Non-Mendelian female sterility in *Drosophila melanogaster*: hereditary transmission of reactivity levels. *Heredity*, 40: 207–223.

Bussey, H. and Fields, M.A. (1974) A model for the stably inherited environmentally induced changes in plants. *Nature*, 251: 708–709.

Campbell, J.H. (1982) Autonomy in Evolution. In R. Milkman (Ed.), *Perspectives on Evolution*, Sinauer Assoc., Sunderland, pp. 190–200.

Campbell, J.H. (1983) Evolving concepts of multigene families. *Curr. Top. Biol. Med. Res.*, 10: 401–417.

Campbell, J.H. and Zimmermann, E.G. (1982) Automodulation of genes: a proposed mechanism for persisting effects of drugs and hormones in mammals. *Neurobehav. Toxicol. Teratol.*, 4: 435–439.

Caspari, E. (1948) Cytoplasmic inheritance. *Adv. Genet.*, 2: 1–66.

Csaba, G. (1980) Phylogeny and ontogeny of hormone receptors: the selection theory of receptor formation and hormonal imprinting. *Biol. Rev.*, 55: 47–63.

Csaba, G. and Lantos, T. (1977) An attempt to differentiate selection and amplification in hormone receptor development. The unicellular model. *Differentiation*, 8: 57–59.

Cullis, C.A. (1977) Molecular aspects of the environmental induction of heritable changes in flax. *Heredity*, 38: 129–154.

Cusan, L., Belanger, A., Seguin, C. and Labrie, F. (1980) Impairment of pituitary and gonadal functions in alloxan-induced diabetic male rats. *Mol. Cell. Endocrinol.*, 18: 165–176.

Denenberg, V.H. and Rosenberg, K.M. (1967) Nongenetic transmission of information. *Nature*, 216: 549–550.

Detlefsen, J.A. (1925) The inheritance of acquired characters. *Physiol. Rev.*, 5: 244–278.

Echols, H. (1981) SOS functions, cancer and inducible evolution. *Cell*, 25: 1–2.

El-Etr, M., Schorderet-Slatkine, S. and Baulieu, E.E. (1979) Meiotic maturation in *Xenopus laevis* oocytes initiated by insulin. *Science*, 205: 1397–1399.

550

El-Etr, M., Schorderet-Slatkine, S. and Baulieu, E. E. (1980) Reply. *Science*, 210: 929–930.

Foglia, V. G., de Paralta Ramos, M. C. and Ibarra, R. (1970) Alteracion hidrocarbonada en ratas hijas de madres prediabeticas. *Congr. Int. Diabetic Assoc. Prog. Abstr.*, 7: 62.

Fried, P. A. and Charlebois, A. T. (1979) Cannabis administered during pregnancy: first- and second-generation effects in rats. *Physiol. Psychol.*, 6: 307–310.

Friedler, G. (1974) Long-term effects of opiates. In J. Dancis and J. C. Hwang (Eds.), *Perinatal Pharmacology: Problems and Priorities*, Raven Press, New York, pp. 207–219.

Friedler, G. (1978) Pregestational administration of morphine-sulfate to female mice: long-term effects on the development of subsequent progeny. *J. Pharmacol. Exp. Ther.*, 205: 33–39.

Friedler, G. and Cochin, J. (1972) Growth retardation in offspring of female rats treated with morphine prior to conception. *Science*, 175: 654–655.

Friedler, G. and H. S. Wheeling (1979) Behavioral effects in offspring of male mice injected with opioids prior to mating. *Pharmacol. Biochem. Behav.*, 11(s): 23–28.

Fujii, T. (1978) Inherited disorders in the regulation of serum calcium in rats raised from parathyroidectomised mothers. *Nature*, 273: 236–237.

Fujii, T. and Morita, K. (1978) Transmission of the hypocalcemia resistant-trait through male gamete in rats. *Jpn. J. Pharmacol.*, 28: 172P.

Fujii, T. and Yamamoto, N. (1983) Delayed onset of persistent estrus in aged rats raised from parathyroidectomized mothers. *Exp. Aging Res.*, 9: 129–133.

Fujii, T., Morimoto, S. and Ikeda, H. (1980) Hypersensitivity to lethal effect of injected calcium chloride in the third generation rats raised from parathyroidectomized mothers. *Biomed. Res.*, 1: 432–434.

Fujii, T., Yamamoto, N., Shirakur, Y. and Komura, T. (1985) Inherited functional alterations in hypothalamus-pituitary-thyroid system in rats raised from parathyroidectomized mothers. *Proc. Jpn. Acad.*, 61B: 229–232.

Gellert, R. J., Bakke, J. L. and Lawrence, N. L. (1971) Delayed vaginal opening in the rat following pharmacologic doses of T4 administered during the neonatal period. *J. Lab. Clin. Med.*, 77: 410–416.

Gept, W. (1965) Discussion. In B. S. Leibel and G. A. Wranshell (Eds.), *On the Nature and Treatment of Diabetes*, Excerpta Medica Foundation, Amsterdam p. 640.

Glick, S. D., Strumph, A. J. and Zimmerberg, B. (1977) Effect of in utero administration of morphine on the subsequent development of self-administered behavior. *Brain Res.*, 132: 194–196.

Goldner, M. G. and Spergel, G. (1972) On the transmission of alloxan diabetes and other diabetogenic influences. *Adv. Metabol. Disorders*, 6: 57–72.

Goldschmidt, R. (1938) *Physiological Genetics*, McGraw-Hill, New York.

Goldsmith, R. E., McAdams, A. J., Larsen, P. R., MacKenzie, M. and Hess, E. V. (1973) Familial autoimmune thyroiditis: maternal-fetal relationship and the role of generalized autoimmunity. *J. Clin. Endocrinol. Metab.*, 37: 265–275.

Gorczynski, R. M. and Steele, E. J. (1980) Inheritance of acquired immunological tolerance to foreign histocompatibility antigens in mice. *Proc. Natl. Acad. Sci. USA*, 77: 2871–2875.

Gorczynski, R. M. and Steele, E. J. (1981) Simultaneous yet independent inheritance of somatically acquired tolerance to two distinct H-2 antigenic haplotype determinants in mice. *Nature*, 289: 678–681.

Gorczynski, R. M., Kennedy, M., MacRae, S. and Ciampi, A. (1983) A possible maternal effect in the abnormal hyporesponsiveness to specific alloantigens in offspring born to neonatally tolerant fathers. *J. Immunol.*, 131: 1115–1120.

Guttman, R. D. and Aust, J. B. (1963). A germplasm-transmitted alteration of histocompatibility in the progeny of homograft tolerant mice. *Nature*, 197: 1220–1221.

Guyer, M. F. and Smith, E. A. (1918) Studies on cytolysins. I. Some prenatal effects of lens antibodies. *J. Exp. Zool.*, 26: 65–82.

Guyer, M. F. and Smith, E. A. (1920) Studies on cytolysins. II. Transmission of induced eye-defects. *J. Exp. Zool.*, 31: 171–215.

Hammond, G. L., Lai, Y.-K. and Markert, C. L. (1982) Diverse forms of stress lead to new patterns of gene expression through a common and essential metabolic pathway. *Proc. Natl. Acad. Sci. USA*, 79: 3485–3488.

Huxley, J. S. and Carr-Saunder, A. M. (1923) Absence of prenatal effects of lens-antibodies in rabbits. *Br. J. Exp. Biol.*, 1: 215–248.

Jackson, W. P. U. (1954) The prediabetic syndrome. Large babies and the prediabetic father. *J. Clin. Endocrinol.*, 14: 177–183.

Jackson, W. P. U. (1960) The present status of prediabetes. *Diabetes*, 9: 373–378.

Jinks, J. L. (1964) *Extrachromosomal Inheritance*, Prentice-Hall, Englewood Cliffs, New Jersey.

Joffe, J. M. (1979) Influence of drug exposure of the father on perinatal outcome. *Clin. Perinatol.*, 6: 21–36.

Joffe, J., Peterson, J. M., Smith, D. J. and Soyka, L. (1978) Sublethal effects on the offspring of male rats treated with methadone before mating. *Res. Commun. Chem. Pathol. Pharmacol.*, 13: 611–621.

Kahn, A. J. (1982) Alterability of development of hemoglobin concentration in mice: transmission of changes to the next generation. *Growth*, 46: 247–258.

Kanazawa, K. and Imai, A. (1974) Parasexual-sexual hybridization – heritable transformation of germ cells in chimeric mice. *Jpn. J. Exp. Med.*, 44: 227–234.

Kilpatrick, D. L. and Millette, C. F. (1986) Expression of proenkephalin messenger RNA by mouse spermatogenic cells. *Proc. Natl. Acad. Sci. USA*, 83: 5015–5018.

Koestler, A. (1971) *The Case of the Midwife Toad*, Random House, New York.

Koloss, E.I. (1966) On the changes of iris muscles of white mice during long-term experiments. *Zh. Obshch. Biol.*, 27: 117–127.

Korec, R. (1981) Observations on the progeny of alloxan- or streptozotocin-diabetic rats cured by pancreatic transplantation. *Diabetologia*, 20: 678.

Kusano, K., Miledi, R. and Stinnakre, J. (1977) Acetylcholine receptors in the oocyte membrane. *Nature*, 270: 739–741.

Lewin, R. (1981) Lamarck will not lie down. *Science*, 213: 316–321.

Lints, F.A. and Lints, C.V. (1965) Depression, heterosis and carry-over effects after many generations of inbreeding with *Drosophila melanogaster. Genetica*, 36: 183–207.

Lotan, I., Dascal, N., Cohen, S. and Lass, Y. (1982) Adenosine-induced slow ionic currents in the *Xenopus* oocyte. *Nature*, 298: 572–574.

Lutwak-Mann, C., Schmid, K. and Keberle, H. (1967) Thalidomide in rabbit semen. *Nature*, 214: 1018–1020.

Mampell, K. (1965) Gene expression and developmental rate. *Genetica*, 36: 135–146.

Mampell, K. (1966) Genetic and environmental control of melanotic tumors in *Drosophila. Genetica*, 37: 449–465.

Mampell, K. (1968) Differentiation and extragenic transmission of modified gene expression. *Genetica*, 39: 553–566.

McClintock, B. (1984) The significance of responses of the genome to challenge. *Science*, 226: 792–801.

McLaren, A., Chandler, P., Buehr, M., Fierz, W. and Simpson, E. (1981) Immune reactivity of progeny of tetraparental male mice. *Nature*, 290: 513–514.

Milner, R.D.G. and Sheffrin, R.A. (1982) Vertical transmission of diabetes in the rat. *J. Dev. Physiol.*, 4: 39–51.

Mullbacher, A., Ashman, R.B. and Blanden, R.V. (1983) Induction of T-cell hyporesponsiveness to Bebaru in mice, and abnormalities in the immune responses of progeny of hyporesponsive males. *Aust. J. Biol. Med. Sci.*, 61: 187–191.

Neel, J.V. (1962) Diabetes mellitus: A 'thrifty' genotype rendered detrimental by 'progress'. *Am. J. Hum. Genet.*, 14: 353–362.

Nisbett-Brown, E. and Wegmann, T.G. (1981) Is acquired immunological tolerance genetically transmissible? *Proc. Natl. Acad. Sci. USA*, 78: 5826–5828.

Ohno, K. (1969) Electron microscopic study on beta cells of the islet of Langerhans in the rats under an experimentally induced prediabetic state. *Kumamoto Med. J.*, 22: 41–53.

Okamoto, K. (1965) Apparent transmittance of factors to offspring by animals with experimental diabetes. In B.S. Liebell and G.A. Wrenshell (Eds.), *On the Nature and Treatment of Diabetes*, Excerpta Medica Foundation, Amsterdam, pp. 627–640.

Oksanen, A. (1975) Testicular lesions of streptozotocin diabetic rats. *Horm. Res.*, 6: 138–144.

Ratner, V.A. and Tchuraev, R.N. (1978) Simplest genetic systems controlling ontogenesis: organization, principles and models of their function. *Prog. Theor. Biol.*, 5: 81–127.

Ritossa, F. (1976) The *bobbed* locus. In M. Ashburner, and D. Novitski (Eds.), *The Genetics and Biology of Drosophila, Vol. 1b*, Academic Press, London, pp. 801–846.

Rubin, A. (1958) Studies in human reproduction. II. The influence of diabetes mellitus in men upon reproduction. *Am. J. Obstet. Gynecol.*, 76: 25–29.

Sakamoto, M. and Fujii, T. (1980) Changes in the functional differentiation of the testis of F1 offsprings from parathyroid-transplanted rats. *Jpn. J. Pharmacol.*, 30(S): 158P.

Sastry, B.V.R., Janson, V.E., Owens, L.K. and Tayeb, O.S. (1982) Enkephalin-like and substance P-like immunoreactivity of human sperm and accessory sex glands. *Biochem. Pharmacol.*, 31: 3519–3522.

Smith, A.A., Hui, F.W. and Crofford, M.J. (1977) Inhibition of growth in young mice treated with d,l-methadone. *Eur. J. Pharmacol.*, 43: 307–314.

Smith, D.J. and Joffe, J.M. (1973) Increased neonatal mortality in offspring of male rats treated with methadone or morphine before mating. *Nature*, 253: 202–203.

Smith, R.N. (1981) Inability of tolerant males to sire tolerant progeny. *Nature*, 292: 767–768.

Sonderegger, T. and Zimmermann, E. (1978) Adult behavior and adrenocortical function following postnatal morphine treatment in rats. *Psychopharmacologia*, 56: 103–109.

Sonderegger, T., O'Shea, S. and Zimmermann, E. (1979a) Consequences in adult female rats on neonatal morphine pellet implantation. *Neurobehav. Toxicol.*, 1: 161–167.

Sonderegger, T., O'Shea, S. and Zimmermann, E. (1979b) Progeny of male rats addicted neonatally to morphine. *Proc. West. Pharm. Soc.*, 22: 137–139.

Soyka, L.F. and Joffe, J.M. (1980) Male mediated drug effects on offspring. In R.H. Schwartz and S.J. Yaffe (Eds.), *Drug and Chemical Risks to the Fetus and Newborn*, Alan R. Liss, New York, pp. 49–66.

Spergel, G., Levy, L.J. and Goldner, M.G. (1971) Glucose intolerance in the progeny of rats treated with single subdiabetogenic dose of alloxan. *Metabolism*, 20: 401–413.

Spergel, G., Khan, F. and Goldner, M.G. (1975) Emergence of overt diabetes in offspring of rats with induced latent diabetes. *Metab. Clin. Exp.*, 24: 1311–1319.

Steele, E.J. (1981a) *Somatic Selection and Adaptive Evolution: On the Inheritance of Acquired Characters*, 2nd edn., University of Chicago Press, Chicago.

Steele, E.J. (1981b) Lamarck and immunity: a conflict resolved. *New Scientist*, 90: 360–361.

Steele, E.J. (1984) Acquired paternal influence in mice. Altered serum antibody response in the progeny population of immunized CBA/H males. *Aust. J. Exp. Biol. Med. Sci.*, 62: 253–268.

Steele, E.J., Gorczynski, R.M. and Pollard, J.W. (1984) The somatic selection of acquired characters. In J.W. Pollard (Ed.) *Evolutionary Theory: Paths into the Future*, J. Wiley & Sons, London, pp. 217–236.

Strand, D.J. and McDonald, J.F. (1985) *Copia* is transcriptionally responsive to environmental stress. *Nucleic Acids Res.*, 13: 4401–4410.

Svetlof, P.T. and Korsakova, G.F. (1972) Inheritance of changes in expressivity of eyeless *Drosophila melanogaster* caused by temperature effects in critical periods of ontogenesis. *Sov. J. Dev. Biol.*, 2: 279–285.

Vuillaume, M. and Berkaloff, A. (1974) LSD treatment of *Pieris brassicae* and consequences on the progeny. *Nature*, 251: 314–315.

Waddington, C.H. (1952) Selection of the genetic basis for an acquired character. *Nature*, 169: 278.

Waddington, C.H. (1957) The *Strategy of the Genes*, MacMillan Press, New York.

Wallace, E., Calvin, H.I. and Cooper, G.W. (1983) Progressive defects observed in mouse sperm during the course of three generations of selenium deficiency. *Gamete Res.*, 7: 377–387.

Wallace, R.A. and Misulovin, Z. (1980) The role of zinc and follicle cells in insulin-initiated meiotic maturation of *Xenopus laevis* oocytes. *Science*, 210: 928–929.

Wehmer, F., Porter, R.H. and Scales, B. (1970) Pre-mating and pregnancy stress in rats affects behavior of grandpups. *Nature*, 227: 622.

Weismann, A. (1893) *The Germ-plasm: A Theory of Heredity*, Tr. by W.N. Parker and H. Rönnfeldt, Scribner, New York.

Zamenhof, S. and Marthens, E.V. (1978) Nutritional influences on prenatal brain development. In G. Gottlieb (Ed.), *Studies on the Development of Behavior and the Nervous System, Vol. 4, Early Influences*, Academic Press, New York, pp. 149–186.

Zamenhof, S., van Martens, E. and Grauel, L. (1972) DNA (cell number) and protein in rat brain: second generation (F2) alterations by maternal (F0) dietary protein restriction. *Nutr. Metab.*, 14: 262–270.

Zimmermann, E. and Sonderegger, T. (1980) A syndrome of drug-induced delay of maturation. In H. Parvez and S. Parvez (Eds.), *Biogenic Amines in Development*, Elsevier/North-Holland Biomedical Press, Amsterdam, pp. 591–606.

Discussion

W. Lichtensteiger: As far as the thyroid axis and its regulation are concerned, there has been a characteristic deficit in humans, i.e. cretinism. This condition disappeared completely after preventive administration of iodine. This rather appears to speak against a genetic fixation of the setpoint sensitivity.

J.H. Campbell: This is an interesting observation. Insufficient dietary iodine in various parts of the world is extreme enough to cause cretinism, and more generally goiter, but obviously has not induced a permanent continuation of this pathology. You're probably right to add a caveat about interpreting this observation in humans. It would be interesting to know if, indeed, there are residual functional or histological abnormalities in the thyroids of people today with a long suspected family history of iodine insufficiency. Of course, even if this were the case it would be hard to draw any definite conclusions. We really need controlled studies on experimental animals. Even so, your point is important: past widespread iodine deficiency has not imperiled the human gene pool to any detected degree.

M. Mirmiran: Does showing that small mouse offspring produce small offspring in the following generations allow you to conclude that any receptor set point is determined genetically?

J.H. Campbell: If mice made small by neonatal exposure to morphine, or with an induced thyroid imbalance, generate offspring with related defects there must be a mechanism for this. A small size might be transmitted through the female line due to a small placenta or inadequate milk supply but it is trickier to devise an epigenetic mechanism for inheritance through the male line. I doubt that small mice produce small sperm and therefore cause the F*1 progeny to grow more slowly after birth. Bakke et al. (1974, 1976) have characterized the altered phenotype of the F*1 progeny from thyroidectomized male mice. The changes are multifold, as one might expect for an alteration in a hormone system with diverse roles in development and adult metabolism. With respect to the effects of thyroid balance a change in the set point of the thyrostat would explain the changes.

M. Mirmiran (Comment): I can understand your sympathy for genes. However, your conclusion that a carry-over effect occurs for receptor set point is largely speculative with no data. In this regard, I am afraid you neglected the dynamic interactions between neurotransmitters and receptors during development, and our belief that the set point develops largely as a function of neurotransmitter availability on the synaptic level.

V.R. Sara: A receptor is a protein translated from a gene. One way to regulate the threshold of sensitivity would therefore be via changes in the promotor regions of the gene. Any such structural change would provide a means for genetic transmission of a 'hormonostat'. The techniques are now available to map the structure of the gene suspected of being altered in the germ cells.

J.H. Campbell: Yes, the basic prerequisite techniques are available. Moreover, they have been used to prove that various chemicals and drugs can induce specific heritable alterations in relevant genes of simple organisms. However, the amount of work needed to pinpoint changes in a complex gene of mammals should not be underestimated. You make a good point when you state that sequences regulating a receptor gene might be changed instead of the structural gene itself.

G. J. Boer (addition to V. R. Sara): Before we go into DNA technology, however, we should be sure about the transgenerational characteristics of the effect.

J. H. Campbell: Absolutely.

G. J. Boer: If, indeed, DNA changes are underlying the effect you described, what do you think should be our attitude towards experimentally approaching this.

J. H. Campbell: The obvious approach would be firstly to demonstrate conclusively that a persisting, heritable alteration can be induced reproducibly by a simple experimental manipulation on the male parent. This has not been done as yet. Secondly, it is necessary to characterize the syndrome of changes in affected offspring precisely enough to pinpoint fairly definitively the gene that is likely to have been altered.

Only thereafter can one try to isolate, clone and sequence the DNA of that gene in order to prove that a change in structure was induced. Each of these steps is substantial and requires its own sort of work and expertise. To me it seems likely that if certain genes have evolved machinery to modify their structure in response to environmental conditions, the first example to be discovered will probably be in a system that is mainstream in molecular biology. This should perhaps be considered by anyone interested in approaching this problem.

References

Bakke, J. L., Lawrence, N. L. and Wilbur, J. F. (1974) The late effects of neonatal hyperthyroidism upon the hypothalamic-pituitary-thyroid axis in the rat. *Endocrinology*, 96: 406–411.

Bakke, J. L., Lawrence, N. L., Robinson, S. and Bennett, J. (1976) Life long alterations in endocrine function resulting from brief perinatal hypothyroidism in the rat. *J. Lab. Clin. Med.*, 88: 3–13

Subject Index